Proceedings of the IEEE

Workshop on Mathematical Methods in Biomedical Image Analysis

D1373075

Proceedings of the IEEE

Workshop on Mathematical Methods in Biomedical Image Analysis

June 21 – 22, 1996　　　　**San Francisco, California**

Sponsored by
The IEEE Computer Society Technical Committee on Pattern Analysis and
Machine Intelligence

In cooperation with
SIAM

IEEE Computer Society Press
Los Alamitos, California

Washington　　　•　　　Brussels　　　•　　　Tokyo

IEEE Computer Society Press
10662 Los Vaqueros Circle
P.O. Box 3014
Los Alamitos, CA 90720-1314

IEEE Computer Society Press Order Number PR07367
ISBN 0-8186-7367-2
Library of Congress Number 96-77115

IEEE Order Plan Catalog Number 96TB100056
IEEE Order Plan ISBN 0-8186-7368-0
Microfiche ISBN 0-8186-7369-9

Additional copies may be ordered from:

IEEE Computer Society Press
Customer Service Center
10662 Los Vaqueros Circle
P.O. Box 3014
Los Alamitos, CA 90720-1314
Tel: + 1-714-821-8380
Fax: + 1-714-821-4641
E-mail: cs.books@computer.org

IEEE Service Center
445 Hoes Lane
P.O. Box 1331
Piscataway, NJ 08855-1331
Tel: + 1-908-981-1393
Fax: + 1-908-981-9667
mis.custserv@computer.org

IEEE Computer Society
13, Avenue de l'Aquilon
B-1200 Brussels
BELGIUM
Tel: + 32-2-770-2198
Fax: + 32-2-770-8505
euro.ofc@computer.org

IEEE Computer Society
Ooshima Building
2-19-1 Minami-Aoyama
Minato-ku, Tokyo 107
JAPAN
Tel: + 81-3-3408-3118
Fax: + 81-3-3408-3553
tokyo.ofc@computer.org

Editorial production by Mary E. Kavanaugh
Cover by Alexander Torres
Printed in the United States of America by KNI Inc.

 The Institute of Electrical and Electronics Engineers, Inc.

Table of Contents

Session 4: Medial Axes

Keynote II — "Deformable Models in Medical Image Analysis" 171

Session 5: Deformable Models I

Panel Discussion

Session 6: Deformable Models II

Session 7: Shape

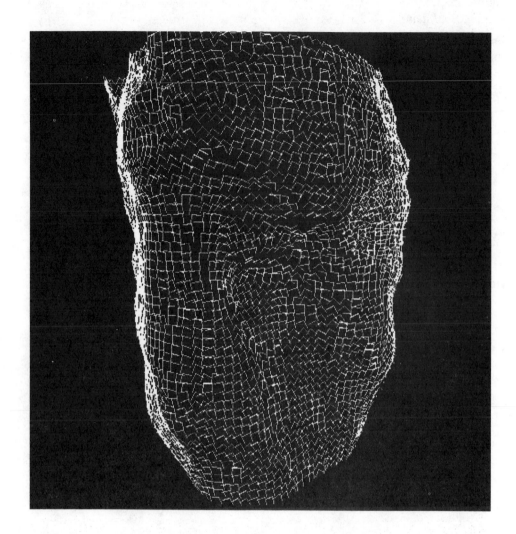

Cover image —

The above graphic represents analysis done on the endocardial wall of the left ventricle of the heart from images generated by the Mayo clinic's Dynamic Spatial Reconstructor. Arrowheads represent directions of principal curvature on the surface of the endocardium. Green represents minimum principal curvature directions. Magenta represents the maximum principal curvature directions. This graphic was produced by an algorithm developed by Amir Amini.

Preface

It has been a great pleasure for us to put together the program for the Workshop on Mathematical Methods in Biomedical Image Analysis (MMBIA), being held at the Hotel Nikko, San Francisco, on June 21 and 22, 1996. The idea for holding this meeting was rooted in the Mathematical Methods in Medical Imaging meetings previously held under SPIE sponsorship and at the Workshop on Biomedical Image Analysis held in Seattle in 1994. MMBIA is an attempt to provide a forum for representatives of both communities.

In addition to electronic dissemination, our Call-for-Papers was published by Rangachar Kasturi and Michael Vannier in IEEE-PAMI and IEEE-TMI. It also appeared in several SIAM and mathematical community publications. Of the 50 papers received for review, we accepted 32 for presentation. Most papers were reviewed by three members of the Program Committee, and the recommendations were compiled to produce the list of papers appearing in these proceedings.

The themes for the submitted papers correspond to the titles of the sessions: Medical Image Registration, Deformable Models, Medial Axes, Bayesian Methods, and Shape. Some of these areas have traditionally received a good deal of attention within the more mathematically-minded segment of the medical image analysis community; others, considerably less. Collectively we often meditate about the factors underlying this degree of (im)balance. Some of it understandably derives from the needs of our clinical colleagues or the power of today's magnificent hardware. But some certainly derives from the capabilities of the associated mathematical manipulations, and some simply from the timing of our realization of these capabilities. Indeed, most of our current research areas entail not so much applications of recent fundamental breakthroughs in applied mathematics as rediscoveries of techniques that have resided in the mathematical literature for a considerable period of time. Branches of mathematics fundamental to our discipline include geometry, linear algebra, functional analysis, partial differential equations, optimization theory, and graph theory; other disciplines that contribute to our thinking include medical physics and statistics. The papers in this volume develop computational methods based on these sources in many clever ways, providing interesting solutions to medical image analysis problems.

Our two keynote addresses focus on the theme of Shape, which is being paid a steadily increasing attention across a wide range of medical image analyses. They approach this core from two strikingly different mathematical points of view — the formalization of shape (Bookstein) and the formalization of deformation of shape (Terzopoulos).

We thank the entire Program Committee for their meticulous reviews of all the submitted manuscripts. We also thank the IEEE Computer Society and the PAMI Technical Committee for sponsoring MMBIA, as well as SIAM, which has been a cooperating society. Special thanks are due the organizers of CVPR '96 and the IEEE Computer Society staff. Finally, thanks to Dmitry Goldgof and Kevin Bowyer for constructive comments on organizational aspects of MMBIA.

We look forward to an exciting meeting. Welcome!

Amir Amini, Fred Bookstein, and David Wilson
Program Co-Chairs

Program and Organizing Committees

General Co-Chairs

Thomas S. Huang
University of Illinois
huang@uicsl.csl.uiuc.edu

Stephen M. Pizer
University of North Carolina
smp@cs.unc.edu

Program Co-Chairs

Amir A. Amini
Yale University
amini@minerva.cis.yale.edu

Fred L. Bookstein
University of Michigan
fred@brainmap.med.umich.edu

David C. Wilson
University of Florida
dcw@math.ufl.edu

Program Committee

Raj Acharya – *State University of New York*

Nicholas Ayache – *INRIA*

Kevin Bowyer – *University of South Florida*

Chin-Tu Chen – *University of Chicago*

Laurent Cohen – *University of Paris*

Steve Collins – *University of Iowa*

Edward Delp – *Purdue University*

James Duncan – *Yale University*

Guido Gerig – *ETH*

Dmitry Goldgof – *University of South Florida*

William Green – *University of Michigan*

Eric Grimson – *Massachusetts Institute of Technology*

Alok Gupta – *Siemens*

David Hawkes – *UMDS - London*

Eric Hoffman – *University of Iowa*

Ramesh Jain – *University of California, San Diego*

Takeo Kanade – *Carnegie Mellon University*

Benjamin Kimia – *Brown University*

Nick Lange – *National Institutes of Health*
Richard Leahy – *University of Southern California*
Zhi-Pei Liang – *University of Illinois*
Murray Loew – *George Washington University*
Dimitri Metaxas – *University of Pennsylvania*
Bahram Parvin – *Lawrence Berkeley Lab*
Sandy Pentland – *Massachusetts Institute of Technology*
Jerry Prince – *Johns Hopkins University*
Christian Roux – *Telecom Bretagne*
Ajit Singh – *Siemens*
Ernest Stokely – *University of Alabama*
Massimo Tistarelli – *University of Genoa*
Demetri Terzopoulos – *University of Toronto*
Bart ter Haar Romeny – *Utrecht University*
Baba Vemuri – *University of Florida*
Max Viergever – *Utrecht University*
Sandy Wells – *Brigham and Women's Hospital*

Local Arrangements Chair

Bahram Parvin
Lawrence Berkeley Lab
parvin@george.lbl.gov

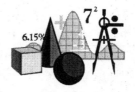

Keynote I

"Shape and the Information in Medical Images: A Decade of the Morphometric Synthesis"

Speaker

Fred L. Bookstein

Shape and the Information in Medical Images:
A Decade of the Morphometric Synthesis

Fred L. Bookstein
University of Michigan, Ann Arbor, Michigan
fred@brainmap.med.umich.edu

Abstract

This keynote address reviews several techniques from morphometrics (the multivariate biometrics of shape) developed mainly in the context of medical image analysis over the last decade. The new techniques provide powerful tools for geometric tasks that arise in the course of most analyses of medical images in groups. These tasks include standardizing against Euclidean similarity transformations or shear transformations, encoding informative prior knowledge about shape variation, and detecting, testing, and visualizing linear statistical patterns of variation within or between groups. I review the features of the present toolkit, the standard underlying data models entailed, and some of the extensions that reach out to the additional information content of medical images for common clinical or scientific applications.

1. Introduction

Over the last decade there has been a remarkable convergence of several disciplines in one shared core of techniques, a **morphometric synthesis,** for the handling of biometric shape information as data.

The speed of this development caught most of us by surprise. The first announcement of the mathematical foundation (the Riemannian geometry of Kendall's shape space) came only in 1984 [1], via a long and difficult exposition making no reference at all to medical images. The initial publication of what is now taken to be the obvious associated multivariate statistical method [2] made no reference to this fundamental geometry except in one sentence of a contributed discussion. A crucial technique from interpolation theory, the thin-plate spline, was borrowed in 1987 [3] without reference to this or any other statistical context. (The same technique had already been applied by Terzopoulos and several colleagues to problems in image processing and computer graphics quite separate from this statistical arena.) In 1989 that multivariate statistics of shape was combined with the spline [4] for describing and decomposing group differences, still without acknowledgement of the geometric foundation. My full-length monograph [5] of 1991 continued to overlook the geometric roots of the relation between the spline and the statistics. As recently as five years ago, we still did not understand why the splines were so effective for the visualization of statistical effects on shape.

Only since then has the community of interested statisticians agreed on the source of this efficacy: the (elementary) theorem that the eigenfunctions of the spline are orthonormal in the Procrustes geometry of shape. This observation did not appear in the technical literature until 1995 [6–7], and is only now being broadcast to readers not expert in mathematical statistics [8–10]. The most persuasive examples by which it is bought to the attention of these larger audiences, nevertheless, remain those drawn from the domain of medical image analysis: specifically, analyses of human brain shape variability in normal forms and in diagnosed disease states. Even though the canonical examples are thus medical image data sets, this keynote address is the first exposition of this synthesis for the professional community having the greatest use for it.

2. The geometric foundation

The core of the morphometric synthesis deals with *landmark data*, labelled points that correspond from instance to instance across all the images of a data set. Identification of landmarks is a strenuous and complex procedure requiring considerable prior anatomical understanding. The effort involved is justified afterward by the leverage that the information in their locations affords for subsequent scientific analyses. At present landmarks are almost always located manually; but work underway at Washington University and McGill suggests that it may soon be possible to locate them automatically.

Proceedings of MMBIA '96

2.1. Procrustes shape distance

In ordinary language, the *shape* of an object is described by words or quantities that do not vary when the object is moved, rotated, enlarged, or reduced. The translations, rotations, and changes of scale we thereby ignore constitute the *similarity group* of transformations of the plane. When the "objects" are landmark sets, it turns out to be useful to say that their shape simply *is* the set of all point sets that "have the same shape." That is, we have formally defined *the shape* of a set of points as the *equivalence class* of that point set, within the collection of all point sets of the same cardinality, under the operation of the similarity group. (The more general linear groups SL_2 and SL_3 will concern us in Section 3.1.)

We need a distance measure for landmark shapes that have been defined in this way. Were it not for that complication of the similarity group, the obvious formula would involve the usual Pythagorean sum of squared distances between corresponding landmarks. It proves reasonable to define the squared distance between two shapes (that is, two equivalence classes) as the *minimum* of these sums of squares over representatives of the equivalence classes—over the operation of the group of similarities that shape is supposed to ignore. That is, the squared shape distance between one landmark set A and another landmark set B is the minimum summed squared Euclidean distances between the landmarks of A and the corresponding landmarks in point sets C as C ranges over the whole set of shapes equivalent to B. For this definition to make sense, we have to fix the scale of A. The mathematics of all this is most elegant (see [1]) just when the sum of squares of the points of A around their center-of-gravity is constrained to be exactly 1. A small adjustment of the definition, required for symmetry between A and B, need not concern us here.

The steps in this computation follow down the rows of Figure 1. At the top are two quadrilaterals of landmarks presumed to arise from real images. Connect each landmark to the centroid of its own form and, for each form, rescale the sum of squares of the distances shown to unity (second row). Then (third row) translate one of the forms so that its centroid directly overlies the centroid of the other form. Finally, identify the rotation (third row right) that minimizes the sum of squares of the residual distances between matched landmarks; it can be computed analytically [5]. The squared Procrustes distance between the forms (fourth row) is the sum of squares of those residuals at its minimum. It is (approximately) the total area of the circles shown at the lower right, divided by π.

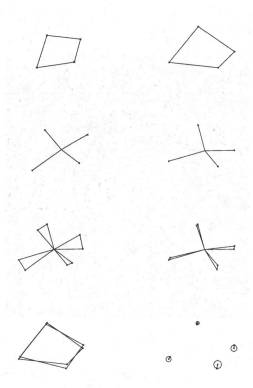

Figure 1. Procrustes shape distance for two quadrilaterals of landmarks (top row). Each form is scaled separately (second row) to sum of squares 1 around its own centroid. After the centroids are superimposed (third row left), either form is rotated about the other (right) until the sum of squared distances between matched landmarks is minimized. (fourth row) The squared Procrustes distance between the original quadrilaterals is this minimum sum of squared distances between corresponding points; it is proportional to the sum of the areas of the circles drawn here.

Figure 2 typifies how landmark data arise from medical images. It is one image from a data set of 28 nearly midsagittal sections of human brains (14 schizophrenic and 14 not). The ten landmark points represent some reliable anatomical structures that intersect this plane.

2.2. Averaging shapes

The average of an ordinary list of numbers is their sum divided by their count. For averaging equivalence classes like these, we have recourse to a different characterization of that ordinary average: the *least-squares fit* to those numbers, the quantity about which they have the least sum of squared differences. From a distance between shapes, then, we inherit *this* notion of average shape directly. The necessary minimization is not too

3

difficult [11]—for two-dimensional data, it comes from a closed-form eigenanalysis [12].

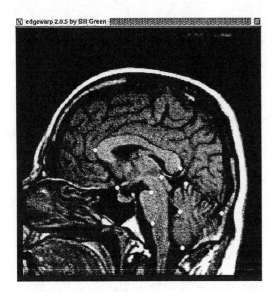

Figure 2. Landmark data ordinarily arise from the identification of particular named points in routine biomedical images. Here we identify ten landmarks in a parasagittal magnetic resonance image of a normal brain. Bottom to top: bottom of cerebellum, bottom of pons at medulla, tentorium at dura, obex of fourth ventricle, top of pons, optic chiasm, top of cerebellum, superior colliculus, splenium of corpus callosum, genu of corpus callosum.

For instance, for a data set of shapes like that of the dots in Figure 2, the average (Figure 3, left) looks just like a template for some landmark location scheme applicable to any case in particular. After we've computed the average, we can put each individual shape down over the average using the similarity transformation that made the sum-of-squares from the average a minimum for that particular case. There results the diagram at the right in Figure 3.

This tactic, far from being a mere graphical aid, is in fact the most crucial step in the geometric computations. The set of shapes construed as equivalence classes in this wise actually make up a Riemannian manifold, the **Kendall shape manifold,** with Procrustes distance as metric [1]. The manifold is of dimension $2k-4$: $2k$ original Cartesian coordinates, decremented by the four degrees of freedom (two for translation, one for rotation, one for scale) of the similarity group of the plane. The tangent space to this manifold is likewise of dimension $2k-4$ at every point. We will attend only to one of those tangent spaces, the one that is tangent at the sample average shape. The

construction at the right in Figure 3 actually represents the projection of each shape of our sample onto the tangent space to that manifold at the sample average shape. Such a projection preserves the metric (in the small, in the vicinity of the sample average): for each pair of specimens, the summed squared distance between the representatives of the cases in Figure 3 is the same as their Procrustes shape distance. The k coordinate pairs of that figure actually serve as a set of $2k$ redundant coordinates for this $(2k-4)$–dimensional tangent space.

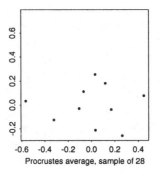
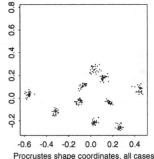

Procrustes average, sample of 28　　　Procrustes shape coordinates, all cases

Figure 3. How Procrustes shape coordinates arise. (left) The Procrustes average of 28 shapes like that of the set of ten landmark points in Figure 2. (right) Procrustes shape coordinates come from fitting every individual case back over the sample average (left) by the procedure of Figure 1. These actually represent the orthogonal projection of the sample onto the tangent space to Kendall's shape manifold at the shape on the left (see text). The diagram is scaled to sum-of-squares 1 around $(0,0)$; then both axes are in units of Procrustes distance per se.

2.3. Multivariate statistical analysis

An alternate way of construing tangent spaces provides the conceptual link to the next theme of the synthesis. The same tangent space to a Riemannian manifold that one initially intuits as a higher-dimensional plane touching a curving hypersurface, rather as a sphere rests on the ground, can be construed instead [13] as the space of all linear germs of scalar functions along curves through a point of the manifold. To the statistician, these functions are just what we mean by **shape variables.** That is, the tangent space construction of Figure 3 provides the setting for all possible linearized multivariate analyses of the information in the shapes of the landmark configurations. Furthermore, the usual multivariate sum-of-squares metric of that representation is the underlying Procrustes metric of the manifold, and so the multivariate statistics will be commensurate with the original Procrustes geometry. This series of steps is reviewed in more detail in [14].

For shapes that are concentrated in a small region of the full shape space (as any within-species sample of the shape of an organ is likely to be), one can carry out most of the ordinary maneuvers of multivariate statistical analysis—tests of group differences, correlations of shape with causes or effects, principal components analysis with respect to Procrustes distance—directly in terms of this basis for the tangent space. But because the basis is redundant, in this form it does not support techniques like regression that use matrix inversion; we will deal with this at Section 3.2.

At the left in Figure 4, for example, is the computation of two averages for subsets of the 28 cases: one for fourteen patients actually diagnosed schizophrenic, the other for fourteen age- and sex-matched normals. This contrast is computed as a vector in the tangent space to Kendall's manifold. Again, it is drawn here by way of k separate (but not orthogonal) projections onto k planes within that space.

2.4. Visualization via thin-plate spline

There is a way to render that same vector of the tangent plane as one coherent graphical construction: a deformation grid. Imagine one of the averages, say, the normals (the dots), put down on ordinary square graph paper. Deform the paper so that the dots now fall directly over the *other* set of points, the triangles. The right panel in Figure 4 shows one plausible representation of what happens to the grid.

Naturally it matters what deformation one uses. The morphometric synthesis emphasizes one particular choice, the *thin-plate spline*, that minimizes yet another sum-of-squares. In this context, we are minimizing the summed squared second derivatives (integrated over the whole plane) of the map in the figure. Interpreted as the summed squared deviations of the shapes of the little squares from the shapes of their neighbors, it becomes a measure of local information in the mapping. That minimum actually turns out to be a quadratic form in the coordinates of the points of the target shape, with coefficients that depend on the starting shape [4, 8–10]. This quadratic form, the *bending energy*, joins two others, the Procrustes metric and the empirical covariance matrix of the coordinates in Figure 3, to make up the geometrical substrate of the morphometric synthesis. Morphometrics seems unusual among branches of modern applied statistics in the centrality of this set of three quadratic forms rather than the usual two.

Please note that the spline is not claimed to be a realistic model for the correspondence of images between the landmarks. It is, rather, a visualization of directions in the tangent space to the shape manifold defined solely by the shapes of the landmark configurations. What is crucial about it, then, is that it is linear in the coordinates of the landmark shapes after projection, the coordinates of the right-hand panel in Figure 3. There are many other plausible parametric models for deformations of Euclidean space, but none of them seem to be linear in landmark coordinates in this same way. I will return to this concern of realism of deformations in Section 4.4.

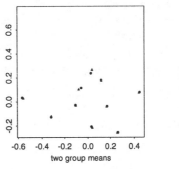 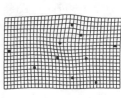

two group means   thin-plate spline, dots to triangles

Figure 4. Statistics and visualizations in the tangent space to Kendall's manifold. (left) Example of statistical analysis in the tangent space: Average shapes for the two subgroups making up our original sample. Triangles, schizophrenics; dots, normals. The most striking discrepancy is at upper center. (right) The thin-plate spline is an interpolation function from one point set to another having the minimum variation (over the whole plane) of affine derivative. In the synthesis, it serves to visualize vectors in the tangent space at left. The grid here, the spline from the dots to the triangles at left, directly leads the eye to a local characterization of the shape difference under study. In other applications [7–9] an equally obvious signal may appear at much larger scale.

2.5. Testing a group difference

The journals in which our typical clients publish are often overly concerned with statistical significance, improbability on a conventional "null hypothesis." For the simple two-group design here, there is a standard statistic owing to Goodall [15; see also 9] that often serves to reassure anxious reviewers and editors. Goodall's statistic, which applies equivalently to the two presentations paired in Figure 4, is based in the ratio between the squared Procrustes distance between group means (sum of squares of the distances between dots

5

and triangles at the left in Figure 4) and the total of the squared Procrustes distances from each specimen to the grand mean (sum of the squares of the distances of the points from their landmark-specific centroids at the right in Figure 3). While the exact distribution of this ratio is a tabulated F under one very symmetric set of assumptions, it is often more realistically taken as a permutation test [16]. For this computation, the observed value of the ratio I just mentioned is calibrated against the cumulative distribution of analogous ratios computed after group is assigned by (hundreds of) random permutation of the truth rather than according to the actual diagnosis case by case.

By either approach, the average shapes of schizophrenics and normals here differ at about the 2% level of statistical significance. (That is, we have a finding to report.) The consequences of such a verification for comparison of functional images will concern us presently.

2.6. Three dimensions

All this geometry goes over to three-dimensional data without any essential changes (except that things are much harder to draw). The characterization of Procrustes distance between shapes is the same (minimum sum-of-squares over the Euclidean similarity group when one form is constrained to sum-of-squares unity), and likewise the definition of the average shape. The dimension of the shape manifold, likewise the tangent space, is now $3k - 7$, and the Procrustes residuals (analogues to the points in Figure 3, right) now have 7 redundant coordinates, not 4. The formalism of the spline goes over to three-dimensional data almost unchanged [5], and likewise all the multivariate statistical strategies.

3. Shape variation between subjects

The main import of this Morphometric Synthesis for medical image analysis is the praxis it supplies for coping with the non-invariance of the meaning of individual pixels—with shape variation between subjects. In this section I review the remaining statistical and graphical tools that apply to these problems.

The thin-plate spline applies to unwarp a data set of images to the average landmark configuration. Introduced in 1990, the splined unwarping uses the *inverse* of the thin-plate spline interpolant from sample mean landmark shape to each specimen of the sample. Image by image, pixel values are pulled back to the coordinate system of the mean landmark configuration, where they may be subjected to various further

manipulations. Figure 5 shows the unwarping of the case of Figure 2 to the mean landmark configuration of the normal subgroup (dots in Figure 4). The averages by group of these unwarped images are presented in Figure 6.

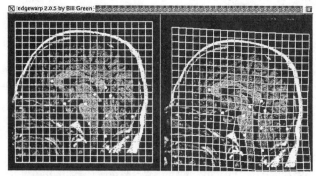

Figure 5. Unwarping of the image in Figure 2 to the normal average landmark configuration. Grid: thin-plate spline mapping, left→right. Unwarping: pixel pullback, right→left.

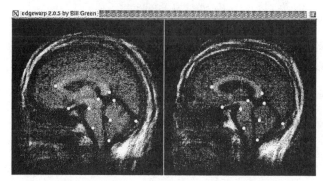

Figure 6. Average unwarped images, 14 per group. Each specimen is unwarped as in Figure 5 to its own average landmark configuration, and the resulting images summed pixelwise. Note the difference in shapes at the averages of splenium (right end of arch at center).

The import of the morphometric synthesis for medical image analysis follows mainly from the scientific power of these straightforward geometric maneuvers. The $2k$-vector of landmark shape from Figure 3 behaves just like any other classic vector-valued **biometric covariate**, a list of associated values by which effects on the primary datum (in this case, the entire image) can be observed more precisely. But, in view of its extremely low dimension, the manipulation is more appropriately considered a relabeling of the pixels of the ground plane than any form of image processing per se. (For instance, the adjustment across Figure 5 does not alter the qualitative properties of any segmentation, but only the Cartesian coordinates at which the segments are located.)

The context in which the morphometric synthesis is applicable to medical image analysis is thus not the consideration of images one at a time, as as for segmentation, or even two at a time, as in some more recent methods of deformable-template analysis, but their consideration in whole stacks of samples, for the extraction of patterns, typologies, forecasts, or causal understandings. The shape information, in other words, is intended from the outset to be *combined with other information outside the image*—group labels, clinical assessments, or coregistered images of another modality—*toward the formulation or testing of quantitative biomedical hypotheses.*

3.1. Empirical components of shape variation

One current community concern that the synthesis immediately resolves is the problem of *uniform standardization.* The same Procrustes geometry that optimally handles the four (in 3d, seven) nuisance parameters of the similarity group (translation, rotation, scale) extends directly to the additional two parameters of the general linear group SL_2 (in three dimensions, the additional five of SL_3). In the Procrustes space of 2d data, the set of forms that derive from the sample average landmark configuration by uniform transformations (simple shears) lie on an ordinary (two-dimensional) plane through the average shape. Every specimen has a *uniform coordinate pair* derived from Procrustes-orthogonal projection onto this subspace, and also a Procrustes-orthogonal *residual* from that projection, which is, rigorously, the geometrically unique *nonuniform part* of shape variation. The Pythagorean Theorem applies to this decomposition: squared Procrustes distance equals squared uniform distance plus squared nonuniform distance, and the two parts can be averaged and tested separately.

As the formulas for this term were not published until 1995, I will repeat them here. Let the Procrustes mean form (Figure 3 left), oriented with principal axes horizontal and vertical (as in the figures here), have coordinates $(x_1, y_1), (x_2, y_2), \ldots, (x_k, y_k)$, and let $\alpha = \Sigma x_i^2$ and $\gamma = \Sigma y_i^2$ be the principal moments along those axes. Then the two elements of this two-vector may be taken as dot products of the Procrustes fit coordinates (Figure 3, right), treated as a 20-vector of real numbers, with the vectors Un_1 and Un_2 where

$$\lambda Un_1^t = ((\alpha y_1, \gamma x_1), (\alpha y_2, \gamma x_2), \ldots, (\alpha y_k, \gamma x_k)),$$

$$\lambda Un_2^t = ((-\gamma x_1, \alpha y_1), (-\gamma x_2, \alpha y_2), \ldots, (-\gamma x_k, \alpha y_k)).$$

Here λ is the scaling factor $\sqrt{\alpha\gamma}$. The first of the vectors corresponds to Cartesian shears aligned with the x-axis, the second to Cartesian dilations along the y-axis.

Notice that these formulas are closed—the Procrustes uniform term is evaluated without further iteration.

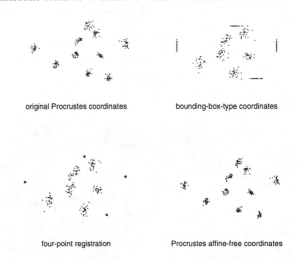

original Procrustes coordinates

bounding-box-type coordinates

four-point registration

Procrustes affine-free coordinates

Figure 7. Counterintuitive behavior of plausible registration rules. (upper left) Original Procrustes-fit coordinates as in Figure 3. (upper right) Ad-hoc attempt to remove the uniform part by alignment of the shape with a "bounding box." (lower left) "Refinement" of the bounding box, generated by nonlinear (inverse-spline) unwarping of the remaining landmarks when those on the bounding box are sent to their mean positions. Either of these innocuous-seeming protocols makes the scatter of registered points considerably *worse* than the original Procrustes registration that allowed no shape adjustments at all. (lower right) Optimal least-squares removal of the uniform term using the formulas in the text. Net Procrustes shape variance (summed moments of the little scatters) is necessarily reduced.

Standardization of the uniform part of shape variation by this least-squares procedure is guaranteed to *optimally* reduce the residual shape variance of any sample (Figure 7, upper left vs. lower right). Plausible-seeming approaches to uniform standardization not couched in this Procrustes geometry, such as the "bounding-box" routine simulated at upper right in the figure, are quite capable of *adding* unwanted shape variance, as they in fact do in this case. The paradox is not evaded, furthermore, by "nonlinear" treatment of the same four bounding landmarks (lower left: think of this as an analogue of Talairach-type registration on an arbitrary selection of scattered points). The error in all the ad-hoc techniques is a consequence of failure to apply least-squares to the information in the landmark configuration as a whole. Should the landmarks be known to have different precisions a priori, it is easy to adjust all these methods [5]. That heteroscedasticity is not particularly pressing here. Figure 8 shows the implications of such partial registrations for the averaged images that result. These and several other fallacies are wholly obscured when one works in units of raw centimeters in the original image space; they become obvious only when one evaluates methodological choices in the appropriate space of shape variation from the outset.

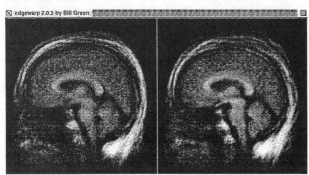

Figure 8. The difference between partial and full registrations is apparent in sharpness all over the averaged images except at shared landmark loci. Left, four-point registration (lower left, Figure 7); right, ten-point registration (average of the two frames in Figure 6 after a further unwarping to the average in Figure 3).

As these plausible partial registrations do not explain much of the shape variation in this actual sample, to what features should we turn? Because the Procrustes metric is retained alongside the sample covariance structure, the synthesis offers an optimal solution to this problem [7, 10–14]: a set of empirical orthogonal components of bending that standardize images as efficiently as possible (in the Procrustes metric) for a given number of components. As Figure 9 shows, the first two of these components are *not* particularly aligned with the uniform part of the transformation. There is thus no good reason for any standardization [of this particular data set, anyway] to begin there, and no justification for *any* method of registration to *end* there. In this data set, while the first relative warp loads substantially on the uniform subspace, it is apparently more efficient to proceed with standardization of one particular small-scale bending term than with the second dimension of the uniform term. As it happens, that bending term is almost exactly aligned with the mean difference of the two samples: it is exactly the supervariance in which we were interested all along.

Principal components supply the optimal lower-dimensional linear reconstructions of empirical shape data vectors just as they do in any other application. In

Figure 10, we compare the ad-hoc four-point spline unwarping of Figure 7 to the optimal Procrustes registration using the same number of parameters.

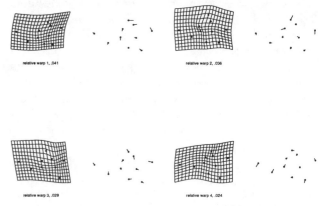

Figure 9. Empirical principal components (relative warps) of the full Procrustes shape scatter. Top row: first and second. Lower row: third and fourth. Each is shown both as a thin-plate spline and as a pattern of displacements in Procrustes space. Notice that the second component is very localized and strongly resembles the group difference in Figure 4.

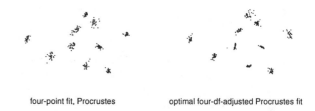

Figure 10. Two four-df adjustments. (left) Procrustes reprojection of the ad-hoc four-point spline unwarping from Figure 7. (right) Optimal four-dimensional adjustment (projection): residual from the first four principal components of the full Procrustes scatter. Only 30% of the original 16-dimensional variance remains.

3.2. Geometric components a priori

Some other approaches to deformable templates invoke a-priori bases for curving forms considered as functions. Sometimes these are copied directly out of textbooks (the Fourier decomposition for closed outlines, the Legendre polynomials for open curves, spherical harmonics for smooth convex blobs). Other bases occasionally suggested are functions of the mean or typical form: for instance, the normal modes of bending of the equivalent surface shells.

The morphometric synthesis includes one such basis, which, for our ten-point brain example, is shown in Figure 11: the eigenfunctions of the bending-energy quadratic form. These landmark displacements are actually orthonormal in the Procrustes metric underlying the geometry of the data. When projected onto *both* the *x*- and *y*-axes of the Procrustes shape space, and supplemented by the uniform term just reviewed, they make up an orthogonal rotation of the original Procrustes residuals, Figure 3 (right), into a basis of the correct rank. Multivariate regressions and MANOVAs, for instance, go forward using this basis, and Procrustes distance is still preserved [14]. The bending energy of each of these normal modes serves as a useful index of its localization in the geometry of the original image plane. It is these features, not polynomials, that constitute the natural extension of the a-priori geometric basis beyond the obvious uniform term. For instance, for the ten-landmark data set here, the next two natural parameters are the *x*- and *y*-projections of the surface at upper left in Figure 11, and the two after that, the projections of the surface to its right.

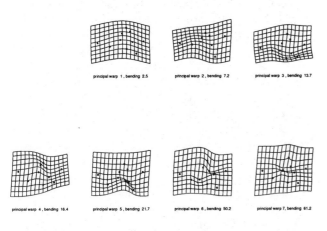

Figure 11. All seven principal warps of the sample average shape (Figure 3, left): eigenfunctions of the bending-energy quadratic form, drawn at Procrustes length 0.16 and interpreted as splined surfaces. Augmented by the uniform component, this basis provides a Procrustes-orthogonal rotation of the 16 nontrivial dimensions of the redundant basis at the right in Figure 3.

Using this basis, we can at last understand why "bounding-box" adjustments like those in Figure 7 almost always make Procrustes scatters worse rather than better. By projecting the full sample of shapes onto the set of eight principal planes arising from the uniform term and these seven surfaces, we arrive at another ordination of which the uniform part is one single term (instead of being distributed over all the panels of the projection as in Figure 3). In this sample of brain

shapes, the uniform term only accounts for only 20% of the total shape variance; the largest-scale nonuniform term (displacement of the center with respect to the anterior and posterior) actually accounts for more variation. The bounding box is a registration on an *unnecessarily noisy estimate* of this term; that noise propagates throughout the registered images, swamping any potential gain from the adjustment.

In some applications [7–8], the uniform or the first couple of nonuniform terms more or less exhaust the variation of shape space. Only in such cases are simplistic nonlinear registrations an efficient use of the algorithm's, or the investigator's, time. I have seen no evidence of any such a-priori low-dimensional statistical structure for brain data in either two or three dimensions. Whenever such structure is lacking, little can be gained by restriction of one's attention to *any* a-priori subspace of the shape tangent space. Still, the first four relative warps, Figure 9, account for 70% of the total shape variation, considerably more than the ad-hoc procedure based on a "bounding box." Of course, this subspace is not known a priori.

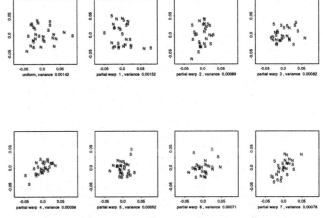

Figure 12. Decomposition of sample variation by partial warps (projections onto the orthonormal basis of Figure 11), together with the uniform component (upper left). Of the total shape variance of .0072, only about 20% is uniform, and less than 25% is aligned with the largest-scale nonlinear bending (Figure 11, upper left). *N*, normals; *S*, schizophrenics. All frames are commensurate in the Procrustes metric. The separation of *N*'s and *S*'s is largest in the panel at lower right, corresponding to the most focused dimension of warping. Axes are in the same units as Figure 3.

Prior knowledge. Incorporating prior knowledge of shape variability is one of the main frontiers of medical image analysis. In the presence of sufficiently many cases, the representation by the full Procrustes landmark shape covariance structure is optimal for most multivariate purposes, such as linear discriminant function analysis. When samples are too small, or landmarks too numerous, to permit exploiting the full covariance matrix, any sublist of the first few empirical components or canonical variates provides an optimal basis of its order. The empirical orthogonal basis is also quite useful for describing the effects of any exogenous predictor of shape, such as group membership; it calls the scientist's attention to features that may suggest mechanisms, for example. In the example here, more than a third of the difference between schizophrenic and normal mean shapes is aligned with the *last* partial warp (Figure 11, lower right), but hardly any on the large-scale features that were adjusted out at the left in Figure 8; this "plausible" partial registration thus made the detection of group differences a good deal more difficult.

The "Procrustes sphere" against which all these distributions are calibrated actually corresponds to a statistical distribution of its own, the "null" of the Goodall F [11]. It is nearly spherical normal in the tangent space, and corresponds to the origin of landmarks by a process of isotropic diffusion (Brownian motion) around their mean positions. In this version, the distribution is even applicable to a case of "all landmarks the same"—diffusion of particles from the same origin, astronomical loci, etc. [1,6].

4. Future applications throughout medical image analysis

The role of the landmark-driven methods in rationalizing registration rules and in generating descriptions of group shape variation and shape differences is well-understood by now. In this section I will sketch extensions, most of them topics of active current research, that probe a wider range of scientific and clinical applications of the same classes of images.

4.1. "Statistical parametric images"

In any structural data set there will be more information about structural differences than can be captured by landmarks. The remaining information can often be unearthed by further consideration of these landmark-driven registrations *as hints about further unwarping.* The difference between images like those in Figure 6, for example, suggests that there is additional information along the lower boundary of corpus callosum, at the roof of the third ventricle. The bulb of the averaged schizophrenic splenium appears considerably thinner in

an anteroposterior direction, as if it has been eroded from the front.

Such differences, because they pertain to already-sharp boundaries of named structures, should be interpreted "horizontally"—as loci at which unwarping is evidently inadequate—rather than "vertically" as differences of mean gray level to be analyzed by t-ratio or another geometry-free statistic. Because the unwarping methods so very effectively concentrate the information from these very low-dimensional parameter spaces, the efficiency by which they extract additional geometric signals is far higher than anything available from analysis of pixel values "in place," which only deblurs rather than relabeling. In last year's Proceedings [17] I introduced a method for improving the spatial precision of unwarping by comparison of group mean images in this way, an example that will appear shortly [10] in a more expository context; I will not repeat the demonstration here.

A structure-driven unwarping can be applied as well to any other image that has been placed in register with the structural image: for instance, fMRI. In this context, the same language of "covariate correction" applies that I have already introduced. The landmark-driven unwarping serves to substantially increase the precision of clinically or scientifically interesting comparisons arrived at with its aid. Increase in precision of unwarping can be translated into increased precision of regression slopes inferred or into reduction in sample size required for statistical significance of the patterns detected, whichever you, your reviewers, or the bureaucrats who fund you prefer. Unlike the usual biometric covariate adjustment, however, these covariates do not adjust the "dependent variable" (the functional image) linearly in its own (pixelwise) function space. The adjustment is, rather, a *highly* nonlinear manipulation in that space—a pixel relabeling—that has been made linear only by the powerful Procrustes machinery of the synthesis.

4.2. "Endophrenology" (structure-function covariance)

When structure is used as a covariate of function in this way, as with any other covariate adjustment, there may be group differences in the covariate (shape) and in the adjusted outcome (function) at the same time. In many studies, too, there will be very interesting correlations *between* structure and function. The permutation test for group difference introduced in Section 2.5 is a special case of a quite general approach to the testing of covariance structures relating landmark locations to any outside feature vectors, such as image contents or clinical aspects of a diagnosis. The pivotal statistic for the generalization is the first singular value of the matrix of covariances between the Procrustes shape coordinates and the vector of exogenous measurements. The same computation can be used to test the association of normalized image contents with putative causes or effects [18]. In that application, the amplitude of an image variation pattern substitutes for the Procrustes length of a shape change.

These two styles of analysis can be combined to analyze landmark shape, normalized image contents, and function in one omnibus least-squares procedure. Because this computation (which comes under the general heading of Partial Least Squares) is invariant against rotation of any block separately, findings in the shape space can be visualized equivalently as Procrustes shifts or as splines, whichever seems more congenial. Rotation of vectors of image contents (e.g., counts by regions-of-interest) or of exogenous vectors is ordinarily much more difficult to reify; typically, these are interpreted as "profiles" or "contrasts" instead.

4.3. When structure is "missing"

Perhaps the most important application of these cross-correlation methods will be to the task of registering functional images. One often hears the argument that most functional images (e.g., PET images from cognitive studies of normals) are not accompanied by structural images, and hence must be unwarped using only parameters that are available from the functional image itself: in practice, only the very most reliable loci where source intensity drops to zero (cerebrospinal fluid, skull). But the crosscorrelation methods of Partial Least Squares [18] can be applied to a training set of landmarks from two images in adequate rigid registration—structure and function of the same cases—to produce a hierarchy of covariances of anatomical structure with the "landmarks" of the functional image. Regressions driven by those covariances, applied to new functional images, produce "expected" landmark locations that can, in turn, drive the usual unwarping to an average shape (using only the information in the functional image). In this way we may be able to simulate the power of single-subject z-pixel analyses for studies that actually pool normal subjects in large numbers. I am very eager to help someone try this approach soon.

4.4. Information from curving form

Landmarks are image features, but as a set they constitute a stringent abstraction of the information from that medical image. There is considerably more to

be learned about shape and shape normalization from parts of boundaries between landmarks: curves in two dimensions, curves or surfaces in three. Elsewhere in this volume [19] I introduce a joint modification of the two main methods of the synthesis, Procrustes projections and the thin-plate spline, that seems to handle this extended class of data with striking effectiveness. The spline is used to relax claims of point-correspondence along the smooth manifolds upon which homologues are actually bound [20]; the Procrustes procedures continue to apply to describe interesting dimensions of the resulting feature spaces and to provide optimal detection of scientifically important differences.

I put forward these new models as a novel experimental link between multivariate statistics of actual sample differences, statistics that must be in low-dimensional spaces, and the enormously higher dimension of the warping representations produced by spatially distributed lattices. Models of that class appear to minimize mismatch energies (the Miller approach) or maximize correlation (the Evans approach) under a different geometry not apposite, as this one is, to linear statistical description of group differences or to structure-function correlations. In my view, the *statistical* interplay between vertical and horizontal analyses— analysis of deformation vs. analysis of levels of gray— will be the next great theme of the morphometric toolkit. It might be possible, for instance, to set a scale for accuracy of the spatially parameterized warps when they are viewed as residuals from globally specified spline schemes. At the next of these Workshops I look forward to being able to report far less tentatively on this new class of methods.

5. Envoi

The morphometric synthesis for landmarks and landmark-like data is now a nearly mature branch of applied statistics. These powerful new linearized procedures represent *all* the information content of an important abstraction from the image: the shapes of landmark configurations. The techniques, some optimal and some canonical, are all characterized or defended by theorems. Their importance corresponds to the growing importance of the aspect of medical image science with which they directly articulate: analyses of groups, types, or causes and effects—large data sets of images, over multiple subjects, considered all at once. The Human Brain Project, for instance, is particularly interested in this nexus, and supports Miller's work and Evans's alongside mine.

In this context of irreducible intersubject variation, the shape representations afforded by the synthesis, and the splines that visualize the linear space they span, are meant to be borrowed for medical informatics in the same respectful but routine way that one borrows the Cramér-Rao inequality, or the singular-value decomposition, or Student's t. These are constructs and formulas, not software modules and certainly not "black boxes." The basic tools I have reviewed—the Riemannian shape manifold, Procrustes tangent space, Goodall's F and its permutation test, the spline visualization, the affine subspace, relative warps, Partial Least Squares—are optimal solutions, on hand in advance, for a host of informatic problems. There is usually no longer any gain to be had by speculating on these matters in the course of other studies. Occasionally one can do better in particularly problematic contexts, to be sure, but this basic toolkit is sturdy enough for most scientific applications and clinical typologies.

The techniques I have sketched here, accompanied by a greater variety of examples than I can yet supply, ought to become part of future textbooks in medical image analysis. I look forward, too, to equally canonical breakthroughs in the extended applications—statistical images, structure-function correlations, information from curving form—on which I speculated at the close.

Acknowledgement. Preparation of this contribution was supported by NIH grants DA–09009 and GM–37251 to Fred L. Bookstein. The former grant is jointly supported by the National Institute on Drug Abuse, the National Institute of Mental Health, and the National Institute on Aging as part of the Human Brain Project. Images were analyzed by Bill Green's program package `edgewarp`, available by FTP from the directory `pub/edgewarp` on `brainmap.med.umich.edu`.

References

[1] D. G. Kendall. Shape-manifolds, procrustean metrics, and complex projective spaces. *Bull. London Mathematical Society* 16:81–121, 1984.

[2] F. L. Bookstein. Size and shape spaces for landmark data in two dimensions. *Statistical Science* 1:181–242, 1986.

[3] F. L. Bookstein. Toward a notion of feature extraction for plane mappings. Pp. 23–43 in C. de Graaf and M. Viergever, eds., *Proceedings of the Tenth International Conference on Information Processing in Medical Imaging.* New York: Plenum, 1988.

[4] F. L. Bookstein. Principal warps: Thin-plate splines and the decomposition of deformations. *I.E.E.E. Trans. Pattern Analysis and Machine Intelligence* 11:567–585, 1989.

[5] F. L. Bookstein. *Morphometric Tools for Landmark Data.* Cambridge University Press, 1991.

[6] K. V. Mardia. Shape advances and future perspectives. Pp. 57–75 in K. V. Mardia and C. A. Gill, eds., *Proc. Current Issues in Statistical Shape Analysis*, Leeds University Press, 1995.

[7] F. L. Bookstein. Metrics and symmetries of the morphometric synthesis. Pp. 139–153 in K. V. Mardia and C. A. Gill, eds., *Proc. Current Issues in Statistical Shape Analysis.* Leeds University Press, 1995.

[8] F. L. Bookstein. The Morphometric Synthesis for landmarks and edge-elements in images. *Terra Nova* 7:393–407, 1995.

[9] F. L. Bookstein. Biometrics, biomathematics, and the morphometric synthesis. *Bulletin of Mathematical Biology* 58:313–365, 1995.

[10] F. L. Bookstein. Biometrics and brain maps: the promise of the Morphometric Synthesis. To appear in S. Koslow and M. Huerta, eds., *Neuroinformatics: An Overview of the Human Brain Project. Progress in Neuroinformatics*, vol. 1. Hillsdale, NJ: Lawrence Erlbaum, 1996.

[11] F. J. Rohlf and D. Slice. Extensions of the Procrustes method for the optimal superposition of landmarks. *Systematic Zoology* 39:40–59, 1990.

[12] J. T. Kent. Current issues for statistical inference in shape analysis. Pp. 167–175 in K. V. Mardia and C. A. Gill, eds., *Proc. Current Issues in Statistical Shape Analysis.* Leeds University Press, 1995.

[13] J. Koenderink. *Solid Shape.* Cambridge, MA: M.I.T., 1990.

[14] F. L. Bookstein. Combining the tools of geometric morphometrics. Pp. 131–151 in L. Marcus et al., eds., *Proceedings of the NATO Advanced Study Institute on Morphometrics.* New York: Plenum, 1996.

[15] C. R. Goodall. Procrustes methods in the statistical analysis of shape. *J. Royal Statistical Society* B53:285–339, 1991.

[16] P. Good. *Permutation Tests.* New York: Springer-Verlag, 1994.

[17] F. L. Bookstein. How to produce a landmark point: the statistical geometry of incompletely registered images. Pp. 266–277 in R. Melter et al., eds., *Vision Geometry IV. S. P. I. E. Proceedings*, v. 2573, 1995.

[18] McIntosh, A. R., F. Bookstein, J. Haxby, and C. Grady. Multivariate analysis of functional brain images using Partial Least Squares. *NeuroImage*, in press.

[19] F. L. Bookstein. Landmark methods for forms without landmarks. This volume.

[20] W. D. K. Green. Spline-based deformable models. Pp. 290–301 in R. Melter, A. Wu, F. Bookstein, and W. D. K. Green, eds., *Vision Geometry IV.* S. P. I. E. *Proceedings*, vol. 2573, 1995.

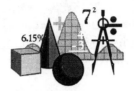

Session 1

Registration I

Multi-Modality Image Registration by Maximization of Mutual Information

Frederik Maes,* André Collignon, Dirk Vandermeulen, Guy Marchal, Paul Suetens
KU Leuven, Laboratory for Medical Imaging Research
Radiologie-ESAT, UZ Gasthuisberg, Herestraat 49, B-3000 Leuven, Belgium
Frederik.Maes@uz.kuleuven.ac.be

Abstract

Mutual information of image intensities has been proposed as a new matching criterion for automated multi-modality image registration. In this paper, we give experimental evidence of the power and the generality of the mutual information criterion by showing results for various applications involving CT, MR and PET images. Our results illustrate the large applicability of the approach and demonstrate its high suitability for routine use in clinical practice.

1. Introduction

Voxel similarity based (VSB) registration methods have recently captured a lot of interest for multi-modality image registration and have been shown to allow for robust retrospective registration by an automated algorithm without interaction or segmentation requirement [21]. VSB methods optimize a functional measuring the similarity of all geometrically corresponding voxel pairs for some feature. Feature calculation is straightforward or even absent when only grey-values are used. The registration accuracy is not limited by segmentation errors as with surface based registration methods and does not depend on the accurate indication of corresponding landmarks as with point landmark based methods.

For *intra-modality* registration multiple VSB methods have been proposed that rely on the assumption that the intensities of the two images are linearly correlated, which is generally not satisfied in the case of *inter-modality* registration. Cross-correlation of feature images derived from the original image data has been applied to CT/MR matching using geometrical features such as edges [13] and ridges [18] or using especially designed intensity transformations [19]. But feature extraction may introduce geometrical errors and requires extra calculation time, while

correlation of sparse features like edges and ridges may have a very peaked optimum at the registration solution, but at the same time be rather insensitive to misregistration at larger distances, as all non-edge or non-ridge voxels correlate equally well. A multi-resolution optimization strategy is therefore required.

In the approach of Woods et al. [22] and Hill et al. [8, 9] misregistration is measured by the dispersion of the two-dimensional (2-D) histogram of the image intensities of corresponding voxel pairs, which is assumed to be minimal in the registered position. But the dispersion measures they propose are largely heuristic and require segmentation of the images or delineation of specific histogram regions to make the method work [15]. Moreover, Woods' criterion is based on additional assumptions concerning the relationship between the grey-values in the different modalities, which reduces its applicability to some very specific multi-modality combinations (PET/MR).

The use of the much more general notion of *Mutual Information* (MI) or relative entropy [4, 16] to describe the dispersive behavior of the 2-D histogram has been proposed independently by Collignon et al. [3, 11] and by Viola et al. [20]. Mutual information is a basic concept from information theory, measuring the statistical dependence between two random variables or the amount of information that one variable contains about the other. The MI registration criterion states that the mutual information of the image intensity values of corresponding voxel pairs is maximal if the images are geometrically aligned. Because no limiting constraints are imposed on the nature of the relation between the intensities in the images to be registered and no assumptions are made regarding the image content of the modalities involved, the mutual information criterion is very general and powerful. It allows for robust and completely automated registration of multi-modal images without prior segmentation, feature extraction or other preprocessing steps, which makes this method very well suited for clinical applications.

In this paper we give experimental evidence for the power of the mutual information approach by showing re-

---

*Frederik Maes is Aspirant of the Belgian National Fund for Scientific Research (NFWO).

sults for various clinical applications. In sections 2 and 3, we first describe the algorithm and discuss some implementation issues. Section 4.1 presents results for CT/MR and PET/MR registration of brain images, validating the sub-voxel accuracy of the method. The same method has been used successfully for the rigid body registration of MR brain images of different patients to correlate functional MRI data (section 4.2) and for the registration of spiral CT images of a hardware phantom to its geometrical description to assess the accuracy of spiral CT imaging (section 4.3). Section 5 discusses our current findings, while section 6 gives some directions for further work.

2. The mutual information matching criterion

The image intensity values a and b of a pair of corresponding voxels in the two images that are to be registered can be considered to be random variables A and B respectively. A and B are related through the geometric transformation T_α defined by the set of registration parameters α. Estimations for the joint and marginal distributions $p_{AB}(a, b)$, $p_A(a)$ and $p_B(b)$ can be obtained by simple normalization of the joint and marginal image intensity histograms of the overlapping parts of both images.

Mutual information (MI) $I(A, B)$ of two random variables A and B measures the degree of dependence between A and B by the Kullback-Leibler distance [16] between the joint distribution $p_{AB}(a, b)$ and the distribution associated to the case of complete independence $p_A(a).p_B(b)$:

$$
\begin{aligned}
I(A, B) &= \sum_{a,b} p_{AB}(a, b) \log \frac{p_{AB}(a, b)}{p_A(a).p_B(b)} & (1) \\
&= H(A) - H(A|B) & (2) \\
&= H(B) - H(B|A) & (3) \\
&= H(A) + H(B) - H(A, B) & (4)
\end{aligned}
$$

with $H(A)$ and $H(B)$ being the entropy of A and B respectively, $H(A, B)$ their joint entropy and $H(A|B)$ and $H(B|A)$ the conditional entropy of A given B and of B given A respectively. The entropy $H(A)$ is known to be a measure of the amount of uncertainty about the random variable A, while $H(A|B)$ is the amount of uncertainty left in A when knowing B. Hence, $I(A, B)$ is the reduction in the uncertainty of the random variable A by the knowledge of another random variable B, or, equivalently, the amount of information that B contains about A. If A and B are statistically independent, then $p_{AB}(a, b) = p_A(a).p_B(b)$ and $I(A, B) = 0$, while if A and B are maximally dependent, they are related by a one-to-one mapping T such that $p_A(a) = p_B(T(a)) = p_{AB}(a, T(a))$ and $I(A, B) = H(A) = H(B) = H(A, B)$.

The mutual information registration criterion states that the images are geometrically aligned by the transformation T_{α^*} for which $I(A, B)$ is maximal. This criterion assumes that the amount of information that A contains about B is maximal in the registered position. When applied to images of the brain, for instance, the skull is high intense in CT images and low intense in MR images. If both images are correctly aligned, the uncertainty about the MR voxel intensity is therefore largely reduced if the corresponding CT voxel is known to be high intense and thus likely to be part of the skull. This correspondence is lost in case of misregistration. However, the mutual information criterion does not rely on limiting assumptions regarding the nature of the relation between corresponding voxel intensities in different modalities, which is highly data-dependent, and no constraints are imposed on the image content of the modalities involved. From equation 4, the mutual information matching criterion can be interpreted as follows [20]: "maximizing mutual information will tend to find as much as possible of the complexity that is in the separate datasets (maximizing the first two terms) so that at the same time they explain each other well (minimizing the last term)".

3. Implementation issues

Let $(f(s), r(T_\alpha s))$ be a pair of image intensity values in the images $\mathbf{F}$ and $\mathbf{R}$ to be registered at corresponding sites s in $\mathbf{F}$ and $T_\alpha s$ in $\mathbf{R}$ with T_α a geometric transformation with parameters α. Let $p_F(f)$, $p_R(r)$ and $p_{FR}(f, r)$ be the marginal and joint probability distributions of $f(s)$ and $r(T_\alpha s)$. The mutual information registration criterion can then be summarized by the following equations:

$$
\begin{aligned}
I(\alpha) &= \sum_{f,r} p_{FR}(f, r) \log \frac{p_{FR}(f, r)}{p_F(f)\, p_R(r)} & (5) \\
\alpha^* &= \arg \max_\alpha I(\alpha) & (6)
\end{aligned}
$$

with $I(\alpha)$ the mutual information of $\mathbf{F}$ and $\mathbf{R}$ at registration position α and α^* the position at which $I(\alpha)$ is maximal.

One of the images is selected to be the *floating* image $\mathbf{F}$ from which samples $s \in S$ with intensity $f(s)$ are taken and transformed into the *reference* image $\mathbf{R}$. The set of sample points S usually is the set of grid points of $\mathbf{F}$, although sub-sampling of the floating image can be used to increase speed performance. Each sample taken from $\mathbf{F}$ is transformed into $\mathbf{R}$ by the transformation T_α. For each value of the registration parameter α only those values $s \in S_\alpha \subset S$ are retained for which $T_\alpha s$ falls inside the volume of the reference image $\mathbf{R}$.

The joint image intensity histogram $h(f, r)$ is computed by binning the image intensity pairs $(f(s), r(T_\alpha s))$. In or-

15

der to do this efficiently, the floating and the reference image are first linearly rescaled to the range $[0, n_F - 1]$ and $[0, n_R - 1]$ respectively, $n_F \times n_R$ being the total number of bins in the joint histogram. Typically, we use $n_F = n_R = 256$. Normalization of $h(f, r)$ yields estimations for the marginal and joint image intensity distributions $p_F(f)$, $p_R(r)$ and $p_{FR}(f, r)$ of the overlapping volume of the images:

$$p_{FR}(f, r) = \frac{h(f, r)}{\sum_{f,r} h(f, r)} \qquad (7)$$

$$p_F(f) = \sum_r p_{FR}(f, r) \qquad (8)$$

$$p_R(r) = \sum_f p_{FR}(f, r) \qquad (9)$$

In general, $T_\alpha s$ will not coincide with a grid point of $\mathbf{R}$ and interpolation of the reference image is needed to obtain the image intensity value $r(T_\alpha s)$ at the position $T_\alpha s$ in the reference image. *Nearest neighbor* (NN) interpolation of $\mathbf{R}$ is generally insufficient to guarantee subvoxel accuracy, as it is insensitive to translations up to 1 voxel. Other interpolation methods, such as *trilinear* (TRI) interpolation, may introduce new intensity values which are originally not present in the reference image, leading to unpredictable changes in the marginal distribution $p_R(r)$ for small variations of α. To avoid this problem, we have proposed to use *trilinear partial volume distribution* (PV) interpolation to update the joint histogram for each voxel pair $(s, T_\alpha s)$. Instead of interpolating new intensity values in $\mathbf{R}$, the contribution of the image intensity $f(s)$ of the sample s of $\mathbf{F}$ to the joint histogram is distributed over the intensity values of all 8 nearest neighbors of $T_\alpha s$ on the grid of $\mathbf{R}$, using the same weights as for trilinear interpolation. Each entry in the joint histogram is then the sum of smoothly varying fractions of 1, such that the histogram changes smoothly as α is varied.

The optimal registration parameters α^* are found by maximization of $I(\alpha)$ using Powell's direction set method [14]. The images are positioned initially such that their centers coincide and that the floating and reference image coordinate axes corresponding to the same patient axis (i.e. right to left, anterior to posterior, and inferior to superior) are properly aligned, which assumes that the orientation of each of the images with respect to the patient is known.

The algorithm has been implemented[1] on an IBM RS6000/3AT workstation (58 MHz, 185 SPECfp92, AIX 4.1.3). The complexity of one evaluation of the MI registration criterion was found to vary linearly with the number of samples taken from the floating image. While trilinear or

---

[1]Object-oriented C++ source code available on request.

partial volume interpolation have about the same complexity, nearest neighbor interpolation is about twice as efficient (1.36 vs. 0.60 CPU seconds per million samples for one evaluation of the criterion). The number of evaluations performed during optimization depends on the initial orientation of the images and on the convergence parameters specified for the Powell algorithm. All experiments described in this paper typically required between 300 and 500 criterion evaluations.

4. Results

In this section, we show registration results obtained by using the mutual information criterion for various applications. These include the registration of CT, MR and PET brain images of the same patient, the registration of MR brain images of different patients and the registration of a mathematical model of a hardware phantom to its CT image. For all experiments discussed in this paper, we have restricted the geometric transformation T_α to rigid body transformations only, although it is clear that the mutual information criterion can be applied to more general transformations as well. The rigid body transformation T_α is a superposition of a 3-D rotation and a 3-D translation and the registration parameter α is a 6-component vector consisting of 3 rotation angles and 3 translation distances.

4.1. Registration of CT, MR and PET brain images

The performance of the MI registration criterion has been evaluated extensively for rigid body registration of MR, CT and PET images of the brain of the same patient. The rigid body assumption is well satisfied inside the skull in 3-D scans of the head, if abstraction is made of scanner calibration problems and problems of geometric distortions, both of which can be minimized by careful calibration and scan parameter selection respectively.

The accuracy of the matching criterion was validated within the framework of the Retrospective Registration Evaluation Project (RREP) conducted by Fitzpatrick et al. at Vanderbilt University [6]. In total, 76 CT/MR and PET/MR registrations were performed on 9 patient datasets provided by Vanderbilt. Each dataset consisted of axial CT, MR and PET images which were acquired stereotactically using the same protocol for each patient, but the images were edited to remove the stereotactic markers (figure 1). 6 different MR images were acquired: proton density (PD), T1- and T2-weighted images and the corresponding images corrected for geometric distortion (PDr, T1r, T2r) [21]. The slice thickness was 4 mm for the CT and MR images and 8 mm for the PET images (table 1).

Registration of these images using the mutual information criterion was performed fully automatically on an IBM

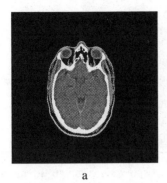 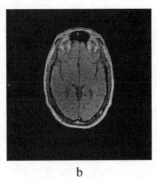 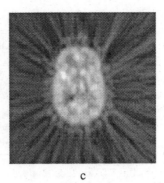 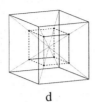

a   b   c   d

Figure 1. a,b,c: Typical axial slices of the CT, MR and PET images used in the experiments of section 4.1. d: The bounding box of the innermost eighth of the floating image defines 8 points near the brain surface at which registration accuracy is evaluated.

	Dimensions	Voxelsizes (in mm)
MR	256×256×25	1.25×1.25×4.00
CT	512×512×30	0.65×0.65×4.00
PET	128×128×15	2.59×2.59×8.00

Table 1. Typical dimensions and voxelsizes of the images used in the experiments of section 4.1.

RS6000/3AT workstation using PV interpolation in about 20 minutes for MR to CT matching and in only about 2 minutes for PET to MR matching. The recovered rotational transformation parameters were generally smaller than 5 degrees, while the translational parameters varied up to 30 millimeter.

For each registration result separately, the difference between the stereotactic reference transformation and the registration solution as obtained with the mutual information matching criterion was evaluated by considering 8 points near the brain surface in the CT or PET image (defined as the 8 cornerpoints of the bounding box of the innermost eighth of the image, figure 1d), transforming these into the MR image using either of both transforms and taking the mean over all 8 points of the norm of the transformation difference vector ($|\Delta|$) and of the absolute value of its three coordinate components separately ($|\Delta x|$, $|\Delta y|$, $|\Delta z|$). These error values are summarized in table 2 and in table 3 by the mean and the maximal value respectively over all patient datasets. The x, y and z direction correspond to the patient's right to left, anterior to posterior and inferior to superior direction respectively.

The mean errors are all subvoxel accurate for each of the modality combinations with respect to the largest voxelsize of the images. The maximal error values show that errors are subvoxel for almost all 41 CT/MR and 35 PET/MR

	N	$|\Delta x|$	$|\Delta y|$	$|\Delta z|$	$|\Delta|$
CT/PD	7	0.5301	1.3527	1.2952	2.2041
CT/T1	7	0.5104	1.2746	1.5321	2.2577
CT/T2	7	0.5808	1.1779	1.4569	2.1919
CT/PDr	7	0.3588	0.5748	0.9360	1.3004
CT/T1r	6	0.2977	0.5633	1.1708	1.4662
CT/T2r	7	0.3760	0.6746	1.3699	1.7496
PET/PD	7	1.5232	2.8007	3.4607	5.1995
PET/T1	7	0.9105	1.9351	4.6114	5.5750
PET/T2	7	0.8930	1.9682	2.7568	3.9311
PET/PDr	5	1.1752	1.7516	2.7908	3.9214
PET/T1r	4	0.9002	1.0050	2.4337	3.1128
PET/T2r	5	0.9115	1.7599	2.6957	3.7094

Table 2. Registration error (in mm) evaluated at 8 points near the brain surface: mean values over all N cases.

	N	$|\Delta x|$	$|\Delta y|$	$|\Delta z|$	$|\Delta|$
CT/PD	7	1.1894	2.7498	2.8421	3.2472
CT/T1	7	0.8425	2.7716	3.5301	4.7798
CT/T2	7	1.4095	2.2235	2.7453	3.5607
CT/PDr	7	0.6449	0.8322	1.4986	1.9723
CT/T1r	6	0.4347	1.0065	2.6635	2.7929
CT/T2r	7	0.7475	1.5521	3.8785	4.5174
PET/PD	7	2.4587	6.2855	6.6968	10.1254
PET/T1	7	1.6536	3.3762	11.0182	11.1916
PET/T2	7	1.6703	4.7235	4.4445	6.2122
PET/PDr	5	1.4953	2.6593	4.6017	5.7440
PET/T1r	4	1.5704	1.9126	2.9016	4.0556
PET/T2r	5	1.7895	4.3078	5.4507	7.9527

Table 3. Registration error (in mm) evaluated at 8 points near the brain surface: maximal values over all N cases.

registrations, while in at least 2 cases for PET to MR registration errors were clearly larger than a PET voxel. The largest errors occur in the z direction, while we also noted that the optimization proved to be more robust if the inplane parameters t_x, t_y and ϕ_z were optimized first, before optimizing the out-of-plane parameters ϕ_x, ϕ_y and t_z. Both observations can be explained by the lower resolution of the images in the z direction and by the fact that the registration is less well conditioned for translation in the cranio-caudal direction as these images do not include the top of the skull. When comparing the results for the MR images that were corrected for geometric distortion with those for the uncorrected images, there is a clear tendency towards lower registration errors for the corrected images [21].

4.2. Patient-to-patient MR registration

Correlation of functional MRI data obtained from different patients was done by registration of the corresponding anatomical MR images with a template image of the brain, obtained by segmentation of an original MR image[2]. The template has been mapped into Talairach space, such that after registration of each of the patient images to the template, functional measurements from different patients can be compared within the Talairach frame.

The template has 2 mm cubic voxels and size $64 \times 87 \times 64$. The patient MR MPRAGE images have a voxelsize of $1 \times 1 \times 1.25$ mm and dimensions $256 \times 256 \times 128$. Registration was done from the template to the patient image using a rigid body transformation, but allowing for anisotropic scaling factors around the center of the template in the 3 axis directions. Figure 2 shows overlays of an axial, coronal and sagittal slice of the template on the registered MR image. Because of the variability of the brain topology, the rigid body assumption is not satisfied in this case, but the MI criterion succeeds at finding such a transformation that on average very well matches corresponding structures in both images.

The same method has been applied successfully on 15 other patient images. Visual inspection of the results by clinicians showed superior performance of the MI criterion compared to the registration technique that is used in the SPM package of Friston et al. [7], which is based on intensity correlation of segmented white and grey matter regions.

4.3. Image-to-model registration

To validate the geometric accuracy of various spiral CT imaging protocols for orthopedic applications [17], spiral CT images were acquired from a hardware phantom of the spine [10]. This phantom is a geometric abstraction of

---

[2]Template image provided by Friston et al [7].

three vertebrae, consisting of different vertebrae components. Different components are modeled by different tissue substitute materials, which appear with a distinct intensity in the image. A mathematical model was constructed from the geometrical description of the phantom by assigning each structure a different label (32 in total, including background). The CT images were registered with this model using the mutual information criterion on the intensity of each voxel in the CT image and its corresponding label in the model. After registration, edges segmented from the image are compared with the corresponding edges in the model, which allows to assess the acquisition accuracy, provided that registration and segmentation errors can be assumed to be small.

The result of the registration is illustrated in figure 3, showing the midsagittal plane through the model and the corresponding plane in the image after registration for a 1/1 spiral CT acquisition reconstructed at 0.5 mm slice distance. The original voxelsizes are $0.16 \times 0.16 \times 0.5$ mm, but the images of figure 3 were resampled into 0.16 mm square voxels for the purpose of visualization. Overlay of the contours of the model on the CT image allows visual inspection of the registration accuracy. The segmentation result shown in figure 3d was obtained automatically using the method described in [12].

5. Discussion

The mutual information matching criterion is based on the assumption that the statistical dependence between corresponding voxel intensities is maximal if both images are geometrically aligned. Mutual information measures statistical dependence by comparing the complexity of the joint distribution with that of the marginals. Both marginal distributions are taken into account explicitly, which is an important difference with the measures proposed earlier by Hill et al. [9] (third order moment of the joint histogram), Woods et al. [22] (variance of intensity ratios) and Collignon et al. [2] (entropy of the joint histogram). In appendices 1 and 2, we discuss the relationship between these measures and the MI criterion.

Because no assumptions are made regarding the nature of the dependence between corresponding voxel intensities, the MI criterion is highly data independent and allows for robust and completely automated registration of multimodality images in various applications without any prior segmentation or other pre-processing steps. The results of section 4.1 demonstrate that subvoxel registration accuracy can be obtained for CT/MR and PET/MR matching without using any prior knowledge about the grey-value content of both images and the correspondence between them. The generality of the approach is demonstrated by the results of sections 4.2 and 4.3. Although in all experiments discussed

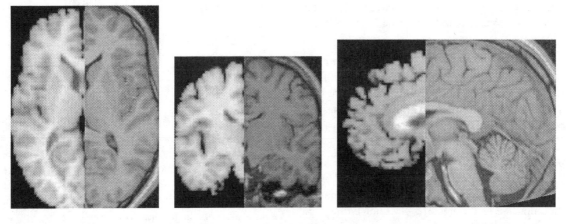

Figure 2. Registration of a template MR brain image to patient MR images of the head. Overlay of an axial, coronal and sagittal slice of the template on the registered patient image.

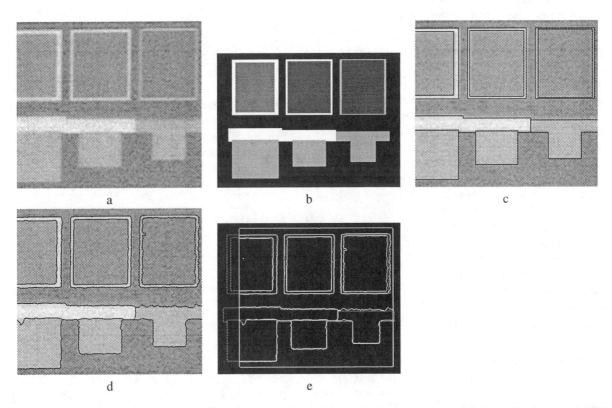

a   b   c

d   e

Figure 3. Registration of the mathematical model of a hardware phantom with its CT image. a) Mid-sagittal cross section through the CT image (resampled into square voxels). b) Corresponding slice through the model. c) Overlay of model contours on the registered CT image. d) Contours extracted from the CT image. e) Overlay of model and image contours allows validation of acquisition accuracy.

in this paper a rigid body transformation was used, it is clear that the MI criterion can as well be applied to more general transformations.

Partial volume interpolation was introduced to make the joint and marginal distributions and their mutual information vary smoothly for small changes in the registration parameters. Our results indicate that PV interpolation indeed behaves superior with respect to robustness compared to nearest neighbor and trilinear interpolation [11].

Evaluation of the MI criterion requires estimations of the image intensity distributions, which were obtained by simple normalization of the joint histogram. We have not evaluated the influence of the bin size, the choice of a region of interest or the application of non-linear image intensity transformations on the behavior of the MI registration criterion. Other schemes can be used to estimate the image intensity distributions, for instance by using Parzen windowing [5] on a set of samples taken from the overlapping part of both images. This approach was used by Viola et al. [20], who also use stochastic sampling of the floating image to increase speed performance.

The optimization of the MI registration criterion was implemented using Powell's method, which proved to be very reliable and robust. To increase the speed performance of the registration method, optimization efficiency may be increased by decreasing the number of criterion evaluations, for instance by taking into account that small parameter corrections hardly influence registration accuracy. We have also noted experimentally that for high resolution data subsampling of the floating image can be applied without deteriorating optimization robustness. Important speed-ups can thus be realized by using a multi-resolution optimization strategy, starting with a coarsely sampled image for efficiency and increasing the resolution as the optimization proceeds for accuracy. Viola et al. [20] applied a gradient-based optimization method, using explicit expressions for the derivatives of the MI function with respect to the registration parameters. However, it is not clear how registration robustness is affected by such alternative search techniques.

Mutual information is only one of a family of measures of statistical dependence or information redundancy (see appendix 3). We have experimented with $\rho(A, B) = H(A, B) - I(A, B)$, which can be shown to be a metric [4], and $ECC(A, B) = 2I(A, B)/(H(A) + H(B))$, the *Entropy Correlation Coefficient* [1]. In some cases, both measures showed superior performance compared to the original MI criterion, but we could not establish a clear preference for either of these. Furthermore, the use of mutual information for multi-modality image registration is not restricted to the original image intensities only: other derived features, such as edges or ridges, can be used as well. Selection of appropriate features is an area for further research.

6. Conclusion

The mutual information matching criterion allows for accurate, robust and completely automated registration of multi-modality medical images. The method is highly data independent and requires no user interaction, segmentation or pre-processing and is therefore well suited to be used in clinical practice. However, the performance of the method on clinical data needs to be further investigated and compared to that of other registration methods. Further research is also needed to better understand the influence of implementation issues, such as sampling and interpolation, on the registration criterion and to tune the optimization method towards specific applications. Finally, other registration criteria can be derived from the one presented here, using alternative information measures applied on different features.

7. Acknowledgments

This research was supported by IBM Belgium (Academic Joint Study) and by the National Fund for Scientific Research, Belgium, under grant numbers FGWO 3.0115.92, 9.0033.93 and G.3115.92. The authors would like to acknowledge the contributions to this paper of Sylvie Van Oostende and Stefan Sunaert to section 4.2 and of Johan Van Cleynenbreugel to section 4.3. The work on spiral CT accuracy measurement is part of PHIDIAS (laser PHotopolymerisation models based on medical Imaging, a Development Improving the Accuracy of Surgery), project nr. BE/5930 of the BRITE-EURAM programme of the European Commission.

A. Appendix 1

We show the relationship between the multi-modality registration criterion devised by Hill et al. [8] and the joint entropy $H(a, b)$. Hill et al. used the n-th order moment of the scatter-plot h as a measure of dispersion:

$$T_n = \sum_{a,b} (\frac{h(a,b)}{V})^n \qquad (10)$$

with $h(a, b)$ the histogram entries and $V = \sum_{a,b} h(a, b)$ the common volume of overlap. Approximating the joint probability distribution $p(a, b)$ by $p(a, b) = h(a, b)/V$, we get:

$$T_n = \sum_{a,b} p(a,b)^n$$

It turns out that T_n is one-to-one related to the joint Rényi entropy H_n of order n [16]:

$$H_n = \frac{1}{1-n} \log(T_n)$$

with the following properties:

- $\lim_{n\to 1} H_n(p) = \sum_i p_i \log p_i$, which is the Shannon entropy.

- $n_2 > n_1 \to H_{n_2}(p) \leq H_{n_1}(p)$

Hence, the normalized second or third order moment criteria defined by Hill et al. are equivalent to a generalized version of the joint entropy $H(a, b)$.

B. Appendix 2

We show how the multi-modality registration criterion devised by Woods et al. [22] relates to the conditional entropy $H(a|b)$. Denote by A and B the set of possible intensities in the two images. Denote by a_i and b_i the intensities of A and B at the common voxel position i. For each voxel i with value $b_i = b$ in image B, let $a_i(b)$ be the value at voxel i in the corresponding image A. Let $\mu_a(b)$ be the mean and $\sigma_a(b)$ be the standard deviation of the set $\{a_i(b) \mid \forall i : b_i = b\}$. Let $n_b = \#\{i \mid b_i = b\}$ and $N = \sum_b n_b$. The registration criterion that Woods et al. minimize is then defined as follows:

$$\sigma'' = \sum_b \frac{n_b}{N} \frac{\sigma_a(b)}{\mu_a(b)} \quad (11)$$

$$= \sum_b p_b(b) \frac{\sigma_a(b)}{\mu_a(b)} \quad (12)$$

with p_b the marginal distribution function of image intensities B.

It can be shown [4] that for a given mean $\mu_a(b)$ and standard deviation $\sigma_a(b)$

$$H(A|B) = \sum_b p(b) H(A|B = b) \quad (13)$$

$$= -\sum_b p(b) \sum_a p(a|b). \log p(a|b) \quad (14)$$

$$\leq \sum_b p(b) \log(\sigma_a(b)) + \frac{1}{2} \log(2\pi e) \quad (15)$$

with equality if the conditional distribution $p(a|b)$ of image intensities A given B is the normal distribution $N(\mu_a(b), \sigma_a(b))$.

Using Jensen's inequality for concave functions [4] we get

$$H(A|B) \leq \sum_b p(b)(\log(\frac{\sigma_a(b)}{\mu_a(b)}) + \log(\mu_a(b))) \quad (16)$$

$$\leq \log(\sum_b p(b) \frac{\sigma_a(b)}{\mu_a(b)}) + \log(\sum_b p(b) \mu_a(b)) \quad (17)$$

$$= \log(\sigma'') + log(\mu(a)) \quad (18)$$

with $\mu(a) = \sum_b p(b) \mu_a(b)$ the mean intensity of image A.

If $\mu(a)$ is constant and $p(a|b)$ can be assumed to be normally distributed, minimization of σ'' then amounts to optimizing the conditional entropy $H(A|B)$. In the approach of Woods et al., this assumption is approximately accomplished by editing away parts in one data set (in casu the skin in MR) for which otherwise additional modes might occur in $p(a|b)$, while Hill et al. have proposed to take only specifically selected regions in the joint histogram into account.

C. Appendix 3

Mutual Information $I(a; b)$ is only one example of the more general *f-information* measures of dependence $f(P \| P_1 \times P_2)$ [16] with P the set of joint probability distributions $P(a, b)$ and $P_1 \times P_2$ the set of joint probability distributions $P(a).P(b)$ assuming a and b to be independent.

f-information is derived from the concept of *f-divergence*, which is defined as:

$$f(P \| Q) = \sum_i q_i. f(p_i/q_i)$$

with $P = \{p_1, p_2 \ldots\}$ and $Q = \{q_1, q_2 \ldots\}$ with suitable definitions when $q_i = 0$.

Some examples of f-divergence are:

- I_α-*divergence*:

$$I_\alpha = \frac{1}{\alpha(\alpha - 1)} \left[\sum_i \frac{p_i^\alpha}{q_i^{\alpha-1}} - 1 \right]$$

- χ^2-*divergence*:

$$\chi^2 = \sum_i \frac{(p_i - q_i)^2}{q_i}$$

with corresponding f-informations:

- I_α-*information*:

$$I_\alpha(P \| P_1 \times P_2) = \frac{1}{\alpha(\alpha - 1)} \left[\sum_{i,j} \frac{p_{ij}^\alpha}{(p_{i.}.p_{.j})^{\alpha-1}} - 1 \right]$$

with $p_{ij} = P(i, j)$ and $p_{i.} = \sum_j p_{ij}$ and $p_{.j} = \sum_i p_{ij}$

- χ^2-*information*:

$$\chi^2(P \| P_1 \times P_2) = \sum_{i,j} \frac{(p_{ij} - p_{i.}.p_{.j})^2}{p_{i.}.p_{.j}}$$

21

Note that $I_\alpha(P||P_1 \times P_2)$ is the information-measure counterpart of the n-th order moment used by Hill et al. for $n = \alpha = 2, 3$. Furthermore, $I_1(P||P_1 \times P_2) = \sum_{i,j} p_{ij} \log(\frac{p_{ij}}{p_{i.}p_{.j}})$ which is the definition of Mutual Information used in this paper.

References

[1] J. Astola and I. Virtanen. Entropy correlation coefficient, a measure of statistical dependence for categorized data. In *Proc. of the Univ. of Vaasa, Finland*, number 44 in Discussion Papers, 1982. 12 pages.

[2] A. Collignon, D. Vandermeulen, P. Suetens, and G. Marchal. 3d multi-modality medical image registration using feature space clustering. In N. Ayache, editor, *Proc. of the First Int'l Conf. on Computer Vision, Virtual Reality and Robotics in Medicine (CVRMed'95)*, volume 905 of *Lecture Notes in Computer Science*, pages 195–204, Nice, France, April 1995. Springer-Verlag.

[3] A. Collignon, D. Vandermeulen, P. Suetens, and G. Marchal. Automated multimodality medical image registration using information theory. In Y. Bizais, C. Barillot, and R. di Paola, editors, *Proc. of the XIV'th Int'l Conf. on Information Processing in Medical Imaging (IPMI'95)*, volume 3 of *Computational Imaging and Vision*, pages 263–274, Ile de Berder, France, June 1995. Kluwer Academic Plublishers.

[4] T. Cover and J. Thomas. *Elements of Information Theory*. John Wiley & Sons, Inc., New York, 1991.

[5] R. Duda and P. Hart. *Pattern Classification and Scene Analysis*. A Wiley-Interscience Publication, 1973.

[6] J. Fitzpatrick (Principal Investigator). Evaluation of retrospective image registration. National Institutes of Health, Project Number 1 R01 NS33926-01.

[7] K. Friston, J. Ashburner, C. Frith, J.-B. Poline, J. Heather, and R. Frackowiak. Spatial registration and normalisation of images. *Humun Brain Mapping*, 1996. In press.

[8] D. Hill, D. Hawkes, N. Harrison, and C. Ruff. A strategy for automated multimodality image registration incorporating anatomical knowledge and imager characteristics. In H. Barrett and A. Gmitro, editors, *Proc. of the XIIIth Int'l Conf. on Information Processing in Medical Imaging (IPMI'93)*, volume 687 of *Lecture Notes in Computer Science*, pages 182–196, Flagstaff, Arizona, USA, June 1993. Springer-Verlag.

[9] D. Hill, C. Studholme, and D. Hawkes. Voxel similarity measures for automated image registration. In R. A. Robb, editor, *Visualization in Biomedical Computing 1994*, volume 2359 of *Proc. SPIE*, Rochester, Minnesota, USA, October 1994. SPIE, Bellingham, WA.

[10] W. Kalender. A phantom for standardization and quality control in peripheral bone measurements by qct and dxa: Design considerations and specifications. *Medical Physics*, 19:583–586, 1992.

[11] F. Maes, A. Collignon, D. Vandermeulen, G. Marchal, and P. Suetens. Multi-modality image registration by maximization of mutual information. Submitted to IEEE Trans. on Medical Imaging, February 1996.

[12] F. Maes, D. Vandermeulen, P. Suetens, and G. Marchal. Automatic image partitioning for generic object segmentation in medical images. In Y. Bizais, C. Barillot, and R. di Paola, editors, *Proc. of the XIV'th Int'l Conf. on Information Processing in Medical Imaging (IPMI'95)*, volume 3 of *Computational Imaging and Vision*, pages 215–226, Ile de Berder, France, June 1995. Kluwer Academic Plublishers.

[13] J. Maintz, P. Van den Elsen, and M. Viergever. Comparison of feature-based matching of ct and mr brain images. In N. Ayache, editor, *Proc. of the First Int'l Conf. on Computer Vision, Virtual Reality and Robotics in Medicine (CVRMed'95)*, volume 905 of *Lecture Notes in Computer Science*, pages 219–228, Nice, France, April 1995. Springer-Verlag.

[14] W. Press, B. Flannery, S. Teukolsky, and W. Vetterling. *Numerical Recipes in C: The Art of Scientific Computing, Second Edition*. Cambridge University Press, Cambridge, England, 1992. Chapter 10, pages 412–419.

[15] C. Studholme, D. Hill, and D. Hawkes. Multiresolution voxel similarity measures for mr-pet registration. In Y. Bizais, C. Barillot, and R. di Paola, editors, *Proc. of the XIV'th Int'l Conf. on Information Processing in Medical Imaging (IPMI'95)*, volume 3 of *Computational Imaging and Vision*, pages 287–298, Ile de Berder, France, June 1995. Kluwer Academic Publishers.

[16] I. Vajda. *Theory of Statistical Inference and Information*. Kluwer Academic Publisher, 1989.

[17] J. Van Cleynenbreugel, F. Maes, F. Haven, G. Marchal, and P. Suetens. A phantom based approach to assess the geometrical accuracy obtainable from spiral ct imaging. In preparation.

[18] P. Van den Elsen, J. Maintz, E. Pol, and M. Viergever. Image fusion using geometrical features. In R. A. Robb, editor, *Visualization in Biomedical Computing 1992*, volume 1808 of *Proc. SPIE*, pages 172–186, Chapel Hill, North Carolina, USA, October 1992. SPIE, Bellingham, WA.

[19] P. Van den Elsen, E. Pol, T. Sumanaweera, P. Hemler, S. Napel, and J. Adler. Grey value correlation techniques used for automatic matching of ct and mr brain and spine images. In R. A. Robb, editor, *Visualization in Biomedical Computing 1994*, volume 2359 of *Proc. SPIE*, pages 227–237, Rochester, Minnesota, USA, October 1994. SPIE, Bellingham, WA.

[20] P. Viola and W. W. III. Alignment by maximization of mutual information. In *Proc. of the Vth International Conference on Computer Vision*, pages 16–23. Cambridge, Massachusetts, U.S.A, June 1995.

[21] J. West, J. Fitzpatrick, and M. Wang et al. Comparison and evaluation of retrospective intermodality image registration techniques. In M. A. Loew, editor, *Medical Imaging: Image Processing*, volume 2710 of *Proc. SPIE*, Newport Beach, California, USA, February 1996. In press.

[22] R. Woods, J. Mazziotta, and S. Cherry. Mri-pet registration with automated algorithm. *Journal of Computer Assisted Tomography*, 17(4):536–546, July/August 1993.

Incorporating Connected Region Labelling into Automated Image Registration Using Mutual Information

C.Studholme, D.L.G.Hill, D.J.Hawkes
Radiological Sciences
UMDS, Guys Hospital
London SE1 9RT
{cs,dlgh,djh}@umds.ac.uk

Abstract

The information theoretic measure of mutual information has been successfully applied to multi-modality medical image registration for several applications. There remain however, modality combinations for which mutual information derived from the occurrence of image intensities alone does not provide a distinct optimum at true registration. We propose an extension of the technique through the use of an additional information channel supplying region labelling information. These labels, which can specify simple regional connectivity or express higher level anatomical knowledge, can be derived from the images being registered. We show how the mutual information measure can be extended to include an additional channel of region labelling, and demonstrate the effectiveness of this technique for the registration of MR and PET images of the pelvis.

Keywords: Automated Image Registration, Voxel Similarity Measures, Region Labelling, Mutual Information.

1 Introduction

It has been shown that optimisation of voxel similarity based registration measures [5], in particular that of mutual information [8, 1, 4], provides a robust approach to the registration of brain images acquired with MR and PET, or MR and CT.

Experimentally we have found problems can occur when using mutual information to align other modality combinations or images acquired in other regions of the body. In some cases this may be due to a of a lack in differentiation between spatially unconnected regions in one modality which are connected in the other modality. This is a particular problem when the two images are truncated or when the corresponding structures in the images essential in defining the registration are significantly perturbed by noise. Optimisation of mutual information, which can be derived from the joint and separate probability distributions of image intensities, contains no information on either the spatial distribution of intensities or the connectivity of uniform regions.

In principle a complete segmentation of the MR image, in which each distinguishable anatomical structure has a unique label, could be registered by maximising mutual information between the labelled image and the lower contrast, lower resolution image. In practice fully automated, complete and accurate regional labelling is impossible in anatomically complex and noisy images. It is difficult to ensure connectivity of regions of the same anatomical structure or tissue type while maintaining separation of regions corresponding to different structures or tissue types. In particular the identification of truly corresponding anatomical boundaries in different modalities is non-trivial.

In previous work mutual information between two channels, derived from the intensities in a each modality, has been maximised to achieve registration. We propose the introduction of further channels containing information in the form of labelling of distinct regions within the images. An additional channel of region labels allows differentiation of unconnected regions of similar intensity within an image.

In this paper we introduce a formalism for a similarity measure enabling the inclusion of coarse labelling of regions within the high resolution, high contrast image. An information theoretic approach enables the original image and region labelling to be combined in the registration process making use of information provided by both. We discuss how a simple region labelling process introduces additional information into the registration process. The behaviour of the approach is demonstrated in the registration of MR and PET images of the pelvis, conventionally difficult to register, by the addition of a coarsely labelled anatomical map derived from the MR image.

23

2 Mutual Information

2.1 Two Images

Given a pair of images to register and a transformation mapping one set of voxels onto the other, we can find for corresponding voxels, the intensities $m \in M$ in image $\mathbf{m}$, and intensities $n \in N$ in a lower contrast, lower resolution image $\mathbf{n}$. In the example considered in this paper $\mathbf{m}$ is an MR image of the pelvis and $\mathbf{n}$ is a nuclear medicine PET image. The sets M and N therefore depend on the rigid body transformation between the images. We can calculate the probability of occurrence of individual intensities $p\{m\}$ from the image $\mathbf{m}$, and intensities $p\{n\}$ from the image $\mathbf{n}$, and also the probabilities of corresponding intensity pairs $p\{m, n\}$.

The mutual information measure is derived from a statistical analysis of a communication channel, and is a measure of corresponding or mutual information between the transmitted and received signals [3]. This measure is alternatively referred to as relative entropy or transinformation and makes no assumption about the functional form of the channel. Mutual information has been proposed independently for various medical image registration applications by Collignon et al [1] and Viola and Wells [7] [8]. The mutual information between an image $\mathbf{m}$ with intensity m and an image $\mathbf{n}$ with intensity n defined from the 2D probability distribution is:

$$I(M; N) = \sum_{m \in M} \sum_{n \in N} p\{m, n\} \log \frac{p\{m, n\}}{p\{m\}p\{n\}} \quad (1)$$

This can be expressed in terms of the information present in image $\mathbf{m}$ $H(M)$, the image $\mathbf{n}$ $H(N)$, and the combined image $H(M, N)$:

$$I(M; N) = H(M) + H(N) - H(M, N) \quad (2)$$

In other words by maximising mutual information we minimise the information in the combined image with respect to that present in the two component images. If there are any shared features in the two images, at misregistration they are duplicated in the combined image. This duplication of features results in an excess of information in the combined image with respect to that provided by the two images separately. The relationship between the information provided by the images can be illustrated in a set theory form as shown in figure 1. The sets on the left illustrate the entropies of the two images separately. The central diagram represents the joint entropy of the combined image when a transformation maps the intensities of one onto the intensities of the other. The right hand figure shows that the mutual information is the replicated information from the two images.

2.2 Three Images

In our application we introduce further information in the form of a labelling of image $\mathbf{m}$ prior to registration, by creating a third image $\mathbf{l}$ with labels $l \in L$. This is shown graphically in figure 2. The measure of mutual information can be directly extended for this case as the difference between the sum of the information in the three images separately, and the information in the combined image:

$$I(M; L; N) = H(M) + H(L) + H(N) - H(M, L, N) \quad (3)$$

Images $\mathbf{m}$ and $\mathbf{l}$ are inherently registered and we are interested in the information shared between the PET image and these images which is illustrated by the set representation in figure 3.

This can be written algebraically as:

$$I(M, L; N) = H(M, L) + H(N) - H(M, L, N) \quad (4)$$

The entropies $H(M, L)$ $H(N)$ $H(M, L, N)$ can be derived from the probability of occurrence of intensities M and N, and labels L:

$$H(M, L) = \sum_{m \in M} \sum_{l \in L} p\{m, l\} \log \frac{1}{p\{m, l\}} \quad (5)$$

$$H(N) = \sum_{n \in N} p\{n\} \log \frac{1}{p\{n\}} \quad (6)$$

$$H(M, L, N) = \sum_{m \in M} \sum_{l \in L} \sum_{n \in N} p\{m, l, n\} \log \frac{1}{p\{m, l, n\}} \quad (7)$$

and substituted into equation 4 giving:

$$I(M, L; N) = \sum_{m \in M} \sum_{l \in L} p\{m, l\} \log \frac{1}{p\{m, l\}} + \\ \sum_{n \in N} p\{n\} \log \frac{1}{p\{n\}} - \\ \sum_{m \in M} \sum_{l \in L} \sum_{n \in N} p\{m, l, n\} \log \frac{1}{p\{m, l, n\}}$$

Given that $p\{m, l\} = \sum_{n \in N} p\{m, l, n\}$ and $p\{n\} = \sum_{m \in M} \sum_{l \in L} p\{m, l, n\}$,

$$I(M, L; N) = \sum_{m \in M} \sum_{l \in L} \sum_{n \in N} p\{m, l, n\} \log \frac{1}{p\{m, l\}} + \\ \sum_{n \in N} \sum_{m \in M} \sum_{l \in L} p\{m, l, n\} \log \frac{1}{p\{n\}} - \\ \sum_{m \in M} \sum_{l \in L} \sum_{n \in N} p\{m, l, n\} \log \frac{1}{p\{m, l, n\}}$$

this can be rearranged to give a simpler form:

$$I(M, L; N) = \sum_{m \in M} \sum_{l \in L} \sum_{n \in N} p\{m, l, n\} \log \frac{p\{m, l, n\}}{p\{m, l\}p\{n\}} \quad (8)$$

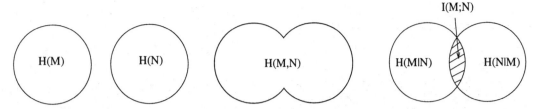

Figure 1. A set theory representation of the entropies involved when combining two images

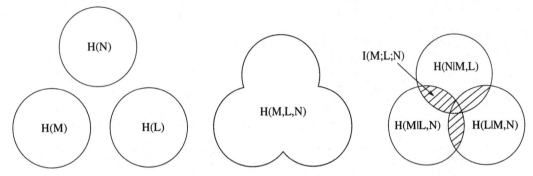

Figure 2. A set theory representation of the entropies involved when combining three images

2.3 Information and Region Labelling

In order to illustrate how extra regional information is being introduced we consider a simple region extraction process. This may consist of a thresholding to distinguish boundaries of interest, followed by a connected component labelling of the identified regions as illustrated in figure 4. Thresholding is effectively combining intensities (symbols) in the image, producing only a subset of the information in the original image. If a binary threshold is used then the image is being reduced to two symbols $T = \{t_0, t_1\}$ where, if there are i intensities in the original image and m_t is the threshold intensity so,

$$t_0 = \{m_0, \dots m_t\} \qquad (9)$$
$$t_1 = \{m_{t+1}, \dots m_i\}. \qquad (10)$$

The information contained in this thresholded image is then given by,

$$H(T) = - \sum_{t \in \{t_0, t_1\}} p\{t\} \log p\{t\}. \qquad (11)$$

Using the additivity property of information measures (see Reza[3], page 84) it can be shown that the information content of a set of symbols cannot be decreased when symbols are partitioned so,

$$H(m_0, \dots m_t, m_{t+1} \dots m_i) \geq H(t_0, m_{t+1}, \dots m_i) \qquad (12)$$

From this we can say that the information content of the thresholded image is always less than or equal to that in the original image,

$$H(T) \leq H(M). \qquad (13)$$

In addition the joint entropy between the image and its thresholded version is given by,

$$H(M, T) = - \sum_{t \in T} \sum_{m \in M} p\{m, t\} \log p\{m, t\} \qquad (14)$$

which can be re-written in terms of the occurrence of the original intensities only,

$$H(M, T) = - \sum_{m \in t_0} p\{m\} \log p\{m\}$$
$$- \sum_{m \in t_1} p\{m\} \log p\{m\}, \qquad (15)$$

giving $H(M, T) = H(M)$. Using this, the mutual information between the image and its threshold,

$$I(M; T) = H(T) + H(M) - H(M, T). \qquad (16)$$

becomes simply $I(M; T) = H(T)$, i.e. the information in the thresholded image $H(T)$ is simply a subset of that provided by the original image $H(M)$.

Labelling unconnected regions differently, effectively repartitions the threshold labels and conversely can only maintain or increase the number of symbols (intensities or labels) present in the image. Applying the additivity property again, this must always maintain or increase the amount of information so that, if the threshold label t_0 is being divided up into unconnected regions $\{l_0 \dots l_k\}$,

$$H(l_0 \dots l_k, t_1) \geq H(t_0, t_1). \qquad (17)$$

If $\{l_0, \dots l_k\}$ is simply a repartitioning of $\{m_0, \dots m_t\}$ (i.e. no regions with the same intensity are spatially unconnected) then $H(M, L) = H(M)$ and so $I(M, L; N) =$

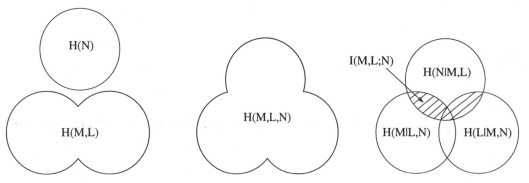

Figure 3. A set theory representation of the entropies involved when combining two images with a third

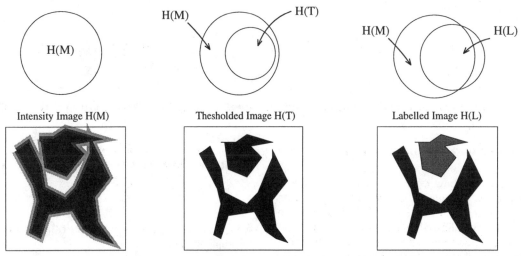

Intensity Image H(M) Thesholded Image H(T) Labelled Image H(L)

Figure 4. Simple image region labelling consisting of thresholding and connected component labelling.

$I(M; N)$. If though, the image contains cases where an intensity $m \in t_0$ is partitioned into more than one label l then,

$$H(M, L) \geq H(M) \qquad (18)$$

and similarly $H(M, L, N) \geq H(M, N)$, so from figure 3,

$$I(M, L; N) \geq I(M; N). \qquad (19)$$

By introducing connected region labelling information we can only maintain or increase the mutual information in the registration process. What we would like is a labelling for which $I(M; L)$ is minimised (there are no duplicated features in the labelling and the image) and $I(L; N)$ is maximised (there is optimum additional shared information with the other modality).

2.4 One Dimensional Example

These concepts can be illustrated with the following simple example. Consider the registration of two one-dimensional signals M and N shown in figure 5. The distance AB and $A'B'$ are equal and the dotted line on the lower figure shows the correct registration solution. The task is to register the two functions by maximising mutual information. In this simple example registration is by lateral translation only. Let the overall length corresponding to intensities m_1 and m_2 in M equal $x(m_1)$ and $x(m_2)$ respectively. Let the length (AB) corresponding to intensity n_2 in N equal $x(n_2)$. In addition we assume that the signal M is truncated as shown, that the signal N has sufficient extent to cover the whole of M for all possible registrations and that the registration solution is constrained so that AB must lie within the field of view of M.

The joint probability distribution is shown on figure 6 at registration. The intensity of each peak is proportional to the values of x indicated on the plot. This distribution and hence the measure of mutual information is identical to that which would occur if the feature AB in N were to overlay any position within $C'D'$ in M. The maximum of mutual

26

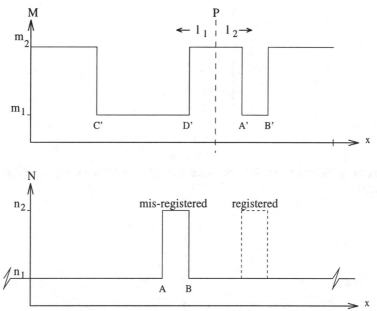

Figure 5. The registration of one dimensional signal m to n with additional labelling of M into $L\{l_1, l_2\}$

information is degenerate. In practice for an image with the addition of noise and other imaging artifacts there may well be an erroneous maximum of mutual information registering regions with similar intensities to those of the correct solution but corresponding to unrelated anatomical structures.

Now consider the addition of labels l_1 and l_2 as shown on figure 5. The partition, P, by the boundary between l_1 and l_2 is arbitrarily located on $D'A'$. The lengths of intensity m_1 and m_2 in region label l_1 are $x(m_1l_1)$ and $x(m_2l_1)$ respectively and in region label l_2, $x(m_1l_2)$ $x(m_2l_2)$ respectively. The joint probability distributions at registration are shown in the upper half of figure 7 and at misregistration with AB overlaying $C'D'$ in the lower half of figure 5. At registration there are only 4 peaks with intensities proportional to the lengths indicated while at misregistration there are 5. A few lines of algebra confirm that the mutual information of the correctly registered functions is now higher than the incorrectly registered functions.

This result holds for all positions of P in $D'A'$. We can therefore consider the partition into l_1 and l_2 as a coarse segmentation of the two regions.

3 Method

3.1 Image Data

A clinically acquired MR-PET image pair of the pelvis was used for the registration tests. Clinically the images were acquired for the localisation and staging of cervical cancer. The PET [18]FDG image of the pelvis was relatively low resolution, sampled with 57 $3.375mm$ slices of 128×128 $3mm \times 3mm$ pixels with a spatial resolution of around $8mm$ F.W.H.M. Regions of uptake usually take the form of small high contrast points in the image. [18]FDG also provides a weak differentiation between intra-abdominal tissues and fat and air but this is of low contrast and is influenced heavily by reconstruction artifacts and noise. Due to the different bed shapes in the the scanners this can also be non-rigidly deformed. The main source of anatomical information shared with MR is provided by [18]F$^-$ which is added as an additional tracer to identify bone structure. These bone landmarks are of greater contrast than the FDG tissue boundary but are still noticeably affected by reconstruction artifact and noise. Example axial and reformatted coronal slices from the PET image used in the test are shown in figure 8.

The MR data set was a clinically acquired T_1 weighted image consisting of 66 $4mm$ slices of 256×256 pixels of size $1.6mm \times 1.6mm$ as shown in figure 8. The MR image is of a much higher spatial resolution and contrast, showing many anatomical features. Many of these features, including marrow and fat, have a similar MR intensity with this sequence, as shown in figure 8.

3.2 Estimate of Registration

The image pair was registered by an experienced clinician interactively locating corresponding anatomical bone landmarks to provide a visually acceptable registration [9].

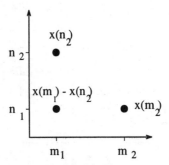

Figure 6. The two dimensional probability distribution of M and N at registration showing the relative intensities of 3 peaks.

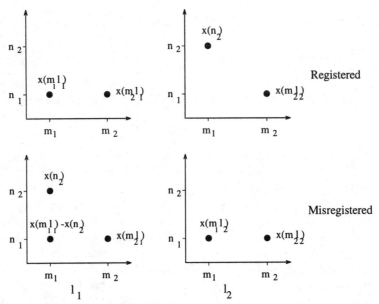

Figure 7. Slices through the three dimensional probability distribution of M (horizontal) and N (vertical) and labels (l_1 left and l_2 right) for registered (top) and unregistered (bottom) signals.

Due to the nature of the images the misregistrations between the modalities generally takes the form of large scale translational differences particularly along the length of the patient. Inspection of a range of manually estimated registration parameters for a number of datasets indicated typical misregistrations up to $90mm$ in translations along this axis.

Automated registration was attempted for the image pair shown in figure 8 by multi-resolution optimisation of mutual information $I(M;N)$ as described in [4]. This produced a poor estimate of the rigid registration parameters with a Z axis (along patient) translational error of greater than $30mm$.

3.3 Region Labelling

The MR image was labelled interactively into four categories:

- Air
- Fat
- Bone Marrow
- Non-Fatty Intra-abdominal tissue

This was carried out using an interactive intensity based region growing algorithm to produce a third image with voxels set to one of four values. Figure 9 illustrates a slice from the labelled volume.

3.4 Evaluation of $p\{m,l,n\}$

The MR image was first re-sampled at the same resolution as the PET image. Linear interpolation was used to increase axial sampling. A Gaussian kernel was used to blur

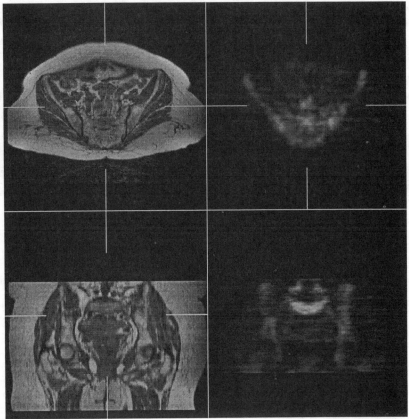

Figure 8. Example manually registered axial (top) and reformatted coronal (bottom) slices through an MR volume (left) and PET volume (right), illustrating the different representation of bone and fat in the two modalities.

the MR to give a similar spatial resolution to the PET. For a given rigid transformation T all voxels in the region of overlap of the two images were used to evaluate $p\{m, l, n\}$. The MR was used as the reference image (m) and corresponding PET (n) intensity was estimated using tri-linear intensity interpolation. MR and PET intensities were binned into 64 levels each and four bins were used for the labels in L to form a discrete distribution. Estimates of $I(M; N)$ and $I(M, L; N)$ were then evaluated from this distribution using equations 4 and 8 respectively.

4 Results

Figure 10 shows a plot of z axis displacement from the manual estimate of mutual information derived from only intensity, and of mutual information including labelling. The lower plot of $I(M; N)$ shows both a poor repose to misalignment and an optimum appreciably displaced from the manual estimate. The addition of labelling into the measure $I(M, L; N)$ increases the overall mutual information for all displacements produces distinct optimum close to the manual estimate.

A multi-resolution optimisation of $I(M, L; N)$ was carried out from a starting orientation defined by the scanner acquisitions, with the centres of the MR and PET volume aligned. The final transformation estimates are shown in table 1 along with those for optimisation of $I(M; N)$ and the manual estimate. The axes are as follows; x is from patient left to right, y is from patient front to back and z is from patient top to bottom. Registration by evaluation and optimisation of $I(M; N)$ derived from intensity only resulted in a visually poor registration. Multi-start of the optimisation and initialisation of the optimisation from the manual estimate confirmed that $I(M; N)$ was providing an incorrect global optimum corresponding to the alignment of bone features in PET with intra-abdominal fat. This resulted in both a large z axis displacement and a rotation around the y axis.

The manual estimate and the final estimate using the labelling approach $I(M, L; N)$ are within the expected accuracy of the manual registration procedure given the resolution of the original images. Interactive visual inspection of the results using colour overlay of PET intensity onto grey level MR in three orthogonal planes confirmed that the two results were visually comparable. Further work needs to be

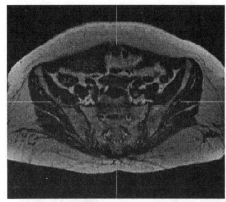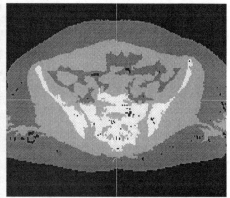

Figure 9. Example slice from MR volume (left) with labels (right).

done in assessing final accuracy.

Method	Translation (mm)			Rotation (deg.)		
	t_x	t_y	t_z	θ_x	θ_y	θ_z
Manual	-6.0	34.5	39.0	2.5	0.0	-2.0
$I(M;N)$	-4.3	34.3	15.6	2.4	-3.0	-0.2
$I(M,L;N)$	-4.9	34.1	37.1	3.9	0.0	0.0

Table 1. Rigid transformation parameters estimated for the test image pair

5   Discussion and Conclusion

In our test example we have interactively labelled voxel values to provide additional information in the registration measure. By using an information theoretic approach which includes these labels the segmentation need not be ideal allowing the possibility of using an automated labelling scheme. Segmentation schemes distinguishing strongly between unconnected regions are favoured. Work is underway in looking at how such schemes can be integrated into the registration process. In particular our current multi-resolution approach to optimising mutual information could be extended to include a multi-resolution region extraction stage.

Further work is required to assess the extent to which labelling can be corrupted before the the final accuracy (location of the global optimum) is affected. The effect of typical errors produced by automated labelling schemes on the registration measure for a range of clinical images needs to be determined.

In our simple 1D example and on the clinical test image we have supplied labelling information to differentiate regions of similar intensity which are distinguished in the other modality. Given a higher level knowledge about the regions it maybe be possible to use the same approach to combine regions of different intensity. This may be useful in reducing the influence of certain tissue boundaries which may have deformed between acquisitions.

This approach is an example of a case where pre-segmentation of images can provide additional information to help in the registration process. Alternatively it is also possible to use the information provided by the process of registration to assist in segmentation or classification.

We have introduced a new type of voxel similarity approach that makes use of voxel label information as well as the original image intensities. Coarse segmentation of the higher resolution image is necessary to provide the label information. Unlike a surface matching approach, eg: [2], this technique does not require identification of corresponding boundaries from both modalities, and we believe our information theoretic approach is more robust to segmentation errors. Van den Elsen et al [6] used an approach to MR and CT registration, in which an intensity mapping technique was used to make CT images "look" like MR images, prior to using cross correlation for registration. Intensity re-mapping in this way is only possible because of the simple relationship between tissue and intensity found in CT. The approach we propose here is more general, and preserves the original image intensities throughout. A possible interpretation of our technique is that the original intensity information is used for the accurate registration, and the labelling provides coarse scale information that removes unwanted optima far from the correct solution.

We have demonstrated this technique for the registration of MR and PET images of the pelvis, which could not be registered using the standard mutual information approach. The registration solution was close to that produced using interactively identified point landmarks and produced a visually acceptable result.

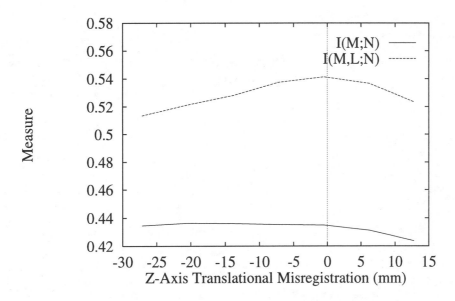

Figure 10. Graph of $I(M;N)$ and $I(M,L;N)$ with respect to axial (z) translation ($z = 0mm$ is the manual estimate).

6 Acknowledgements

This work was funded by the Guy's and St Thomas's NHS trust. We would particularly like to thank Prof. M. N. Maisey and the Clinical PET Centre of Guy's and St Thomas's. We are grateful for the support and encouragement of our clinical colleagues in this work, in particular Dr Joseph Wong (Radiologist), Dr Wai-Lup Wong (Radiologist), and for the technical assistance of the Radiographic staff of Guy's and St. Thomas' Hospitals in London. We would also like to thank Dr John Little of UMDS for mathematical advice and we acknowledge useful discussions with Andre Collignon and Dirk Vandermeulen of KUL, Leuven, Belgium and Sandy Wells and Paul Viola of MIT and Brigham and Women's Hospital Boston, USA, on the subject of mutual information.

References

[1] A. Collignon, F. Maes, D. Delaere, D. Vandermeulen, P. Suetens, and G. Marchal. Automated multimodality image registration using information theory. In B. Y., B. C, and D. P. R., editors, *Proceedings of Information Processing in Medical Imaging*, pages 263–274, 1995. Brest, France.

[2] H. Jiang, R. Robb, and K. Holton. New approach to 3-D registration of multimodality medical images by surface matching. In *Proceedings of Visualisation in Biomedical Computing*, pages 196–213, 1992. Chapel Hill, N.C.,U.S.A.

[3] F. Reza. *An Introduction to Information Theory*. Dover, New York, 1994.

[4] C. Studholme, D. Hill, and D. Hawkes. Automated 3D registration of truncated MR and CT images of the head. In D. Pycock, editor, *Proceedings of the British Machine Vision Conference*, pages 27–36. BMVA, 1995. Birmingham.

[5] C. Studholme, D. Hill, and D. Hawkes. Multiresolution voxel similarity measures for MR-PET registration. In B. Y., B. C., and D. P. R., editors, *Proceedings of Information Processing in Medical Imaging*, pages 287–298, 1995. Brest, France.

[6] P. Van den Elsen, E. Pol, T. Sumanawaeera, P. Hemler, S. Napel, and J. Adler. Grey value correlation techniques used for automatic matching of CT and MR brain and spine images. In *Proceedings of Visualisation in Biomedical Computing*, pages 227–237, 1994. Rochester Mn.,U.S.A.

[7] P. Viola and W. Wells. Alignment by maximisation of mutual information. In *Proceedings of the 5th International Conference on Computer Vision*, pages 15–23, 1995.

[8] W. Wells, P. Viola, and R. Kikinis. Multimodal volume registration by maximization of mutual information. In *Proceedings of the 2nd annual international symposium on Medical Robotics and Computer Assisted Surgery*, pages 55–62, 1995. Baltimore, U.S.A.

[9] W. Wong, C. Studholme, P. Lewis, K. Raju, R. Beaney, K. Tonge, T. Nunan, D. J. Hawkes, and J. Pemberton. Combined MR,CT and PET imaging in oncological patients. *British Journal of Radiology*, 66(suppl):33–34, 1993.

Non-Invasive Functional Brain Mapping Using Registered Transcranial Magnetic Stimulation

G.J. Ettinger[1,6]   W.E.L. Grimson[1]   M.E. Leventon[1]   R. Kikinis[2]   V. Gugino[3]

W. Cote[3]   M. Karapelou[3]   L. Aglio[3]   M. Shenton[4]   G. Potts[4]   E. Alexander[5]

Abstract

We describe a method for mapping the functional regions of the brain using a transcranial magnetic stimulation (TMS) device. This device, when placed on a subject's scalp, stimulates the underlying neurons by generating focused magnetic field pulses. A brain mapping is then generated by measuring responses of different motor and sensory functions to this stimulation. The key process in generating this mapping is the association of the 3D positions and orientations of the TMS probe on the scalp to a 3D brain reconstruction such as is feasible with a magnetic resonance image (MRI). We perform this matching process by (1) registering the subject's head position to an a priori MRI scan, (2) tracking the 3D position/orientation of the TMS probe, (3) transforming the TMS probe position/orientation to the MRI coordinate frame, and (4) tracking movements in the subject's head position to factor out any head motion. The resultant process generates a high resolution, accurate brain mapping which supports surgical planning, surgical guidance, neuroanatomy research, and psychiatric therapy. When compared to other functional imaging modalities, this approach exhibits much lower cost, greater portability, and more direct active control over the functional areas being studied.

1. Introduction

Functional brain mapping, consisting of the association of motor, sensory, and perception functions with different regions of the brain, is currently an active research area with a wide range of potential applications. Sample applications include (1) neuroanatomy research into the structure and functioning of components of the brain, (2) study of neurological disease origination, progression and diagnosis, (3) surgical planning and guidance of biopsy and ablation procedures, (4) treatment monitoring and (5) neurological therapeutic procedures. Current techniques for functional brain mapping utilize 3D medical scanners to image the brain while the subject undergoes an activity aimed at activating the functional area of interest. Scanners currently used for this purpose are single photon emission computed tomography (SPECT), positron emission tomography (PET), and magnetic resonance imaging (MRI). The ability of these scanners to capture brain activity results from their sensitivity to such factors as metabolism rate and blood oxygenation. The benefit of such scanners is their ability to quickly capture 3D snapshots of the complete brain activity. Some of their limitations, however, are:

- High cost limits their use. In addition, the use of radioactive agents in SPECT and PET further limit the frequency of use of those scanners.

- Passive control of functional activation limits the pinpointing of the areas of interest. Ideally, one wants to limit the functional activation of the brain to just the areas of interest and to do so at the same time the image is acquired. Standard methods, such as asking the subject to perform certain activities, or trying to control the environment around the subject, are less than ideal in achieving this since there are many potentially confounding factors that cannot be isolated from the process. For example, it is difficult to ensure that the subject performed only the desired mental activity, and no other related activity, at the time of imaging.

A promising approach to avoiding these limitations is the use of a transcranial magnetic stimulation device (Magstim Company Ltd, England) for actively stimulating different parts of the brain. Such devices consist of a circular or

[1] MIT AI Lab, 545 Technology Sq, Cambridge MA 02139

[2] Dept. of Radiology, Brigham and Womens Hospital, Harvard Medical School, Boston MA 02115

[3] Dept. of Anesthesiology, Brigham and Womens Hospital, Harvard Medical School, Boston MA 02115

[4] Dept. of Psychiatry, Brigham and Womens Hospital, Harvard Medical School, Boston MA 02115

[5] Dept. of Neurosurgery, Brigham and Womens Hospital, Harvard Medical School, Boston MA 02115

[6] email: ettinger@ai.mit.edu

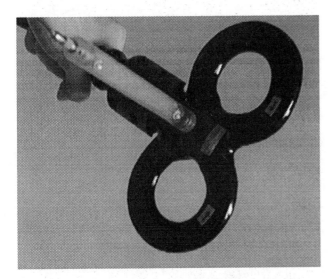

Figure 1. Stimulation coil used for TMS mapping. Note the rod mounted orthogonal to the plane of the coil—two LEDs are fixed on the rod for tracking the position and orientation of the coil.

figure-8 shaped coil, termed the TMS probe, which can deliver single magnetic field pulse stimuli or pulse trains. In our experiments we have only used a figure-8 coil, which delivers a more sharply focused pulse. One such coil is shown in Figure 1. The diameter of each circular component of the figure-8 ranges from about 3 to 10 cm in the different coils used. There is no direct electrical contact with the subject—the device works by inducing small electrical currents (<50 mA) in tissue using brief magnetic pulses that are focused in front of the coil. The magnetic field generated by the coil passes through the scalp and skull without attenuation, but causes excitation of cortical neurons. If the excitation is in the motor cortex, peripheral responses are observed in the affected muscles. If it is in the speech control or vision processing areas, brief disruption and/or inhibition of the affected processes is observed. The peak magnetic fields are similar to those used with MRI scanners, except that magnetic stimulator pulses are very short (<1 msec). Resulting energy dissipation in tissue is minimal (<0.25 mJ). The advantages of such a device are:

- Relatively low cost and ease of use—the device is highly portable with little constraints on its applicability.

- Active functional activation—rather than trying to spot brain activity when the subject performs different actions, the TMS attempts to directly stimulate certain brain regions and monitor their impact. In principle, this leads to functional mapping that is highly localized

both spatially within the brain and temporally for ease of acquisition.

While research is on-going on the biological implications of such a device, the physics of the generated magnetic field, and the development of psychophysical experiments which gauge brain function, we are exploring the technical problems of converting the TMS data, locations of TMS probe, and associated muscular/sensory responses to a 3D functional brain map, similar to ones that are obtained with 3D medical scanners. The heart of our problem is (1) the registration of the subject's MRI scan, the subject position during transcranial magnetic stimulation, and the TMS probe positions/orientations to the same coordinate frame, and (2) the associated tracking problem of maintaining that registration across possible subject movements during the data collection. The following section defines this registration/tracking problem, followed by a description of our registration/tracking system in Section 3. Sample results from the application of our system to a neurosurgery patient are shown in Section 4.

2. Problem Definition

We divide the problem into four parts:

1. Register an MRI scan of the subject's head to the actual subject head position as he is readied for TMS data collection. The goal is to compute a transform from the subject's world coordinate system to the MRI coordinate system to allow us to transform TMS probe points to the MRI scan. The registration should not require any attachment of fiducials to the patient as the time between the MRI scan and TMS data collection may be large.

2. Track the 3D position/orientation of the TMS probe in the world coordinate system and record those locations when it is stimulated. Also record the muscular/sensory responses of each stimulation.

3. Track the subject's head motion in order to maintain the registration of step 1. Head tracking avoids the need to fixate the subject.

4. Combine the TMS probe positions/orientations, TMS responses, subject-to-MRI transform, and head motion to generate a functional brain mapping on any 3D surface rendered from the MRI scan, such as cortical or white matter surface.

While the registration does not necessarily need to be real-time, there are advantages to performing all the steps as the TMS data is collected, particularly to show the technician what regions of the head have already been covered, and

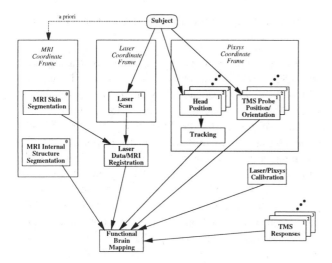

Figure 2. Architecture of functional brain mapping system.

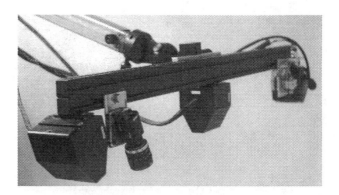

Figure 3. Laser scanner and Pixsys system mounted on movable arm. Devices on bar from left to right are: Pixsys camera 1, laser camera, Pixsys camera 2, laser on stepper motor, Pixsys camera 3.

where maximal responses have been attained. Accuracy requirements are relatively high as many of the active brain centers being studied are on the order of a few mm^3 in volume. Thus the overall accuracy should be within about 1-2 mm, which is generally not much larger than the voxel resolution of the MRI scan.

3. Registration System

The system we have developed to address the problems of Section 2 is shown in Figure 2. We work with three different coordinate systems:

1. MRI: The MRI data is captured in a coordinate frame that is arbitrarily attached to the volume of data. The data itself is segmented into skin surface for registration and internal structures for brain mapping visualization, within this coordinate frame.

2. Laser: The laser scanner provides 3D data of the subject's scalp surface as positioned for transcranial magnetic stimulation. We use a laser striping triangulation system consisting of a laser unit (laser source and cylindrical lens mounted on a stepper motor) and a camera. Here the coordinate frame of the acquired points is centered at a fixed point within the working volume of the laser system.

3. Pixsys: This is a 3D tracking system (IGT Inc., Boulder, Colorado) consisting of 3 linear cameras which localize flashing IR LEDs. The system can track a number of LEDs simultaneously. We mount two LEDs on the TMS coil (specifying its 3D position and orien-

tation with twist the only degree of freedom not measured) and tape five LEDs on the subject's scalp for tracking head motion. Redundant LEDs are used for tracking head position in case motion is great enough to block up to two of the LEDs. The position and orientation information returned by the system are represented in a coordinate frame centered at a fixed point within the working volume of the cameras.

The goal of the system is to integrate all of these coordinate systems into a single reference frame. That is, we need to relate sampled TMS probe points to the corresponding points in the MRI scan, which we do by using the laser coordinate system as an intermediary.

The laser scanner (laser and its associated camera) and Pixsys system (three linear cameras) are mounted on the same bar which is attached to a movable arm for ease of placement, as shown in Figure 3. Since we fixate the laser and Pixsys systems relative to each other, we perform an offline calibration to obtain the Pixsys-to-laser transform. This transform is then constant for all subsequent TMS data collections. The transform from laser data to MRI coordinates, though, must be computed for each TMS data collection since the transformation of the TMS probe positions to the MRI scan requires knowledge of the subject's head position during the stimulation session.

A sample data collection procedure, from the perspective of the subject, is:

1. Acquire an MR image of the subject prior to the TMS session. Segment the scan into desired anatomical structures, such as skin, cortical surface, white matter, etc.

2. Prepare for TMS data collection:

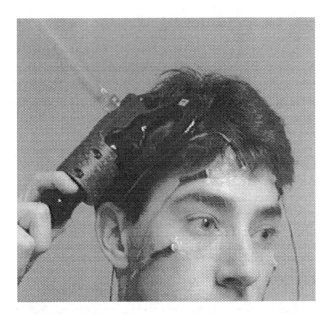

Figure 4. Subject set up for TMS stimulation. LEDs taped to face are used for tracking head motion.

   (a) Place subject on a bed.

   (b) For motor cortex mapping, place muscle activity sensors on muscles of interest. Upon appropriate stimulation, the muscles will contract. Visual or speech suppression can be used to map other functional areas.

   (c) Place Pixsys LEDs on rigid points of the subject's scalp. These LEDs are currently loose LEDs which are taped to the skin such that they will not interfere with the TMS probing, but are spaced widely apart on the head.

3. Laser scan the subject—the laser plane is swept across the subject's head collecting 3D positional data of visible skin surfaces. At the same time the positions of the five LEDs taped to the subject's head are acquired by the Pixsys system.

4. Collect TMS data—the TMS probe is placed at various points on the subject's scalp. At each point, the TMS generates a brief magnetic pulse and the responses from the muscle sensors (or other responses) are recorded. The position and orientation of the TMS probe is also recorded by the Pixsys system at the same time. 3D renderings of the subject's MRI skin superimposed with TMS points may be generated during the data collection to chart progress and guide continued stimulations.

An example of a subject outfitted with the LEDs for tracking and placement of the TMS for stimulation is shown in Figure 4. The processing of the MRI, laser, Pixsys, and TMS data is described in the following sections.

3.1. MRI Segmentation

The MRI data is segmented to extract the skin surface, for use in registration, and the internal structures, for use in visualization. By segmentation, we refer to the process of labeling individual voxels in the MRI scan by tissue type, based on properties of the observed intensities as well as known anatomical information about normal subjects. The labeled voxels are further gathered into connected components whose surfaces are used for registration and rendering.

The functional brain mapping is usually overlaid on both the cortical surface and the white matter surface so at least these two structures are segmented. In addition, ventricles, blood vessels, tumors, or other pathologies may also be segmented. Current segmentation techniques used at Brigham and Women's Hospital include an automatic gain artifact suppression technique based on expectation-maximization [17] in association with a cortical volume isolation technique based on image morphology and active contours [10]. These techniques are complemented by semi-automatic techniques which interactively classify tissue types using high performance rendering algorithms.

3.2. Laser Data / MRI Registration

The MRI segmentation yields a 3D model of the patient's anatomy for visualizing and identifying internal structures. To relate these structures to functional recordings, we need to place the MRI segmentation into correspondence with the actual patient, which we accomplish by registering surface data from the model and the patient. To do this, we need positional information from the patient's skin surface. Here, we have two possibilities available to us. The first uses a laser striping device to acquire positional data from the skin surface of the patient, which we can then register with the segmented skin surface from the MRI. An alternative is to use a Pixsys probe to acquire 3D data of the subject's position by moving the Pixsys probe along the subject's scalp. The laser is preferable due to its high accuracy and avoidance of direct contact with the subject. The Pixsys probe, though, is often useful to supplement the laser data by probing scalp points which are not visible to the laser scanner. In either case, laser data or Pixsys data, the registration algorithm is the same. The basis of the registration algorithm has been previously described in [3, 4, 5, 6]. The algorithm is depicted in Figure 5 and is briefly reviewed below.

3.2.1. Initial Match

Before commencing the matching process we preprocess the laser data to separate data of the subject's head from

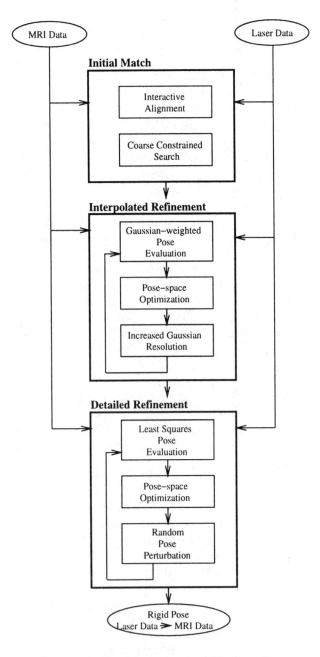

Figure 5. Registration algorithm outline.

active alignment we use a graphical interface to manipulate the MRI and laser data. We use two displays to view our alignment. In one display we view the 3D MRI skin surface superimposed on the laser camera's video image of the subject. This display supports 3D translation and rotation of the MRI head data to achieve close alignment with the video image of the head. The second display consists of three orthogonal projections of sampled points from the MRI skin surface overlaid with the projection of the laser points. To facilitate interpretation of sidedness within each projection, the intensity of the points is made proportional to the normal depth within each projection. In this display we interactively translate and rotate the laser points such that they roughly align with the underlying MRI points. This initial alignment does not need to be very accurate: rotational errors on the order of 20 degrees, and translational errors on the order of centimeters are permissible, since the subsequent matching stage is quite reliable at removing these misalignments.

If we do not want to rely on operator intervention, we can instead use an automated constrained search procedure to find the initial alignment. In this method, we first select a pair of widely separated laser points, and at each point, we estimate the surface normal, by a local least squares fit. We then search over all possible pairs of MRI surface points, at some subsampling, and use those pairs whose distance roughly agrees with the distance between the chosen laser points. For each pair of MRI points and the pair of laser points, we solve for the transformation that aligns the points and the surface normals at the two points, provided such a transformation exists. For those pairings of points with legal transformations, we apply the transformation to all of the laser points, and measure the least squares distance between the transformed laser data and the MRI skin model. We use this measure to rank order the possible alignments. For efficiency purposes, we hash the pairings of MRI points by distance, in a coarse-to-fine manner, thereby saving considerably on the computation required. We keep the n best transformations for use at the next stage. Note that we can accomplish the same constrained search by using triples of points without normal information, if desired.

For each selected alignment transformation, we execute the refinement processes described below.

3.2.2. Interpolated Refinement

We first refine the alignment of the two data sets by minimizing an evaluation function that measures the amount of mismatch between the two data sets. In particular, we sum, for all transformed laser points, a term that is a sum of the distances from the transformed laser point to all nearby MRI points, where the distance is weighted by a Gaussian distribution [18]. This Gaussian weighting roughly interpolates between the sampled MRI points to estimate the

background data. Currently we do this with a simple user interface in which the view obtained from the video camera used in conjunction with the laser is displayed, with the laser data overlaid two dimensionally on top of that view. The user can thus use a simple mouse interface to block out laser points coming from the skin of the subject. Note that this process need not be perfect—the matching process is designed to deal robustly with outliers.

To initiate the matching, we have two options: interactive alignment and coarse constrained search. Under inter-

nearest point on the underlying surface to the transformed laser point. More precisely, if vector ℓ_i is a laser point, vector m_j is an MRI point, and $\mathcal{T}$ is a coordinate frame transformation, then the evaluation function for a particular transformation is

$$E_1(\mathcal{T}) = -\sum_i \sum_j e^{-\frac{|\mathcal{T}\ell_i - m_j|^2}{2\sigma^2}}. \qquad (1)$$

Because of its formulation, the objective function is quite smooth, and thus facilitates "pulling in" solutions from moderately removed locations in parameter space.

In order to minimize this evaluation function we use the Davidon-Fletcher-Powell (DFP) quasi-Newton method [13]. This method requires an estimate of the gradient of the objective function, which is easily obtained in closed form. Solving this minimization problem yields an estimate for the pose of the laser points in MRI coordinates.

We execute this minimization stage with a multiresolution set of Gaussians. A broad Gaussian is used to allow influence over large areas, resulting in a coarse initial alignment, which can be reached from a wide range of starting positions. Then, narrower Gaussian distributions are used to focus on only nearby MRI points to derive the pose.

3.2.3. Detailed Refinement

Starting from the pose obtained with the interpolated refinement stage, we repeat the evaluation process, using a rectified least squares distance measure. We again use the DFP method to minimize the evaluation function:

$$E_2(\mathcal{T}) = \left[\frac{1}{n} \sum_i \min \left[d_{\max}^2, \min_j |\mathcal{T}\ell_i - m_j|^2 \right] \right]^{\frac{1}{2}} \qquad (2)$$

where $d_{\max}$ is some preset maximum distance used to limit the impact of outliers. This objective function acts much like a robust chamfer matching scheme (e.g. [9]). The expectation is that this second objective function is more accurate locally, since it is composed of saturated quadratic forms.

We observe that while this refinement method gets very close to the best solution, it can get trapped into local minima in the minimization of E_2. To improve upon this problem, we take the pose returned by the above step and perturb it randomly, then repeat the minimization. We continue to do this, keeping the new pose if its associated RMS error is better than our current best. We terminate this process when the number of such trials that have passed since the RMS value was last improved becomes larger than some threshold. The final result is a pose, and a measure of the residual deviation of the fit to the MRI surface.

3.3. Pixsys Data Processing

The Pixsys 3D tracking system is a self-contained system which can be used to generate 3D coordinates of LEDs in the system's field of view. The system is based on a straightforward triangulation process, in which a point is observed in three orthogonal linear cameras, whose positions and orientations are known with respect to one another. By identifying the image projection of the same point in each camera, one can back out the projection geometry to determine the position of the point in scene coordinates. To achieve simple and robust identification of the same point in each image, infrared light emitting diodes (IR LEDs) are used, and the pulsing of each diode is synchronized to the imaging process. In this way, there is no possible ambiguity in identifying corresponding image points, and reliable estimation of 3D point positions of the LEDs is possible.

This active triangulation system is highly reliable, with an accuracy of about 1 mm at the 1 m standoff from the 3 linear cameras which we normally use. By mounting three LEDs to a rigid object we can track the object's pose (position and orientation) in three-space. Using two LEDs allow us to solve for five degrees of freedom (all but the twist angle around the axis connecting the two LEDs). Using more than three LEDs provides us with some redundancy, allowing for a least-squares pose solution and wide range of motion in which some LEDs may be blocked from view. We use the Pixsys system for tracking head motion (using five LEDs taped to the head) and localizing the position and orientation of the TMS probe (using two LEDs mounted to the probe).

3.3.1. Head Motion Tracking

In order to track the head motion we record the position of the LEDs taped to the patient's head at the time we perform the laser data/MRI registration. This reference position provides a basis for tracking the head. When the TMS probe is stimulated we record the new position of the head-mounted LEDs and compute the transform necessary to return the head to its reference position. This transform is applied to the position/orientation of the TMS probe at the time of the corresponding stimulation in order to apply the laser data/MRI transformation.

Since we may have up to five LEDs to track we use Horn's closed form least-squares solution based on quaternions [8] for the tracking transform. On the subjects on which we have tested this procedure we taped the LEDs to bony surfaces on which little skin movement (relative to the underlying bone) is expected. Two LED were taped to the cheek bones, two to the sides of the forehead, and one to bridge of the nose or center of the forehead. We need at least three LEDs visible at all times.

3.3.2. TMS Probe Localization

In order to use the Pixsys data obtained for localizing the TMS probe we perform two calibration steps: calibrate the TMS probe to identify the position of the coil's magnetic field hot spot relative to its Pixsys coordinates and calibrate the Pixsys coordinate system to the laser coordinate system. In order to calibrate the TMS probe itself we mount two LEDs on a rigid rod which is rigidly bracketed to the center of the figure-8 coil. The rod is connected to be perpendicular to the coil such that the hot spot of the coil is along the same line as the two LEDs. Experimentation on the exact position and shape of the hot spot relative to the coil is still on-going. The Pixsys system is then calibrated to output the position where the line formed by the two LEDs intersects the surface on which the underside of the coil is resting along with the orientation of that line.

In order to calibrate the Pixsys coordinate system to the laser coordinate system we use a Pixsys probe to record points on a calibration gauge which have known laser co-ordinates. Given the correspondences between Pixsys and laser points we solve for the transformation between the two coordinate systems. Since the three linear Pixsys cameras and laser scanner (laser and camera) are all mounted on the same rigid bar, this calibration remains fixed.

3.3.3. Alternative methods

We are also currently investigating the possibility of using a more passive system to track both head position and probe position and orientation. This method [11] utilizes some simple visual markers placed on the objects of interest, which are then tracked reliably and rapidly by observation in a single camera. The advantage of this system is that the passive markers are less intrusive than the LEDs, and that tracking can in principle be done by any camera in any location, rather than relying on the Pixsys cameras.

3.4. Functional Brain Mapping

We combine the registration and tracking data to obtain the functional brain mapping using the following transforms:

- $\mathbf{P_L}$ — transformation from Pixsys coordinates to laser coordinates; computed from *a priori* calibration.

- $\mathbf{L_M}$ — transformation from laser coordinates to MRI coordinates; computed from dynamic registration procedure.

- $\mathbf{H_r^t}$ — transformation of head from time t to reference position at time 1, computed from calibration of the LEDs at time t to the LEDs at time 1.

We have also collected the following TMS data:

- C_p^t, C_o^t — position and orientation of TMS coil at time t, $t \in [1, T]$, in Pixsys coordinates.

- R_j^t — measured response j to stimulation t. Multiple responses are usually collected such as from several different hand, arm, and leg muscles.

In order to compute the brain mapping we need to map the TMS responses to the brain surface using the measured coil positions/orientations and associated transformations. To perform this mapping, for each stimulation t, we process those MRI surface points, $S[i]$, that are sufficiently close to $\mathbf{L_M P_L H_r^t} C_p^t$ to have been possibly stimulated by the pulse. Note that closeness here can be determined in a number of ways. We can simply use the transformed position of the tip of the probe and gather all MRI points within some predefined distance. Alternatively, if we have a detailed model of the shape of the magnetic field generated by the probe, we can use it, together with information about the orientation of the probe, to select the relevant MRI points. For now, we are simply using Euclidean distance from the position of the probe to select $S[i]$.

For each such $S[i]$ we compute the distance, $d^t[i]$, to the line defined by the point $\mathbf{L_M P_L H_r^t} C_p^t$ and the orientation $\mathbf{L_M P_L H_r^t} C_o^t$. We are currently using a Gaussian weighting function proportional to that distance to "spread" the response R_j^t to the points $S[i]$. The purpose of this (simple) weighting function is to interpolate across the stimulation to obtain a smooth and visible map. If we let $map_j^t[i]$ represent the mapping of response j to stimulation t on the selected surface, then $map_j^t[i] = G(d^t[i], \sigma) R_j^t$, with G being the Gaussian weighting function. We then let $map_j[i]$, the composite mapping from all stimulations, be the maximum $map_j^t[i]$ over all t, which are then normalized over i.

While we generally are most interested in the mapping of the TMS responses to the cortical surface of the brain, we may perform this mapping onto to any underlying segmented surface. The white matter surface is often useful since it highlights some of the major sulci. The skin surface itself is also sometimes useful to examine coverage range of stimulations.

4. Test Results

We have performed the TMS brain mapping on five subjects thus far, two of whom were neurosurgery patients. Although the resultant mappings were positively reviewed by radiology and neurology specialists, it is difficult to validate the results. A qualitative solution is to validate the results in the operating room in the case of craniotomy surgeries. In one of the neurosurgery cases, the patient had a tumor on the surface of the brain near the right motor and sensor strips.

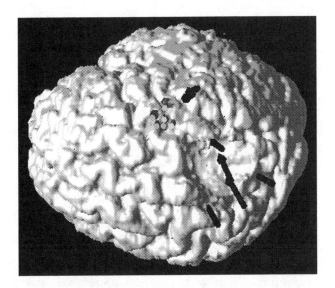

Figure 6. Patient's cortical surface overlaid with TMS probe positions/directions. Black probes elicited no index finger response. The finger response of the remaining probes is coded from light to dark proportional to the strength of the response.

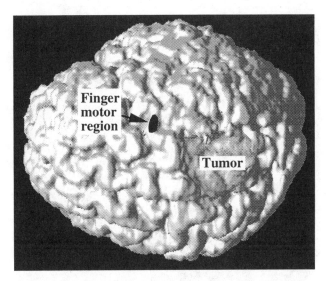

Figure 7. Patient's cortical surface and tumor overlaid with functional mapping of index finger control–region of maximum response is shown in black.

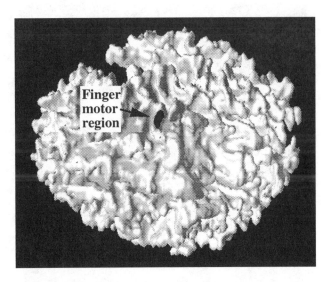

Figure 8. Patient's white matter surface overlaid with functional mapping of index finger control–region of maximum response is shown in black.

We mapped part of the motor cortex by collecting muscular responses of the index finger, forearm, and biceps muscles. These responses were mapped to the surface of the brain as well as to the white matter. Figure 6 shows the brain surface overlaid with the TMS probe positions/directions used. The color coding of the TMS probing vectors and surface indicates the strength of the finger muscle response. In this visualization and the remaining ones, the mapping of the other arm muscles looked very similar to the finger muscle.

Figure 7 shows the finger muscle response overlaid on the brain surface. The hot spot, along with the mapping of the other muscles, identifies the location of the motor strip. This mapping was exploited by the surgeons to appropriately plan the tumor excision. Furthermore, once in surgery, our results were validated using conventional electrical stimulation made directly on the surface of the brain. According to the surgeons, our functional mapping was qualitatively localized in the right place.

For reference, we also generated functional maps on the surface of the white matter, Figure 8. The presence of the hot spot on a gyrus of the white matter is consistent with the location of the hot spot on the cortical surface.

Based on responses from a set of muscles we can perform a more complete mapping of the motor cortex. An example of such an extensive mapping from a volunteer subject in which finger (index), arm (forearm and biceps), and leg (calf) muscle responses were tracked is shown in Figure 9.

5. Related Work

Several other groups have reported registration methods similar to ours, but for different applications. Pelizzari et al [12] have developed a method that matches retrospective data sets, (MRI, CT, PET), to one another. This work also uses a least squares minimization of distances between

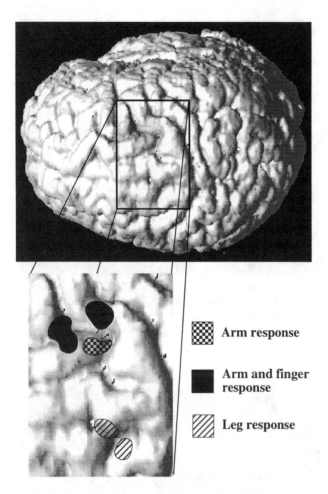

Figure 9. Functional mapping showing combined responses of several muscles. Strongest responses are shown.

Arm response

Arm and finger response

Leg response

6. Potential Applications of TMS-based Functional Mapping

In our discussion above, we have used the example of motor strip stimulation to illustrate our method for registering transcranial magnetic stimulation responses to segmented reconstructions of a patient's brain. There are some natural applications that follow from this scenario.

- **Identification of motor cortex for surgical planning.** Our first demonstration of this technique, as illustrated in the earlier figures, involved mapping out portions of a neurosurgical patient's motor strip, and providing the registered mapping, overlaid onto a segmented MRI reconstruction, to the surgeon for surgical planning. In particular, the surgeon used the registered reconstruction to plan access to a tumor for removal, while avoiding critical structures.

- **Surgical guidance.** Not only is the identification of motor strip useful for planning processes, it can also serve a useful role during the actual surgery. In the case cited above, during the surgical procedure itself, enhanced reality visualizations of the MRI model, registered and overlaid on a live video view of the patient (e.g. [4, 5, 6]), were used to help guide the surgical procedure. This included both guidance for tumor removal while avoiding critical structures and guiding the placement of sensors onto the exposed cortical surface for direct stimulation of the motor cortex. Such stimulation serves both as a check of the noninvasive mapping of cortex, and as a means of monitoring patient status during the surgery.

While mapping of motor cortex is a good motivating example for this approach, many other applications may benefit from the ability to relate noninvasive magnetic stimulation of the brain to MRI reconstructions of the neuroanatomy:

- **Neuroscience.** The method provides the potential for relating functional properties to specific locations in the brain. Examples include detailed mappings of motor or sensory cortex across subject populations. Such mappings could be used in building anatomical atlases, measuring deviations in location, and potentially serving as a base for seeking correlations between functional properties and disease processes. Such functional mapping could extend to other modalities, such as speech and vision, by designing psychophysical protocols that utilize either stimulation or inhibition of percepts via transcranial magnetic stimulation.

- **Diagnostic tools.** The ability to relate induced magnetic stimulation response to anatomical models poten-

data sets, although with a different distance function and with more operator guidance required. One goal of their work was to register MRI/CT data with PET data to obtain functional mappings. Lavallee and Szeliski [15] also perform a least-squares minimization of a distance function to match data sets. Here, the distance is weighted by an estimate of the inverse variance of the measurement noise, and a Levenberg-Marquardt method is used to find the minimum. Once an initial solution is found, points with large errors are removed and the minimization is repeated to refine the pose. They also applied their registration approach to multi-modality registration, in part to obtain functional maps. Other related registration techniques include [2, 7, 14, 16, 19].

tially provides the ability to identify and isolate damage to cortical tissue in a noninvasive manner.

- **Therapy.** Some work has already begun on the utility of TMS as a therapeutic tool [1] in the treatment of depression, akinesia, and related areas. By providing registration tools, we may enable a practitioner to use graphical models and real time registration of a probe to those models and the patient to accurately direct stimulation to desired targets.

7. Summary

We have reported on an initial system combining 3D registration and 3D tracking techniques to generate functional brain maps from transcranial magnetic stimulation responses. In limited testing thus far the system has achieved accurate results which indicate promise to a wide of applications requiring low cost and portable brain mapping. In addition to surgical planning and guidance, this work can benefit growing research efforts into understanding the brain and learning about neurological diseases. Work is continuing in exploring these applications as well as testing and validation of the procedure.

8. Acknowledgments

This report describes research supported in part by ARPA under ONR contract N00014-94-01-0994 and in part by a Scottish Rite Schizophrenia Grant.

References

[1] R.H. Belmaker, A. Fleischmann, "Transcranial Magnetic Stimulation: A potential new frontier in Psychiatry", *Biol. Psychiatry* **38**:419–412, 1995.

[2] P. Besl, N. McKay, "A Method for Registration of 3D Shapes", *IEEE Trans. PAMI*, **14**(2), 1992.

[3] G.J. Ettinger, W.E.L. Grimson, T. Lozano-Pérez, W.M. Wells III, S.J. White, R. Kikinis, "Automatic Registration for Multiple Sclerosis Change Detection", *Proceedings of IEEE Workshop on Biomedical Image Analysis*, Seattle WA, June 1994, pp. 297–306.

[4] W.E.L. Grimson, T. Lozano-Pérez, W.M. Wells III, G.J. Ettinger, S.J. White and R. Kikinis, "An Automatic Registration Method for Frameless Stereotaxy, Image Guided Surgery, and Enhanced Reality Visualization", *Proceedings of IEEE Computer Vision and Pattern Recognition Conference*, Seattle WA, June 1994, pp. 430–436.

[5] W.E.L. Grimson, G.J. Ettinger, S.J. White, P.L. Gleason, T. Lozano-Pérez, W.M. Wells III, R. Kikinis, "Evaluating and Validating an Automated Registration System for Enhanced Reality Visualization in Surgery", *Proceedings of First International Conference on Computer Vision, Virtual Reality and Robotics in Medicine*, Nice France, April 1995, pp. 3–12.

[6] W.E.L. Grimson, G.J. Ettinger, S.J. White, T. Lozano-Pérez, W.M. Wells III, and R. Kikinis, "An Automatic Registration Method for Frameless Stereotaxy, Image Guided Surgery, and Enhanced Reality Visualization", *IEEE Trans. Medical Imaging*, **15**(2), April 1996, pp. 129–140.

[7] A. Gueziec, N. Ayache, "New Developments on Geometric Hashing for Curve Matching", *Proceedings of IEEE Computer Vision and Pattern Recognition Conference*, 1993.

[8] B.K.P. Horn, "Closed-form Solution of Absolute Orientation Using Unit Quaternions", *Journal of the Optical Society of America A*, **4**, April 1987, pp. 629–642.

[9] H. Jiang, R. Robb, K. Holton, "A New Approach to 3D Registration of Multimodality Medical Images by Surface Matching", *Proceedings of Visualization in Biomedical Computing*, 1992.

[10] T. Kapur, W.E.L. Grimson, R. Kikinis, "Segmentation of Brain Tissue from MR Images", *Proceedings of First International Conference on Computer Vision, Virtual Reality and Robotics in Medicine*, Nice France, April 1995, pp. 429–433.

[11] J.P. Mellor, "Realtime Camera Calibration for Enhanced Reality Visualization", *Proceedings of First International Conference on Computer Vision, Virtual Reality and Robotics in Medicine*, Nice France, April 1995, pp. 471–475.

[12] C. Pelizzari, G. Chen, D. Spelbring, R. Weichselbaum, C. Chen, "Accurate three-dimensional registration of CT, PET, and/or MR images of the brain", *Journal of Computer Assisted Tomography* **13**(1), 1989.

[13] W.H. Press, S.A. Teukolsky, S.T. Vetterling, B.P. Flannery, *Numerical Recipes in C, The Art of Scientific Computing, Second Edition*, Cambridge University Press, 1992.

[14] D. Simon, et al. "Techniques for Fast and Accurate Intrasurgical Registration", *Proceedings of First International Symposium on Medical Robotics and Computer Assisted Surgery*, Pittsburgh PA, September 1994.

[15] R. Szeliski, S. Lavallee, "Matching 3D Anatomical Surfaces with Non-Rigid Deformations using Octree-Splines", *Proceedings of IEEE Workshop on Biomedical Image Analysis*, June, 1994, pp. 144–153.

[16] J.P. Thirion, "Extremal Points: Definition and Application to 3D Image Registration", *Proceedings of IEEE Conference on Computer Vision and Pattern Recognition*, June 1994, pp. 587–592.

[17] W.M. Wells, "Adaptive Segmentation of MRI Data", *Proceedings of First International Conference on Computer Vision, Virtual Reality and Robotics in Medicine*, Nice France, April 1995, pp. 59–69.

[18] W.M. Wells, *Statistical Object Recognition*, MIT AI Technical Report 1398, January 1993.

[19] Z. Zhang, "Iterative Point Matching for Registration of Free-form Curves and Surfaces", *International Journal of Computer Vision*, **13**(2), 1994.

Registration of Planar Film Radiographs with Computed Tomography

Lisa M. Gottesfeld Brown *
lisab@watson.ibm.com
I.B.M T.J. Watson Research Center
Hawthorne, NY 10532

Terrance E. Boult
teb6@Lehigh.edu
LeHigh University
Bethlehem, PA 18015

Abstract

In this paper we describe a method to register Computed Tomography (CT) data with planar film radiographs. Previous methods applied to the problem of CT-radiograph registration rely on determining the correspondence between occluding contours of the 3D surface in the CT data with 2D contours in the projection image. These methods implicitly assume that the correspondence is accurate, ignoring fundamental nonlinear differences in the underlying measurements. In contrast, our emphasis has been to directly exploit the relationship between imaging devices. This is performed by registering radiograph data with intensity-corrected simulated radiograph data derived from CT measurements. We will show that by exploiting the physical relationship between CT and radiograph measurements we can significantly improve registration accuracy. Concomitantly, we detail the relationship between CT and radiograph measurements and the primary factors influencing discrepancies between simulated and real radiograph data.

1 Introduction

Registration of medical data from different imaging devices has proven to be an important tool for extracting additional information for diagnosis, therapy, and surgery. For example, high resolution, three dimensional, structural medical images, such as data from X-ray computed tomography (CT) and magnetic resonance imaging (MR), are capable of clearly delineating many anatomical structures. These images may be taken prior to a surgical operation for diagnosis and localization. The surgeon may use such images to plan a surgical procedure. Then during surgery, 2D ultrasound images or fluoroscopy data may be used to guide the surgeon through his plan. To effectively execute the plan, the intra-operative images need to be registered with the pre-operative images. However, the poor resolution of the intra-operative images, the differences in the sensor characteristics, and the changes in the patient's position and state make this a challenging task.

Historically, this registration has been performed using stereotactic frames, external markers, and 3D positioning devices. These interventions pose a burden on the surgeon and patient and limit the accuracy and generality of the registration. The ideal solution is anatomy-based patient registration. Several methods have been proposed to perform this type of image-guided registration, but in general, these methods are sensor-independent and do not address one of the most significant distortions between data sets: distortions due to differences in sensor measurements.

This paper specifically addresses the problem of registering X-ray CT data with planar film radiographs. Our emphasis has been to directly exploit the relationship between imaging devices. This is performed by registering radiograph data with intensity-corrected simulated radiograph data derived from CT measurements. We will show that by utilizing the physical relationship between CT and radiograph measurements we can significantly improve registration accuracy. Concomitantly, we detail the relationship between CT and radiograph measurements and the primary factors influencing discrepancies between simulated and real radiograph data. This relationship is useful, not only in improving registration, but also to enhance our understanding of the measurements of the individual modalities, their distortions and sensor-dependent information. We also intend to use this relationship to aid our understanding of the more complex relationship between CT and fluoroscopic images.

We start off by describing previous work in this area and the strategy we employed to improve the accuracy currently achieved. In Section 3, we describe the acquisition of our data and the calibration procedure we implemented to evaluate our registration technique. In Section 4, we examine the relationship between radiographic and CT data. CT data is used to simulate radiographic data and the factors which influence the differences between real and simulated data are

---

*This work is supported in part by NSF CISE grant #CDA-90-24735, in part by NSF Presidential Young Investigators Awards program #IRI-90-57951, and in part by ARPA contract DACA-76-92-C-007.

discussed.

Sections 5 and 6 describe the registration technique and the results. The registration method uses the results of Section 4 to exploit the full sensor relationship. The transformation between a single radiograph and a 3D CT data set is determined using the simulated radiographs generated from the CT data. The optimal transformation is the X-ray system configuration which generated the simulated radiograph which is maximally correlated with the original radiograph. An error analysis is conducted based on the results of the calibration study. In the last section, we summarize the results of this research and offer suggestions for future work.

2 Related Work

Registration methods designed for determining the X-ray system parameters which relate CT data with one or more X-ray projection images, can be split into two major categories. In the first category, surfaces in the CT data are initially extracted. Then, corresponding features in X-ray images, such as edges or contours, are found. The registration transformation is then found by minimizing a cost function which evaluates the proximity between the projected 3D surface and the 2D contours. This strategy was used by [7] and [3]. In [8] a similar approach was taken except only a small number of anatomical features, namely, boundaries along skull landmarks, were used.

These methods presume the correspondence between CT data and X-ray projection images is inherent, or minimally, that a prior stage has performed some kind of calibration to make this presumption true. The underlying assumption is that surfaces found in the CT data that are tangent to perspective rays of the X-ray system configuration, will correspond to edges in the projection images. There are several limitations of this approach and its general implementation. In particular, the formal ray integral equation is not used. The fact that radiographic data is a negative exponential of an integral is ignored. Similarly, the different sensor resolutions and measurement sensitivities are overlooked. Only the simpler relationship, between occluding contours of 3D surfaces and their projections onto the radiograph image, is used. Information is limited to surface boundaries [7, 3] or feature extraction [8]. Grey value information is only used at the level of 3D segmentation and typically this difficult problem is solved independently to the registration problem. Usually only specific anatomic structures are found. This has advantages that only structures which are known to be rigid are used. However, contours in projection images do not necessarily arise from 3D surface tangents. View-dependent supposition of anatomic structures may effect projection contours in complex ways. When ray integration is not performed, only a small subset of the original grey value information is utilized. In structure/contour matching

methods, outliers are often a significant source of error.

Because the underlying relationship between the two data sets is not exploited, the relationship between the resolution of the two data sets is also not exploited. Typically 3D segmentation is performed without regard to either CT or X-ray detector resolution, or the particular X-ray system configuration. Surfaces are improperly smoothed and simplified. Both over and under-sampling are common and partial volume effects cannot be modeled. Methods are often tested on simulated data or verified by dependent information. In [6] video camera images were used to simulate fluoroscopy. In [3] accuracy is measured in average distance of matched points, which is not necessarily conclusive. These methods are advantageous in that they are potentially fast and less sensitive to changes in patient state or sensor domain. They perform well in applications where the sensor differences between images are minimal. If sensor differences are significant, they may be usefully applied for fast initial estimate prediction.

The other major approach to this problem uses voxel or pixel similarity and includes our method. Methods which use this strategy do not rely on higher level extraction of features or regions. Such extraction is typically application-dependent, sensor-dependent, and often only semi-automated, and therefore subjective. Examples of multimodal registration methods of this kind are given in [12, 5]. In [12] a filtering technique is used to find "sensor-invariant" ridges in image space. Correlation is then used to find the optimal transformation between data sets. This is successfully applied to MR and CT data. In [5] MR and CT data were also registered. Instead of maximizing a correlation function, they minimize the coefficient of variation of intensity ratios between the two images and devise a similarity measure sensitive to this metric. Both investigations attempt to find features and matching metrics which use the full data set but are invariant to sensor differences. However, both investigations are general-purpose; neither exploits the particular sensors or sensor relationship.

In our approach, voxel/pixel similarity is performed by simulating radiographic data and then optimizing the match between simulated and real radiographs. Two other research teams have been investigating this approach concurrently with our own. In [11, 1] image-guided radiosurgery is performed by correlating an orthogonal pair of radiographs with precomputed radiographs. The details of this project have not been published and are proprietary[1a]. In [9] registration was performed of CT data with a stereo pair of radiographs. Their work closely follows our own. However, our objective has been to scrutinize the underlying relationship between the radiographic and CT data, to achieve the maximal accuracy in registration, while the research of [9] was directed more towards achieving a feasible solution which could be implemented and tested more efficiently. They did not directly consider the intensity and resolution relationship between simulated and real radiographs. On the other hand, they present a more elaborate procedure for finding an initial estimate and for more efficiently optimizing the correlation between the CT data and a stereo pair of radiographs.

3 Experimental Setup

In our experiment, planar X-ray film was taken of a dry femur bone rigidly attached to a precisely machined calibration object. The calibration object was composed of two 3/8 inch plexiglass sheets, attached at their ends at a right angle. Each sheet contained a grid of 6x15 embedded stainless steel balls with 5/32 inch (3.97mm) diameter.

X-rays were taken with a Siemens SIRESKOP4 with 125 KV tube voltage, at roughly 40 inches between the X-ray source and the screen film cassette. The film was Fuji Super HR-G 14x17 inch double emulsion and the intensifier screen was a Kyokko GH1 made by Kasei Optonix Ltd. The X-ray film was then digitized using IBM's Time-Delay-and-Integration Imaging System. This system is a high resolution digitizing scanner which can capture images at a spatial resolution of 3072x4096 pixels with a dynamic range of 69.65 DB and state-of-the-art noise suppression. The digitized images were roughly 2000x3000x12-bits (only 8-bits were ultimately used) with pixel sizes on the order of 0.078x0.075 mm^2. X-ray computed tomography data of the same femur/calibration object was taken on a GE9800 scanner. The CT data was stored in a 158x512x512x8-bit matrix, with slice thickness 3mm, and pixel size 0.390625x0.3906525 mm^2.

To test our registration method, the markers of the calibration device were used to determine the parameters of the X-ray system. To perform this registration, we used the calibration procedure described in [8] and detailed for this application in [2]. This calibration determines, in addition to the rigid transformation between the CT and radiograph world, the intrinsic parameters of the X-ray system: the projection image x and y scale factors and offsets. The scale factors are implicitly related to the focal length of the X-ray system, or in other words, the distance between the X-ray source and the film. The root mean square error for the final calibration was less than 0.2 mm for both configurations. Monte Carlo simulations in which the data were perturbed using normal deviates, show that for Configuration 1, the calibration error is greatest along the optical axis. This suggests a possible error in the focal length.

4 The Relationship between Radiographs and Computed Tomography

In order to develop better methods to register radiographs with X-ray CT, we have simulated radiographs from CT data. The details of the radiograph simulation are given in [2]. In this section, we examine the intensity relationship between radiographs and simulated radiographs computed from CT. Understanding this relationship provides an important link which we will exploit to improve the methodology for the registration of radiographic and CT data. Several investigators have studied methods for registering CT and radiographs or X-ray fluoroscopy images but to our knowledge, the empirical relationship has yet to be delineated.

In the outputs shown in the top of Figures 1-2, simulated and real radiographs are shown for two data sets. The intensity values of the real radiograph represent the digitized values of the intensity transmitted by the film. The intensity values of the simulated radiograph represent the ray sum of the CT values along the ray from the X-ray source to the radiograph plane. These were computed from sufficiently small, uniformly spaced samples along the ray through the CT data, using trilinear interpolation. In this initial evaluation, we have not yet exploited the complete physical relationship between CT values and digitized radiograph measurements. Since the film is darkest where the most light strikes it, and the ray sum, by itself, is just the sum of attenuation, the images appear in many ways similar - both are brightest where the least amount of X-rays were transmitted. However, as we will show in this section, there are several important factors that can be modeled to improve this similarity.

We have determined four primary factors effecting the intensity relationship between the simulated and real radiographs. They are from the:

1. formal intensity relationhship: the ray integral equation, linearly-scaled measurements, initial and final intensities, and film characteristics,

2. differences in domain,

3. limitations in CT resolution and partial volume effects,

4. variations in X-ray source spectrum and the Heel Effect.

We will describe each factor, its effect on the intensity relationship, and how it effects the design of a registration method for radiographic and CT images.

4.1 Formal Intensity Relationship

The initial simulations shown in the top right of Figures 1-2 are based on the simple ray sum of the CT values. However this does not fully model the physical generation of digitized film measurements. In particular, assuming a narrow, monochromatic X-ray beam passing along a ray from the X-ray source to the detector, the relationship between the input and output intensity, is the ray integral of the linear attenuation coefficients $\beta(x, y, z)$:

$$I_{out} = I_{in} e^{\{-\int_{source}^{detector} \beta(x,y,z) dx\, dy\, dz\}}$$

Film effectively measures the transmitted intensity, I_t. The optical density (OD) of the film is defined to be the $\log(I_{in}/I_t)$ and this is linearly proportional to the log of the relative exposure, for the straight-line portion of the H-D or characteristic curve of the film. Since exposure is intensity over time, relative exposure is equivalent to the relative intensity for the same exposure time. Thus, $\log(I_{in}^{radiograph}/I_t) \propto \log(I_{out}/I_{in}^{CT})$, where $\propto$ implies linear proportionality. Because of the large bandwidth of our digitizer, we believe our digitized measurements are linearly related to the transmitted intensity of the film. Similarly, lack of CT calibration, bit reduction, and unit conversions from linear attenuation to Hounsfield units, are also all linear. Therefore we can derive the following relationship between the measured radiographic intensities, I_r and the measured attenuation coefficients β_m, of our CT data,

$$\log\left(\frac{1}{a_1 I_r + b_1}\right) = a_2 \log\left(a_3 \exp\left(-\sum_{ray}[a_4 \beta_m + b_4]\right)\right) + b_2$$

$$(4.1)$$

where the constants a_i, b_i are from the following linear relationships:

[a_1, b_1] Optical density is the log of the inverse of the transmitted intensity *relative* to the intensity incident on film, and the digitization is linearly related to transmitted intensity.

[a_2, b_2] For the straight-line portion of the H-D curve of the film, the optical density is linearly related to the log of the relative exposure.

[a_3] The relative exposure, and therefore the relative intensity incident on the film depends on the initial intensity emitted from the source.

[a_4, b_4] The numbers output by the CT scanner are linearly related to the linear attenuation coefficients used in the line integral equation. This may be due to the need for calibration, conversion in units, or bit reduction. The constant offset b_4 can probably be ignored, since β_{air} is zero.

Equation (4.1) can be rewritten as,

$$\ln(I_r + k) \propto \sum_{ray} \beta_m$$

where k is a constant. The derivation and relations between k and the constants of linearity, and the constants a_i, b_i are given in [2].

Furthermore, if we would like to clip intensity values which are nonlinearly related because they are above or below the straight-line portion of the H-D curve, we can add the following cut-offs:

$$\text{if } \sum_{ray} \beta_m > c_l \text{ then } I_{sim} = c_l \text{ else } I_{sim} = \sum_{ray} \beta_m$$

$$\text{if } \sum_{ray} \beta_m < c_u \text{ then } I_{sim} = c_u \text{ else } I_{sim} = \sum_{ray} \beta_m,$$

where I_{sim} replaces $\sum_{ray} \beta_m$ in the previous equation. This is applicable only if we have a suitable signal to noise ratio. Notice, because the sum of the attenuation coefficients is inversely related to the amount of X-ray transmission the lower cut-off operates like an upper bound and similarly, the upper cut-off acts like a lower bound. For our radiographs, i.e., for the H-D curve of our film, only the upper cut-off c_u appears to be relevant.

We have written the equation in terms of a tranformation of our radiographic data to our "simulated" radiograph for two reasons. First, since the resolution of our radiographic data is superior to our CT data, we would like to perform our calculations using the better data. Secondly, from a computational point of view, we would like to perform correction one time on the true radiograph, rather than for each simulation in the correlation tests. On the other hand, for visualization only, it may be useful to perform the inverse transformation, since there is greater familiarity with real radiographs.

4.2 Differences in Domain

A potentially significant difference between simulated and real radiographs can arise because of changes or differences in the patient or environment. Even in our controlled environment, where the environment was fixed, these differences were manifested in Configuration 2. The calibration object was not completely in the field of view of the CT scanner. As a consequence, both ends of the calibration plate are visible in the actual radiograph and not in the simulation. Domain differences are inevitable. Registration methods designed for this application must be able to withstand substantial domain differences to be effective.

4.3 Resolution Limitations

The third factor effecting the intensity relationship between the simulated and real radiographs arises from the limitations in CT resolution and the effect this has on the simulated radiograph. This is pertinent, not only in avoiding the matching of blurred data with data at a higher resolution, but also in needlessly matching more data than can be usefully considered. In the simulated radiographs of the previous section, vertical blurring is apparent because, the vertical image axis, $\vec{v}$, is roughly aligned with the z-axis, or slice dimension, of the CT data.

To compensate, in general, for this type of resolution discrepancy, the resolution limits of the simulated radiograph is determined based on the resolution of the CT data, $(res_x^{ct}, res_y^{ct}, res_z^{ct})$ in mm/pixel, and the initial estimate of the X-ray configuration for computing the simulation. Assuming orthogonal projection, the optimal resolution for an image whose optic axis is aligned with one of the axes of the world, is simply the resolution of the world in this direction. When the image intersects the world along some direction $\vec{u} = (u_x, u_y, u_z)$, we would like the resolution to reflect the projection of the world resolution onto this directional vector. We model this effect by assuming the world resolution is elliptical with principal axes aligned with the sampling axes and whose magnitudes are related to the respective half resolution of each axes. In particular, let the resolution of the 3D world be represented by the ellipsoid:

$$\frac{x^2}{(res_x^{ct}/2)^2} + \frac{y^2}{(res_y^{ct}/2)^2} + \frac{z^2}{(res_z^{ct}/2)^2} = 1.0$$

The resolution in the 2D projection space, is defined to be the diameter of the ellipsoid in each projection direction, $(\vec{u}, \vec{v})$. This can be computed by finding the intrinsic parameters t_u and t_v such that the points $(u_x t_u, u_y t_u, u_z t_u)$ and $(v_x t_v, v_y t_v, v_z t_v)$ are on the ellipsoid. The resolution of the 2D projection space is then the diameters of the ellipsoids at these points,

$$res_{\vec{u}}^{image} = 2 \left\| \frac{1}{\frac{(u_x t_u)^2}{(res_x^{ct}/2)^2} + \frac{(u_y t_u)^2}{(res_y^{ct}/2)^2} + \frac{(u_z t_u)^2}{(res_z^{ct}/2)^2}} \right\|$$

$$res_{\vec{v}}^{image} = 2 \left\| \frac{1}{\frac{(v_x t_v)^2}{(res_x^{ct}/2)^2} + \frac{(v_y t_v)^2}{(res_y^{ct}/2)^2} + \frac{(v_z t_v)^2}{(res_z^{ct}/2)^2}} \right\|$$

where $\| * \|$ is the second norm. An elliptical resolution is reasonable, since the resolution along directions other than the principal axes should reflect the ability to interpolate using the values along both axes. This is similar to the multivariate case in which we know we have white noise with a given standard deviation along each axes; the standard deviation in 2D is elliptical. One might consider the resolution in 2D to be the resolution of the pixel quad. However, when the projection direction runs diagonally between the two resolution axes, this suggests that the resolution actually decreases, since the Euclidean distance of the diagonal of the quad is its largest cross-section. This does not take into account the progressively more information that is obtained by neighboring pixels as the projection direction moves between the original orthogonal sampling directions for the case of trilinear interpolation.

In the real case, we do not have orthogonal projection, although, as previously discussed, the distance between the X-ray source and detector is relatively large compared with distances in the image. More importantly, the distance between rays upon entering the CT-data and exiting must be similar. This depends on the dimensions of CT data relative to the X-ray configuration, and ultimately on the size and location of the body. Generally a patient is placed as close to the detector plane as possible to minimize perspective distortion. We have chosen to ignore these complications and to use the worst case estimate based on orthogonal projection.

We would like to make one comment. This resolution limitation reflects the limitations of the CT data to clearly "see" 3D objects which are smaller than the sampling size. This is evident with our data set; it was difficult to accurately discern the location of the markers whose diameter size was only slightly greater than the slice spacing. This in turn, limits the resolution of the simulated radiograph. However, because the simulated radiograph is composed of ray sums, and these sums pass through the various voxels at different locations, in cases where there are multiple objects or objects whose boundaries are crossed multiple times in any one ray, the radiograph may provide information at a higher resolution than is reflected in the analysis here.

Alternatively, we could attempt to improve the resolution of the simulated radiograph using more sophisticated techniques to interpolate the CT data. Our approach has several advantages. Improving the interpolation requires assumptions that depend on the object characteristics and the acquisition. Furthermore, since our proposed matching scheme relies on simulating many projections, we would like to limit the size and time required to simulate each radiograph. Finally, depending on the assumptions that we are able to make, it is not clear to what extent we can add real information.

Limitations in the resolution of the projections used to reconstruct CT data may cause an artifact known as the partial volume effect[4]. In our domain, this may be the cause of an under-estimation of the intensity of the markers in the CT data, since the marker size is on the order of magnitude of the slice spacing. This should also be corrected for by the limited resolution of the simulated projection which re-enacts the same type of averaging as occurred originally. However, it is also possible, that the marker brightness is due to a greater sensitivity of the film to high attenuation than the CT scanner, or a a consequence of the different energy levels used in the two mediums.

4.4 Variations in X-ray Source and the Heel Effect

The fourth primary factor effecting the intensity relationship between the real and simulated radiographs is apparently due to differences in the energy spectrums of the X-ray sources of the two modalities. This is extremely difficult to quantify. Since the local attenuation coefficient varies with energy, we need more information than we have from a single CT scan to model the effects of different energies. This is further complicated if we would like to consider the full energy spectrum and the changing energy spectrum as the X-rays traverse the medium. It does not appear necessary to model this level of complexity for the purposes of registration.

However, there is significant spatial variation in intensity apparent in the real radiograph that may be more easily explained. In both real radiographs, as compared with their respective simulations, the images appear to get brighter as you move from the bottom to the top of the image. We attribute this to the anode heel effect. In addition to the polychromatic nature of X-ray sources, the intensity of many diagnostic X-ray sources varies from one side of the source to the other. This is a physical property of the X-ray source because of the way it is constructed. Electrons produced by heating a tungsten filament strike a target which absorbs the electrons and emits X-rays. Because the target, or anode assembly, is mounted at an angle to the filament, or cathode assembly, the X-ray intensity decreases from the cathode to the anode side of the beam. This relative decrease may be as large as 25 percent.

This effect is seen vertically throughout the images. It appears more significantly where the bone and markers are present, but it is harder to quantify since its effects depend on the variations in attenuation coefficient with energy. This effect is not evident in the simulated radiograph. We expect that the best way to correct for this phenomena would be through calibration of the X-ray system using film obtained with no objects in the field of view. This information could then be used to replace a_3 in equation[4.1]. However, since our objective is to design registration methods, we note that the effect is, for the most part, monotonic and gradual across the image. This implies that although raw image intensities are effected, metrics such as edge detectors would still be effective since they are invariant to gradual intensity fluctuations.

5 Registration of Radiograph and CT data

In this section, we describe a method to register radiograph and CT data using simulated radiographs. We use the model developed in the previous section to improve the intensity

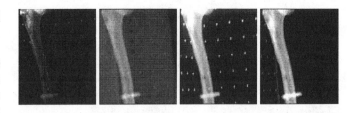

Figure 1: Intensity Matched Real and Simulated Radiographs - Configuration 1, Left image pair is the original and simulated radiographs. Right image pair is corresponding intensity corrected original and simulated radiographs.

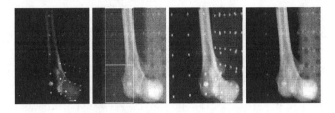

Figure 2: Intensity Matched Real and Simulated Radiographs - Configuration 2

relationship between real and simulated radiographs. We then analyze the accuracy of this approach compared with the calibration results. Finally, we examine the robustness of our approach by testing the sensitivity to intrinsic parameters and resolution and by examining the smoothness of our cost function over the search space.

5.1 Intensity Correction

The right pair of images in Figures 1-2 show the results of correcting the intensity relationship and resolution between the original and simulated radiographs for the two configurations using the formulations described in the previous section. The left pair of images are the original (far left) and simulated (second from left) radiographs as discussed in the previous section. On the right, the intensity matched original and simulated radiographs are shown, including the film cut-off and sampling of the original radiograph. Notice how segmentation performed without intensity matching would have a difficult time matching the femur outlines in both images. Even if adaptive thresholding is capable of finding the femur in the original real radiograph, which is possible, this outline is narrower than the outline in the simulated radiograph because the peak of the intensity gradient is effected by the nonlinear intensity scaling. This is also clearly seen in the marker size, which changes from the original to the intensity-scaled version. In this case, the resolution matching also plays a role, since the vertical resolution in the real radiograph is reduced.

Figure 3 shows 2D histograms of the intensity relationship between the original and simulated radiographs. In these histograms, the intensities in each radiograph are linearly scaled to 8 bits. The two images are matched point-wise and a histogram of the number of points which have each pair of intensities, (I_{orig}, I_{sim}) is computed, where I_{orig} is the intensity in the original radiograph, and I_{sim} is the intensity in the simulation. The plots show this histogram, by indicating with color, the number of points with each intensity pairing. The smallest number is represented as dark blue and the largest by red.

In the top of Figure 3 the 2D histograms for Configuration 1 are shown. The left plot shows the original histogram before intensity correction, while the right shows the histogram after correction. Although significant information is lost due to the relatively poor resolution of the CT data, the corrected histogram is significantly more linear than the original.

In the lower portion of Figure 3 the 2D histograms for Configuration 2 are shown. The middle images show the original and corrected histograms as before. However, because of the differences in domain, the corrected histogram has a "shadow." We verified this by computing the histogram for the part of the image without this problem. The histogram is shown in the lower left; the image section we used is shown by two boxes outlined on the simulated X-ray in Figure 2. The histogram still appears to saturate - the original radiograph seems to have higher intensities which are not represented in the simulation. We hypothesize that this is a manifestation of the Heel Effect. Again, we took only a subset of the images - this time limiting the image to lower box shown in Figure 2, the part of the image near the center of the image detector. The histogram for this subset is shown in the lower right. The results support our hypothesis. It is also interesting to infer from the 2D histogram the relative *intensity* resolutions of the two data sets. Notably, the simulated radiograph contains significantly less information.

5.2 The Similarity Metric

Since domain differences between images are potentially unavoidable, edges are extracted from the intensity matched radiographs. Images are normalized and filtered using a horizontal and vertical 3x3 Sobel filter. The output of this edge detection is two grey values, $[G_x, G_y]$, indicating the gradient in each direction. Gradient correlation is then performed using the following equation,

$$\sum_i (G_x^o(i) * G_x^s(i) + G_y^o(i) * G_y^s(i))$$

where the superscripts indicate (o)riginal or (s)imulated image, and i is a spatial index into the images. It is not correct to take the magnitude of the gradient dot product, since a negative gradient product indicates opposite gradient directions and therefore dissimilarity. On the other hand, since domain differences are expected, we do not want to penalize

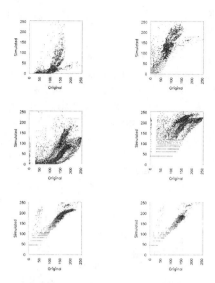

Figure 3: 2D Histograms of Intensity Relationship: Configuration 1, Top: original intensity relationship (left), corrected intensities (right) Configuration 2, Middle: original intensities (left), corrected intensities (right). Bottom: eliminating image portions with different domains (left), eliminating upper image where heel effect occurred (right).

a match because of the degree to which gradients do not agree. Therefore, we accumulate gradient product only if the product is positive indicating some similarity in the gradients at that location. Finally, we normalize our measure based on the sum of the gradient products of each image by itself, to obtain the absolute correlation coefficient.

To find the optimal rigid transformation, the maximum gradient correlation between the original and simulated, intensity-corrected radiographs was searched using Powell's multidimensional direction set method [10]. We assume that a good initial estimate is available. This is reasonable since surface/contour matching techniques and semi-automatic implementations have successfully and efficiently been able to perform this step. In addition, we found that initializing the directions so that the translational parameters are searched along the three axes of the projection space was advantageous. This was implemented using the initial estimate to compute the projection space axes.

An important parameter of Powell's method is the stopping criteria which signals that the algorithm has converged. In this case, failure to decrease the gradient correlation by some fractional tolerance, is used to determine whether to stop. For this reason, the absolute correlation coefficient is used, so that the magnitude of the fractional tolerance is meaningful.

	Pertubation 1			Perturbation 2			Perturbation 4		
	Initial	Final		Initial	Final		Initial	Final	
		.1	.0001		.1	.0001		.1	.0001
Mean	13.0	2.6	.96	25.9	3.00	1.91	51.5	111.4	5.2
x	9.3	0.17	.27	18.3	0.34	0.54	35.6	2.9	1.0
y	9.0	0.70	.83	18.5	2.48	1.71	37.3	20.9	5.1
z	0.8	2.49	.40	1.8	1.67	0.67	4.2	109.4	0.7
Tx	.48	6.0	.89	1.2	14.4	1.8	2.4	64.5	44.7
Ty	.52	8.8	.35	1.0	2.5	0.6	1.6	8.5	2.1
Tz	.65	1.2	.25	1.1	2.0	0.4	2.9	111.9	4.2
θ_x	.018	.001	.0003	.041	.002	.0005	.07	.004	.004
θ_y	.013	.005	.0006	.055	.015	.0001	.06	.048	.048
θ_z	.019	.008	.0006	.034	.004	.0012	.07	.041	.001
Correlation		.9985	1.0000		.9983	.9999		.8597	.9922

Table 1: 3D and Parameter Error for Low Resolution No Noise Case

6 Results

To evaluate the error in the registration, we computed the 3D positional error for random points in the 3D coordinate space viewed by the radiograph. For each configuration, we used a cubic region in CT or world space, centered at the femur at the vertical position in the femur which was in the vertical center in the radiograph. The assumption is that the radiograph used for 3D localization views the object of interest. The cubic region was 10cm on each side. We took 100 random 3D points in the cube and compared these with their locations as estimated by the optimization. Finally, we evaluated the components of these errors with respect to the coordinate axes of the projection space.

We performed two types of tests. To test our implementation, its accuracy, robustness to initial estimate, and tolerance to the stopping condition, we performed tests using a simulated projection instead of the actual radiograph. This is the case with no noise except resolution limitations. The results are shown in Table 1. Three studies of the no noise case were conducted. In each study, we reduced the CT data set to (79x64x64) and the radiograph size to (47x39). This corresponds to a CT resolution of (6.04mm,3.17mm,3.17mm) and a radiograph resolution of (3.8mm,6.07mm). For each study, we performed 5 trials with random initial estimates in the range $\pm 1mm$ for translation parameters and $\pm 1degree$ for rotation parameters, for Perturbation 1, ± 2 mm or degree for Perturbation 2, and ± 3 mm or degree for Perturbation 3. For each study we also computed the results for two different stopping conditions, a fractional tolerance of 0.1 and 0.0001 in the correlation. The table shows the resulting 3D and parameter errors.

First, we point out that the method can tolerate significantly more rotational error than translational error. Although not shown here, the results for the same perturbation cases with reduced error in the initial estimate of the rotational parameters are very similar, except the initial 3D positional errors are much smaller. Notice also, since we have relatively large rotational error, the initial error in X and Y is significantly greater than the error in Z ,the optic axis.

The next observation we would like to make is that the parameter error is not a useful measure in this case. This makes sense, since the origin of the projection space coordinate system lies at the X-ray source, whose position can be moved by a relatively large factor without the same effect on localization error. Lastly, we observe, that the method is very sensitive to the range in the initial estimate and this can be partially overcome by decreasing the fractional tolerance used as a stopping condition. However, this implies that the method is vulnerable to noise in the data, which will make it difficult to obtain the optimal solution as the size of the perturbation of the initial estimate increases. Notice, the error in the 3D components of the localization error for the larger perturbations reflects the resolution limitations in the data - in this case, the y-axes is roughly aligned with the CT slice or vertical radiograph spacing which was on the order of 6mm, and the z-axes is the optical axis for which a single radiograph contains little information.

Table 2 show the results of the registration method applied to the real radiographs and the full CT data set. As we discussed in the study using simulated data, i.e. data with no noise, only small perturbations in the initial estimate are acceptable. Furthermore, high accuracy in the correlation is necessary; for these tests we set the fractional tolerance to 0.001, and the initial estimate perturbation size to ± 2 mm or degrees. For initial estimates greater than ± 4 mm or degrees, the method did not typically reach the optimal solution. We assume here that a good initial estimate is given, either by re-initializing Powell's method, by implementing hierarchical

	Configuration 1		Configuration 2	
	Initial	Final	Initial	Final
Mean	25.3	2.82	25.9	.78
x	20.6	.58	18.3	.61
y	14.1	1.66	18.2	.44
z	3.5	2.20	1.8	.22
Max	26.4	3.2	27.3	.93
x	22.7	.89	19.7	.67
y	14.1	1.91	20.1	.58
z	4.5	2.64	2.6	.27
Correlation		0.7545		0.6115

Table 2: 3D Error for Full Resolution Radiograph/CT Registration

optimization, and/or using contour/surface matching techniques. For this research, we are primarily interested in the accuracy that can be achieved.

The results are mixed. For Configuration 2, the 3D error is less than 1mm. The optimal correlation was within the tolerance of the correlation for the "true" solution. For Configuration 1, however, the correlation for the "true" solution was only 0.7396, while the optimal correlation was 0.7543, indicating that a simulated radiograph was generated which was more highly correlated than the calibrated solution. This has two potential explanations. First, our calibration results may include error in the intrinsic parameters, thereby corrupting the results here. In fact, our calibration results of the intrinsic parameters from Configuration 1, were indeed questionable. This is corroborated by the error components which are greatest along the optic axis. Second, the error along the optic axis and in the vertical direction, are reasonable given the limitations of a single radiograph with a focal length of 1000mm and vertical spacing of 3mm. This was confirmed by visual inspection of the objective function over translation space; a nearly constant-value ridge occurred along the optical axis. This is shown in Figure 4 in which the axes coming out of the page is T_z. In the no-noise case (upper surface), a peak is barely discernible at the appropriate location (0,0), while for the real radiograph (lower surface), the peak is off center, in the fore-ground, i.e. along a different position in the optical axis.

7   Conclusion

In summary, we have verified that by using intensity-corrected simulated radiographs, a single planar film radiograph can be registered to CT data at high accuracy. For our two test radiographs whose vertical axes are nearly aligned with the CT slice dimension and CT data with slice thickness

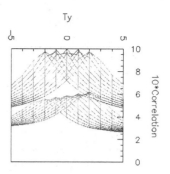

Figure 4: Surface plot of the objective function for Config. 1 over translation space (T_y, T_z). Plot shows the ridge along the optic axis peaking at the calibration solution for the no-noise case (upper surface where absolute correlation values are higher), and peaking at a different position along the optic axis for the real data.

of 3mm, a maximum error of less than 1mm in the horizontal direction, less than 2mm in the vertical direction, and less than 3mm along the optic axis was achieved. We assume intrinsic parameters can be accurately measured and other methods can be used to efficiently find a good initial estimate. Previous methods have relied on multiple radiographs, have been tested only by simulations, and have not exploited the full sensor model.

We have also detailed the relationship between CT and digitized planar radiograph film measurements. We have described a model for simulating radiographs from CT data for registration with real radiographs. To optimize the intensity relationship between simulated and real radiographs the linearity of the measurements, film characteristics, and relations between initial and final intensities are utilized to derive a formal mathematical relationship between measured attenuation and digitized planar film. Other factors influencing the discrepancy between simulated and real radiographs were addressed including the differences in domain, limitations in CT resolution and partial volume effects, and variations in X-ray source spectrum and the Heel Effect.

For future work, we propose to confirm our model and registration method using more test cases including different and more realistic patient data, and other radiographic systems including bi-planar radiographic devices and different film/screen combinations. It would also be useful to corroborate our model with calibration information and possibly pre-calibrate to remove known error sources such as domain and source intensity differences and intensity variations due to the Heel Effect. One interesting potential experiment is to register CT data with scout data from the same scanner.

This eliminates several factors influencing the simulation error such as X-ray source spectrum and some calibration errors but would allow us to evaluate the potential accuracy of the radiograph simulation.

Our ultimate objective is to combine this type of highly accurate but inefficient registration method with a classical contour/surface approach. In this way, we would be able to achieve both the computational speed and accuracy necessary for clinical applications. Lastly, we would like to use the relationship derived for CT and radiographic film to derive the more complex relationship between CT and fluoroscopy.

8 Acknowledgements

We would like to thank Professor Gerald Q. Maguire of the Royal Institute of Technology(KTH)/Teleinformatik, Stockholm, Sweden for significant contributions to this work.

References

[1] J. R. Adler, "Image-Based Frameless Stereotaxy," in *Interactive Image-Guided Neurosurgery*, ed. R. J. Maciunas, 1993, 81-98.

[1a] Correspondence with J. R. Adler.

[2] L. G. Brown, *Multi-Modal Medical Image Registration - Exploiting Sensor Relationships*, Ph.D. Dissertation, Columbia University, 1996.

[3] J. Feldmar, N. Ayache, F. Betting, "3D-2D Projective Registration of Free-Form Curves and Surfaces," Institut National de Recherche en Informatique et en Automatique, Sophia-Antipolis, France, Rapport de Recherche, No. 2434, December 1994.

[4] G. T. Herman, *Image Reconstruction from Projections*, Academic Press, Orlando, FL, 1980.

[5] D. L. G. Hill and D. J. Hawkes, "Medical Image Registration using Voxel Similarity Measures," *AAAI Applications of Computer Vision in Medical Image Processing*, March 21-23, 1994, 34-37.

[6] S. Lavallée, J. Troccaz, P. Sautot, L. Brunie, P. Cinquin, P. Merloz, and J. Chirossel, "Robot Assisted Spine Surgery," *IEEE Trans. on Robotics and Automation*.

[7] S. Lavallée, J. Troccaz, P. Sautot, P. Sautot, B. Mazier P. Cinquin, P. Merloz, and J. Chirossel, "Computer Assisted Spine Surgery," *Proc. of 1st Int'l Symp. on Medical Robotics in Computer Assisted Surgery,*, Vol I, Pittsburgh, PA, 1994.

[8] B. Lee, *Stereo Matching of Skull Landmarks* Ph.D. Dissertation, Stanford University, 1991.

[9] L. Lemieux, R. Jagoe, D. R. Fish, N. D. Kitchen, and D. G. T. Thomas, "A Patient-to-Computed-Tomography Image Registration Method based on Digitally Reconstructed Radiographs," *Medical Physics*, **21**, No. 11, November 1994, 1749-1760.

[10] W. H. Press, S. A. Teukolsky, W. T. Vetterling, B. P. Flanner, *Numerical Recipes in C*, Cambridge University Press, 1992.

[11] A. Schweikard, R. Tombropoulos, J. R. Adler, and J-C. Latombe, "Planning for image-guided radiosurgery," *Applications of Computer Vision in Medical Image Processing*, March 21-23, 1994, 96-101.

[12] P. A. van den Elsen, "Retrospective Fusion of CT and MR Brain Images Using Mathematical Operators," *AAAI Applications of Computer Vision in Medical Image Processing*, March 21-23, 1994, 30-33.

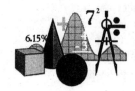

Session 2

Bayesian Analysis

Hierarchical Bayesian Classification of Multimodal Medical Images

K.V.Mardia, T.J.Hainsworth, J.Kirkbride
Department of Statistics,
The University of Leeds,
Leeds LS2 9JT.
sta6kvm@amsta.leeds.ac.uk, tim@amsta.leeds.ac.uk, jayne@amsta.leeds.ac.uk

M.A.Hurn
School of Mathematical Sciences,
The University of Bath,
Bath BA2 7AY.
mah@maths.bath.ac.uk

E. Berry
Department of Medical Physics,
Wellcome Wing, LGI,
Leeds LS1 3EX.
e.berry@leeds.ac.uk

Abstract

It has gradually been recognised that Bayesian algorithms are more widely applicable and reliable than ad-hoc algorithms. Advantages include the use of explicit and realistic stochastic models making it easier to understand the working behind the algorithm and allowing confidence statements about conclusions. We propose a method, within a Bayesian framework, to assimilate information from images obtained from different modalities at different resolutions. The algorithm is used with a pair of images, from which a fused high resolution image and improved data reconstructions are simultaneously obtained. We illustrate our method by two examples, the first fuses a pair of SPECT and CT phantom images and the second a pair of MR brain scan images, obtained from different acquisition techniques. We provide a pseudo-comparison of the latter example with a commercially available package called ANALYZE. However, the phantom images from physical experiment given here provide a true validation and performance of the model.

1. Introduction

Medical images are obtained using a range of modalities and techniques. As the images provide complementary information it is advantageous to combine the information from the images in a manner analogous to the techniques used in computer vision and signal processing when data is available from multiple sources. The process is sometimes known as "data fusion"; methods used in machine vision are reviewed by Abidi and Gonzalez (1992) [1], while medical applications are covered by Viergever *et al* (1995) [22]. Although data fusion can concern the combination of images from different fields of view, or from completely different media, in this presentation we are interested in data fusion of images from different types of sensor with the same field of view. An example outside the field of medicine is scene analysis from multispectral satellite images, in medicine the analysis may involve a pair of images acquired using different techniques one of which gives anatomical detail, the other providing information about metabolic function. For example, consider the problem of matching anatomy and function (blood perfusion) from registered CT and SPECT scans of the same patient's brain. The higher resolution CT image uses the attenuation properties of the body to show anatomical structure, defining areas of bones and tissues of differing density. In contrast, the SPECT image is of relatively low spatial resolution but clearly shows areas of functioning tissue, by imaging a radioactive tracer carried by blood.

One interpretation of data fusion is the registration of the two data sets to allow the physician to compare the matching slices by eye; the images may be displayed side by side or overlaid. However, in this work we propose to obtain a single image representing the synthesis of important details from two or more modalities, rather than simply this simultaneous display of a set of registered images. It is intended that the result of this data fusion will be a parsimonious representation of the most important information from all the source images. Previous investigators (Kohn *et al*, 1991) [14] have achieved this by performing segmentation in "feature space", that is a histogram representing the population distribution of pixel values in the various images available.

Here, an alternative approach utilising a Bayesian hierarchical technique is used, as described in the Bayesian formulation of Clark and Yuille (1990) [6] which aims to provide a unifying mathematical foundation for data fusion for sensory information processing systems in terms of constraint based models. It is proposed that there exists a super population which is modelled by a Markov Random Field (MRF), from which the observed images are drawn, duly modified by the imaging process and introducing blurring and noise. There are two broad categories of model (Geman & Geman, 1984) [7] and (Marr & Poggio, 1976) [18]. The first is the weakly coupled model, in which it is assumed that the imaging modalities are independent. The second is the strongly coupled model, in which there is dependence between imaging modalities. The dependence between the modalities is modelled, for example, by using a Gibbs prior (Geman & Geman, 1984) [7]. The weakly coupled approach is likely to be most appropriate for fusion of modalities such as CT and SPECT which image different properties of the tissue. In this work, low-level pixel-based methods of data fusion using Markov Random Field models using both weakly and strongly coupled constraints between the imaging modalities are used. MRF models have previously been used for data fusion of images of the same resolution in colour image segmentation (Wright, 1989) [23], and for temporal image sequences (Hainsworth & Mardia, 1993) [11]. An iterative algorithm is applied which generates images intermediate in the hierarchy to the data and the MRF model, these incorporate features of both modalities. A fused classification image is also produced.

Two aspects of our approach are worth noting. The first is that the image sets must be spatially registered, so that perfectly matching slices are used. The registration of various image sources is an area of active research which is already showing promising results; for a review of registration methods see Brown (1992) [5]. Within the field of medical imaging there exists an interest in the processing of pre- registered images (Gindi et al, 1993) [9]. The second aspect is that the SPECT and CT data used in our first example have been generated by the commonly-used filtered back projection method: the use of alternative statistical reconstruction is discussed.

In section 2, we propose a Bayesian framework to the problem of estimating the classification (segmentation) of a scene given image data from two or more modalities. In section 3, we describe the method of Maximum A Posteriori (MAP) image reconstruction and the concurrent estimation of model parameters. section 4 demonstrates the method with applications to two example image pairs. An illustrative comparison is made with one of the multispectral classification routines available in the biomedical image processing package ANALYZE(TM). We conclude with a discussion in section 5.

2. Bayesian Framework

The framework within which we intend to work is that of Bayesian hierarchical models. There will be three levels to our hierarchy. The first level is a model for the underlying classification of the object of interest, Z. Under ideal conditions, observing Z under M different modalities would give rise to the second level, M ideal observed images, $X_1, ..., X_M$. A model for how the $\{X\}$ depend on Z should utilise information about how the different imaging modalities respond to the different Z categories. The third level of the hierarchy, that of the actual observed data $Y_1, ..., Y_M$, represents the unavoidable degradations inherent for whatever reason in the recording process. Our aim is to make inferences on Z, and as a by-product the $\{X\}$, based on the observed $\{Y\}$. The use of such a hierarchical framework mirrors the inherent structure of the problem.

2.1. A Model For The Classification

Suppose that the object contains L distinct classes, arbitrarily labeled $\{1, ..., L\}$. For example, if the scene were a planar cross-section through a head, the labels might represent "bone", "tissue", "tumour", and so on, possibly with subdivisions according to functionality of the material, "active" and "inactive". The continuous real-world scene is approximated by a discrete representation; let $Z = (Z_j)$ denote this pixellated image, where Z_j is the class of pixel j on an $N_0 \times N_0$ regular lattice. We shall model the true image as a realisation of a Markov Random Field (MRF) with prior probability density function in the form of an Ising model with parameter β. This model associates relatively high probability to images with few mismatching neighbouring pixels, which is appropriate when the object is expected to contain relatively large regions of the same type.

$$P(Z;\beta) \propto \exp\{-\beta \sum_{<i,j>} I_{[Z_i \neq Z_j]}\}, \qquad \beta \geq 0, \qquad (1)$$

$$\text{where} \qquad I_{[Z_i \neq Z_j]} = \begin{cases} 1 & \text{if } Z_i \neq Z_j \\ 0 & \text{otherwise} \end{cases} \qquad (2)$$

and $< i, j >$ indicates that the summation in equation (1) is to be taken over all nearest neighbour pairs of pixels i and j in the Z lattice. For a general introduction to this strategy, we refer to Mardia and Kanji (1993) [16] and Mardia (1994) [17].

2.2. A Model For The Intermediate $\{X\}$

We model the relationship between the observed data $\{Y\}$ and the underlying classification Z using intermediate ideal response images $X_i = (X_{ij})$, one for each modality i, $(i = 1, ..., M)$, where X_{ij} is the ideal response at pixel location j on the $N_i \times N_i$ pixel lattice. We shall be mainly concerned with the case $M = 2$, motivated by our practical examples. Note that, in general, different modalities will produce observed images of different resolution; for example, for reasons of patient safety, SPECT images are usually of relatively low resolution (for example, 64×64 pixels, with an inherent resolution of approximately 3mm), whereas CT images have relatively high resolution (for example, 512×512 pixels, with an inherent resolution of under 1mm). In the case of synthetic images, the resolution of the true pixel image Z is known by construction. With real data, the choice of N_0 is rather more arbitrary, although for the purposes of our model we shall always use $N_0 > N_i$ for all $i = 1, \cdots, M$, (typically with $N_0 = 2 \times \max_i N_i$) so that the true image is of higher resolution than either of the observed images. We shall also assume that these different image modalities are registered so that the correspondence between pixel positions in Z, Y_1 and Y_2 is known. We justify this assumption by noting that the registration of images from different modalities is an active research area.

We model the $\{X\}$ as conditionally independent of one other given Z, so that the joint conditional probability density function of $\{X_i\}$ given Z can be written, $P(X_1, ..., X_M | Z) = \prod_{i=1}^{M} P(X_i | Z)$. This is reasonable when the classification Z determines the behaviour under each modality; for example, given that a particular region is classified as bone, the ideal CT and SPECT responses for this region will not affect one another.

The form of $P(X_i | Z)$ will contain both a deterministic transformation modelling the reduction in pixel resolution over an appropriate area of the real-world region and a stochastic model to generate texture. One of the simpler, but still effective, models which could be used is that the X_i response at a pixel j follows a Gaussian distribution, with mean given by the average of the equivalent location typical Z responses. Denote the vector containing the typical responses of the L different classes of Z under modality i by $\mu_i(\ )$. Let $K_i(\ )$ be the aggregation operator which reduces the resolution of an $N_0 \times N_0$ grid to an $N_i \times N_i$ grid by simple local averaging. Then the mean response of modality i is given by $K_i(\mu_i(Z))$. Under this simple model, given Z the ideal responses X_{ij}, are distributed as independent Gaussians with means $K_i(\mu_i(Z))$ and variance γ_i^2,

$$P(X_i | Z) \propto \exp\left\{-\frac{1}{2\gamma_i^2}|X_i - K_i(\mu_i(Z))|^2\right\}, \quad (3)$$

where $|\ |$ indicates Euclidean distance.

2.3. A Model For The Data $\{Y\}$

In the next stage of the hierarchical model, considering the dependencies of the M observed data sets, both on each other, and on $\{X\}$ and Z , it seems reasonable to assume that the data Y_i recorded for modality i depend only upon the ideal response X_i. That is,

$$P(\{Y_i\} | \{X_i\}, Z) = \prod_{i=1}^{M} P(Y_i | X_i). \quad (4)$$

The next issue is determining a suitable form for $P(Y_i | X_i)$. It is well known, for example (Green, 1990) [10], that count data arising in emission recording processes have a Poisson type noise structure. However, the CT and SPECT data which we have available for this study are not the raw count information, but rather the widely used filtered back projection (FBP) reconstructions. We intend to use another Gaussian form for (4), justifying this approximation by the following reasoning: it is hoped that the filtered back projection is allocating many of the counts back, if not to exactly the correct pixel locations, then at least to within some small region of them. As a result, the typical value of Y_{ij} will be some locally blurred average of the X_i values around pixel j. Since the Y_i value at pixel j is generated by superimposing filtered count contributions from a number of detectors, we resort to a Normal approximation, assuming independent noise with variance σ_i^2 at each pixel.

$$P(Y_i | X_i) \propto \exp\left\{-\frac{1}{2\sigma_i^2}|Y_i - H_i \circ X_i|^2\right\}, \quad (5)$$

where $(H_i \circ X_i)$ represents the mean grey-level of Y_i, obtained by blurring the intermediate X_i image using a blurring operator H_i.

2.4. The Full Model

Under our assumptions of conditional independence, the joint probability distribution for the variables Z, $\{X_i\}$ and $\{Y_i\}$ may be written, $P(Z, \{X_i\}, \{Y_i\})$ = $\prod_{i=1}^{M} P(Y_i | X_i) \times \prod_{i=1}^{M} P(X_i | Z) \times P(Z)$. We will be interested in drawing inferences about Z and $\{X_i\}$, conditioned on the observed data $\{Y_i\}$. The required posterior conditional distribution is

$$P(Z, \{X_i\} | \{Y_i\}) \propto \prod_{i=1}^{M} P(Y_i | X_i) \times \prod_{i=1}^{M} P(X_i | Z) \times P(Z)$$

$$\propto \exp\{-\sum_{i=1}^{M} \frac{|Y_i - H_i \circ X_i|^2}{2\sigma_i^2} - \sum_{i=1}^{M} \frac{|X_i - K_i(\mu_i(Z))|^2}{2\gamma_i^2}$$

$$- \beta \sum_{<i,j>} I_{[z_i \neq z_j]}\}. \quad (6)$$

The particular specification up to proportionality of distributions (1), (3) and (5) now allows us to define (7) up to a constant of proportionality not depending on the $\{X_i\}$ or Z. Each term in this posterior probability can be interpreted. The first term is the likelihood, it sums over the discrepancy between each of the noisy data images and its corresponding blurred ideal image. The second term models the relationship between each pixel in the ideal image with corresponding groups of pixels in the super-population image mapped by K. The last term penalises pixel pairs which are not of the same type in the super-population. For a diagram showing the hierarchical form of the model, see Figure 1.

We shall refer to (7) as the coupled model since it incorporates dependencies between the modalities via the classification Z.

3. Estimation Issues

We are interested in estimating the classification Z and the ideal observed images $\{X_i\}$ based on the data $\{Y_i\}$. We have chosen to use the *maximum a posteriori* (MAP) estimates, that is those values of Z and $\{X_i\}$ which maximise the posterior distribution (7) and so are most likely under that model. Since it is computationally infeasible to obtain these MAP estimates exactly, we shall use an iterative numerical approximation, Iterated Conditional Modes (ICM) proposed by Besag (1986) [3], which is guaranteed to find at least a local optimum.

The model (7) also contains several unknown parameters: β, $\{\mu_i\}$, $\{\gamma_i^2\}$ and $\{\sigma_i^2\}$. The aggregation operators $\{K_i(\ )\}$ which match the dimensions of Z and $\{X_i\}$ will be assumed known by construction. In addition, we will also assume the $\{H_i\}$ to be known, specifying them to be uniform blurring kernels. The approach to estimating the unknown parameters will be iterative, estimating them based on the data and the current estimates of the classifications and ideal responses. As a result, the two sets of estimation problems will be run in alternating steps, an update of the parameter estimates given the current images, followed by an update of the images given the current parameter estimates. Initial estimates of all quantities are required; these could be obtained by a variety of means including prior expert information, simple thresholding, or from test data.

3.1. Estimation Of Classification Z And Ideal Response Images $\{X_i\}$

The desired estimates of Z and $\{X_i\}$ are those images which are most likely under model (7) given the data $\{Y_i\}$. Clearly this is a very high dimensional optimisation problem which cannot be solved exactly. The approach we will adopt here is an iterative, strictly uphill search procedure, Iterated Conditional Modes or ICM, (Besag, 1986) [3]. This procedure is guaranteed to converge, at least to a local optimum of the posterior (7).

Suppose that we are considering the case $M = 2$, and that provisional estimates of X_1, X_2 and Z are available. We wish to update X_{ij}, the value of the ideal response at pixel j at modality i ($j \in \{1, \cdots, N_i^2\}$), by maximising (7)

with respect to X_{ij} while holding everything else fixed. The Markov random field nature of (1), combined with the local structure of (3) and (5), lead to very considerable simplifications in computing these updates. Substituting (1), (3) and (5) into equation (7), it can be seen that the posterior probability of X_{ij} given the rest, i.e. everything excluding X_{ij}, takes the form

$$P(X_{ij}|rest) \propto \exp\{-\frac{\sum_{k\in\psi_{ij}}(Y_{ik} - (H_i \circ X_i)_k)^2}{2\sigma_i^2}$$
$$- \frac{(X_{ij} - (K_i(\mu_i(Z))_j)^2}{2\gamma_i^2}\}, \quad (7)$$

where ψ_{ij} is the set of Y_i pixels whose values are influenced by the value of X_i at pixel j. The updated value of X_{ij} is chosen to maximise the value of this penalty while all other values are held fixed. Similarly, the posterior probability of Z_j given the rest, i.e. everything excluding Z_j, can be seen to take the form

$$P(Z_j|rest) \propto \exp\{-\sum_i \sum_{k\in\zeta_{ij}} \frac{(X_{ik} - (K_i(\mu_i(Z))_k)^2}{2\gamma_i^2}$$
$$- \beta \sum_{k\in\partial_j} I_{[z_k \neq z_j]}\}, \quad (8)$$

where ζ_{ij} is the set of modality i pixels which are formed by the aggregation of an area of the Z grid including Z-pixel j, and ∂_j is the set of Z-pixels which are neighbours of j, ie those k for which a $<k, j>$ interaction exists in (1).

In practice, the final solutions are slightly dependent upon the order in which both the images and the pixels are visited, and also upon the initial parameter values. However, the performance of the algorithm is reasonable provided that the data are not too heavily degraded, and good starting values are available. There are several possible update strategies: we adopt the following four-stage approach.

1) Estimate parameters β and $\{\mu_i, \gamma_i, \sigma_i\}$, $i = 1, 2$ using the methods to be described in this section;

2) Update X_1: Visit each pixel $j = 1, \cdots, N_1^2$ in turn and choose X_{1j} to maximise the local conditional posterior density $P(X_{1j}|rest)$ given by (8);

3) Update X_2: Visit each pixel $j = 1, \cdots, N_2^2$ in turn and choose X_{2j} to maximise the local conditional posterior density $P(X_{2j}|rest)$ given by (8);

4) Update Z: Visit each pixel $j = 1, \cdots, N_0^2$ in turn and choose Z_j to maximise the local conditional posterior density $P(Z_j|rest)$ given by (9).

3.2. Estimation Of Typical Responses $\{\mu_i\}$

The mean response of each of the classification types $1, ..., L$ under the different modalities is estimated by averaging the current X_i values over pixels corresponding purely to that single classification type. Mixed X_i pixels were excluded from the estimation procedure because of the usual modelling weaknesses associated with them. $\hat{\mu}_i(k) = \frac{1}{n_{ik}} \sum_{j \in S_{ik}} X_{ij}$, $k = 1, ..., L$ where S_{ik} is the set of X_i pixels corresponding purely to pixels of classification k in Z, and n_{ik} is the number of elements of this set.

3.3. Estimation Of Variabilities $\{\gamma_i^2\}$ And $\{\sigma_i^2\}$

The noise parameters could be estimated by a maximum likelihood approach using the current estimates of the ideal responses $\{X_i\}$ and Z. However, one feature of the models (3) and (5) is that the total variability in the system, that between the data $\{Y_i\}$ and the values which would be predicted from the classification, $\{H_i \circ K_i(\mu_i(Z))\}$, is difficult to partition between the two levels of the hierarchy without additional expert advice. For this reason, γ_i^2 is taken equal to σ_i^2, with an estimate formed by halving the total variability, $\hat{\gamma}_i^2 = \hat{\sigma}_i^2 = \frac{1}{2N_i^2} |Y_i - H_i \circ K_i(\mu_i(Z))|^2$.

3.4. Estimation Of The Classification Model Parameter β

The prior model for the classification Z is an Ising model (1) with parameter β. As such, β influences the extent to which the classification forms itself into homogeneous regions. It is an important parameter, but difficult to estimate. Maximum likelihood estimation of β is infeasible because of the intractable normalising constant in (1). Besag (1975, 1986) [2], [3] proposes an alternative estimation approach, Maximum Pseudo-Likelihood Estimation (MPLE), which we adopt here.

Suppose that a provisional estimate, $\tilde{Z}$, of the classification is available, possibly from a previous iteration. Then the MPLE of β is that value of β which maximises $\prod_j P(\tilde{Z}_j \mid \tilde{Z}_{\partial_j}; \beta)$. Recall that Z follows the Ising model, (1); hence, the local conditional probability density function takes the following form:

$$P(Z_j \mid Z_{\partial_j}; \beta) = P(Z_j; \beta) / \sum_{Z_j' = 1}^{L} P(Z_j'; \beta)$$
$$= \exp\{-\beta \overline{u}_j(Z_j)\} / \sum_k \exp\{-\beta \overline{u}_j(k)\} \quad (9)$$

where $\overline{u}_j(k)$ denotes the number of neighbours of pixel j not having class k. Note that if $u_j(k)$ denotes the number of neighbours of pixel j with class k, then $u_j(k) + \overline{u}_j(k) = |\partial_j|$ independent of k. Hence (9) can be written in the form $P(Z_j \mid Z_{\partial_j}; \beta) = \exp\{\beta u_j(Z_j)\} / \sum_k \exp\{\beta u_j(k)\} = 1/\sum_k \exp\{-\beta \delta_j(Z_j, k)\}$ where $\delta_j(Z_j, k) \equiv u_j(Z_j) - u_j(k)$. Therefore, the pseudo-likelihood takes the form $L_P(\beta) = \prod_j (\sum_k \exp\{-\beta \delta_j(Z_j, k)\})^{-1}$, and the log-pseudo-likelihood is

$$\ln\{L_P(\beta)\} = -\sum_j \log\left[\sum_k \exp\{-\beta \delta_j(Z_j, k)\}\right]. \quad (10)$$

The MPLE of β maximises (10); taking derivatives of equation (10) twice with respect to β yields

$$\ln\{L_P(\beta)\}' = \sum_j \frac{\sum_k \delta_j(Z_j, k) \exp\{-\beta \delta_j(Z_j, k)\}}{\sum_k \exp\{-\beta \delta_j(Z_j, k)\}}$$

$$\ln\{L_P(\beta)\}'' = \sum_j \left\{ -\frac{\sum_k \delta_j^2(Z_j, k) \exp\{-\beta \delta_j(Z_j, k)\}}{\sum_k \exp\{-\beta \delta_j(Z_j, k)\}} + \left(\frac{\sum_k \delta_j(Z_j, k) \exp\{-\beta \delta_j(Z_j, k)\}}{\sum_k \exp\{-\beta \delta_j(Z_j, k)\}}\right)^2 \right\}$$

The log-pseudo-likelihood (10) is maximised numerically using a Newton-Raphson method:

$$\beta_{[n+1]} = \beta_{[n]} - \frac{\ln\{L_P(\beta_{[n]})\}'}{\ln\{L_P(\beta_{[n]})\}''} \quad (11)$$

where $\beta_{[n]}$ is the value of β at iteration n. Note that in this implementation, the initial estimate of β is $\beta_{[0]} = 0$, which corresponds to a prior belief of no spatial interaction in the classification Z.

4. Assessment With Medical Images

In this section, we present the results of our proposed approach in two scenarios. The first is the fusion of phantom images from two types of scan, SPECT and CT. The second example is the assimilation of information gathered by the same modality, in this case MR, but from two different sequences with different contrast properties. Various additional validation studies have been carried out.

4.1. Example 1 — Fusing phantom CT and SPECT images

Figure 2(a) shows a 256×256 CT image of a cross-section through a phantom consisting of a cylindrical perspex container containing several perspex spheres supported on perspex rods and surrounded by water treated with radioactive tracer. Figure 2(b) shows a 64×64 SPECT image of the same phantom cross-section.

Identifying CT as Modality 1, and SPECT as Modality 2, we choose to use 3 classes: Air, Perspex and Liquid. A visual inspection of the pixel values in the two data images suggests the use of $\mu_1 = (0.0, 200.0, 100.0)$ and $\mu_2 = (0.0, 30.0, 210.0)$ as initial parameter estimates. As described in section 3, we take $\sigma_i = \gamma_i$, for $i = 1$ and 2. The blurring operators H_1 and H_2 are assumed to be 1×1 and 3×3 uniform kernels respectively.

ICM converges after around 23 sweeps to give the classification and reconstructions shown in Figure 2. Figure 2(c) shows the 512×512 classification with the region boundaries depicted in Figure 2(d). The CT reconstruction is shown in Figure 2(e) and the SPECT reconstruction is given in Figure 2(f). Note that the segmentation in Figure 2(c) contains all the main features from the CT image (Figure 2(e)); the contribution from the SPECT image (Figure 2(f)) is not clear. Taking a closer look at the SPECT reconstruction it can be seen that all six spheres are visible whereas, at best only five can be seen in the original SPECT data image, this information is obtained from the CT image. The CT reconstruction in Figure 2(e) does not seem to contain any information from the SPECT image, however it is smoother than the original data. This is due to the fact that the SPECT image does not contain features which differ to those in the CT image hence, no information is propagated from the SPECT to the CT image. The SPECT data image indicates functional material in the region of the smallest ball (because of the low resolution) whereas the reconstruction (correctly in this case) indicates no function. Further, the SPECT reconstructions of the spheres are less blurred than in the original image.

4.2. Example 2 — Fusing two MR Scans

Figure 3(a) shows a 256×256 (with pixel sizes 0.9mm $\times$ 0.9mm) cross-sectional MR scan through a subject's brain, we will identify this as Modality 1. Figure 3(b) shows the matched 256×256 (with pixel sizes 0.9mm $\times$ 0.9mm) MR scan of the same cross-section, we will identify this as Modality 2. The image acquisition sequence for Modality 1 was T_1 weighted spin echo acquisition, and for Modality 2 T_2 weighted spin echo acquisition. There are clear differences between the two scans. For example, in Modality 1, the cerebro-spinal fluid (CSF) gives a low signal, whereas this signal is high in Modality 2. The contrast between White Matter and Grey Matter is different in the two images. Previous work on segmenting major tissue components of MR images has been reported by Mowforth (1990) [21], Kohn et al (1991) [14] and Hillman et al (1995)[12], for example.

The results obtained using the new technique with the coupled model (7) are compared with the classification given by a feature-space segmentation method in the commercially available biomedical image processing package ANALYZE(TM) [20]. It is assumed that there are five distinct populations: air, white matter, grey matter, skull and cerebro-spinal fluid (CSF). First, we will consider the Bayesian fusion method. A 512×512 grid is be used for the classification Z. The blurring operators H_1 and H_2 are both assumed to be 1×1 uniform kernels. For the initial $\mu_1 = (7.0, 180.0, 160.0, 20.0, 50.0)$ and

$\mu_2 = (1.0, 71.0, 103.0, 32.0, 138.0)$, the estimated variances are $\hat{\gamma}_1^2 = \hat{\sigma}_1^2 = 606.50$ and $\hat{\gamma}_2^2 = \hat{\sigma}_2^2 = 24.96$, with $\hat{\beta} = 1.42$; these variance estimates are different, confirming the differing variation between the two scans. The final estimated means for each modality are $\hat{\mu}_1 = (14.4, 173.6, 144.3, 114.9, 81.1)$ and $\hat{\mu}_2 = (6.3, 75.9, 99.3, 21.4, 141.9)$. Figure 3(c), (d) and (e) show the corresponding estimated Z, X_1 and X_2 respectively. It can be seen that the different sequence MR reconstructions are influenced by features from each other. For example, reconstruction of Modality 2 now shows a slight increase in definition of the CSF boundary and the Modality 1 reconstruction shows better contrast between white and grey matter than in the original data. As would be expected, inaccuracies in the classification Z mainly appear to be along boundaries, or in identifying classes with relatively low occurrence rates. This can be observed in Figure 4, which gives a breakdown of the individual populations; it can be seen that parts of the skull are classified as air, and vice versa. Note that subcutaneous fat has also been classified within the skull population which explains the difference between the initial and estimated means. **It must be noted that no direct comparison is possible to any existing methods , hence we resort to a pseudo comparison with *ANALYZE*.** For example, all images used within *ANALYZE* must be of size 256×256 and as a result images may need to be reduced or enlarged. In this case, images of the required size have been used. For an illustrative comparison of classification results, the use of *ANALYZE(TM)* version 7.5 is now considered. For a description of the fusion methods available in *ANALYZE(TM)* see [19]. For this example, the classification technique used was the K-Nearest Neighbour algorithm. A population sample is manually obtained by outlining a small area of a chosen population and the intensity values for each sample are represented on the vector-histogram with different colours. This is used a starting point and each region in the vector-histogram is "grown" such that pixels become classified according to the constraints of the method. Once the individual classes have been identified the K-Nearest neighbour method assigns a population label to the voxels nearest the initial starting point of that particular population. The maximum distance that each class can 'grow 'in the vector histogram is specified. Values used were K=3 and maximum distance = 15.

The vector histogram showing the intensity relationship between Modality 1 and Modality 2 can be seen in Figure 5 (a) and the classification on the vector histogram Figure 5 (b). The final classified image is shown in Figure 5 (c). A comparison of the populations generated by the two techniques can be seen in Figure 6 for each of the five classes. Mid-grey represent pixels assigned to the same class by both methods, lighter pixels were assigned to the class only by Analyze(TM), and dark grey only by the Coupled model.

Note that for this comparison the 512×512 super-population image had to be reduced to 256×256. The coupled model has generated similar classifications to the established technique, but in addition has produced improved intermediate modality reconstructions and a higher resolution classified image. We discuss below more exhaustive testing of the coupled model.

5. Discussion

In this paper, we have presented a Bayesian approach to data fusion based on the existence of an underlying, unobservable classification Z, and ideal response images $\{X_i\}$. A hierarchical model for the distribution of these quantities given the observed data $\{Y_i\}$ is formulated (7). Parameter estimation issues for this model have been addressed. Maximum a posteriori estimates of the Z and $\{X_i\}$ are then sought using a numerical technique (Besag, 1986) [3]. The methods used in this paper fall into the general category of Bayesian models for data fusion using Gibbs probability density functions; see for example Clark and Yuille (1990) [6]. Methods which involve minimisation of a smooth energy function are a special case of the Bayesian formulation; see the review in Clark and Yuille (Chapter 3, 1990) [6].

In the medical examples in section 4, the approach has been shown to be effective, providing classifications comparable with existing techniques, but with the additional advantage of propagating information between the ideal response images. The method has shown promising results, but further development including the measurements of known volumes and validation of the tissue classification is required to establish how effective the methods are in practice. There are several possibilities to improve the model:

(1) We could construct a strongly coupled model to reconstruct X_1 and X_2 without Z as follows: Suppose that there are two modalities recorded at different resolutions and, as before, assume that the images from the two modalities are registered. Let Y_i denote the observed image for modality i, with corresponding ideal response image X_i, for $i = 1, 2$. Suppose that X_1 is of higher resolution than X_2, that is $N_1 > N_2$. We now model interdependence between the X_i using an appropriate conditional probability density $P(X_2|X_1)$, rather than through an underlying image Z as in previous models. Assuming that Y_1 and Y_2 are conditionally independent given X_1 and X_2 and using Bayes' Theorem,

$$
\begin{aligned}
P(X_1, X_2 \mid Y_1, Y_2) &\propto P(Y_1, Y_2|X_1, X_2)P(X_1, X_2) \\
&\propto P(Y_1 \mid X_1)\, P(Y_2 \mid X_2)\, P(X_2|X_1)\, P(X_1)
\end{aligned}
$$

under the assumptions given in section 2. For example, we could use models of the form

$$
P(Y_i \mid X_i) \propto \exp\left\{ -\frac{1}{2\sigma_i^2}|Y_i - H_i \circ X_i|^2 \right\}, \quad (12)
$$

$$
P(X_2 \mid X_1) \propto \exp\left\{ -\Phi(X_2 - K(\mu(X_1))) - \Phi_2(X_2) \right\}, \quad (13)
$$

$$
P(X_1) \propto \exp\left\{ -\Phi_1(X_1) \right\}, \quad (14)
$$

where $H_i, i = 1, 2$ are appropriate blurring operators, K is an appropriate operator to convert the $N_1 \times N_1$ image into an $N_2 \times N_2$ image, and μ represents the conversion of typical response values from one modality to the other. The smoothness function $\Phi(\ )$ could take the form of a Geman-Reynolds (Geman & Reynolds, 1992) [8] prior, and $\Phi_1(\ )$ and $\Phi_2(\ )$ could be those for the Ising model. There is an issue of normalising constants for these distributions. This model may be more useful for combining several modalities which all provide the same type of information (for example, all anatomical, or all functional) rather than for superimposing functional information on anatomical detail. The reconstructions of a particular modality would contain elements from other modalities, but would be biased in favour of the characteristics of that modality.

(2) The SPECT data used have been produced by filtered back-projection of count data. If we were working on the count data itself, then either the EM or OSL algorithms (Green, 1990) [10] could be used instead to improve the restorations. In this case, anatomical information via the classification of the CT image could be usefully incorporated in estimating the attenuation weights on a patient-by-patient basis.

(3) The pixel-based methods are relatively simple to implement, but such methods are low-level and do not incorporate prior knowledge of object shape or structure. In medical applications, more detailed knowledge of the contents of the image is often available. For example, consider the problem of locating a tumour in an image of a bone. The bone shape could be extracted using deformable template methods from an anatomical CT image and this information incorporated into the prior models before fusion with the functional information of the tumour location from the SPECT image. For further details of such a technique see Bookstein (1989) [4] and Mardia and Hainsworth (1993) [15].

(4) The model we have used for Z is a hard classification model, but there may be a case for using a fuzzy membership model, for example, following Kent and Mardia (1988) [13] for "functionality", with tissues having a proportion of functionality which would allow modelling of abnormal or partially functioning tissue.

Acknowledgements

The authors are grateful to Bill Crum, Ian Driver and John Ridgway (CoMIR, The University of Leeds) for providing CT and SPECT phantom images and an MR registered pair of brain scans. We would also like to thank Ian Dryden, David Hogg, John Kent, John Little and Alistair Walder for their helpful comments. This work has been carried out under an initial grant from The University of Leeds to the Centre of Medical Imaging Research (CoMIR) and the research studentship from EPSRC to Jayne Kirkbride. One of the authors (Prof. K.V.Mardia) benefited from the participation in the Isaac Newton Institute programme.

References

[1] Abidi, M.A. and Gonzalez, R.C. (1992). *Data Fusion in Robotics and Machine Intelligence*, Academic Press Inc., Boston.

[2] Besag, J.E. (1975). Statistical analysis of non-lattice data, *The Statistician*, **24**, 179–195.

[3] Besag, J.E. (1986). On the statistical analysis of dirty pictures (with discussion), *Journal of the Royal Statistical Society*, **B48**, 259–302.

[4] Bookstein, F.L. (1989). Principal warps: Thin plate splines and decomposition of deformations, *IEEE Transactions on Pattern Analysis and Machine Intelligence*, **PAMI-11**, 567–585.

[5] Brown, L.G. (1992). A survey of image registration, *ACM computing surveys*, **24**, 4, 325–376.

[6] Clark, J.J. and Yuille, A.L. (1990). *Data Fusion for Sensory Information Processing Systems*, Kluwer Academic Publishers, Boston.

[7] Geman, S. and Geman, D. (1984). Stochastic relaxation, Gibbs distributions and the Bayesian restoration of images, *IEEE Transactions on Pattern Analysis and Machine Intelligence*, **PAMI-12**, 609–628.

[8] Geman, D. and Reynolds, G. (1992). Constrained estimation and the recovery of discontinuities, *IEEE Transactions on Pattern Analysis and Machine Intelligence*, **PAMI-14**, 367–383.

[9] Gindi, G., Lee, M., Rangarajan, A. and Zubal, I.G. (1993). Bayesian reconstruction of functional images using anatomical information as priors, *IEEE Transactions on Medical Imaging*, **12**, 670–680.

[10] Green, P.J. (1990). Bayesian reconstruction from emission tomography data using a modified EM algorithm, *IEEE Transactions on Medical Imaging*, **9**, pp.84–93.

[11] Hainsworth, T.J. and Mardia, K.V. (1993). A Markov Random Field restoration of image sequences. In: R.Chellappa and A.Jain, eds, *Markov Random Fields: Theory and Applications*: 409–446. Academic Press Inc., Boston.

[12] Hillman, G.R., Chang, Chih-Wei., Ying, H., Kent, T.A. and Yen,. J. (1995). Automatic system for brain MRI analysis using a novel combination of fuzzy rule-based and automatic clustering techniques, *Proceedings of the international society for optical engineering, SPIE*, **Vol 2434**, 16-25.

[13] Kent, J.T. and Mardia, K.V. (1988). Spatial Classification using fuzzy membership models, *IEEE Pattern Analysis and Machine Intelligence*, **PAMI-10**, 659–671.

[14] Kohn, M.I., Tanna N.K., Herman G.T., Resnick S.M., Mozley P.D., Gur R.E., Alavi A., Zimmerman R.A. and Gur R.C. (1991). Analysis of Brain and cerebro-spinal fluid volumes with MR imaging, *Radiology*, **178**, 115–122.

[15] Mardia, K.V. and Hainsworth, T.J.(1993). Images warping in Bayesian reconstruction with grey-level templates. In: Mardia, K.V. and Kanji, G.K., eds, *Statistics and Images*: Vol I, 257-280. Carfax, Oxford.

[16] Mardia, K.V. and Kanji, G.K., eds,(1993). *Statistics and Images*:Vol. I, 336pp, Carfax Publishing Co., Abingdon.

[17] Mardia, K.V.(1994). *Statistics and Images*:Vol. II, Carfax Publishing Co., Abingdon.

[18] Marr, D. and Poggio, T. (1976). Cooperative computation of stereo disparity, *Science*, **194**, 283–287.

[19] Mayo Biomedical Imaging Resource (1986- 1993). *ANALYZE* Reference Manual, 199-209.

[20] Robb, R.A.(1990). A software system for interactive quantitative analysis of biomedical images. In: K.H.Hohne, H.Fuchs and S.M.Pizer, eds, *3D Imaging in Medicine*:Vol F60, 333-361. NATO ASI Series.

[21] Mowforth, P.H. and Zhengping, J. (1990). Model based tissue differentiation in MR brain images, *Revista d Neuroradiologica*, **3**, 95-103.

[22] Viergever, M.A., Maintz, J.B.A., Stokking, R., van den Elsen, P.A. and Zuiderveld, K.J. (1995). Matching and integrated display of brain images from multiple modalities, *Proceedings of the international society for optical engineering, SPIE*, **Vol 2434**, 2-13.

[23] Wright, W.A. (1989). A Markov Random Field approach to Data Fusion and colour segmentation, *Image and Vision Computing*, **7**, 144–150.

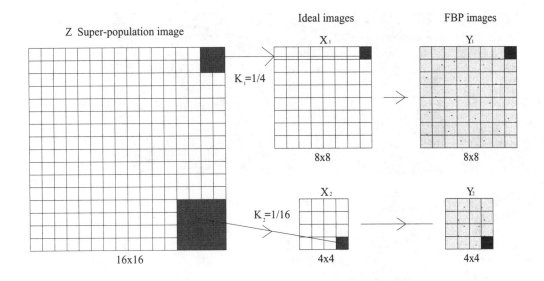

Figure 1. A diagram showing the hierarchical format of the model and the role of K_i

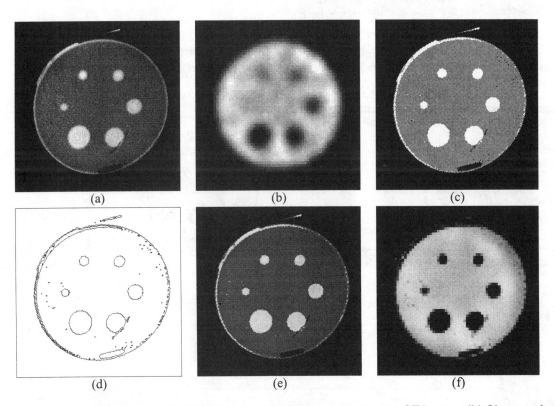

Figure 2. Phantom CT and SPECT images: (a) Observed 256×256 CT image; (b) Observed 64×64 SPECT image; (c) Estimated classes; (d) Estimated class boundaries; (e) Reconstruction for first modality (CT); (f) Reconstruction for second modality (SPECT).

61

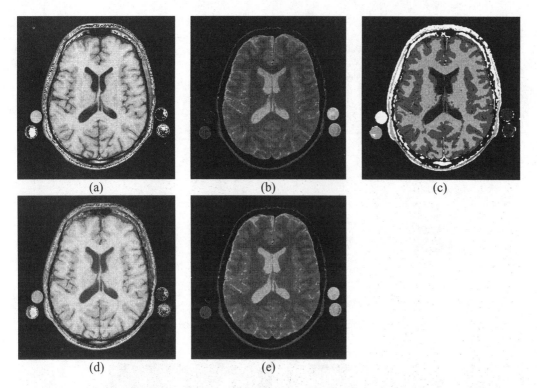

Figure 3. Observed MR images: **(a)** Observed 256×256 **MR image; (b)** Observed 256×256 **MR image; (c)** Final classification; **(d)** Reconstruction for first modality; **(e)** Reconstruction for second modality;

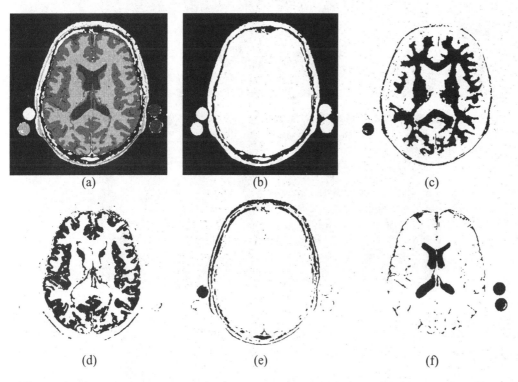

Figure 4. Classification showing breakdown of individual classes: **(a)** Classes Z $(512 \times 512$ **pixels); (b)** "Air"; **(c)** "Skull"; **(d)** "CSF"; **(e)** "Grey Matter"; **(f)** "White Matter".

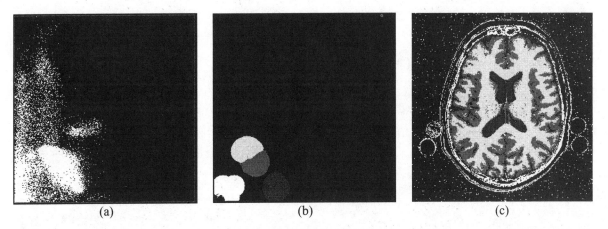

Figure 5. Classification of the MR images in Figure 3 (a) and (b) using *ANALYZE(TM)*:. **(a) Vector Histogram (Modality 1 on y axis Modality 2 on x axis); (b) Vector Histogram showing classification in feature-space; (c) Final Classification, Z** (256×256 **pixels).**

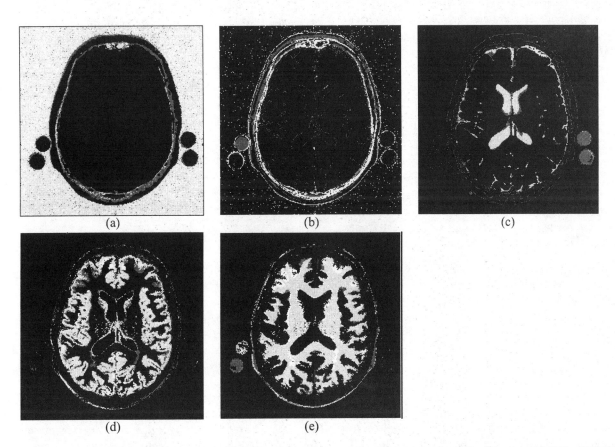

Figure 6. Comparison of classes found by the two methods: **(a) "Air"; (b) "Skull"; (c) "CSF"; (d) "Grey Matter"; (e) "White Matter". Mid-grey represent pixels assigned to the same class by both methods, dark grey pixels were assigned to the class only by the Coupled model, and lighter pixels only by Analyze(TM).**

Optimal Linear Transformation for MRI Feature Extraction

Hamid Soltanian-Zadeh[1,2], Joe P. Windham[1], Donald J. Peck[1]

[1]Medical Image Analysis Laboratory of Henry Ford Hospital, Detroit, MI 48202, USA
[2]Elec. & Comp. Eng. Department of the University of Tehran, Tehran 14399, Iran

Abstract

This paper presents development and application of a feature extraction method for magnetic resonance imaging (MRI), without explicit calculation of tissue parameters. A three-dimensional (3-D) feature space representation of the data is generated in which normal tissues are clustered around pre-specified target positions and abnormalities are clustered elsewhere. This is accomplished by a linear minimum mean square error transformation of categorical data to target positions. From the 3-D histogram (cluster plot) of the transformed data, clusters are identified and regions of interest (ROIs) for normal and abnormal tissues are defined. These ROIs are used to estimate signature (feature) vectors for each tissue type which in turn are used to segment the MRI scene. The proposed feature space is compared to those generated by tissue-parameter-weighted images, principal component images, and angle images, demonstrating its superiority for feature extraction. The method and its performance are illustrated using MRI images of an egg phantom and a human brain.

Key words: *Image Segmentation; Image Analysis; Feature Extraction; Pattern Recognition; Linear Transformation; Magnetic Resonance Imaging; and Image Processing.*

1 Introduction

The ultimate goal of medical image analysis is to extract important clinical information that would improve diagnosis and treatment of disease. In the past few years, magnetic resonance imaging (MRI) has drawn considerable attention for its possible role in tissue characterization. The image gray levels in MRI depend on several tissue parameters including: proton density (N(H)); spin-lattice (T1) and spin-spin (T2) relaxation times; flow velocity (ν); and chemical shift (δ).

A sequence of MRI images of the same anatomical site (an MRI scene sequence) contains information pertaining to the tissue parameters. This implicit information may be used for image analysis.

Image analysis can be accomplished using an appropriate feature space method. Feature space methods can be useful for all three steps of image analysis: (1) identification of objects (feature extraction); (2) segmentation of objects; and (3) quantitative measurements on objects, to obtain information that can be used in decision making (diagnosis, treatment planning, and evaluation of treatment). Basics of image processing and the interrelationship of the above three steps in image analysis are discussed in [1]-[4]. This paper focuses on MRI feature extraction through an optimal feature space method.

Methods of preparing data for an MRI feature space representation can be classified into three categories: (1) generation of tissue-parameter-weighted images [5]-[6]; (2) explicit calculation of tissue parameters [7]-[8]; and (3) linear transformations (e.g., principal component analysis [9]) and non-linear transformations (e.g., angle images [10]). Both categories (1) and (2) require acquisition of several images using specific MRI protocols. A difficulty with category (1) is its limitation to using at most three MRI images, where more than three images may be needed to extract different biological properties of tissues. A difficulty with category (2) is that it requires protocols which are usually different from those routinely used in clinical studies. In addition, noise propagation, through the required nonlinear calculations, combines with the model inaccuracies and yields unsatisfactory results [11]-[13]. The decision boundaries based on the calculated tissue parameters are also different from the correct statistical boundaries [14]. Category (3) can be applied to any MRI scene sequence. It can improve the clustering properties of the data for the feature space representation while reducing its dimensionality. However, as will be explained later, previous transformations are not optimally designed for MRI. For instance, a difficulty with the feature space generated by principal component images is its limitation to the size of the objects in the scene. Small objects make slight contributions to the covariance matrix and thus are not enhanced and visualized in the first few principal component images. The first few principal component images are normally used for the feature space representation, since they have the best signal-to-noise ratios (SNRs). A concern with angle images is the nonlinearity of the transformation which generates curves, rather than lines, for partial volume regions, in the cluster plot; this complicates the distinction between clusters for partial volume regions and those for heterogeneous tissues. We have therefore devoted our effort towards the derivation of an *optimal linear* transformation to prepare MRI data for feature space analysis.

The next step after data preparation is feature identification. A sensible method for feature identification is looking at the multi-dimensional histogram (cluster plot) of the data. We restrict our attention to feature spaces with dimensions less than four, so that they can be easily visualized and used by radiologists for diagnosis. We therefore want to reduce the dimensionality of the data to three while improving its clustering properties. Further, for easy distinction between normal and abnormal tissues, we would like to cluster each of the normal tissues around a pre-specified location; this should result in clustering abnormal tissues around different locations. The optimal transformation should therefore project the data into a three-dimensional subspace, subject to the constraints of: clustering normal tissues around pre-specified locations; and minimizing the intraset Euclidean distance for each of the normal tissues to improve distinguishability among them. We arrange the output of the optimal transformation as three composite images, each illustrating a projection of the features in the scene into the direction of a normal tissue.

At this point, each pixel is represented by a three-dimensional vector. We generate a two-dimensional view of the cluster plot for these three-dimensional pixel vectors. From the cluster plot, we are able to define several cluster centers corresponding to different features (tissue types), and segment the scene into these features using a Euclidean distance classifier. Feature localization and measurement can then be easily performed using the segmented scenes for several slices through the desired volume.

Application of the technique to feature extraction of a human brain with a tumor makes it possible to extract several different tissues, including white matter, gray matter, cerebrospinal fluid (CSF), muscle, cartilage, the orbit of the eye, tumor, and cyst, as well as partial volumes between normal and abnormal tissues. We make a comparison of the proposed method to other techniques including tissue-parameter-weighted images, principal component analysis, and angle images. The foundations and new developments for the proposed feature space method are explained in Section 2. Applications to an egg phantom and a clinical brain study as well as a comparison to the above techniques are presented in Section 3. Conclusions are given in Section 4.

2 Methods and Materials

2.1 Spatial and Feature Space Representations

An MRI scene sequence shows spatial locations of different tissues, with a different contrast in each image. It can therefore be considered as a *spatial domain* representation of tissues. In a spatial domain representation, pixels corresponding to a specific tissue are locally connected but may be distributed over different sections of the image. A *feature space (domain)* representation of tissues can be generated from an MRI scene sequence. In a feature space representation, pixels corresponding to a specific tissue are connected as clusters, even though their spatial locations in the image domain may be far apart. For an MRI scene sequence consisting of n images, a feature space representation is generated by defining an n-dimensional pixel vector for each pixel in the image (spatial) domain, using pixel gray levels of the same location from different images in the sequence as elements of this vector.

A major ingredient of a feature space technique is visualization of the generated feature space, i.e., visualization of the multi-dimensional histogram of the data, which we call a cluster plot. This constrains the dimensionality of the feature space. As the dimensionality of the feature space increases, its visualization becomes more difficult. One- and two-dimensional (1-D or 2-D) feature spaces can easily be visualized using a conventional histogram, and an image whose pixel intensity is proportional to the number of data points in a certain range, i.e., a 2-D cluster plot. With a little bit more effort, we may generate a 3-D cluster plot, by drawing three axes of an orthogonal coordinate system in an image, for 3-D perception, and making image pixel gray levels proportional to the number of data points in certain ranges (see Figure 2.a). Further, we may generate a 4-D feature space, by creating 3-D feature spaces and showing them in a loop, i.e., using time as the fourth axis. This visualization will however be limited in that the operator can not easily draw regions of interest (ROIs) on it and find the corresponding pixels in the image domain. More difficulties will be involved with visualizing feature spaces of dimensions higher than four. Therefore, we restrict our attention to feature spaces with dimensions not larger than three.

2.2 Optimal Transformation

We derive a linear transformation that maps all the pixel vectors from each tissue in the original feature space to tightly clustered regions in the transformed subspace (e.g., a three-dimensional subspace). We restrict our attention to linear transformations, since they preserve geometric properties between clusters, i.e., partial volume pixels cluster along a *straight* line connecting centers of the clusters for the corresponding pure pixels. This is useful for distinguishing partial volume clusters from other clusters in the final feature space representation.

In the derivation of the transformation, we use the following notation: (1) calligraphic letters, such as $\mathcal{V}$, to refer to a vector space; (2) uppercase italic letters, such as V, to refer to a matrix each of whose columns is a point in $\mathcal{V}$; and (3) lower case boldface letters, such as $\mathbf{v}$, to refer to the vector coordinates of a point in $\mathcal{V}$.

Let $\mathcal{V}$ and $\mathcal{W}$ be n-dimensional and p-dimensional real vector spaces, respectively. Then points in $\mathcal{V}$ and $\mathcal{W}$ are vectors in $\mathcal{R}^n$ and $\mathcal{R}^p$, respectively. Further assume that a collection of data can be classified or categorized in terms of M pre-defined groups, with data points in a group more *similar* to other data points in that group than to the data points in other groups. Let each data category have a target position in $\mathcal{W}$ about which transformed data are expected to be well clustered. Denote the number of data points (samples) in each category as $NS(j)$, $j = 1, \cdots, M$. A linear transformation T is desired which maps points in $\mathcal{V}$ to points in $\mathcal{W}$ as follows.

$$\mathbf{c} = T\mathbf{v} \qquad (1)$$

The transformation matrix T is to be found such that the ratio of interset distance (IED) to intraset distance (IAD) is maximized (The ratio of IED to IAD is a standard criterion for quantifying clustering properties of data [15].). This problem can be formulated as the following constrained optimization problem.

$$\text{Maximize:} \quad \frac{IED}{IAD} \qquad (2)$$
$$\text{subject to:} \quad \mathbf{c}_j = T\bar{\mathbf{v}}_j, \quad 1 \leq j \leq M \qquad (3)$$

where $\mathbf{c}_j$ is the target position for the average vector

of the jth group ($\bar{\mathbf{v}}_j$) defined by

$$\bar{\mathbf{v}}_j = \frac{1}{NS(j)} \sum_{l=1}^{NS(j)} \mathbf{v}_j^l \qquad (4)$$

with $\mathbf{v}_j^l$ being the lth data point in the jth group.

The IED reflects the average distance between different data groups. It is defined as the average of distances between each pairs of the average vectors from different groups in the transformed domain:

$$IED^2 = \frac{2}{M(M-1)} \sum_{j=1}^{M} \sum_{i=j+1}^{M} \| T\bar{\mathbf{v}}_j - T\bar{\mathbf{v}}_i \|^2 \qquad (5)$$

where $\bar{\mathbf{v}}_j$ and $\bar{\mathbf{v}}_i$ are the average vectors for the jth and ith groups, respectively, and $\| \cdot \|$ represents the Euclidean norm. This definition makes the interset distance independent of the number of points in each data group. This is an important property in that it avoids dependency of the transformation to the object size, in contrast to principal component analysis. The IAD reflects the average variance of the data points in each group. It is defined as the average of distances between each vector in a group and the average vector from the same group, again in the transformed domain:

$$IAD^2 = \frac{1}{M \sum_{j=1}^{M} NS(j)} \sum_{j=1}^{M} \sum_{i=1}^{NS(j)} \| T\mathbf{v}_j^i - T\bar{\mathbf{v}}_j \|^2 \qquad (6)$$

where $\mathbf{v}_j^i$ is the ith data point in the jth group.

To attain easy distinction between normal and abnormal tissues, we may project the average vectors of the normal tissues onto pre-specified locations, e.g., on the axes of the new subspace. This is sometimes referred to as projection of categorical data to target positions. Once target positions are specified, IED is fixed. Therefore, maximizing the ratio of IED to IAD will be equivalent to minimizing IAD. Minimizing IAD will be similar to minimizing the mean-square error between specified target positions in $\mathcal{W}$ and projections of the measurement data [16]. The general solution is obtained by taking partial derivatives of IAD^2 with respect to elements of T and numerically solving the resultant system of equations. Here we consider a special case which has an analytical solution.

2.2.1 Special Case

A special case is defined if $M = p$ and we decide to assign the target positions for normal tissues to be on the axes of the new subspace, i.e.,

$c_i = [0, \cdots, 0, c_i, 0, \cdots, 0]^T$ in the ith row (Interestingly, $c_i = 1$ provides an MRI signal decomposition in terms of normal tissues' signals.). This requires for $1 \leq i, j \leq M$

$$t_i \cdot \bar{v}_j = \begin{cases} c_i & \text{if } j = i \\ 0 & \text{otherwise} \end{cases} \qquad (7)$$

where t_i is an $n \times 1$ vector whose elements are identical to that of the ith row of the $M \times n$ transformation matrix T and $\cdot$ represents the usual inner product. For this case, it can be shown that IED^2 simplifies to

$$IED^2 = \frac{2}{M} \sum_{i=1}^{M} c_i^2 \qquad (8)$$

which is a constant. Using the Gaussian white noise model with standard deviation σ for MRI noise simplifies IAD^2 to

$$IAD^2 = \frac{\sigma^2}{M} \sum_{i=1}^{M} \|t_i\|^2 = \frac{\sigma^2}{M} \sum_{i=1}^{M} t_i \cdot t_i. \qquad (9)$$

Considering (7)-(9), the objective function as well as the constraints are separable and the formulated problem by Equations (2) and (3) can be written as the following set of constrained optimization problems (as previously stated, IED and σ are constants).

Minimize: $\qquad t_i \cdot t_i, \quad 1 \leq i \leq M \qquad (10)$

subject to: $\qquad t_i \cdot \bar{v}_j = 0, \quad 1 \leq j \leq M, \ j \neq i, \ \text{and}$

$$t_i \cdot \bar{v}_i = c_i. \qquad (11)$$

Further, Equations (10) and (11) can be re-formulated as (since $t_i \cdot \bar{v}_i = c_i$ is a constant)

Maximize: $\qquad \dfrac{t_i \cdot \bar{v}_i}{\sigma [t_i \cdot t_i]^{\frac{1}{2}}}, \quad 1 \leq i \leq M \qquad (12)$

subject to: $\qquad t_i \cdot \bar{v}_j = 0, \quad 1 \leq j \leq M, \ j \neq i, \ \text{and}$

$$t_i \cdot \bar{v}_i = c_i. \qquad (13)$$

We have derived analytical solutions to a class of optimization problems which are similar to that given in Equations (12) and (13) (see Appendix of [17]). With a slight modification of that analytical solution, we find the optimal transformation matrix and the resulting transformed images. We then generate a 3-D cluster plot for the transformed images, which we use to extract features from the scene and to segment the scene into the corresponding features.

2.3 Feature Extraction Method

The steps of the proposed approach for MRI feature extraction are summarized below.

1. **Noise Suppression:** We use a multi-dimensional non-linear edge-preserving restoration filter to suppress the MRI noise [18]-[19]. The filter uses both inter-frame and intra-frame information, along with the Euclidean distance discriminator, to suppress the noise while preserving edge and partial volume information.

2. **Data Preparation:** Using an MRI scene sequence with n images ($n \geq 3$), we define an n-dimensional vector for each pixel, by using the corresponding image gray levels as elements of this vector. We refer to such a vector as a pixel vector. Similarly, we define n-dimensional signature vectors for three of the normal tissues, by using the mean values of the image gray levels in *sample* regions of interest (ROIs) corresponding to these tissues. A sample ROI does not need to cover every pixel from the corresponding tissue in the image. It should cover a pure region from the tissue type (the bigger the ROI the better).

3. **Transformation:** We find the optimal transformation matrix T and apply it to the MRI scene sequence to generate three composite images. For brain studies, we generate composite images for white matter, gray matter, and CSF. Using these composite images, each pixel is now represented by a three-dimensional pixel vector.

4. **Cluster Plots:** We generate a two-dimensional view of the cluster plot for the three-dimensional pixel vectors generated in step 3. An image gray level in this cluster plot represents the number of pixel vectors whose components fell in a certain range; this range depends on the location of the pixel in the cluster map. For brain studies, white matter, gray matter, and CSF are clustered around $(1,0,0)$, $(0,1,0)$, and $(0,0,1)$, respectively. Other normal tissues as well as all abnormal tissues are clustered around different locations. This facilitates feature extraction and identification.

5. **Scene Segmentation:** From the cluster plot, we define several cluster centers (ROIs) corresponding to different features (tissue types). These ROIs actually define a volume of interest from the 3-D cluster plot. We call them ROIs since they are drawn on a 2-D view of the 3-D cluster plot. New signature vectors are defined by averaging image gray levels, from the original or transformed data set, which correspond to the ROIs drawn on the cluster plot. Using these signature vectors and the Euclidean distance classifier, the scene is segmented. Feature localization and measurement

may be performed using the segmented scenes for several slices through the desired volume.

2.4 Comparisons

We compare the proposed feature space method to other methods of MRI feature space representation including tissue-parameter-weighted images, principal component images, and angle images. We do not consider explicit calculations of tissue parameters, since as stated previously: (1) this requires data using several specific pulse sequences; (2) the results are prone to noise propagation through the nonlinear calculations involved; and (3) the boundaries in the resulting feature space do not match with correct statistical decision boundaries. The three conventional techniques are described below.

2.4.1 Tissue Parameter Weighted Images

Using a multiple spin-echo pulse sequence with a short echo time (e.g., TE=25 msec) and a long repetition time (e.g., TR=2500 msec), a sequence of four images can be acquired. The contrast in the first image is mainly due to the proton density difference between tissues, thus called proton density weighted. The contrast in the third and fourth images is mainly due to the T2 relaxation difference between tissues, thus called T2-weighted. Likewise, using a single spin-echo pulse sequence with a short echo time (e.g., TE=20 msec) and a short repetition time (e.g., TR=500 msec), a T1-weighted image can be acquired. These three images define a three-dimensional feature space representation of the tissues. Alternatively, a T1-weighted image can be acquired using an inversion recovery pulse sequence, with a short echo time (e.g., TE=12 msec), a moderate inversion time (e.g., TI=519 msec), and a relatively long repetition time (e.g., TR=2000 msec).

2.4.2 Principal Component Images

Principal component analysis (PCA) is a linear transformation which has been applied in a variety of fields including MRI. It has been employed in digital image processing as a technique for image coding, compression, enhancement, and feature extraction. For MRI feature space representation, PCA generates linear combinations of the acquired images which maximize the image variance. The weighting vectors for these linear combinations are the normalized eigenvectors of the sample covariance matrix estimated using all of the acquired images. The number of principal component images equals the number of acquired images, but the variance (equivalently, SNR) of the principal

component images sharply decreases from the first image to the last. The first three principal component images contain most of the information and hence may be used to define a three-dimensional feature space representation of the tissues.

2.4.3 Angle Images

Angle images are defined by calculating a set of parameters for each pixel vector in an orthogonal subspace defined by the constant vector ($\vec{\mathbf{cv}} = [1, 1, \cdots, 1]^T$) and the signature vectors for normal tissues ($\vec{s}_i$, $i = 1, \cdots, M$, where M is the number of normal tissue types) that are encountered in a study, e.g., white matter, gray matter, and CSF for the brain. The orthogonal subspace is defined by inputing $\vec{\mathbf{cv}}$ and $\vec{s}_i$ into the Gram-Schmidt orthogonalization process.

Among all the possibilities for a three-dimensional feature space, it has been found that the feature space generated by: (1) the Euclidean norm of each pixel vector; (2) the angle between each vector and the constant vector; and (3) the angle between each pixel vector and the orthogonal complement of white matter to the constant vector, best separates normal and abnormal tissues in a brain study [10]. We therefore consider this three-dimensional feature space representation of the brain tissues for our comparison.

3 Experimental Results

The steps of the proposed feature space method are illustrated using an egg phantom. Fig. 1 shows acquired (original), restored, and transformed images of the egg phantom. Acquired images are shown in the first row, the restored images (after noise suppression according to Step 1 in Section 2.3) are shown in the second row, and the transformed images (after transformation into a three-dimensional subspace according to Steps 2 and 3 in Section 2.3) are shown in the third row. Fig. 2 shows the cluster plot for the transformed images (generated according to Step 4 in Section 2.3) and the boundaries of the ROIs defined for different features. It also shows the segmented scene (extracted features according to Step 5 in Section 2.3).

Application of the method to an actual brain study is illustrated in Figures 3 through 7. Acquired, restored, and transformed images of a human brain with a tumor are shown in Fig. 3. The optimally transformed images are compared to images generated by other methods (tissue-parameter-weighted, PCA, and angle images) in Fig. 4. The cluster plots generated for images in each row of Fig. 4 are shown in Fig. 5. The boundaries of ROIs for features' clusters are also shown in Fig. 5. The extracted features using these ROIs are shown in Figs. 6 and 7. It is observed that the optimal method correctly extracts all of the features in the scene. Except for this method, none of the techniques could correctly segment both zones of the lesion (tumor and cyst) from each other and from the normal tissues. For example, the PCA method included part of the tumor in the feature called gray matter.

4 Summary and Conclusions

After a brief explanation of spatial and feature space representations, we presented a feature extraction method for MRI. We restricted our attention to a 3-D feature space, since it can be easily visualized and used by radiologists for feature extraction, scene segmentation, and diagnosis. For applications in which visualization is not important, one can consider higher dimensional feature spaces and use unsupervised clustering algorithms for feature extraction and scene segmentation. We utilized a vector space approach for data preparation and mathematical development.

A major part of the proposed method was reducing the dimensionality of data while improving its clustering properties. This can generally be accomplished by maximizing the interset-to-intraset Euclidean distance ratio for normal tissues, using an optimal (linear minimum mean square error) transformation of categorical data to target positions. We considered a special case for which we derived an analytical solution; the general case has no analytical solution. Another nice feature of the special case is that it decomposes the MRI signal in terms of a basis generated by *normal* tissues.

The optimal method was illustrated through its applications to phantom and brain studies. Its performance was compared to that of three other feature space methods, namely tissue-parameter-weighted images, principal component images, and angle images. It outperformed others in correctly extracting all of the features in the scene.

The proposed method seems promising for distinguishing abnormal tissues from normal tissues, and different abnormalities from each other. Therefore, it may serve as a tissue characterization tool in MRI and help radiologists to achieve a more accurate diagnosis.

5 Acknowledgment

This work was supported in part by NIH grant R29-CA61263. The authors would like to thank Lucie Bower and Linda Emery from the Medical Image Analysis Laboratory of Henry Ford Hospital for their help with programming, data collection, and analysis.

6 References

[1] W.K. Pratt, *Digital Image Processing.* New York: John Wiley & Sons, Inc., 1978.

[2] K.R. Castleman, *Digital Image Processing.* Englewood Cliff, New Jersey: Prentice-Hall, Inc., 1979.

[3] R.C. Gonzalez, P. Wintz, *Digital Image Processing.* 2nd Ed., Reading, Massachusetts: Addison-Wesley Publishing Company, Inc., 1987.

[4] A.K. Jain, *Fundamentals of Digital Image Processing.* Englewood Cliffs, New Jersey: Prentice Hall, 1989.

[5] H.K. Brown, T.R. Hazelton, J.V. Fiorica, A.K. Parsons, L.P. Clarke, M.L. Silbiger, "Composite and Classified Color Display in MR Imaging of the Female Pelvis," *Magn. Reson. Imaging*, vol. 10, No. 1, pp. 143-145, 1992.

[6] H.K. Brown, T.R. Hazelton, M.L. Silbiger, "Generation of Color Composite for Enhanced Tissue Differentiation in Magnetic Resonance Imaging of the Brain," *American Journal of Anatomy*, vol. 192, No. 1, pp. 23-24, 1991.

[7] P.H. Higer, B. Gernot, *Tissue Characterization in MR Imaging: Clinical and Technical Approaches.* New York: Springer-Verlag, 1990.

[8] M. Just, M. Thelen, "Tissue Characterization with T1, T2, and Proton Density Values: Results in 160 Patients with Brain Tumors," *Radiology,* vol. 169, pp. 779-785, 1988.

[9] H. Grahn, N.M. Szeverenyi, M.W. Roggenbuck, F. Delaglio, P. Geladi, "Data Analysis of Multivariate Magnetic Resonance Images: I. A Principal Component Analysis Approach," *Chemometrics and Intelligent Laboratory Systems*, vol. 5, pp. 311-22, 1989.

[10] J.P. Windham, H. Soltanian-Zadeh, and D.J. Peck: "Tissue Characterization by a Vector Subspace Method." *Presented at the 33rd Annual Meeting of the American Association of Physicists in Medicine (AAPM)*, San Francisco, CA, July 1991, *Abstract Published in Med. Phys.*, vol. 18, No. 3, pp. 619, 1991.

[11] J.N. Lee, S.J. Riederer, "The Contrast-to-Noise in Relaxation Time, Synthetic, and Weighted-Sum MR Images," *Magn. Reson. Med.*, vol. 5, pp. 13-22, 1987.

[12] U. Schmiedl, D.A. Ortendahl, A.S. Mark, I. Berry, L. Kaufman, "The Utility of Principle Component Analysis for the Image Display of Brain Lesions: A Preliminary, Comparative Study," *Magn. Reson. Med.*, vol. 4, pp. 471-86, 1987.

[13] J.R. MacFall, S.J. Riederer, H.Z. Wang, "An Analysis of Noise Propagation in Computed T2, Pseudodensity, and Synthetic Spin-Echo Images," *Med. Phys.*, vol. 13, No. 3, pp. 285-292, 1986.

[14] E.R. McVeigh, M.J. Bronskill, R.M. Henkelman, "Optimization of MR Protocols: A Statistical Decision Analysis Approach," *Magn. Reson. Med.*, vol. 6, pp. 314-333, 1988.

[15] J.T. Tou, R.C. Gonzalez, *Pattern Recognition Principles.* 2nd Edition, Reading, Massachusetts: Addison-Wesley Publishing Company Inc., 1977.

[16] S.A. Zoharian, A.J. Jarghaghi, "Minimum Mean-Square Error Transformation of Categorical Data to Target Positions," *IEEE Trans. Signal Proc.*, vol. 40, No. 1, pp. 13-23, 1992.

[17] H. Soltanian-Zadeh and J.P. Windham: "Novel and General Approach to Linear Filter Design for CNR Enhancement of MR Images with Multiple Interfering Features in the Scene," *Journal of Electronic Imaging*, vol. 1, No. 2, pp. 171-182, April 1992.

[18] H. Soltanian-Zadeh, J.P. Windham, and A.E. Yagle: "A Multi-Dimensional Non-Linear Edge-Preserving Filter for Magnetic Resonance Image Restoration." *Presented at and Published in the Proceedings of the IEEE Medical Imaging Conference*, San Francisco, CA, Nov. 1993.

[19] H. Soltanian-Zadeh, J.P. Windham, and A.E. Yagle: "Magnetic Resonance Image Restoration Using a New Multi-Dimensional Non-Linear Edge-Preserving Filter." *IEEE Trans. Imag. Proc.*, vol. 4, No. 2, pp. 147-161, Feb. 1995.

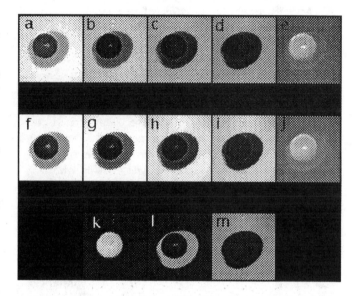

Figure 1. Acquired, restored, and transformed images of a hard-boiled egg, with its shell removed, in gelatin. **a-e**: Four T2-weighted multiple spin echo images (TE/TR = 25-100/2500 msec) and a T1-weighted spin-echo image (TE/TR = 20/500 msec). **f-j**: Restored images generated using the restoration filter described in Section 2.3. **k-m**: Transformed images created by applying the optimal transformation explained in Section 2.2.1, using the egg-yolk, egg-white, and gelatin signature vectors.

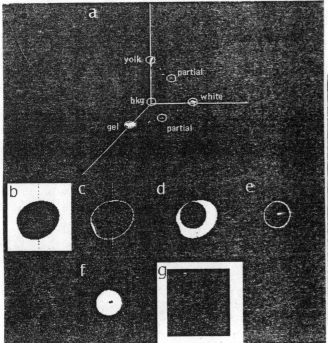

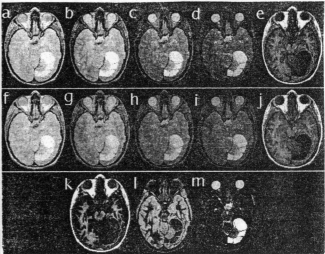

Figure 2. **a**: Three dimensional cluster plot of the pixel intensities of the transformed images in Fig. 1.**k-m**, with clusters identified. Image 1.**k** corresponds to the z-axis, image 1.**l** corresponds to the y-axis, and image 1.**m** corresponds to the x-axis (according to the right hand method). **b-g**: Segmented features (gelatin, egg-white, egg-yolk, partial volumes between adjacent objects, and background) using cluster plot 2.**a**

Figure 3. Acquired, restored, and transformed images of a brain with a tumor. **a-e**: Four T2-weighted multiple spin echo images (TE/TR = 19-76/1500 msec) and a T1-weighted inversion recovery image (TE/TI/TR = 12/519/2000 msec). **f-j**: Restored images generated using the restoration filter described in Section 2.3. **k-m**: Transformed images created by applying the optimal transformation explained in Section 2.2.1, using the white matter, gray matter, and CSF signature vectors.

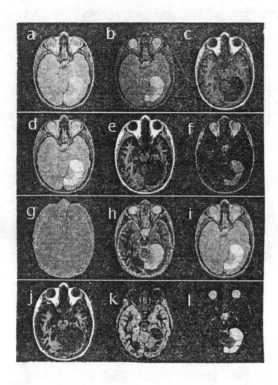

Figure 4. Comparison of images used for four different feature spaces, using the brain data. **a-c:** Tissue-parameter-weighted images. **d-f:** Principal component images. **g-i:** Angle images. **j-l:** Optimally transformed images.

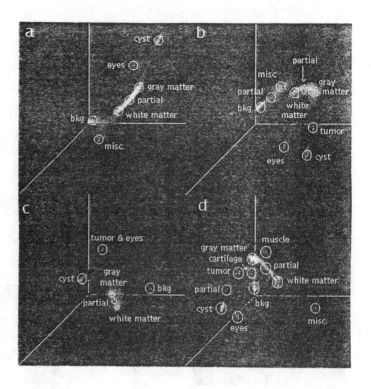

Figure 5. Comparison of cluster plots for feature spaces defined by images in Fig. 4. **a:** Using images 4.a-c. **b:** Using images 4.d-f. **c:** Using images 4.g-i. **d:** Using images 4.j-l. The first image corresponds to the y-axis, the second image corresponds to the z-axis, and the third image corresponds to the x-axis (according to the right hand method). Note the superiority of the clustering properties (number of clusters identified and the interset-to-intraset Euclidean distance ratio between them) using the optimal method.

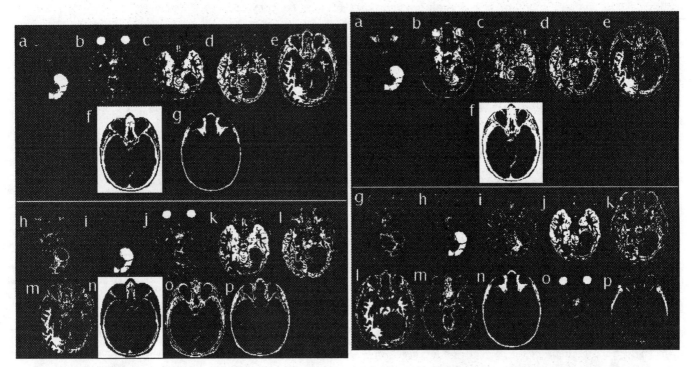

Figure 6. Comparison of the segmented features using cluster plots for tissue-parameter-weighted and PCA images. **a-g**: Segmented features (cyst, eyes, gray matter, partial volume between white and gray matters, white matter, background, and misc.) using cluster plot 5.**a**. **h-p**: Segmented features (tumor, cyst, eyes, gray matter, partial volume between white and gray matter, white matter, background, partial volume between background and misc., and misc.) using cluster plot 5.**b**.

Figure 7. Comparison of the segmented features using cluster plots for angle and optimally transformed images. **a-f**: Segmented features (cyst, tumor & eyes, gray matter, partial volume between white and gray matters, white matter, and background) using cluster plot 5.**c**. **g-p**: Segmented features (partial volume between tumor and cyst, cyst, tumor, gray matter, partial volume between white and gray matters, white matter, cartilage, misc., eyes, and muscles; background is not shown due to the space limitation.) using cluster plot 5.**d**.

Fractal Analysis of Bone Images

Vivek Swarnakar, Raj S. Acharya
Biomedical Imaging Group
Electrical & Computer Engineering Department
SUNY Buffalo, Buffalo, NY, 14260

Adrian Le Blanc, Harlan Evans, Chen Lin   E. Hausman
Baylor College of Medicine   Department of Oral Biology, SUNY Buffalo

Linda Schakelford
Nasa Johnson Space Center

Abstract

Osteoporosis, an age related bone disorder, is a major health concern in the United States and worldwide. Most of the current techniques to monitor bone condition use bone mass measurements. However, bone mass measurements do not completely describe the mechanisms to distinguish between osteoporotic and normal subjects. Structural parameters such as trabecular connectivity have been proposed as features for assessing bone conditions. As such, structure can be seen as an important feature in assessing bone condition. In this article, the trabecular structure is characterized with the aid of the fractal dimension. Existent fractal dimension estimation approaches assume the image to be a Fractional Brownian Motion process. Also, these methods fail when applied to small image samples. A new approach, Continuous Alternating Sequential Filter pyramid (CASF) based fractal dimension estimation is presented. This approach assumes only the self similarity property of fractals, and is applicable to small image sizes, as such it is less constrained. Experimental results demonstrate the efficacy of the fractal dimension model in discriminating normal from osteoporosis cases. The methodology was employed on animal models of osteoporosis and on human data.

Keywords: Fractal Analysis, Morphology, Osteoporosis, Measurement of Anatomical Structures.

1. Introduction

Osteoporosis is a major health concern in the United States and worldwide [1][2][3][4]. It is responsible for at least 1.3 million fractures each year in the United States [3][5][6][7]. About 20 % of women over the age of 60 show symptoms of osteoporosis. Considered as an age related bone disorder, osteoporosis is characterized by decreasing bone mass and strength resulting in an increased susceptibility to fracture [6][8]. Two types of osteoporosis can be broadly distinguished [6]. Postmenopausal osteoporosis found in older women, is related to rapid changes in hormonal balance in the bone metabolism which occur during menopause [9]. Senile Osteoporosis can be seen in men and women 75 years and older. Senile osteoporosis can exhibit both trabecular and cortical bone loss.

Much of the current techniques to monitor bone condition use bone mass measurements. However bone mass measurements do not completely describe the mechanisms to distinguish osteoporotic and normal subjects [10]. It has been shown that the overlap between normals and osteoporosis is found for all of the bone mass measurement technologies: single and dual photon absorptiometry, quantitative computed tomography and direct measurement of bone area/volume on biopsy as well as radiogrammetry. A similar discordance is noted in the fact that it has not been regularly possible to find the expected correlation between severity of osteoporosis and degree of bone loss.

Structural parameters such as trabecular connectivity have been proposed as features for assessing bone conditions [10]. It has been shown that in vertebral crush fracture patients, elements such as vertical trabeculae are retained more or less intact, while elements such as horizontal bracing trabeculae are resorbed entirely [12][13]. This results in disconnection of large number of trabecular elements. However, in

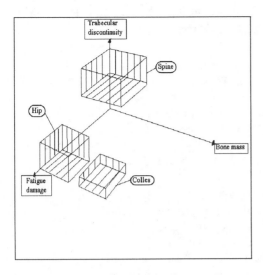

Figure 1. Three-dimensional fracture space, with suggested locations for Colles' fracture, vertebral compression fracture, and hip feature.

non-fracture patients, connections between elements were preserved. Long vertical trabeculae are subject to buckling under loading. When they lose their lateral connections to adjacent trabeculae, the degree of buckling may exceed the inherent strength of the bone. Robert Heaney has proposed a three dimensional osteoporotic fracture space [10]. The three axes (features) of the fracture space correspond to bone mass, trabecular discontinuity and fatigue damage (Figure 1). A classification scheme which uses the integrated features provides a better classification than a scheme which uses individual features.

Structure can be seen as an important feature in assessing bone condition. In this article, we review the use of fractals to model the trabecular bone structure. The research to relate local trabecular structural information to osteoporosis is an important initial step in understanding the effect of osteoporosis and countermeasures on bone condition and strength.

1.1. Random Fractals and dimension

Most natural textures we encounter, such as clouds, mountains and trabecular bone can be modeled as random fractals. Random fractals exhibit statistical *self similarity* which means that their statistical properties are invariant with respect to scaling. A self similar object retains it's statistical properties at all additive and multiplicative scale changes. When one or more scale factors are involved, *self affinity* property is obtained. The ideal function one seeks to model random fractals with should exhibit structured randomness. The continuous Brownian motion diffusion or Weiner process $B(t)$ are examples of random fractals.

An important aspect of a fractal object is it's *fractal dimension*. In order to understand the concept of a fractal dimension, let us consider the approximate length of a smooth curve. The length $L(r)$ is obtained by the product $N \cdot r$, where N is the number of straight line segments of length r needed to span the curve from one end to the other. As the length size r goes to zero, $L(r)$ approaches a finite limit, the length L of the curve.

However, the above does not hold true for fractals as the product $N \cdot r$ diverges to ∞. This is due to the fact that for fractals as r goes to zero, finer and finer wiggles are obtained. There is a critical exponent $D_H > 1$ such that the product $N \cdot r^{D_H}$ stays finite. For exponents smaller than D_H, the product diverges to infinity, while for larger exponents the product will tend to zero. This critical exponent is called the fractional dimension or the *Hausdorff Dimension*. For fractals D_H can be non-integer.

Mandelbrot [26] defined fractals as functions whose dimensions are strictly greater than their topological dimensions. A fractal object can be characterized by it's dimension which may be interpreted as the quantity of space occupied by the object between the m and $m + 1$ dimensional manifolds. Various alternative definitions of dimension have been proposed in the literature. For a detailed discussion of these different definitions the reader is referred to [27][28][29][25].

1.2. Fractals and image analysis

There are number of ways in which fractal geometry can be applied to the analysis of image texture. Pentland et al [19] used a method related to the co-occurrence matrix technique of texture classification based on fractal dimension. They found the standard deviations of the difference of gray levels separated by a given vector and plotted it against the vector lengths as a log-log graph. Maragos has used Morphological Covers to estimate Fractal dimension of Synthetic Images [34]. In another technique [14] a two dimensional gray level image is represented as a three-dimensional surface whose height at each point represents the gray level at that point and the surface area is measured at different scales. It has also been shown that [15] an n-dimensional fractal object can be characterized by the fractional Brownian motion of n variables and that the relationship between the power spectral density and r are independent of the projection [23]. This makes the fractal dimension computed from the projections of an n-dimensional fractal object represent the original object.

Fractal analysis can distinguish between dental radiographs of pre and post menopausal women [31]. Analyses of dental radiographs have shown to be independent of imaging conditions involved in taking the radiographs (such as the angle between x-ray collimator and anatomical structure of interest) to a significant extent [18]. These preliminary studies also suggest that the fractal measure is to a major extent, independent of the anatomical site being analyzed. Another study used fractal dimensions to attempt predicting osseous changes in ankle fractures [22]. The impact of the choice of the structuring element on fractal analysis of radiographs was studied by Lynch [24].

A variety of methods have been proposed to estimate the fractal dimension of trabecular bone structures [20][30][31][32][33]. In the present work a new method is proposed to estimate fractal dimension accurately and robustly. The method is based on using continuous pyramids of Alternating Sequential Filters. Unlike some of the other methods [20][30][31] we do not assume the image to be represented as a Fractional Brownian Motion process. Only the fundamental property of self-similarity is assumed. Another motivation for the development of this new method was the inability of the existing methods to process small image samples. In many bone image analysis cases, the image sizes were in the order of 16 pixels square. Most of the existent methods fail to provide accurate estimates of fractal dimension on such small images.

1.3. Outline

This article is organized as follows: In section 2, we will briefly present the Continuous Alternating Sequential Filter (CASF) theory. Some relevant concepts of measure theory are presented in section 3. Sections 2 and 3 expose the relevant mathematical theory, which are linked together in order to develop the CASF based fractal dimension estimation method described in section 4. Section 5 contains preliminary experimental results obtained from analyzing simulated and real world data. We show the efficacy of the CASF approach on simulated data, when compared to some other most commonly employed methods. This performance justifies the methods applicability towards analysis of real world image data. We have applied the methodology on animal models of osteoporosis and on human data. Finally some conclusions and discussions with respect to future work are presented.

2. Continuous Alternating Sequential Filter Pyramids

This section is divided into two sub-sections. The first one contains a brief overview of the ASF filters and their relevant properties. The second contains the description of continuous mappings and the method employed to obtain continuous ASF pyramids.

2.1. Alternating Sequential Filters

A brief review of Alternating Sequential Filters and some of their properties follows. For further details on the morphological concepts presented here the reader is referred to [33].

Two basic operations in morphology are dilation and erosion. The definition for these operations are as follows. Let $\mathfrak{L}$ be a complete lattice and let X and $\mathbf{B}$ be subsets of $\mathfrak{L}$.

Definition 1 *(Dilation)*

The dilation of X by $\mathbf{B}$ is denoted by $X \oplus \mathbf{B}$ and is given by

$$X \oplus \mathbf{B} = \{z \in \mathfrak{L} \mid z = x + b, \text{ for some } x \in X \text{ and } b \in \mathbf{B}\}.$$

Definition 2 *(Erosion)*

The erosion of X by $\mathbf{B}$ is denoted by $X \ominus \mathbf{B}$ and is given by

$$X \ominus B = \{z \in \mathfrak{L} \mid z + b \in X \text{ for every } b \in B\}.$$

Consider the set X to be a 2-dimensional surface. For instance X can be the surface generated by gray level intensities of biomedical images. Then, in essence, erosion covers the set X from below and dilation covers the set X from above. Based on these operations, two compound operations, opening and closing, can be defined.

Definition 3 *(Opening)*

The opening of X by $\mathbf{B}$ is denoted by $X \circ \mathbf{B}$ and is given by

$$\gamma_\lambda = X \circ \mathbf{B} = (X \ominus \mathbf{B}) \oplus \mathbf{B}.$$

Definition 4 *(Closing)*

The closing of X by $\mathbf{B}$ is denoted by $X \bullet \mathbf{B}$ and is given by

$$\phi_\lambda = X \bullet \mathbf{B} = (X \oplus \mathbf{B}) \ominus \mathbf{B}.$$

The opening operation smooths X by suppressing "sharp caps". While the closing operation smooths by filling "valleys" of X.

Alternating Sequential Filters (ASF) appeared initially in the work of Sternberg [35]. These were employed to restore noise corrupted images. A corrupted image X is filtered by a closing operation ϕ_1 and then an opening operation γ_1, then it is filtered again by a larger closing ϕ_2 and a larger opening γ_2, etc..., which in essence produces the operator

$$M_i(X) = \phi_i \gamma_i \ldots \phi_1 \gamma_1(X) \qquad (1)$$

Note that λ in the closing operation ϕ_λ and the opening operation γ_λ is indexed over a size distribution with $1 < \lambda < i$ and represents the size of the structuring element **B**.

A more rigorous definition of ASF can be given as follows. Define two mappings, from $\mathbb{R}^+ \times \mathfrak{L}$ into $\mathfrak{L}$, a pair of primitives, $(\lambda, X) \to \gamma_\lambda(X)$ and $(\lambda, X) \to \phi_\lambda(X)$ where for all $\lambda > 0$, γ_λ is an opening and ϕ_λ is a closing such that

$$\lambda \geq \mu \Rightarrow \gamma_\lambda < \gamma_\mu \text{ and } \phi_\lambda > \phi_\mu \qquad (2)$$

Now let m_λ be an operator defined as:

$$m_\lambda = \gamma_\lambda \phi_\lambda. \qquad (3)$$

Then for pairs $\lambda, \lambda' \in \mathbb{R}^+$ with $\lambda < \lambda'$ a morphological filter called an Alternating Sequential Filter M, of primitives γ and ϕ and bounds λ and λ' is defined to be:

$$M = M_\lambda^{\lambda'} = \wedge M_k(\lambda, \lambda') \qquad (4)$$

where M is the infimum ($\wedge$)over all M_k given by:

$$M_k = M_k(\lambda, \lambda') = m_\lambda \ldots m_{\lambda + i2^{-k}(\lambda' - \lambda)} \ldots \qquad (5)$$

$$\ldots m_{\lambda + 2^{-k}(\lambda' - \lambda)} m_{\lambda'} , \ 0 \leq i \leq 2^k$$

The mapping M is increasing or $M_{\lambda'} \subset M_\lambda$ for $\lambda' > \lambda$. It is also idempotent or $M(M(X)) = M(X)$. Besides these, two other properties are of direct relevance to the CASF fractal dimension estimation method and are stated next.

CONTINUITY: In order to obtain the continuity property the lattice $\mathfrak{L}$ must be given a topological status. Let the lattice $\mathfrak{L}$ be the set $\mathcal{F} = \mathcal{F}(E)$ of the closed sets of a locally compact and Hausdorff topological space E. It is assumed that the primitives λ and ϕ are both upper-semicontinuous from $\mathbb{R}^+ \times \mathcal{F} \to \mathcal{F}$. Since the mapping $(\lambda, \lambda') \to \lambda + i2^{-k}(\lambda - \lambda')$ from $\mathbb{R}^+ \times \mathbb{R}^+ \to \mathbb{R}^+$ is continuous, the mapping $(\lambda, \lambda') \to m_{i2^{-k}(\lambda - \lambda')}(X)$ is upper semicontinuous and consequently the product $M_k(\lambda, \mu, X)$, composed

of a finite number of factors of type m, is also upper-semicontinuous. In other words, continuity states that ASF operation continuously approaches a limit as the structuring element λ size is reduced continuously.

ABSORPTION LAW: In (5) the segment $[\lambda, \lambda']$ is divided into two, four, eight, ..., etc. equal parts at every step. It can be shown that when the mappings $\lambda \to \gamma_\lambda(X)$ and $\phi \to \phi_\lambda(X)$ from $\mathbb{R}^+$ into $\mathcal{F}(E)$ are upper-semicontinuous for all $X \in \mathcal{F}(E)$, any division procedure performed on the segment $[\lambda, \lambda']$ leads to the same ASF M_λ with primitives γ_λ and ϕ_λ, provided that the division is a dense sampling of the segment $[\lambda, \lambda']$.

2.2. Continuous ASF Pyramids

Gaussian pyramids and the resulting scale-space theory has been widely employed in multiresolution image analysis schemes. However, as pointed out by Perona and Malik Gaussian blurring" does not respect the natural boundaries of objects". Objects that are better left unmerged are merged. Furthermore edge junctions (corners) are destroyed. In order to overcome these difficulties the present paper resorts to the use of morphological pyramids. Use of erosions and dilations and openings to construct morphological pyramids has been reported earlier [41][42]. It has also been shown that analogous to the Gaussian pyramids, morphological pyramids preserve *causality in the resolution domain* [37], in the sense that moving towards larger scales does not result in new details being introduced. Transformations that apply products of openings and closing in general introduce less distortions than individual operation such as dilations and erosions. These operations, openings or closing, tend to better preserve the 'rough' nature of the image X. As such Alternating Sequential Filter are employed here to generate morphological pyramids [38].

As discussed above the lattice $\mathfrak{L}$ is assumed to be a locally compact Hausdorff topological space. Let $X \in \mathfrak{L}$ and **B** be a structuring element of size λ. Through the remainder of this manuscript, $\overline{W}$ represents the ASF filtered version of W, for any arbitrary $W \in \mathfrak{L}$. Let $\overline{X}$ be a set such that

$$\overline{X} = M_\lambda(X) \qquad (6)$$

For increasing sizes $\lambda = \lambda_j \in I$, $j = 1, \ldots, n$ the set's $\overline{X}_j$ generate an ASF pyramid. Although $\lambda \in \mathbb{R}^+$, digital implementation of ASF requires the use of $\lambda \in I$. It has been shown [38] that an ASF pyramid can be obtained by re-sampling the set X between scale values $\epsilon_0 < \epsilon_i < \epsilon_k$ instead of varying λ. This implementation is advantageous as it removes the $\lambda \in I$ restriction imposed due to digital implementation. However some considerations need to be made with respect to the re-sampling procedure.

Let X be the sampled version of an arbitrary s-dimensional function G. Where $m < s$ is the topological dimension of G. Multiresolution pyramids assume that the characteristics of G are available at all scale levels. If X is the only available set then, all characteristics of G at higher resolutions have to be estimated from X. In order to reconstruct G we assume that it is a smooth function with known number of continuous derivatives[36]. Let $\mathcal{B}$ be a family of regular, strictly convex functions [39]. Then, using a structuring element $\mathbf{B} \in \mathcal{B}$ and the continuity property of ASF's, the function $\overline{X} = M_\lambda(X)$ satisfies the assumption above. Now let f be a C^n continuous mapping. Then $G' = f(\overline{X})$ is a reconstruction of G within some bounded error range. If the function $G \in \mathfrak{L}$ is a fractal function then globally it is not a manifold, although on a arbitrarily small neighborhood G has the characteristics of an m-dimensional manifold [28]. As such locally G' is an estimate of G. Let f be given by

$$f : \mathfrak{L} \times [0,1] \to \mathfrak{L} \qquad (7)$$

such that

$$\left. \begin{array}{l} f\left(\overline{X},0\right) = G_0 \\ f\left(\overline{X},1\right) = G_1 \end{array} \right\} \ \forall \ \overline{X} \in \mathfrak{L} \qquad (8)$$

where $\overline{X} = M_\lambda(X)$. Then $\overline{G_\epsilon} = M_\lambda(G_\epsilon)$ generate a *continuous* ASF (CASF) pyramid for $G_\epsilon = f\left(\overline{X}, \epsilon\right)$, $\epsilon \in [0,1]$. The pyramid, formed by $\overline{G_\epsilon}$, is a continuous ASF pyramid with the structuring element $\mathbf{B} \in \mathcal{B}$ maintained at a constant size λ. The absorption law property above guarantees that, as long as the sampling of the scale between ϵ_0 and ϵ_k is dense, the ASF operation should be the same as employing varying $\lambda \in \mathbb{R}^+$.

3. Fractal dimension estimation

Although there is not a rigorous and universal definition of a *fractal*, fractals do posses some characteristic properties. Many fractals are known to obey the self-similarity property. Another characteristic of a fractal is the dimension. Again, different definitions of dimension have been proposed in the literature. One of these definitions is the *Hausdorff* dimension. Before the CASF method for fractal dimension estimation is presented, some relevant nomenclature is considered [40].

Let E be a metric space, endowed with distance $d(x,y)$. For $s > 0$ let

$$|\mathcal{A}|_s = \sum (\ \mathrm{diam}\ X)^s$$

$$\rho(\mathcal{A}) = \sup_{X \in \mathcal{A}} (\ \mathrm{diam}\ X).$$

For a given $A \subset E$, $\mathcal{C}(A)$ denotes the set of countable coverings of A, namely the set of the sets $\mathcal{A}$ of subsets of E which are at most countable and such that

$$A \subset \bigcup \mathcal{A}$$

The Hausdorff outer measure $H^s(A)$ is defined as

$$H^s(A) = c_s \lim_{\substack{\mathcal{A} \in \mathcal{C}(A) \\ \rho(\mathcal{A}) \to 0}} \inf |\mathcal{A}|_s \qquad (9)$$

where c_s is a normalization constant and s is the fractal dimension. For non-euclidean metric spaces E, s can be non-integer.

Let G_ϵ be a sampled version of an s-dimensional G set at some scale ϵ where $\epsilon_0 < \epsilon < \epsilon_k$. Here ϵ_0 is the lowest scale and ϵ_k is the highest scale at which the original set G has to be reconstructed. For non integer s, G is a fractal. Fractal dimension estimates on G_ϵ are approximations to estimates on the original set G. The following theorem supports this assertion.

A collection of sets $\mathcal{V}$ is called a *Vitali class* for E if for each $x \in E$ and $\delta > 0$ there exists $U \in \mathcal{V}$ with $x \in U$ and $0 < U \leq \delta$.

Theorem 1 *(Vitali covering theorem)*

- (a) Let E be H^s- measurable subset of $\mathbb{R}^n$ and let $\mathcal{V}$ be a Vitali class of closed sets for E. Then a (finite or countable) disjoint sequence $\{U_i\}$ can be selected from $\mathcal{V}$ such that either $\sum |U_i|^s = \infty$ or $H^s(\bigcup_i E \setminus Ui) = 0$.

- (b) If $H^s(E) < \infty$, then given $\epsilon > 0$, it can be required that

$$H^s(E) \leq \sum_i |U_i|^s + \epsilon. \qquad (10)$$

4. CASF based fractal dimension estimation

As described earlier, the continuous ASF pyramid for some set X is constructed as follows. Initially X is filtered through an ASF filter with a structuring element $\mathbf{B} \in \mathcal{B}$. Next the set is reconstructed to the highest desired resolution, achieved at scale ϵ_0, using a continuous mapping f to obtain the reconstructed set X_{ϵ_0}. Then the sets X_ϵ, $\epsilon_0 < \epsilon_j < \epsilon_k$ are obtained by subsampling the set G_{ϵ_0}. Note that ϵ_k is the coarsest scale or lowest resolution at which X has to reconstructed.

These in turn are filtered through the ASF filter to obtain the sets $\overline{X_\epsilon}$. The sets $\overline{X_\epsilon}$ form a multiresolution representation of the original signal X. When X is a random fractal it should be self-similar. Statistical properties of X should be maintained at all scale values. As we are dealing with images, one property of interest is the area of the image surface. Note that the surface area represents a measure on the minimal cover of the set X. In the case of one dimensional signals one would use length. Here the image surface is given by the gray level intensities. As the scale values change the area changes proportionally. From the definition given above (9), Hausdorff dimension is the value s for which the relation between the area and scale remains constant.

Following the notation of section 3, Let $N(\epsilon, A)$ be the minimum number of m-dimensional covers A required to cover the filtered sets $\overline{X_\epsilon}$. The quantity $N(\epsilon, A)$ is given by:

$$\mathcal{C}(A) = N(\epsilon, A) = \sum_p \alpha A_{\overline{X_\epsilon}} \qquad (11)$$

where α is proportional to the scale ϵ at which X is being observed and A is the smallest m-dimensional cover that contains the pth element of $\overline{X_\epsilon}$. The sum above is taken over all, smallest possible, compact, closed, neighborhoods A of $\overline{G_\epsilon}$. For instance in the case of images, we have selected A to be a triangle, comprised of the values $\overline{G_\epsilon}(i,j), \overline{G_\epsilon}(i+1,j), \overline{G_\epsilon}(i,j+1), 0 < i < M$ and $0 < j < N$, for a sampled image $\overline{G_\epsilon}$ of size $M \times N$. The fractal dimension estimate s is computed by performing a least squares fit to the following equation

$$\log \sum_A N(\epsilon_j, A) = s \log \epsilon_j \qquad (12)$$

for scale values $\epsilon_0 < \epsilon_j < \epsilon_k$. The fractal dimension s calculated via this method is an estimate of the true value for the original set G. However, the Vitali theorem above (10) guarantees that an upper bound on the error between the real and the estimated value of the fractal dimension can be set.

5. Preliminary Experimental Results.

5.1. Mathematical Simulation Results

In order to evaluate the performance of the various Fractal Dimension Estimators, a series of synthetic fractal images (random midpoint displacement method[11]) of known Fractal Dimension were generated. As the fractal dimension of 2D images lies between 2 and 3, we generated synthetic images whose fractal dimension varied between 2 to 3 in steps of .01.

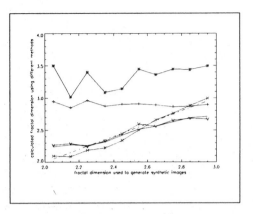

Figure 2. Plot of estimated fractal dimension versus real fractal dimension as a function of method employed. (+) Wavelet; (*) Power Spectra; (v) CASF-32; (-) CASF-64; (x) CASF-512

5.1.1. Evaluation of Different Methods for Fractal Dimension Estimation

Fractal dimensions of the synthetic images were estimated using, Power Spectrum, Wavelets, Morphology and Alternating Sequential Filter methods. The size of the window chosen was large enough so that all the above methods could be used. Figure 2 shows the results obtained from each of the methods. We can see that the ASF method perform better than the Power Spectrum, and Wavelet methods. A direct implementation of the Power Spectrum and the Wavelet methods was employed here, as such a more complex Maximum Likelihood Estimation scheme was not used.

5.1.2. Effect of Window Size in the CASF Method

Fractal dimension was estimated using windows of different sizes. Figure 3 shows results obtained by using 16x16, 32x32 and 64x64 window sizes with the CASF method and 64 x 64 ASF method. We see that for smaller window sizes, between 16 x 16 and 64 x 64, CASF method provides good results. Due to it's superior performance, fractal analysis of real data, shown below was carried on using only the CASF method.

5.2. Animal Models

We have demonstrated the efficacy of fractal analysis to distinguish osteoporotic rats from normal rats. Fractal analysis was carried out on animal models of

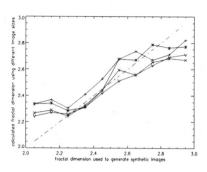

	CASF-64	
	Normal	Osteoporotic
1	2.588	2.549
2	2.665	2.602
3	2.747	2.612
4	2.739	2.627
5	2.752	2.706
6	2.782	2.591

Table 2. Faxitron image analysis results for normal and osteoprotic cases. Paired T=2.685, p =0.023.

Figure 3. Plot of estimated fractal dimension as a function of mask size used in the CASF method. (+) 12x12; (*) 16x16; (x) 32x32; (v) 64x64.

	Control Limb		Immobilized Limb	
Animal	Av. FD	Var.	Av. FD	Var.
1	2.398	0.003	2.397	0.005
2	2.423	0.014	2.315	0.003
3	2.424	0.005	2.239	0.016
4	2.520	0.010	2.460	0.004
5	2.371	0.004	2.292	0.010
6	2.396	0.004	2.330	0.004

Table 1. Experiment 3: Fratal dimension of radiographs of normal and imobilized rat femurs. Paired T =2.16, p =0.06

5.3. Faxitron Bone Images of Osteoporotic and Normal Subjects

Faxitron bone images of normal and osteoporotic human subjects were obtained. A total of six images fo size 110x110 pixels were analysed, one for each patient. Fractal dimension was computed using the CASF method with a window size of 64 x 64 pixels each of the slices. Resutls are shown in table 2. The fractal dimension computed on the osteoporotic subjects was smaller than the fractal dimension computed with the normal subjects. Results of the standard T-test evaluation, performed on the fractal dimension estimates, show that the two groups are statistically different.

6. Summary and Conclusions

In this article, the trabecular bone structure is characterized with the aid of fractal dimension. A new approach, CASF based fractal dimension estimation, is proposed here to estimate fractal dimension accurately and robustly. We show that the new approach needs only a rudimentary assumption of image self similarity and can be applied to relatively small image sizes. The most commonly employed Fourier (Power Spectrum) and Wavelet based methods assume an intrinsic FBM model and are not applicable. With mathematical simulations, we have shown that the CASF method outperforms other commonly employed methods for fractal dimension estimation.

Experimental results prove that the fractal model is appropriate for trabecular bone structure characterization. We have shown that the fractal dimension of osteoporotic subjects is lower than that of the normal subjects. In animal models, we have shown that the fractal dimension of osteoporotic rats was consistently lower than that of the normal rats. This suggests that an automated non-invasive method can be developed to be used towards diagnosis of osteoporosis.

osteoporosis. Radiographs of femurs were analyzed by fractal analysis. Male Sprague-Dawley rats weighing 150-160 g were used. Under ether anesthesia, all animals underwent a unilateral hind-limb immobilization by sciatic neurectomy by resecting 2-3 mm of the sciatic nerve on the posterior aspect of the proximal femur. This was done through a small incision in the skin which was immediately closed with wound clips. The contralateral leg was left intact. Animals were sacrificed 10 days post-surgery. Radiographs were made of isolated femurs at 90 KVP, 1 min exposure on Dupont NDT-35 film. Fractal dimension was calculated on 16 different locations on each of the radiographs of the immobilized and normal limbs. A window size of 32x32 pixels was employed. Average values of fractal dimension and their variances are shown in table 1. Fractal dimension of the two groups of 6 radiographs were shown to be statistically different using the paired-T test.

Further experimental work needs to be done to solidify the discrimination results presented here for bone structure analysis. Also it is conceivable that other measures, along with the area computation can be employed to further improve the robustness of the fractal model and consequently the ability to discriminate between normal and osteoporotic cases.

7. Acknowledgment

The authors would like to acknowledge the help of several colleagues and students from the Methodist Hospital, Houston , Texas, NASA Johnson Space Center and SUNY Buffalo. The present work was partially sponsored through a full Ph.D. scholarship from the Conselho Nacional de Pesquisa (CNPq), Brasil.

References

[1] Urist, M.R. et al, "Long term observations on aged women with pathologic osteoporosis", *Osteoporosis*, pp 3-37, NY, Grune and Stratton, 1970.

[2] A.P. Iskrant et al, "Osteoporosis in women, 45 years and over related to subsequent fractures during 30 years", *Calcified Tissue International*, 42:292-6, 1988.

[3] L. J. Melton et al, "Epidemiology of vertebral fractures in women", *American Journal of Epidemiology*, 129:1000-11, 1989.

[4] B. E. Nordin, "Osteoporosis", *Metabolic Bone and Stone Disease*, pp. 1-70, Edinburgh Churchill Livingston, 1984.

[5] R.B. Martin, "Linear calibration of radiographic mineral density using video digitization methods", *Calcified Tissue International*, 47:82-91, 1960.

[6] B. L. Riggs, "Changes in bone mineral density of the proximal femur and spine with aging", *J. Clin. Invest.*, 70:716-23, 1982.

[7] B.L.Riggs et al, "Involutional osteoporosis", *New England Journal of Medicine*, 314: 1676-86, 1986.

[8] P. Steiger et al, "Age related decrements in bone mineral density in woman over 65", *Journal of Bone and Mineral research*, 7: 625-32, 1992.

[9] P. J. M. Elders et al, "Accelerated vertebral bone loss in relation to the menopause: a cross sectional study of lumbar bone density in 286 women of 46 to 55 years of age", *Bone and Mineral* 5, 11-19 (1988).

[10] R. P. Heaney, "Osteoporotic Fracture Space: An Hypothesis", *Bone and Mineral*, vol 6, pg. 1-13, 1989.

[11] A. Fournier et al, 'Computer rendering of stochastic models', Communication of ACM, 25 pg. 371-384, 1982.

[12] E. Kleerekoper et al, "Calcaneus Bone Architecture and Bone Strength", *Editor: Christinsen C, Osteoporosis* 1987, Viborg, Denmark: Norhaven A/s-1987, pg. 289-300.

[13] J. E. Aaron et al, "The Microanatomy of Trabecular Bone Loss in Normal Aging Men and Women", *Clin Orthop. Res.*, vol 215, pg. 260-271, 1987.

[14] S. Peleg et al, "Multiple Resolution Texture Analysis and Classification", *IEEE-PAMI*, vol 6, No 4, pg. 518-523, July 1984.

[15] T. Lundhal et al, "Fractional Brownian Motion: A Maximum Likelihood Estimator and It's Application to Image Texture", *IEEE Trans. MI*, vol 5, pg. 152-161, Sep 86.

[16] P. Flandrin, "On the spectrum of Fractional Brownian Motion", *IEEE Trans. on Information Theory*, 35(1):197-199, 1989.

[17] C. Fortin et al, "Fractal Dimension in the Analysis of Medical Images", *IEEE Eng. in Medicine and Biology Magazine*, vol 11, pg. 65-71, 1992.

[18] R. L. Webber et al, "Evaluation of Site Specific Differences in Trabecular Bone Using Fractal Geometry", *J. of Dent. Res.*, Abstract no 2095, 1991.

[19] A. Pentland, "Fractal Based Description of Natural Scenes", *IEEE-CVPR*, pp209-210, June 1983.

[20] S. Majumdar et al, "Application of Fractal Geometry Techniques to The Study of Trabecular Bone", *Med. Phys.* 20 (6), Nov/Dec 1993.

[21] S. R. Sternberg, "Morphology for Grey Tone Functions", *Computer Vision Graphics and Image Processing*, Vol. 35, 1986.

[22] R. L. Webber et al, "Predicting Osseous Changes in Ankle Fractures", IEEE Engineering in Medicine and Biology, pg. 103-110, March 1993.

[23] W. S. Kulinski et al, "Application of Fractal Texture Analysis to Segmentation of Dental Radiographs", vol 1092, Medical Imaging-3, SPIE Proceedings, 1989.

[24] J. A. Lynch et al, 'Analysis of texture in microradiographs of osteoarthritic knees using fractal signatures', Phys Med Biol, Vol 36, No 6, 709-722, 1991.

[25] A. N. Kolmogorov, "A New Invariant for Transitive Dynamical Systems", *Dokl. Acad. Nauk SSSR*, pg. 861-864, No. 119, 1958.

[26] B. B. Mandelbrot, *Fractals: Form, Chance and Dimension*, San Francisco, CA: Freeman, 1977.

[27] J. D. Farmer, E. Ott, J. A. Yorke, "The Dimension of Chaotic Attractors", *Physica 7D*, pg. 153 -180, North-Holland Publishing Company, 1983.

[28] T. S. Parker and L. O. Chua, *Practical Numerical Algorithms for Chaotic Systems*, pg. 167-199, Springer-Verlag 1989.

[29] A. Lasota and M. C. Mackey, *Chaos, Fractals and Noise*, pg. 432-437, Second Edition, Springer-Verlag, 1994.

[30] S. G. Mallat, "A theory for multiresolution signal decomposition: the wavelet representation", *IEEE-PAMI*, Vol. 11, No. 7, pg. 674-693, Jul. 1989.

[31] U. E. Ruttiman and J. A. Ship, "The Use of Fractal Geometry to Quantitate Bone Structure From Radiographs", *J. Dent. Res.*, pg. 69, 1990. Abstract no. 1431.

[32] J. Samarabandu, R. Acharya, E. Hausmann, and K. Allen, "Analysis of Bone X-Rays Using Morphological Fractals", *IEEE Trans. on Medical Imag.*, Vol. 12., No. 3. Sept. 1993.

[33] J. Serra, *Image Analysis and Mathematical Morphology*, Vol. 2, New York, Academic Press, 1988.

[34] Petros Maragos and Fang-Kuo Sun, "Measuring the Fractal Dimension of Signals: Morphological Covers and Iterative Optimization", *IEEE Trans. on Signal Processing*, Vol. 41 NO.1. January 1993.

[35] S. R. Sternberg, "Morphology for grey tone functions", *Computer Vision Graphics and Image Processing*, Vol. 35, 1986.

[36] A. P. Korostelev and A. B. Tsybakov, *Minimax Theory of Image Reconstruction*, Springer- Verlag, 1993.

[37] J. J. Koenderink, "The structure of images", *Biological Cybernetics*, vol. 50, no. 363-370, 1984.

[38] A. Morales and R. Acharya, "An Image Pyramid with Alternating Sequential Filters", *IEEE Trans. on Image Proc.*, vol 4, No 7, pp965-977, July 1995.

[39] R. V. den Boomgaard and A. Smeulders, "The Morphological Structure of Images: The Differential Equations of Morphological Scale-Space", *IEEE-PAMI*, Vol. 16, No. 7, pg. 1101-1113, November 1994.

[40] K. J. Falconer, *The Geometry of Fractal Sets*, London, Cambridge University Press, 1985.

[41] M. H. Chen and P. F. Yan, "A multiscaling approach based on morphological filtering", *IEEE-PAMI*, Vol. 11, no. 7. pg. 694-700, 1989.

[42] Paul T. Jackway and Mohamed Deriche, *Scale-Space Properties of the Multiscale Morphological Dilation-Erosion*, IEEE-PAMI, Vol. 18 NO. 1, January 1996

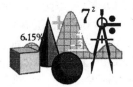

Session 3

Registration II

Extension of the ICP Algorithm to Non-Rigid Intensity-Based Registration of 3D Volumes

Jacques Feldmar, Grégoire Malandain, Jérôme Declerck and Nicholas Ayache
INRIA SOPHIA, Projet EPIDAURE
2004 route des Lucioles, B.P. 93
06902 Sophia Antipolis Cedex, France.
Email : Jacques.Feldmar@sophia.inria.fr
Tel: (33) 93-65-79-27, Fax: (33) 93-65-76-69

Abstract

We present in this paper a new registration and gain correction algorithm for 3D medical images. It is intensity based. The basic idea is to represent the images by 4D points (x_j, y_j, z_j, i_j) and to define a global energy function based on this representation. For minimization, we propose a technique which does not require to compute the derivatives of this criterion with respect to the parameters. It can be understood as an extension of the Iterative Closest Point algorithm [4, 37] or as an application of the formalism proposed in [9]. Two parameters allow us to have a coarse to fine strategy both for resolution and deformation. Our technique presents the advantage to minimize a well defined global criterion, to deal with various classes of transformations (for example rigid, affine and volume spline), to be simple to implement and to be efficient in practice. Results on real brain and heart 3D images are presented to demonstrate the validity of our approach.

1. Introduction

Registration is a key problem in medical imaging. Indeed, the physician must often **compare** or **fuse** different images. The problem is as follow: *given two 3D images, find the geometric transformation that best superposes them, with respect to some constraints.* If the two images come from the same patient and from a rigid anatomical organ, then the problem is *rigid registration*. Otherwise it is *non-rigid registration*.

The registration techniques can be classified into two classes: 1) techniques using additional artificial markers and 2) techniques without additional artificial markers. The fixation of markers can be very invasive or can produce unacceptable constraints. This paper is related to the second class of techniques.

Different methods have been proposed to try to solve the registration problem without additional markers. Usually, registration is based on a representation computed from the 3D images. This representation can be high level (graphs, crest points, crest lines), middle level (surfaces, contours) or low level. We do not review in this paper registration methods based on high and middle level representations. They are quite numerous. A complete review can be found in [2, 5, 33, 16] : we just quote the most recent papers.

The registration method presented in this paper is related to intensity based techniques. Most of them are for 3D-3D rigid registration and try to maximize the correlation [36, 20] or the mutual information [28, 11, 34] between the two images. The basic idea is that a high or middle level representation can be difficult to compute either because of the image acquisition modality or because the organs do not have well defined contours in the images.

Brain images are a good example of images difficult to segment. A lot of research has been done to try to solve this problem [21, 35, 24]. However, matching of two MR brain images coming from two different patients has an important application. Indeed, we have access to a brain image which has been manually segmented (or labeled) (courtesy of Ron Kikinis, at the Brigham and Women's hospital, Boston) and we use it as an anatomical atlas. Hence, non rigid inter-patient registration allows us to label automatically an MR image of a new patient into anatomical regions thanks to the knowledge of voxel to voxel correspondence.

Some interesting research has been done to compute this matching based on crest lines, surfaces or contours [29, 27, 16, 31] or based directly on the intensities in the images [3, 8, 18, 32, 12]. These techniques are either **physics based** or are based on **local information** and do not minimize a global criterion. The algorithm presented in this paper is different: we compute a global **geometric transformation**

84

Proceedings of MMBIA '96

minimizing an **explicit global criterion**. Note that this idea to deform an atlas towards an image can be criticized [23]. However we believe that our method can be useful at least as a preprocessing step before a more sophisticated approach is applied.

One of the difficulties is to segment (for point based techniques) or to correct the intensity (for intensity based techniques) of the images to register. This is because of the shape of the brain but also because of the gain problem in the MR images. We present in this paper a new registration and gain correction algorithm which is intensity based. This algorithm has numerous applications. Indeed, it should allow us to perform registration when contour (or higher level features) extraction is difficult. It is an extension of the ICP algorithm [4, 37, 25, 7, 6]. Our technique presents the advantage to minimize a well defined global criterion, to deal with various classes of transformations (for example rigid, affine and volume spline), to be simple to implement and to be efficient in practice.

In this paper, we first present the representation on which the algorithm is based and the corresponding minimized criterion (section 2). Then, we describe the minimization algorithm (section 3) and the computation of the representation (section 4). Finally, we present the first results obtained with brain which demonstrate the validity of our approach (sections 5 and 6). We conclude by presenting the future directions of this work.

2 A global correlation criterion

2.1 The classical criterion

The most straightforward idea for registering two images i_1 and i_2 with intensity functions $I_1(x, y, z)$ and $I_2(x, y, z)$ is probably to minimize the criterion:

$$C(f) = \sum_{M_i \in i_1} (I_2(f(M_i)) - I_1(M_i))^2,$$

where f is a 3D-3D geometric transformation.

If it is necessary to correct the intensity to register the two images, one can minimize the following criterion:

$$C'(f, g) = \sum_{M_i \in i_1} (I_2(f(M_i)) - g(I_1(M_i), M_i))^2,$$

where f is a 3D-3D geometric transformation and g is an intensity correction function. But these formulations have a drawback: they search for an exact superposition of the two images although this might not always be possible with the considered class of transformations or deformations. We want to bring nearer the points with close intensity but we want to keep a constrained deformation.

2.2 Our criterion

In our formulation, we consider 3D images as surfaces in a 4D space. Hence, an image corresponding to a function $i = I(x, y, z)$ is represented by a set of 4D points (x_j, y_j, z_j, i_j). The first three coordinates are spatial coordinates and the fourth one is an intensity coordinate[1].

We propose to minimize a global criterion measuring the correlation between the two images by deforming the scene image into the model image. In our formulation, it means that we deform the 4D surface. Then, we both correct the geometry and the intensity in the image[2]. The minimized energy function is as follows:

$$E(\mathbf{f}, g) = \sum_{(\mathbf{x}_j, i_j) \in IMAGE SCENE}$$
$$d((\mathbf{f}(\mathbf{x}_j), g(\mathbf{x}_j, i_j)), \quad \mathbf{PPP}_{4D}(\mathbf{f}(\mathbf{x}_j), g(\mathbf{x}_j, i_j)))^{1/2} \quad (1)$$

where

- $\mathbf{x}_j$ denotes the three spatial coordinates of point M_j, i.e. (x_j, y_j, z_j).

- $\mathbf{f}$ is a function which associates a 3D point with a 3D point: it is the geometric transformation of the scene image. Note that it does not depend on the intensity.

- g is a function which associates a scalar value with a 4D point: it associates a new intensity to a point in the image depending on its position and its current intensity.

- $\mathbf{PPP}_{4D}$ is the function which associates to a 4D point its closest point among the points describing the model image.

- Finally, d is a function such that given two 4D points $M = (\mathbf{x}, i)$ and $N = (\mathbf{x}', i')$,

$$d(M, N) = (\alpha_1(x - x')^2 + \alpha_2(y - y')^2 + \alpha_3(z - z')^2 + \alpha_4(i - i')^2)^{1/2},$$

where the α_i are coefficients normalizing each coordinate between 0 and 1.

Of course, a key point is to choose the definition domain of the function E: this constraints the functions $\mathbf{f}$ and g. For example, if two images come from the same anatomical object and if the voxel intensities correctly represent the associated tissues, then the searched function $\mathbf{f}$ will be a **rigid displacement** and g will be fixed to be the **identity function**.

---

[1] More details about the choice of these 4D points to represent the images will be given in section 4.1.

[2] Of course, we choose a very global function for intensity correction otherwise registration would not make sense.

When the two anatomical regions do not come from the same patient, or when the anatomical region is deformable, the function $\mathbf{f}$ can be an **affine** or **spline** function (see appendix A). When the intensity in the images is perturbed by a distortion, one can also search g as an affine, polynomial or spline function, depending on the physical analysis of the pertubation.

2.3 Smoothing

When $\mathbf{f}$ and g are deformation functions, it is often necessary to add a smoothing term to E. In these cases, the new energy function E_{smooth} is:

$$E_{smooth}(\mathbf{f}, g) = E(\mathbf{f}, g) + \lambda \sum_{(\mathbf{x}_j, i_j) \in IMAGESCENE} Smoothness(\mathbf{f}, g, (\mathbf{x}_j, i_j)),$$

where $Smoothness(\mathbf{f}, g, (\mathbf{x}_j, i_j))$ is the sum of the norm of the second derivatives of $\mathbf{f}$ and g with respect to each of their coordinates ("bending energy") respectively at points $(\mathbf{x}_j)$ and $(\mathbf{x}_j, i_j)$.

2.4 Use of the gradient information

Even if the algorithm deals directly with intensities in the images, it can be desirable to enhance the importance of areas where the intensity varies a lot. These are the areas where the norm of the gradient is high. To obtain this result, we weight each term of the energy E with the norm of the gradient at the corresponding point:

$$E(\mathbf{f}, g) = \sum_{(\mathbf{x}_j, i_j) \in IMAGESCENE} \|\vec{\nabla}_{IMAGESCENE}(\mathbf{x}_j)\|. \quad d((\mathbf{f}(\mathbf{x}_j), g(\mathbf{x}_j, i_j)), \\ \mathbf{PPP}_{4D}(\mathbf{f}(\mathbf{x}_j), g(\mathbf{x}_j, i_j)))^{1/2} \quad (2)$$

Note that it is possible to use the information of gradient direction. In this case, the points representing the images are no longer 4D points. They are 7D points: three spatial coordinates, one intensity coordinate and three gradient coordinates. Hence, the distance between two points is a compromise between the spatial distance, the difference of gradient norm and orientation and the difference of intensity. The minimization of the corresponding energy tends to minimize this difference between the two sets of points describing the images. This way of using the gradient information is similar to the use of surface normals presented in [17] for rigid surface registration.

3 Minimization technique

To minimize the energy function E or E_{smooth}, we developed a technique which does not require to compute the

derivatives of these functions with respect to the parameters. It can be understood as an extension of the Iterative Closest Point algorithm [4, 37] or as an application of the formalism proposed in [9].

3.1 The algorithm

The minimization algorithm is iterative. At each iteration i, we compute two new estimates $\mathbf{f}_i$ and g_i of $\mathbf{f}$ and g in two stages.

- Stage 1: we build a set of pairs of 4D points $Match_i$ by associating with each point M_j in the scene image the point N_j such that:

$$N_j = \mathbf{PPP}_{4D}([\mathbf{f}_{i-1}(\mathbf{x}_j), g_{i-1}(M_j)]),$$

where $\mathbf{x}_j$ are the three spatial coordinates of M_j. $Match_i$ is made of the pairs (M_j, N_j).

- Stage 2: we simply compute in the least square sense the best transformations $\mathbf{f}_i$ and g_i corresponding to $Match_i$. These are $\mathbf{f}_i$ and g_i minimizing the criterion:

$$\sum_{(M_j, N_j) \in Match_i} d((\mathbf{f}(\mathbf{x}_j), g(M_j)), N_j)^2 + \\ \sum_{(M_j, N_j) \in Match_i} Smoothness(\mathbf{f}, g, M_j).$$

For the rigid, affine and spline transformations classes and for the smoothing terms which we are using, this criterion is quadratic and the least square estimation turns out to be the resolution of a linear system.

The fact that this algorithm minimizes the defined energy and the convergence is easy to demonstrate[3]. Let us define the energy function E':

$$E'(\mathbf{f}, g, Match) = \\ \sum_{M_j \in IMAGESCENE} d((\mathbf{f}(\mathbf{x}_j), g(M_j)), Match(M_j))^2 + \\ \sum_{M_j \in IMAGESCENE} Smoothness(\mathbf{f}, g, M_j).$$

At stage 1 of our algorithm, the variables $\mathbf{f}$ and g are fixed and E' is minimized with respect to $Match$. Indeed, in this case, the function $Match$ minimizing E' is such that:

$$Match(M_j) = \mathbf{PPP}_{4D}((\mathbf{f}(\mathbf{x}_j), g(M_j))).$$

At stage 2, the variable $Match$ is fixed and E' is minimized with respect to $\mathbf{f}$ and g. Thus, at each stage, E' decreases.

---

[3]Of course, it does not guarantee that we are going to find the global minimum. We are minimizing a non convex function and we can just prove the convergence towards a potentially local minimum.

Because E' is positive, the convergence is guaranteed, even if one can converge towards a local minimum and if the convergence can require an infinite time.

This minimization technique is very efficient. Contrary to the classical minimization techniques, it is not "local" (the transformation parameters can vary a lot between two successive iterations) and it does not require either the computation of the derivative of E with respect to the parameters or the tuning of some parameters. On the other hand, it assumes that each point in the scene image has a correspondent in the model image.

3.2 The occlusion problem

However, some points in one image do not have any correspondent in the other one because of potential occlusions. Another reason can come from the evolution of a pathology (a tumor for example).

It is very important to deal explicitly with this occlusion problem to get an accurate transformation. One could do it thanks to a robust criterion (in the sense of the statistics) like in [19, 10] for rigid surface registration. But stage 2 of the algorithm would not be a linear system resolution anymore and the algorithm would not be so efficient. We prefer the approach proposed in [37] for 3D-3D rigid surface registration. For each match (M_j, N_j) in $Match_i$, we decide if it is plausible or not. This point is very important because if we accept erroneous matches, the solution will be biased and if we reject correct matches, the solution will not be accurate.

For each pair (M_j, N_j) in $Match_i$, we compute the 4D Euclidean distance:

$$\delta_j = d(M_j, N_j).$$

One can suppose that if the registration was correct, this variable δ_j would follow a χ^2 law. Thus, we can compare the statistics of this variable δ_j with a χ^2 with 4 degrees of freedom and decide that a pair (M_j, N_j) is plausible looking at a χ^2 table with a confidence value of say 95 % or 99 %.

Stage 2 of the minimization algorithm is simply modified so that the least square criterion takes into account only the plausible matches in $Match_i$[4].

4 The representation of the images

4.1 Computing the representation

A fundamental point for this registration algorithm is to choose the 4D points representing the images. One can associate with each voxel V a point $M = (x, y, z, i)$, where

x, y, z are the spatial coordinates of the voxel's center and i its intensity. Let us call M the point representing the voxel V. One could use the representing points but the minimization algorithm would be inefficient because of the data volume.

To avoid this problem, we developed an algorithm to compute a more compact representation of the images. The basic idea is to split recursively the image into "quadrilaterals" until each "quadrilateral" contains only voxels of which the representative points can be approximated by a 4D hyperplan with an error smaller than ϵ, where ϵ is a parameter of the splitting algorithm[5].

The details of this algorithm can be found in [22]. As a result, the image is represented by a set of "quadrilaterals" with different sizes containing relatively homogeneous voxels. A 4D centroid and a 4D hyperplan are attached to each "quadrilateral".

The points M_j used to describe the scene image in the minimization algorithm are simply the centroid attached to the "quadrilaterals" obtained by recursively splitting this image. To compute the function $\mathbf{PPP}_{4D}$ in an efficient way, the model image is also splited into "quadrilaterals". A 4D kd-tree [26] is calculated based on the centroids B_j resulting from the recursive split. During minimization, given a 4D point M, $\mathbf{PPP}_{4D}(M)$ is computed as follows (see figure 1).

- Thanks to the kd-tree, we first find the centroid B_j the closest to M. This centroid corresponds to a "quadrilateral" Q_j.

- $\mathbf{PPP}_{4D}(M)$ is the closest point to M onto the hyperplan H_j approximating the "quadrilateral" and lying in this "quadrilateral".

4.2 A coarse to fine multi-resolution strategy

The parameter ϵ of the image splitting algorithm allows us to control the quality of the approximation. The smaller ϵ, the better the approximation. However, when ϵ is large, the number of points/hyperplans describing the image is small. Thus, ϵ allows us to control **the resolution**.

It is also important to control the "quantity" of accepted deformation. We compute first rigid displacements, then affine transformations and finally spline deformations. For this last class of transformations, we can also choose the number of control points and the parameter λ controlling the importance of the bending term in the criterion definition in order to control **the "quantity" of allowed deformation**.

The strategy that we propose to try to avoid the local minima during the minimization uses these two properties.

---

[4] Just note that it would be possible to weight the criterion with a quantity inversely proportional to δ_j and our minimization algorithm would still converge.

[5] The error can be the maximum of the points to plane distances or the average of these distances.

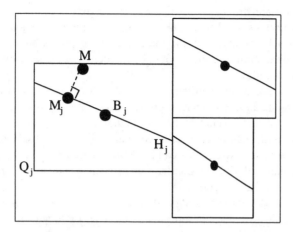

Figure 1. The computation of PPP_4D is done in two stages. First, we compute the centroid B_j the closest to M and then, we project M onto H_j.

At the beginning, we choose a low resolution and we compute rigid displacements. The biggest structures are then first registered. Then, progressively during the minimization process, we decrease ϵ in order to enhance the quality of the approximation of the images and we allow more and more deformation from affine transformations to spline deformations.

Of course, this description of the strategy is very qualitative. In practice, the choice of the functions controlling these resolution and deformation parameters depends on the anatomical regions to register. But they have not been difficult to find in practice.

5   Results on brain data

We present in this section two examples of application of our volume registration algorithm with 3D brain MR images.

5.1   Rigid registration with intensity correction

The top two images of figure 2 are two slices of same index of two MR images of the same brain. One can observe that (1) geometric registration is necessary since the two slices do not correspond to each other (for example the eyes are visible in one image and are not visible in the other one) (2) the left image is much brighter than the right one.

The algorithm described in this paper allows us to compute at the same time a rigid displacement to superpose the two images and a multiplication coefficient to correct the intensity. The bottom image of figure 2 shows the slice corresponding to the slice of the top left image after registration

and resampling of the 3D image corresponding to the top right image.

For the registration, approximately 50000 points are used to describe the images. The resolution does not vary during the iterations. The CPU time is 5 minutes. After registration, the average mean distance between matched 4D points is 0.8 mm and the average difference of intensity is 2.8 (the intensity in the images is between 0 and 255). One can observe that after registration the two slices look much more similar both from the geometric and intensity viewpoints.

5.2   Matching with an atlas

Figures 3, 4 et 5 show an example of spline registration of two MR images of two different brains. In fact, one of the two images has been manually segmented into anatomical regions (courtesy of Ron Kikinis, at the Brigham and Women's hospital, Boston). It can be used as an anatomical atlas. Indeed, the matching allows us to label automatically the second image thanks to the knowledge of the voxel to voxel correspondence.

Registration uses in each image approximatively 50000 points. The computed deformation is a volume spline function (see appendix A) with $15 \times 15 \times 15$ control points. There is no intensity correction. The CPU time is 25 minutes. The resolution varies linearly from 10000 points to 50000 points during the deformation process and λ (the parameter controlling the smoothing term of the criterion) varies linearly from 5 to 2.

The registration is not perfect, even if it is not bad. This is due to two reasons:

- we should use more 4D points to describe the images at the end of the process,

- the spline deformation is not local enough ($15 \times 15 \times 15$ control points is the maximum that we can use because of memory limitations).

We believe that these two problems should be fixed in the future thanks to more powerful workstations (we use a DEC alpha). Another possibility for fixing this problem may be to use radial bases functions [1] or adaptative splines [31]. We just want to note that our deformation seems to be better than the one based on Talairach atlas techniques. Moreover, because our deformation is quite global, we can guarantee that the result of our non rigid registration makes sense. Note also that before registration, it was quite difficult to identify in the two images the corresponding structures while it is quite easy after registration.

If a more local registration was necessary, the output of our algorithm could be a good input for techniques like [32, 8] which are maybe more sensitive to their initialization but which are more local.

6 Results on heart data

A common examination for detection of cardiac ischemia is the stress-rest comparison in myocardial perfusion studies provided by Nuclear Medicine. Experiments on a 40 patients' database of such data are presented in [15].

7 Conclusion

We have presented in this paper a new and efficient algorithm for registration-intensity correction of 3D images. This algorithm is an extension of the original ICP algorithm to volume registration and deals explicitly with the occlusion problem. The computed transformations are rigid, affine or spline. The experiments demonstrate the validity of our approach even if a complete clinical validation is necessary.

For future work, the technique presented in this paper has at least three very interesting extensions. The first problem is the use of another transformation class for non-rigid registration. It could be radial bases functions [1]. The learning-based deformations are also very interesting [13, 30]. It should be possible to perform some statistics (thanks to a database) on the positions of the control points to constraint the possible deformations.

The second problem is the use of volume spline registration for motion tracking in sequences of 3D images (MR, SPECT or f-MRI). Indeed time sequences of 3D images will probably be more and more common and we believe that analysis of such images is a challenge.

The third problem is "atlas building". The problem is as follow: *given a set of images with known diagnosis, assuming that one is able to perform non rigid registration, build a data structure which will allow us, given an image not present in the database, to provide a predicted diagnosis.* We would like to show that our spline registration improves the quality of the results with respect to the affine registration techniques used in most of the papers dealing with this problem.

We hope that some first results for these three problems will be available at the time of the workshop.

A 3D-3D volume spline deformations

We have chosen to implement the algorithm presented in this paper with spline deformations. It is the class of functions get by tensor product of spline bases functions:

$$f(x, y, z) = (\quad \sum_{i,j,k} C^x_{ijk} B_i(x) B_j(y) B_k(z),$$
$$\sum_{i,j,k} C^y_{ijk} B_i(x) B_j(y) B_k(z),$$
$$\sum_{i,j,k} C^z_{ijk} B_i(x) B_j(y) B_k(z)),$$

where the $C_{ijk} = (C^x_{ijk}, C^y_{ijk}, C^z_{ijk})$ are the control points and the B_i are 1-D B-spline functions with regularly distrib-

uted knots. In our formulation, the class of 3D-3D spline function is only described by moving the control points.

In the definition of the criterion, a smoothing energy is added to the least square term on the position in order to control the regularity of the solution. This energy is expressed as a second order Tikhonov stabilizer. The criterion is the sum of the two energies, a multiplying weight λ ponderates the importance of the smoothing energy with respect to the position energy.

Because the criterion is quadratic in C^x_{ijk}, C^y_{ijk} and C^z_{ijk}, the least square minimization at stage 2 of the algorithm presented in this paper is a linear system resolution, which is quite efficient in practice.

We have chosen the 3D-3D spline functions for efficiency but also because they have interesting geometric properties:

- the 3D-3D spline functions and their derivatives are easy to compute thanks to the "de Casteljau" algorithm,

- the intrinsic rigidity properties of B-splines provide regular 3D-3D functions,

- a data point has a local influence: to evaluate a spline function at a given point, only $(K + 1)^3$ control points are necessary, where K is the spline order.

For more details about spline functions, see [14].

References

[1] N. Arad and D. Reisfeld. Image warping using few anchor points and radial functions. *Computer Graphics Forum*, 14(1):35–46, March 1995.

[2] N. Ayache. Medical computer vision, virtual reality and robotics. *Image and Vision Computing*, 13(4):295–313, May 1995.

[3] R. Bajcsy and S. Kovacic. Multiresolution elastic matching. *CVGIP*, 46:1–21, 1989.

[4] P. Besl and N. McKay. A method for registration of 3−D shapes. *IEEE Transactions on Pattern Analysis and Machine Intelligence*, 14(2):239–256, February 1992.

[5] L. G. Brown. A survey of image registration techniques. *ACM Computing Surveys*, 24(4):325–375, December 1992.

[6] G. Champleboux, S. Lavallée, R. Szeliski, and L. Brunie. From accurate range imaging sensor calibration to accurate model-based 3−D object localization. In *Proceedings of the IEEE Conference on Vision and Pattern Recognition*, Urbana Champaign, June 1992.

[7] Y. Chen and G. Medioni. Object modeling by registration of multiple range images. *Image and Vision Computing*, 10(3):145–155, 1992.

[8] G. Christensen, R. Rabbit, M. Miller, S. Joshi, U. Grenander, T. Coogan, and D. VanEssen. Topological properties of smooth anatomic maps. In *Information Processing in Medical Imaging (IPMI '95)*, Brest, June 1995.

[9] L. Cohen. Use of auxiliary variables in computer vision problems. In *Proceedings of the Fifth International Conference on Computer Vision (ICCV '95)*, Boston, June 1995.

[10] A. Colchester, J. Zhao, C. Henri, R. Evans, P. Roberts, N. Maitland, D. Hawkes, D. Hill, A. Strong, D. Thomas, M. Gleeson, and T. Cox. Craniotomy simulation and guidance using a stereo video based tracking system (vislan). In *Visualization in Biomedical Computing*, Rochester, Minnesota, October 1994.

[11] A. Collignon, F. Maes, D. Delaere, D. Vandermeulen, and P. S. ang G. Marchal. Automated multi modality image registration using information theory. In *Information Processing in Medical Imaging (IPMI '95)*, Brest, June 1995.

[12] D. Collins, A. Evans, C. Holmes, and T. Peters. Automated 3d segmentation of neuro-anatomical structures. In *Information Processing in Medical Imaging (IPMI '95)*, Brest, June 1995.

[13] T. Cootes, A. Hill, and C. Taylor. Rapid and accurate medical images interpretation using active shape models. In *Information Processing in Medical Imaging (IPMI '95)*, Brest, June 1995.

[14] J. Declerck, G. Subsol, J. Thirion, and N. Ayache. Automatic retrieval of anatomical structures in 3d medical images. In *First International Conference on Computer Vision, Virtual Reality and Robotics in Medicine (CVRMed '95)*, Nice, April 1995.

[15] J. Feldmar. *Recalage rigide, non rigide et projectif d'images medicales tridimensionnelles*. PhD thesis, Ecole Polytechnique-INRIA, December 1995.

[16] J. Feldmar and N. Ayache. Rigid, affine and locally affine registration of free-form surfaces. *The International Journal of Computer Vision*. Accepted for publication. Published in two parts in ECCV'94 (rigid and affine) and CVPR'94 (locally affine). Also INRIA Research Report 2220.

[17] J. Feldmar, N. Ayache, and F. Betting. 3d-2d projective registration of free-form curves and surfaces. *The Journal of Computer Vision and Image Understanding*. Published in three parts: CVRMed'95, ICCV'95 and IPMI'95. Also INRIA Research Report 2434.

[18] J. Gee, L. Lebriquer, C. Barrillot, and D. Haynor. Probabilistic matching of brain images. In *Information Processing in Medical Imaging (IPMI '95)*, Brest, June 1995.

[19] W. Grimson, T. Lozano-Perez, W. W. III, G. Ettinger, S. White, and R. Kikinis. An automatic registration method for frameless stereotaxy, image guided surgery, and enhanced reality visualization. In *IEEE Proceedings of Computer Vision and Pattern Recognition 1994 (CVPR'94)*, Seattle, USA, June 1994.

[20] F. Hemler, P. V. D. Elsen, T. Sumanaweera, S. Napel, J. Drace, and J. Adler. A quantitative comparison of residual errors for three different multimodality registration techniques. In *Information Processing in Medical Imaging (IPMI '95)*, Brest, June 1995.

[21] G. Malandain. *Filtrage, topologie et mise en correspondance d'images médicales multidimensionnelles*. PhD thesis, Ecole Centrale de Paris, Septembre 1992.

[22] G. Malandain. Reprsentation des images par des arbres binaires. Research report, INRIA, 1995. To appear.

[23] J. Mangin, V. Frouin, I. Bloch, B. Bendriem, and J. Lopez-Krahe. Fast Nonsupervised 3D Registration of PET and MR Images of the Brain. *Journal of Cerebral Blood Flow and Metabolism*, 14(5):749–762, 1994.

[24] J. Mangin, F. Tupin, V. Frouin, I. Bloch, R. Rougetet, J. Regis, and J. Lopez-Krahe. Deformable topological models for segmentation of 3d medical images. In *Information Processing in Medical Imaging (IPMI '95)*, Brest, June 1995.

[25] Y. H.-T. Menq, C.-H. and G.-Y. Lai. Automated precision measurement of surface profile in cad-directed inspection. *IEEE Trans. RA*, 8(2):268–278, 1992.

[26] F. P. Preparata and M. I. Shamos. *Computational Geometry, an Introduction*. Springer Verlag, 1985.

[27] S. Sandor and R. Leahy. Towards automated labelling of the cerebral cortex using a deformable atlas. In *Information Processing in Medical Imaging (IPMI '95)*, Brest, June 1995.

[28] C. Studholme, D. Hill, and D. Hawkes. Multi-resolution voxel similarity measures for mr-pet registration. In *Information Processing in Medical Imaging (IPMI '95)*, Brest, June 1995.

[29] G. Subsol. *Construction automatique d'atlas anatomiques partir d'images mdicales tridimensionnelles*. PhD thesis, Ecole Centrale, 1995.

[30] G. Szekely, A. Kelemen, C. Brechbler, and G. Gerig. Segmentation of 3d object from mri volume data using constrained elastic deformations of flexible fourrier surface models. In *First International Conference on Computer Vision, Virtual Reality and Robotics in Medicine (CVRMed '95)*, Nice, April 1995.

[31] R. Szeliski and S. Lavallée. Matching 3-d anatomical surfaces with non-rigid volumetric deformations. In *Proceedings of the IEEE Workshop on Biomedical Images Analysis (WBIA'94)*, Seattle, Washington, June 1994. Also in AAAI 1994 Spring Symposium Series. Application of Computer Vision in Medical Image Processing, Stanford University, 1994.

[32] J.-P. Thirion. Fast non-rigid matching of 3d medical images. In *Medical Robotics and Computer Aided Surgery (MRCAS'95)*, pages 47–54, Baltimore, November 1995.

[33] P. van den Elsen, E. Pol, and M. Viergever. Medical image matching. a review with classification. *IEEE Engineering in Medecine and Biology*, 12(4):26–39, 1993.

[34] P. Viola and W. M. W. III. Alignment by maximisation of mutual information. In *Proceedings of the Fifth International Conference on Computer Vision (ICCV '95)*, Boston, June 1995.

[35] W. Wells, E. Grimson, R. Kikinis, and F. Jolesz. Adaptative segmentation of mri data. In *First International Conference on Computer Vision, Virtual Reality and Robotics in Medicine (CVRMed '95)*, Nice, April 1995.

[36] R. Woods, S. Cherry, and J. Mazziotta. Rapid automated algorithm for aligning and reslicing PET images. *Journal of Computer Assisted Tomography*, 16(1):1–14, 1992.

[37] Z. Zhang. Iterative point matching for registration of free-form curves and surfaces. *the International Journal of Computer Vision*, 13(2):119–152, 1994. Also Research Report No.1658, INRIA Sophia-Antipolis, 1992.

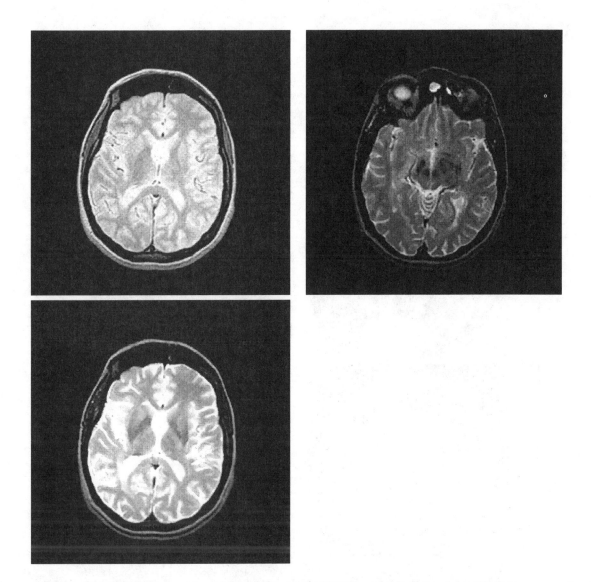

Figure 2. Top: two axial slices of same index of two MR images (left A, right B) of the same brain before registration. We thank Pr. Ron Kikinis, Brigham and Women's Hospital (Boston) for these images. Bottom, left: the slice of image B after registration, resampling and intensity correction corresponding to the slice of the top-left image. One can compare pixel by pixel the left two images.

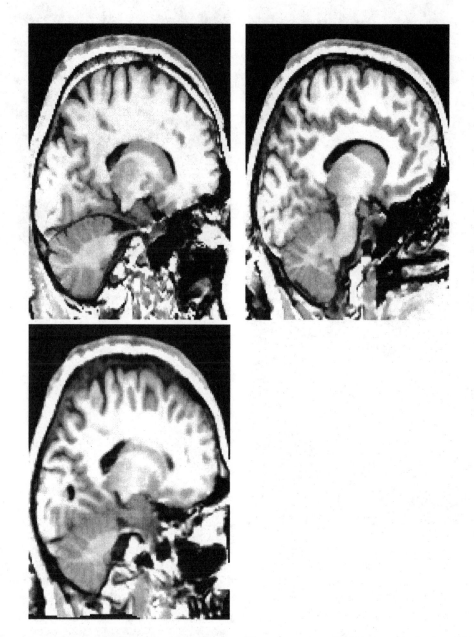

Figure 3. Top: two slices sagittal of same index coming from two MR images of two different brains before registration (left C, right the atlas). We thank Pr. Ron Kikinis, Brigham and Women's Hospital (Boston) for these images. Bottom, left: the slice of the resampled atlas corresponding to the top left image after non rigid spline registration. The two left images can be compared voxel by voxel.

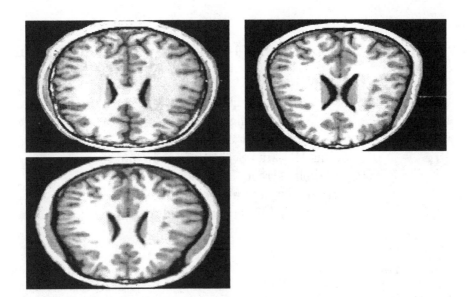

Figure 4. Top: two axial slices of same index coming from the same images than the ones shown figures 3 and 4 (left C, right the atlas). Bottom, left: the slice of the resampled atlas corresponding to the top left image after non rigid spline registration.

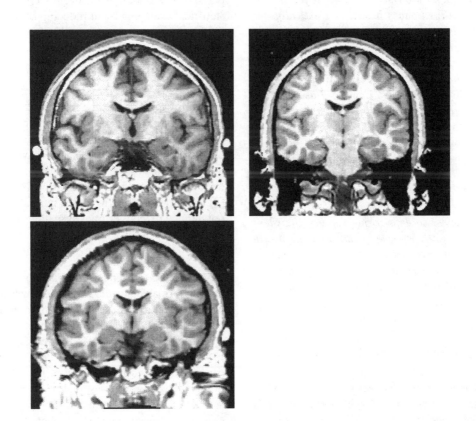

Figure 5. Top: two frontal slices of same index coming from the same images than the ones shown figures 3 and 4 (left C, right the atlas). Bottom, left: the slice of the resampled atlas corresponding to the top left image after non rigid spline registration.

Nonlinear Registration of Brain Images Using Deformable Models

Christos Davatzikos
Neuroimaging Laboratory
Department of Radiology
Johns Hopkins School of Medicine
600 N. Wolfe street, Baltimore MD 21287
hristos@welchlink.welch.jhu.edu
http://ditzel.rad.jhu.edu

Abstract

A key issue in several brain imaging applications, including computer aided neurosurgery, functional image analysis, and morphometrics, is the spatial normalization and registration of tomographic images from different subjects. This paper proposes a technique for spatial normalization of brain images based on elastically deformable models. In our approach we use a deformable surface algorithm to find a parametric representation of the outer cortical surface and then use this representation to obtain a map between corresponding regions of the outer cortex in two different images. Based on the resulting map we then derive a three-dimensional elastic warping transformation which brings two images in register. This transformation models images as inhomogeneous elastic objects which are deformed into registration with each other by external force fields. The elastic properties of the images can vary from one region to the other, allowing more variable brain regions, such as the ventricles, to deform more freely than less variable ones. Finally, we use prestrained elasticity to model structural irregularities, and in particular the ventricular expansion occuring with aging or diseases. The performance of our algorithm is demonstrated on magnetic resonance images.

1 Introduction

A main problem in the cross-subject analysis of brain images is morphological variability. Spatial normalization is a geometric transformation of images which reduces inter-subject differences in brain shape, thereby improving the accuracy of the analysis of superimposed images from different individuals. This paper describes a spatial normalization technique, based on deformable models.

Spatial normalization plays an important role in image guided neurosurgery, since it allows the accurate superposition of multiple anatomical atlases over patient data, thereby assisting in the planning and execution of a surgical procedure. Also, it is important in structural [6] and functional [9] stereotaxis, in which the accurate localization of structural and functional regions of interest depends largely on whether or not images from different subjects are *in register*. Morphological variability can severely confound the results of statistical averaging by introducing an artificial variance in the location and shape of specific functional regions of interest.

Several methodologies for spatial normalization have been proposed in the literature. In [1, 2] a number of landmarks in two images to be registered is defined manually, and a spline transformation matching these landmarks is used to register the images. Normalization techniques based on maximizing similarity measures have been developed by the groups in the University of Pennsylvania [10], Washington University [13], and Montreal Neurological Institute [3]. Other approaches to spatial normalization are based on polynomial or Fourier transformations [7, 8]. Also related is the work in [17] which uses a sequence of increasingly localized transformations to register the surface of the skull.

The approach proposed in this paper is based on elastically deformable models with inhomogeneous elastic properties. Specifically, we first use a deformable surface algorithm to obtain a parametric representation of the outer cortical surface. Based on this representation, geometric features of the cortical surface, such as various curvatures, can be determined and used for the identification and matching of sulci, gyri, fissures, and other distinct cortical characteristics. We then use this mathematical representation to establish a one-to-one map between the three-dimensional images of two individuals, which is subsequently used to obtain a 3D warping of one image into registration with another, by solving the equations governing the deformation of an inhomogeneous elastic object. An internal uniform strain causes the expansion of the ventricles, a phenomenon typically found in elderly individuals.

94

2 Methods

2.1 Overview

Elastic warping transformations have several features which make them suitable to the problem of spatial normalization. Most importantly, they are smooth transformations which tend to preserve the relative positions of anatomical structures, while offering a high flexibility to allow for considerable inter-subject variability. The warping transformation described herein is driven by an external force field defined on a number of distinct anatomical surfaces, which can be either open or closed. In this paper we will use two such surfaces: the outer cortical boundary and the ventricular boundary. In Section 4 we discuss the extension of our method to include additional surfaces (see also [18]). In our approach, each of these surfaces in one of two images to be registered is warped toward its configuration in the other image. This surface deformation then drives a three-dimensional elastic warping of the rest of the image.

In Section 2.2 we focus on the outer cortical surface. In order to define the external forces that deform the outer cortical surface in one image to that in another, we first establish a map between the outer cortex in the two images. We do this by first finding a parametric representation of the outer cortex using a deformable surface algorithm, and then finding the deformation that brings two outer cortical surfaces into registration. We decompose this deformation into two components. The first is a *homothetic map* consisting of a uniform stretching or shrinking followed by an arbitrary bending; this component accounts for overall shape differences and brings the outer cortex in gross correspondence across subjects. The second component is a nonuniform stretching or shrinking, which does not alter the overall outer cortical shape; this component accounts for inter-subject variability of the cortical folds and attempts to bring individual features (sulci, gyri, lobes, etc.) into better registration.

2.2 Outer Cortical Mapping

Our deformable surface algorithm, which finds a map between the outer cortical surfaces in two images, is described below. A more detailed description of the algorithm can be found in [4].

2.2.1 Deformable Surface Algorithm

Throughout our development we will assume that the tomographic images have been preprocessed. Resulting from this preprocessing is a *mass function* $m(\mathbf{x}) \in [0, 1]$, which has high value on the boundary of a structure of interest. In the experiments herein we use a binary mass function, which

is determined via a threshold-based seeded region growing, in conjunction with an erosion and a conditional dilation which extract the brain tissue and strip off tissues which are not of interest (e.g. skull, skin, fat, etc). The region growing is initialized in the interior of a structure of interest (e.g. parenchyma, ventricles, etc.) and terminates on the boundary of the structure where the mass $m(\cdot)$ is set equal to unity.

Having described the mass function, we now turn our attention to the deformable surface. It is a closed surface, denoted $\mathbf{x}(u,v) = (x(u,v), y(u,v), z(u,v))$, where as customary in the differential geometry literature [14] the variables u and v are defined on a planar domain $\mathcal{D}$. The deformable surface is initialized at a spherical configuration surrounding the cortex, and shrinks like an elastic balloon wraping around the cortex, being attracted by the outer cortical mass described above. In its final configuration, the deformable surface provides a parametric description of the outer cortical surface which will be used in the following sections.

2.2.2 Overall Shape Matching

Consider two volumetric images to be registered, referred to as $\mathcal{V}_1$ and $\mathcal{V}_2$. By applying the deformable surface algorithm to each image separately we obtain a parameterization of the outer cortex in the two images, denoted $\mathbf{x}_1(u,v)$ and $\mathbf{x}_2(u,v)$, respectively. We next determine a deformation of the outer cortical surface in $\mathcal{V}_1$ which brings it into correspondence with that in $\mathcal{V}_2$. We decompose this deformation into two components: the first is described in this section and the second is described in Section 2.2.3. The first component is a nearly homothetic map between the two outer cortical surfaces (i.e. an isometry together with a global scaling). This map consists of a uniform stretching or shrinking of the outer cortex in $\mathcal{V}_1$ followed by an arbitrary bending which changes its overall shape. This component matches the overall shape of the brains in $\mathcal{V}_1$ and $\mathcal{V}_2$, but it does not match individual features such as sulci and gyri.

A 2D analog of a homothetic deformation is shown in Fig. 1. In this example, a uniform stretching followed by

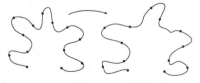

Figure 1. A homothetic deformation consists of a uniform stretching or shrinking followed by an arbitrary bending.

an arbitrary bending was applied to the left curve in Fig. 1

and deformed it to the right curve in Fig. 1. If a number of points, $p_1, p_2, \ldots, p_N$, are evenly spaced along the left curve in Fig. 1, and an equal number of points, $q_1, q_2, \ldots, q_N$, are evenly spaced along the right curve in Fig. 1, then a map corresponding $p_i, i = 1, \ldots, N$, to $q_i, i = 1, \ldots, N$, is a homothetic map between the two curves. Analogously in 3D, if a regular grid[1], $p_{ij}, i, j = 1, \ldots, N$, is placed on one surface and a regular grid, $q_{ij}, i, j = 1, \ldots, N$, is placed on a second surface, then the map that corresponds $p_{i,j}$ to q_{ij} is a homothetic map between the two surfaces (see, for example, Fig. 6).

The motivation behind seeking a homothetic map between the outer cortex in two brain images is that, although different brains have different shapes, their underlying structure is similar, i.e. the relative positions of sulci and gyri with respect to each other are fairly consistent. For example, in Fig. 1 the two curves, which can be viewed as hypothetical cortical folds, have a very similar structure, although the orientations of their folds differ. Therefore, the homothetic map brings homologous regions in the two curves in register.

We find a nearly-homothetic map between two outer cortical surfaces using an iterative procedure which minimizes metric and angular distortion (see [4] for details). In the experiments in Section 3.1 we demonstrate that homothetic mapping accounts for the overall differences in the shape of the brain, and brings images from different subjects into a gross anatomical correspondence. It should be noted, however, that it does not account for inter-subject variability in the relative position of individual cortical folds. In order to account for this variability, in the following section we describe a procedure which refines the homothetic map, by matching individual cortical features.

2.2.3 Curvature matching

In order to match individual cortical features between the outer cortex in $\mathcal{V}_1$ and the outer cortex in $\mathcal{V}_2$, we use the curvature and depth maps of the cortex at various scales, which provide complementary information about the cortical structure, as it was shown in [4]. For example, global features, such as the cortical fissures, the temporal lobes, and the occipital poles, can be identified along the outer cortex from the minimum, maximum, and Gaussian curvatures, respectively, at a coarse scale. Cortical sulci and gyri can be identified from the minimum and maximum curvatures, respectively, at a finer scale.

In order to obtain a match between the curvatures of $\mathbf{x}_1(\cdot, \cdot)$ and $\mathbf{x}_2(\cdot, \cdot)$ that is better than that resulting from the homothetic map, we seek a *reparameterization*, $\mathbf{r}(u, v)$, of $\mathbf{x}_1(\cdot, \cdot)$, which brings its geometric structure into better agreement with that of $\mathbf{x}_2(\cdot, \cdot)$. Let κ_M, κ_m, and κ_G denote

the maximum, minimum, and Gaussian curvatures, respectively. The reparameterization $\mathbf{r}(u, v)$ is a smooth map of the domain $\mathcal{D}$, on which the deformable surface is defined, onto itself (see, for example, Fig. 9c which shows the curvature of a reparameterization of Fig. 9a). We find this reparameterization by elastically deforming $\mathcal{D}$ under the influence of an external force field comprised of two components, $\mathbf{f}_1$ and $\mathbf{f}_2$. The first component attempts to minimize the squared difference between the curvatures, at the coarse scale, of the reparameterized surface $\mathbf{x}_1(\mathbf{r}(u, v))$ and the target surface $\mathbf{x}_2(u, v)$:

$$\iint_{\mathcal{D}} \left\{ \left[\kappa_1^M(\mathbf{r}(u,v)) - \kappa_2^M(u,v) \right]^2 + \left[\kappa_1^m(\mathbf{r}(u,v)) - \kappa_2^m(u,v) \right]^2 \right.$$
$$\left. + \left[\kappa_1^G(\mathbf{r}(u,v)) - \kappa_2^G(u,v) \right]^2 \right\} du\, dv\, .$$

Accordingly, $\mathbf{f}_1$ is defined as follows:

$$\begin{aligned} \mathbf{f}_1(u, v) = \ & -\nabla_{\mathbf{r}} \kappa_1^M(\mathbf{r}(u,v)) \left[\kappa_1^M(\mathbf{r}(u,v)) - \kappa_2^M(u,v) \right] \\ & -\nabla_{\mathbf{r}} \kappa_1^m(\mathbf{r}(u,v)) \left[\kappa_1^m(\mathbf{r}(u,v)) - \kappa_2^m(u,v) \right] - \\ & \nabla_{\mathbf{r}} \kappa_1^G(\mathbf{r}(u,v)) \left[\kappa_1^G(\mathbf{r}(u,v)) - \kappa_2^G(u,v) \right]\, . (1) \end{aligned}$$

The second component, $\mathbf{f}_2$, of the external force field attempts to match fine cortical features, such as sulci and gyri, which are identified using the curvature and depth cortical maps at finer scale. In our current formulation we use the minimum curvature, which reflects the shape and location of the cortical sulci. In particular, we first obtain a flattened representation (two-dimensional image) of the minimum curvature of the outer cortex. This image is defined in the domain $\mathcal{D}$. The location and shape of the sulci are easily identified on this 2D cortical map since the minimum curvature has high value (see, for example, Fig. 9). Based on the curvature map we then manually outline a number, N, of sulci and fissures. Subsequently, these outlines are parameterized by constant speed parameterizations [14], or by piece-wise constant speed parameterizations if sulcal landmarks can be identified. Let $\mathbf{s}_1^i(l)$ and $\mathbf{s}_2^i(l)$, $i = 1, \ldots, N$, be the N pairs of the resulting parametric representations of corresponding sulci on the two outer cortical surfaces to be matched. Here, as l sweeps the unit interval, $\mathbf{s}_1^i(l) \in \mathcal{D}$ and $\mathbf{s}_2^i(l) \in \mathcal{D}$ sweep the two corresponding sulci. The force $\mathbf{f}_2$ attempts to minimize the following measure:

$$\sum_{i=1}^{N} \int_0^1 \| \mathbf{r}(\mathbf{s}_1^i(l)) - \mathbf{s}_2^i(l) \|^2 dl\, .$$

Effectively, $\mathbf{f}_2$ seeks a reparameterization $\mathbf{r}(u, v)$ of the domain $\mathcal{D}$ that satisfies the N sulcal maps:

$$\mathbf{r}(\mathbf{s}_1^i(l)) \longrightarrow s_2^i(l), \ i = 1, \ldots, N, \ l \in [0, 1]\, .$$

Accordingly, $\mathbf{f}_2$ is defined as

$$\mathbf{f}_2(\mathbf{s}_1^i(l)) = -\sum_{i=1}^{N} [\mathbf{r}(\mathbf{s}_1^i(l)) - \mathbf{s}_2^i(l)] \qquad (2)$$

---

[1]A regular grid has points evenly spaced and its horizontal and vertical curves intersect at right angles.

along the N sulci, and zero elsewhere in $\mathcal{D}$.

Having defined the external force fields, $\mathbf{f}_1$ and $\mathbf{f}_2$, we are now in position to write the equations governing the elastic deformation of $\mathcal{D}$ onto itself (see also [5]):

$$\lambda_r \Delta \mathbf{r}(u,v) + (\lambda_r + \mu_r)\nabla \mathrm{Div} \mathbf{r}(u,v) + \mathbf{f}_1(u,v) + \mathbf{f}_2(u,v) = 0, \tag{3}$$

where λ_r and μ_r are the Lame moduli in this (2D) elastic deformation. These equations are discretized and solved using successive overralaxation with Chebyshev acceleration.

Resulting from the procedures described in Sections 2.2.2 and 2.2.3 is a map, $\mathcal{X}$, from the outer cortical surface in $\mathcal{V}_1$ to the outer cortical surface in $\mathcal{V}_2$:

$$\mathcal{X} : \mathcal{V}_1 \ni \mathbf{x}_1(\mathbf{r}(u,v)) \longrightarrow \mathbf{x}_2(u,v) \in \mathcal{V}_2, \tag{4}$$

with

$$\mathbf{r}(u,v), (u,v) \in \mathcal{D}.$$

This map will be used in the following section to derive a 3D transformation of $\mathcal{V}_1$ to $\mathcal{V}_2$.

2.3 3D Elastic Warping

General Framework. We now describe our spatial normalization procedure which uses the outer cortical map $\mathcal{X}$, derived as described in the previous section, to obtain a full 3D normalization transformation. In this procedure, we first deform the outer cortex $\mathcal{V}_1$ to its corresponding configuration in $\mathcal{V}_2$, as prescribed by $\mathcal{X}$. We then let the remaining image warp, following the equations governing the deformation of an elastic body under an external force field. By varying the elasticity properties throughout the images we allow certain structures to deform more freely than others. Moreover, by using a nonzero strain energy at the reference configuration we allow certain structures (e.g. ventricles) to naturally expand. The details of this transformation are described below.

A spatial normalization transformation is a function $\mathbf{U}(\cdot)$ which maps a point $\mathbf{x}$ in $\mathcal{V}_1$ to a point $\mathbf{U}(\mathbf{x})$ in $\mathcal{V}_2$. Let $q(\mathbf{x})$ be an indicator function being unity on the outer cortex in $\mathcal{V}_1$ and zero everywhere else. Let, also, $\mathbf{g}(\mathbf{x})$ be the point on the outer cortex in $\mathcal{V}_2$ to which a point $\mathbf{x}$ on the outer cortex in $\mathcal{V}_1$ is mapped through $\mathcal{X}$. In our algorithm we obtain the transformation $\mathbf{U}(\cdot)$ everywhere in $\mathcal{V}_1$ by solving the equations governing the deformation of an inhomogeneous elastic body with nonzero initial strain, which are derived below.

Let λ and μ be the (spatially varying) elasticity parameters (known as the Lame moduli [12]), and let $\mathbf{E}$ denote the strain tensor[2]. In linear elasticity, $\mathbf{E}$ is given by

$$\mathbf{E} = \frac{1}{2}(\nabla \mathbf{u} + \nabla \mathbf{u}^{\mathrm{T}}) + \mathbf{E}_0, \tag{5}$$

---

[2] As customary in the continuum mechanics notation, we will omit the dependencies of the functions and the tensors on $\mathbf{x}$.

where $\mathbf{u} = \mathbf{u}(\mathbf{x}) = \mathbf{U}(\mathbf{x}) - \mathbf{x}$ is the displacement field from the reference configuration to the deformed configuration. The purpose of the reference strain $\mathbf{E}_0$, which is nonzero in the ventricles, is to cause a uniform ventricular expansion of the reference image, and it is explained in detail later in this section. The strain tensor $\mathbf{E}_0$ is precisely given by

$$\mathbf{E}_0 = \epsilon(\mathbf{x})\mathbf{I}, \tag{6}$$

where

$$\epsilon(\mathbf{x}) = \begin{cases} \epsilon_0 & , \quad \mathbf{x} \text{ belongs to the ventricles}, \\ 0 & , \quad \text{otherwise}. \end{cases}$$

The indicator function of the ventricles is found by the same procedure as the one used in Section 2.2.1 for extracting the mass function $m(\cdot)$.

Under linear elasticity, the Piola-Kirchhoff stress tensor is given by

$$\mathbf{S} = 2\lambda\mathbf{E} + \mu \, tr(\mathbf{E})\mathbf{I}, \tag{7}$$

and the equations governing the deformation of $\mathcal{V}_1$ are [12]

$$\mathbf{F} + \mathrm{Div}\mathbf{S} = 0. \tag{8}$$

Here, Div denotes the divergence of a tensor in the reference configuration, and $\mathbf{F}$ is the total external force field acting on $\mathcal{V}_1$ and is described later in this section.

In order to find $\mathrm{Div}\mathbf{S}$ we use (7) and the fact that

$$\mathrm{Div}(\phi\mathbf{S}) = \phi\mathrm{Div}\mathbf{S} + \mathbf{S}\nabla\phi, \tag{9}$$

where ϕ is a scalar function and $\mathbf{S}$ is a tensor. Inserting (7) into (8), using (9), and after some algebra, we obtain the following equilibrium equations:

$$\mathbf{F} + \lambda\Delta\mathbf{U} + (\lambda + \mu)\nabla\mathrm{Div}\mathbf{U} \quad + $$
$$(\nabla\mathbf{U} + \nabla\mathbf{U}^{\mathrm{T}} - 2\mathbf{I})\nabla\lambda + (\mathrm{Div}\mathbf{U} - 3)\nabla\mu \quad + $$
$$\epsilon(2\nabla\lambda + 3\nabla\mu) + (2\lambda + 3\mu)\nabla\epsilon \quad = \quad 0. \tag{10}$$

The first row in (10) is identical to the left hand side of the Navier equations [12], the second row results from the material inhomogeneity, and the third row results from the strain $\mathbf{E}_0$. The equations in (10) are discretized and solved using successive overrelaxation [11].

External Forces. We now turn our attention to the external force field, $\mathbf{F}$, acting on the reference image. It is comprised of two components. The first component is equal to

$$\mathbf{g}(\mathbf{x}) - \mathbf{U}(\mathbf{x}), \tag{11}$$

and it is applied to the outer cortical surface in $\mathcal{V}_1$ deforming it to its homologous in $\mathcal{V}_2$; this component favors 3D deformations which satisfy the outer cortical map $\mathcal{X}$. The second component, denoted by $\mathbf{b}(\cdot)$, is an internal force field which is active in the interior of the brain and its purpose is to bring internal brain structures in better alignment. In our current formulation, $\mathbf{b}(\cdot)$ is applied to the ventricular boundaries, and it tends to align the ventricular boundaries of the warped $\mathcal{V}_1$ image and the target image $\mathcal{V}_2$. Specifically, the force applied to a point $\mathbf{x}$ on the ventricular boundary in $\mathcal{V}_1$ is equal to (see Fig. 2)

$$\mathbf{b}(\mathbf{U}(\mathbf{x})) = w(\mathbf{x})\left[\mathbf{c}_v(\mathbf{U}(\mathbf{x})) - \mathbf{U}(\mathbf{x})\right] , \quad (12)$$

where $\mathbf{c}_v(\mathbf{U}(\mathbf{x}))$ is the center of the ventricular boundary mass in $\mathcal{V}_2$ included in the neighborhood of the point $\mathbf{U}(\mathbf{x})$. The weight $w(\cdot)$ is given by

$$w(\mathbf{x}) = \langle \mathbf{N}_1(\mathbf{U}(\mathbf{x})), \mathbf{N}_2(\mathbf{U}(\mathbf{x})) \rangle ,$$

on the ventricular boundaries in $\mathcal{V}_1$ and zero elsewhere. Here, $\mathbf{N}_1(\cdot)$ is the outward normal along the ventricular boundary of the deformed reference image $\mathcal{V}_1$ and $\mathbf{N}_2(\cdot)$ is the outward normal of the ventricular boundary of $\mathcal{V}_2$. The weight $w(\cdot)$ measures the co-orientation of the deformed and the target ventricular boundaries; boundaries that are similarly oriented tend to be attracted more strongly to each other. The radius of the neighborhood in (12) is determined

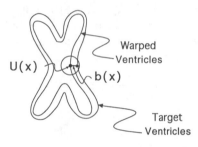

Figure 2. The ventricular force tends to align the warped and the target ventricular boundaries.

by adaptively growing a spherical neighborhood around a point on the ventricular boundary of the deformed reference image until it intersects enough ventricular boundary points of the target image. The ventricular boundary points in both images are obtained as described in Section 2.2.1.

The ventricular force $\mathbf{b}(\cdot)$ in (12) vanishes when the two ventricular boundaries are coincident, and therefore it tends to bring them into alignment.

Material Inhomogeneity. We propose the use of inhomogeneous elastic material primarily because different brain structures tend to have different variability. Accordingly, more variable structures should be allowed to deform more freely than less variable ones. To illustrate the effect of material inhomogeneities on the elastic transformation, we created two synthetic images with two hypothetical cortical folds, shown in Fig. 3. The two images in Figs. 3a and

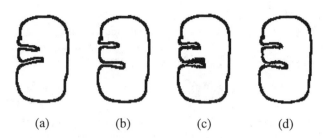

Figure 3. A demonstration of the effect of material inhomogeneity. (a), (b) Two synthetic images. (c), (d) The elastic warping of (a) towards (b) using homogeneous material (c), and inhomogeneous material (d) with higher elasticity in the white region.

3b are identical except for the difference in the orientation of the two folds. We warped Fig. 3a to Fig. 3b using a homogeneous elastic material throughout the brain, and we obtained the result shown in Fig. 3c. We then warped Fig. 3a to Fig. 3b using an inhomogeneous elastic material and obtained the result shown in Fig. 3d. The apparent stretching of the cortex in Fig. 3c was eliminated in Fig. 3d by using a more flexible elastic material in the white region, which allowed the folds to deform more freely.

Ventricular Strain. The ventricular forces in Fig. 2 align the ventricular boundaries, provided that they are in proximity to each other. This is not always the case, however, especially in elderly or diseased brains in which often dramatic ventricular enlargements are present. The uniform strain $\mathbf{E}_0$ accounts for such gross morphological irregularities. To demonstrate this, in Fig. 4 we show a cross-sectional MR image from an elderly individual with considerable ventricular enlargement (left) and its transformation after applying a uniform ventricular strain (right).

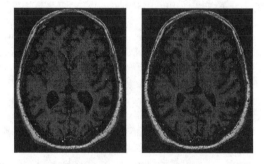

Figure 4. An MR image from an individual with ventricular enlargement (left) and its transformation after applying a uniform strain within the ventricles (right).

The volumetric change imposed by a uniform strain depends, in general, on the shape of the ventricles and on their volume relative to the brain tissue. However, we have determined experimentally from images with a wide variety of ventricular sizes and shapes that the volumetric change is approximately linear, as shown in Fig 5. Based on this relationship and on the ratio of ventricular volumes of the reference and target images we determine the appropriate strain magnitude. We note that the further fine alignment

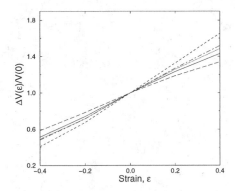

Figure 5. The volumetric change resulting from the application of a uniform strain of magnitude ϵ in the ventricles, for five randomly selected images with a variety of ventricular sizes and shapes.

of the ventricular boundaries is obtained through the force $\mathbf{b}(\cdot)$.

3 Experiments

Homothetic Mapping In our first experiment we test our hypothesis thated homothetic mapping brings homologous cortical regions in rough correspondence. In this experiment we randomly selected six MR volumetric images and applied the procedures of Section 2.2.1 and 2.2.2. A 3D rendering, viewed from the bottom and the top, of the resulting surfaces is shown in Fig. 6. Corresponding regions in the surfaces in Fig. 6 are found using the grid shown superimposed on the surfaces. A subset of the grid lines has been assigned letters so that the reader can identify individual corresponding points.

Fig. 6 shows that homothetic mapping results in a good correspondence of the cortical regions. Landmarks such as the interhemispherical fissure, the anterior-most part of the frontal lobe, the occipital poles, the bottom part of the temporal lobes, the central sulcus and adjacent gyri, the superior frontal sulcus, and others, fall in consistent locations in the grid. Therefore, homothetic mapping does not only match the overall shape of the brain (by mapping outer cortex to outer cortex), but provides a reasonably good correspondence of features as well.

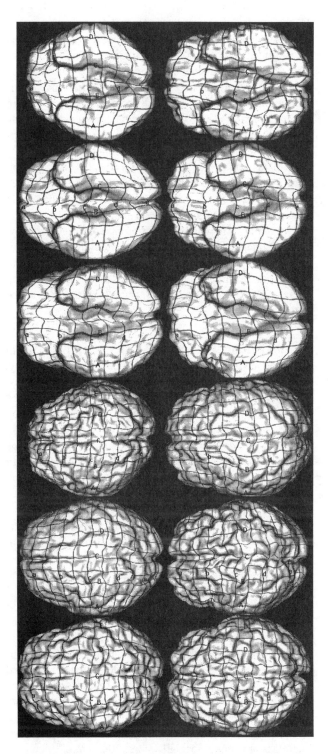

Figure 6. The result of the deformable surface algorithm applied to six randomly selected individuals, viewd from the bottom and from the top. The superimposed labeled grid shows that homothetic mapping brings the cortical regions into rough correspondence.

Elastic Warping. In our second experiment we tested the performance of our elastic warping transformation by registering two MR volumetric images. One of the images was taken from an elderly individual with considerable ventricular enlargement. We applied the deformable surface algorithm obtaining a map from the outer cortex of the individual without ventricular enlargement to the one with ventricular enlargement (target dataset). We then applied the elastic warping procedure using the external force field of (11) and (12), and using $\lambda = 2\mu = 10^{-1}$ everywhere except for the ventricles in which the lower values $\lambda = 2\mu = 2.5 \times 10^{-2}$ were used. The ventricular strain was $\epsilon_0 = 0.3$ (causing an outward expansion). The result is shown in Fig. 7, in which four different cross-sections of the original image, of the warped image, and of the target image are shown superimposed on the cortical and ventricular outlines of the target image. Notable is the good registration in the peri-ventricular region, despite the difference in the ventricular size.

Manual Sulcal Matching. In our third experiment we tested the procedure for curvature-based sulcal matching, described in Section 2.2.3. In this experiment we registered two MR volumetric images, by first using only homothetic mapping, as in the previous experiment. A cross-section of the warped MR image, showing the central sulcus, using only homothetic mapping is shown superimposed on the cortical outline of the target MR image in Fig. 7a. Although a good overall registration is apparent, the central sulcus and the adjacent gyri are mismatched by several millimeters (see arrows in Fig. 8a).

We next calculated the minimum curvature along the outer cortex of each of the two images, which we show in Fig. 9a and Fig. 9b superimposed on the flattened outer cortical surface. In this figure, the outer cortex is viewed from above; the top of the images corresponds to the anterior of the brain and the bottom to the posterior. Based on these curvature maps, and assisted by the 3D rendering of the curvature superimposed on the non-flattened cortex, shown in Fig. 10, we outlined the central sulcus and the interhemispherical fissure. We then elastically deformed the flattened outer cortex in Fig. 9a by matching the outlined central sulcus and interhemispherical fissure, as described in Section 2.2.3. The deformed curvature map is shown in Fig. 9c. A better agreement between the curvatures in Fig. 9b and Fig. 9c is apparent, especially around the central sulcus and the inter-hemispherical fissure (the thick vertically oriented bright curve in the images in Fig. 9).

Finally, we applied our 3D elastic warping transforming the first dataset to the second (target) dataset. A cross-section of the resulting image, taken from the same level as in Fig. 8a, is shown in Fig. 8b. This figure shows a better match of the regions around the central sulcus. It is worth

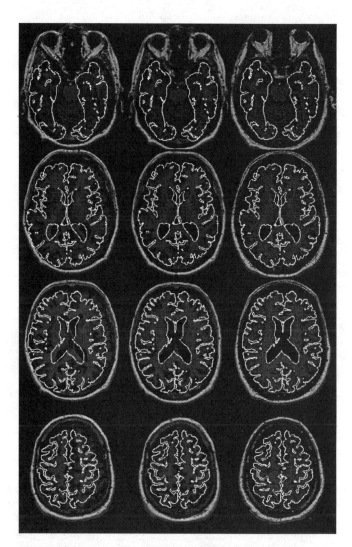

Figure 7. Cross sections from four different levels of the brain. On the left the cross-sections of the unwarped image are shown superimposed on the cortical and ventricular outlines of the target image and in the middle the cross-sections of the warped image are shown superimposed on the same outlines. For comparison purposes, on the right the same outlines are shown superimposed on the cross-sections of the target image, from which they were extracted.

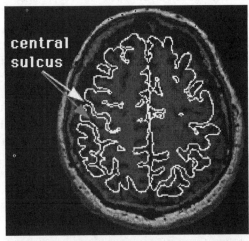

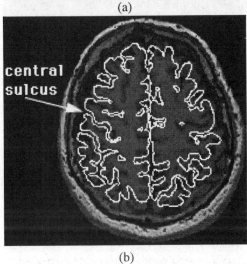

Figure 8. A cross-section from the top of the brain including the central sulcus. The cross-section in (a) is from the warped MR image using only homothetic mapping. The cross-section in (b) is from the warped image using homothetic mapping followed by curvature-based matching of the central sulcus and the interhemispherical fissure. A considerable improvement in the region around the central sulcus is apparent. Note that besides the central sulcus, the pre- and post-central sulci and adjacent gyri are also aligned much better in (b) than in (a).

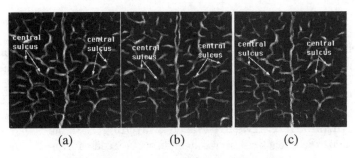

Figure 9. The curvature maps of the outer cortex (the minimum curvature superimposed on the flattened outer cortical surface) for (a) the first and (b) the second (target) image used in the third experiment in Section 3. In (c) we show the elastically warped map in (a) obtained by matching the central sulcus and the interhemispherical line (shown as thick vertically oriented curve in all images). A better agreement of the curvatures in (c) and (b) is apparent, compared to that between (a) and (b).

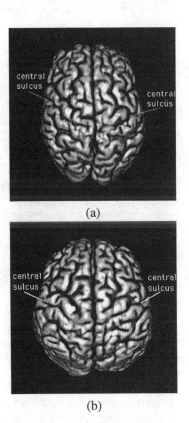

Figure 10. The minimum curvature of the outer cortex shown (dark) superimposed on the outer cortex: (a) corresponds to the map in Fig. 9a and (b) corresponds to the map in Fig. 9b.

101

noting that not only the central sulcus, but the adjacent sulci and gyri are better matched in Fig. 8b. This is because the elastic warping of the curvature maps allowed the sulci and gyri neighboring the central sulcus to "slide" along the outer cortical surface and match their counterparts in the target image.

Automatic Curvature-Based Matching. In our final experiment we show results from our procedure for automatic curvature-based reparameterization of the outer cortical surface. In this experiment we randomly selected two MR volumetric images, we applied the deformable surface algorithm, and calculated the minimum and the maximum curvatures at coarse scale (the deformable surface was sampled with 5,000 points). The top row in Fig. 11 shows the maximum curvature for the bottom half of the cortex (left), and the minimum curvature for the top half (middle) and bottom half (right) of the cortex, for the first image (the top of the images corresponds to the anterior of the cortex and the bottom to the posterior). The analogous curvatures for the second image are shown in the bottom row. The max-

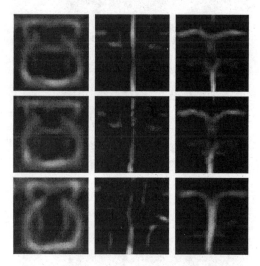

Figure 11. Top and bottom rows: Minimum and maximum curvatures of the outer cortex from two volumetric images. Middle row: the same curvatures of the reparameterized surface corresponding to the top row.

imum curvature reflects the shape of the "rim" formed by the bottom parts of the temporal and occipital lobes, and the anterior part of the frontal lobes. The minimum curvature of the top half shows the interhemispherical fissure (bright vertically oriented curve in Fig. 11, middle column) and the minimum curvature of the bottom shows the gap between the left and right temporal lobes where the cerebelum is located (bright vertically oriented region, right column) and the anterior edge of the Sylvian fissure for the two hemispheres (the two horizontally oriented bright curves, right

column).

We used these three curvatures to find a reparameterization according to the procedure described in Section 2.2.3. The curvatures of the reparameterized surface corresponding to the top row are shown in the middle row of Fig. 11. It is apparent that the shapes of the curvatures of the top row have now adapted to better match those of the bottom row. Notable is the adaptation of the posterior part of the interhemispherical fissure (bottom part of the bright region in the middle and right images, middle row). We note that the reparameterization was derived by combining all these curvatures (see Equation (1)).

4   Discussion

We have presented a new technique for spatial normalization of images. Our methodology is based on an outer cortical mapping between two images to be registered, which is used to drive a three-dimensional elastic warping of the images. An internal force applied to the ventricular boundaries brings the ventricles and the surrounding structures in better correspondence. The spatially varying elasticity allows certain structures, such as the ventricles, to deform more freely than others. Finally, a uniform strain applied to the ventricles causes their expansion, allowing the external forces to better align the ventricular boundaries.

We tested our technique by registering MR images. In particular, we showed that homothetic mapping brings homologous outer cortical regions in good correspondence, thereby determining a large number of corresponding regions in a highly automated way. We obtained such a map by using a deformable surface algorithm, which yields a mathematical representation of the outer cortical surface. We used the correspondences determined by homothetic mapping to elastically warp images into register with each other.

Despite the overall good registration obtained using homothetic mapping, there is still a considerable localization error, which is largely due to anatomical variability in individual brain features. Specifically, although homothetic mapping accounts for an arbitrary bending of the brain boundary, it allows only a uniform expansion or contraction of the outer cortical surface. Equivalently, it accounts for any overall shape differences of the brain but it assumes that an observer sitting on the outer cortical surface sees the same cortical folding pattern in all individuals. This assumption is the main limitation of homothetic mapping, given the inter-subject variability of the cortical folding pattern.

To overcome this limitation we developed a procedure which refines the homothetic map, and allows a non-uniform stretching or shrinking of the outer cortical surface by matching features identified through the curvature maps. By using the resulting map in our 3D elastic warping, we demonstrated a considerable improvement in the registration accuracy in the neighborhood of the features used. More notable was the improvement in the registration around the central sulcus (improvement of $\sim$ 5mm). The non-uniform mapping allowed the central sulcus and the neighboring sulci and gyri to slide along the outer cortical surface and match their counterparts in the target image.

In our experiments we also tested the performance of our spatial normalization technique on pathological cases, obtaining a good registration around the ventricles through an elastic stretching of the ventricular boundaries. An accurate registration in the peri-ventricular region of the brain, and especially in the thalamic region, is of great importance in computer-aided neurosurgery. It is also important in the analysis of data from elderly populations [15, 19, 16], which often have substantial ventricular enlargement.

Several extensions of our basic technique are possible. In particular, in this paper we focused on the alignment of the outer cortical and the ventricular boundaries. In addition to these surfaces, internal cortical features, such as the sulcal surfaces, can be used for matching of the deep parts of the cortex. Current research in our laboratory in that direction focuses on the modeling the deep sulcal surfaces as ribbons, which can be matched based on their differential geometric properties, and are reported in a separate paper [18].

Extensions to our procedure for sulcal matching are also possible. In particular, a main focus of our current and future research is the development of an automatic sulcal identification and matching technique, assisted by prior probability distributions reflecting our expectation about the location and shape of the cortical folds.

5 Acknowledgements

The author would like to thank Nick Bryan for his support to this work, Meiyappan Solaiyappan from ISS for providing the surface rendering software, and Wayne Lawton and Tim Poston from ISS for their insightful discussions on elasticity theory. This work was partially supported by the NIH grants NIH-AG-93-07 and 1R01 AG13743-01.

References

[1] F. Bookstein. Principal warps: Thin-plate splines and the decomposition of deformations. *IEEE Trans. on Pattern Analysis and Machine Intelligence*, 11(6):567–585, 1989.

[2] F. Bookstein. Thin-plate splines and the atlas problem for biomedical images. *Proc. of the 12th Int. Conf. on Inf. Proc. in Med. Imaging*, pages 326–342, 1991.

[3] D. Collins, P. Neelin, T. Peters, and A. Evans. Automatic 3D intersubject registration of MR volumetric data in standardized Talairach space. *J. of Comp. Ass. Tomography*, 18:192–205, 1994.

[4] C. Davatzikos and R. Bryan. Using a deformable surface model to obtain a mathematical representation of the cortex. *Proc. of the IEEE Comp. Vision Symp.*, pages 212–217, Nov. 1995.

[5] C. Davatzikos, J. Prince, and R. Bryan. Image registration based on boundary mapping. *IEEE Trans. on Med. Imaging*, 15(1):112–115, Feb. 1996.

[6] C. Davatzikos, M. Vaillant, S. Resnick, J. Prince, S. Letovsky, and R. Bryan. A computerized approach for morphological analysis of the corpus callosum. *J. of Comp. Assisted Tomography*, 20:88–97, Jan./Feb. 1996.

[7] J. Declerck, G. Subsol, J. Thirion, and N. Ayache. Automatic retrieval of anatomical structures in 3D images. *Proc. of the Conf. on Comp. Vis., Virtual Reality, and Rob. in Med.*, pages 153–162, 1995.

[8] K. Friston, J. Ashburner, C. Frith, J. Poline, J. Heather, and R. Frackowiak. Spatial registration and normalization of images. *Human Brain Mapping*, 1995.

[9] K. Friston, A. Holmes, K. Worsley, J. Poline, C. Frith, and R. Frackowiak. Statistical parametric maps in functional imaging: a general linear approach. *Human Brain Mapping*, pages 189–210, 1995.

[10] J. Gee, M. Reivich, and R. Bajcsy. Elastically deforming 3D atlas to match anatomical brain images. *J. Comp. Assist. Tomogr.*, 17:225–236, 1993.

[11] G. H. Golub and C. F. Van Loan. *Matrix Computations*. The Johns Hopkins University Press, Baltimore, Maryland, 1983.

[12] M. Gurtin. *An Introduction to Continuum Mechanics*. Orlando: Academic Press, 1981.

[13] M. Miller, G. Christensen, Y. Amit, and U. Grenander. Mathematical textbook of deformable neuroanatomies. *Proc. of the National Academy of Sciences*, 90:11944–11948, 1993.

[14] R. Millman and G. Parker. *Elements of Differential Geometry*. Prentice Hall, 1977.

[15] R.N. Bryan et.al. A method for using MR to evaluate the effects of cardiovascular disease of the brain: the cardiovascular health study. *Am. J. Neuroradiology*, 15:1625–1633, 1994.

[16] N. Shock, R. Greulich, R. Andres, D. Arenberg, P. Costa, Jr., E. Lakatta, and J. Tobin. Normal human aging: The Baltimore Longitudinal Study of Aging. *(U.S. Public Health Service Publication No. NIH 84-2450). Washington, D.C.: United States Government Printing Office*, 1984.

[17] G. Subsol, J. Thirion, and N. Ayache. A general scheme for automatically building 3D morphometric anatomical atlases: application to a skull atlas. *INRIA Technical Report N° 2586*, 1995.

[18] M. Vaillant, C. Davatzikos, and R. Bryan. Finding 3D parametric representations of the deep cortical folds. *Proc. of the IEEE Workshop on Mathematical Methods in Biomedical Image Analysis*, June 1996.

[19] S. Whitehead, R. Bryan, S. Letovsky, C. Paik, J. Miller, and J. Gerber. A database for brain structure/function analysis. *Proc. of the Am. Soc. of Neuroradiology Conf.*, page 166, 1994.

Deformations Incorporating Rigid Structures

J. A. Little, D. L. G. Hill & D. J. Hawkes
Division of Radiological Sciences
3rd Floor Guy's Tower
Guy's Hospital
London Bridge
London SE1 9RT
email: {jl,dlgh,djh}@ipg.umds.ac.uk

Abstract

Medical image registration can provide useful clinical information by relating images of the same patient acquired from different modalities, or from serial studies with a single modality. Current algorithms invariably assume that the objects in the images can be treated as a rigid body. In practice, some parts of a patient, usually bony structures, may move as rigid bodies while others may deform. To address this, we have developed a new technique that allows identified objects in the image to move as rigid bodies, while the remainder smoothly deforms. Euclidean distance transforms calculated from the rigid objects are used to weight a linear combination of pre-defined linear transformations, one for each rigid body in the image, and also to form a modified radial basis function. This ensures that the non-linear deformation tends to zero as we move towards the rigid body boundary. The resulting deformation technique is valid in any dimension, subject to the choice of the basis function. We demonstrate this technique in two dimensions on a pattern of rigid square structures to simulate the vertebral bodies of the spine, and on sagittal magnetic resonance images collected from a volunteer.

Keywords: Splines, kriging, radial basis functions, distance transforms, deformable models, image registration.

1. Introduction

In recent years it has become increasingly common to register images of a patient acquired either at different times on the same imaging modality or using multiple imaging modalities for the purposes of clinical evaluation. The majority of methods focus on the head as it is usually valid to assume that the brain will behave as if it is a single rigid body (see [13],[23],[20]). This is, however, rarely the case when matching anatomy outside of the head. Here there is quite often patient deformation between scans and a non-linear approach is more appropriate (see [15]). Even in the head there are cases where the rigid body assumption is not valid, such as that discussed in [10]. Here there was a significant change in the shape of the brain after a surgical procedure to implant subdural electrodes and neither a rigid body nor a non-linear thin-plate spline transformation were satisfactory. A composite approach was used in which the image was segmented into two parts and one part of the image deformed while the other was kept rigid. This led to an improvement but added the problem of discontinuity at the segmented object borders.

Using images to guide interventional procedures is a rapidly growing field. At present the interventionalist usually performs the procedure with only a two dimensional image, typically fluoroscopy, ultrasound or a single slice of computed tomography (CT), for guidance. Often a pre-operative three dimensional scan, either CT or magnetic resonance (MR), is acquired for planning purposes and displaying this matched to the two dimensional image would be advantageous. Between the acquisition of the 3D image and the interventional procedure the patient will almost certainly have moved and may even be lying in a different position and so in order to match the images accurately a deformation must take place.

In principle we could build a model of the patient's anatomy which incorporates sufficient detail on mass, elasticity and viscosity to compute the effect of any distortion to arbitrary accuracy, see for example, [22]. In practice these calculations are very demanding on computational resources and unlikely to provide a solution of sufficient accuracy in the time scale required for interventional work. We therefore have concentrated our efforts on using interpolation to estimate motion and deformation.

At present most deformation techniques assume that all parts of the image being transformed are deformable, in

Proceedings of MMBIA '96

practice, however, this is rarely the case. Medical images, in particular, usually contain some bony material which will not change shape under normal conditions. This has led us to develop an algorithm which allows us to constrain parts of an image to move subject to independent rigid body constraints, while allowing the remainder of the image to deform due to both the rigid body transformations and a deformation due to the transformation of user specified landmark points. We define the rigid structures, or objects, by a segmentation of the image. This is at present a user defined segmentation but the method of segmentation has no bearing on the deformation algorithm. Once the objects are defined, their transformation can be constrained to be any linear transformation, (normally a rigid body).

2. Background theory

This algorithm is formed by the adaptation and combination of three well known methods into one composite form which allows us to constrain portions of an image to move due to a user defined linear transformation. These methods are landmark based interpolation using kriging [14], thin-plate splines [3],[5], or radial basis functions [1],[2], inverse distance weighted interpolation, [19] and distance transforms (DT), [7], in particular a Euclidean distance transform (EDT), [9].

2.1. Point based interpolation

Point based interpolation is useful when we are given sparse data from a multidimensional scalar field and we wish to estimate the value of the field at other spatial locations. For example let us have n sites, $\mathbf{t}_i = (t_i[1], \ldots, t_i[d])^T$, $i = 1, \ldots, n$, in d dimensional space, at each of which we have an observed value x_i. For an interpolating solution we require a function, $f(\mathbf{t})$ say, which maps from $\mathbb{R}^d$ to $\mathbb{R}$ and is exact at the measurement sites, that is that $f(\mathbf{t}_i) = x_i$. There are three methods which have been widely used and lead to the same functional form for the interpolator despite using different underlying assumptions about the form of the scalar field. These are the kriging, thin-plate spline and radial basis function approaches. These solutions are arrived at by using different constraints on the behaviour of the interpolator away from the sites, see [17]. Kriging is a method which provides a best linear unbiased estimate of the solution [8],[14], thin-plate splines minimise a bending energy function [3] and radial basis functions simply provide an exact interpolator at the sites without any minimisation constraints [16].

A general solution for a multi-dimensional scalar field has two components, see [21],[8], a linear combination of monomials and a linear combination of basis functions, $\sigma(\mathbf{t}, \mathbf{t}_i)$ say. The monomials represent an underlying drift or

mean in kriging and the null space of an energy functional in splines. We can form the basis of this drift in the following manner, first define $\mathbf{p} = (p[1], \ldots, p[d])$ to be a multi-index of non-negative integers with size given by $|\mathbf{p}| = p[1] + \cdots + p[d]$ and $\mathbf{t}^{\mathbf{P}} = t[1]^{p[1]} \ldots t[d]^{p[d]}$. The rth order monomial drift is spanned by $\mathbf{t}^{\mathbf{P}}$ for $|\mathbf{p}| \leq r$. We can represent these as $M = \binom{d+r}{d}$ functions, $g_1(\mathbf{t}), \ldots, g_M(\mathbf{t})$. For example for $d = 2$ and a linear drift, $r = 1$, we have $M = 3$ and,

$$g_1(\mathbf{t}) = 1, \ g_2(\mathbf{t}) = t[1], \ g_3(\mathbf{t}) = t[2]. \tag{1}$$

We can write the general form for our interpolating solution as follows, (see [21] page 31),

$$f(\mathbf{t}) = \sum_{j=1}^{M} a_j g_j(\mathbf{t}) + \sum_{j=1}^{n} b_j \sigma(\mathbf{t}, \mathbf{t}_j), \tag{2}$$

Given the constraints, $f(\mathbf{t}_i) = x_i$, the coefficients of (2) are given by the solution to the following set of linear equations,

$$\begin{pmatrix} \Sigma & D \\ D^T & 0 \end{pmatrix} \begin{pmatrix} \mathbf{b} \\ \mathbf{a} \end{pmatrix} = \begin{pmatrix} \mathbf{x} \\ 0 \end{pmatrix}, \tag{3}$$

where

$$\mathbf{x}^T = (x_1, \ldots, x_n),$$
$$\Sigma_{ij} = \sigma(\mathbf{t}_i, \mathbf{t}_j), \ i, j = 1, \ldots, n,$$
$$D_{ij} = g_j(\mathbf{t}_i), \ i = 1, \ldots, n, \ j = 1, \ldots, M$$
$$\mathbf{a}^T = (a_1, \ldots, a_M), \ \mathbf{b}^T = (b_1, \ldots, b_n) \tag{4}$$

The function $\sigma(\mathbf{t}, \mathbf{t}_i)$ can be either a valid kriging covariance which is dependent on a smoothing parameter α and is given by (see [14]),

$$\sigma_\alpha(\mathbf{t}, \mathbf{t}_i) = \begin{cases} |\mathbf{h}|^{2\alpha}, \ \alpha \text{ not an integer} \\ |\mathbf{h}|^{2\alpha} \log |\mathbf{h}|, \ \alpha \text{ an integer} \end{cases} \mathbf{h} \in \mathbb{R}^d,$$

where $\mathbf{h} = \mathbf{t} - \mathbf{t}_i$, or a spline function, see [21] for a list of valid choices for $\sigma(\mathbf{t}, \mathbf{t}_i)$. An important special case is the thin-plate spline (see [3]) which in two dimensions has $\sigma(\mathbf{t}, \mathbf{t}_i) = |\mathbf{h}|^2 \log |\mathbf{h}|$ and for three dimensions has $\sigma(\mathbf{t}, \mathbf{t}_i) = |\mathbf{h}|$. Further, if no assumptions are made about the field then there are a large number of radial basis functions which ensure the conditionally positive definiteness of Σ and hence a solution to (3), see [16].

For image deformation we require a multi-dimensional transformation defined by a set of points or landmarks. Landmarks are points which have a meaning in the context of the problem under study. Homologous landmarks are pairs of points which can be picked accurately from different images of the same or a similar scene. They are usually one of three types either, biological, mathematical or pseudo-landmarks. See [4] for a more detailed discussion of landmark definitions and selection. We now wish to define a deformation based on two sets of homologous landmarks, one on our original image and one on our target or destination image. Our deformation needs to be exact at these landmarks and a smooth transformation elsewhere.

Instead of sites let us have n landmarks $\mathbf{t}_i = (t_i[1], \ldots, t_i[d])^T$ which we wish to transform to new positions $\mathbf{u}_i = (u_i[1], \ldots, u_i[d])^T$ respectively. We can define a general d-dimensional deformation by using d independent interpolators, as defined in (1)-(4), in the following manner,

$$\mathbf{f}(\mathbf{t})^T = (f_1(\mathbf{t}), \ldots, f_d(\mathbf{t})), \tag{5}$$

with constraints,

$$f_1(\mathbf{t}_i) = u_i[1], \ldots, f_d(\mathbf{t}_i) = u_i[d], \ i = 1, \ldots, n, \tag{6}$$

so for any point in the plane we have a deformation given by

$$\mathbf{t} \to (u[1], \ldots, u[d])^T = \mathbf{f}(\mathbf{t}). \tag{7}$$

Where the individual interpolators are given by

$$f_l(\mathbf{t}) = \sum_{j=1}^{M} a_j[l] g_j(\mathbf{t}) + \sum_{j=1}^{n} b_j[l] \sigma(\mathbf{t}, \mathbf{t}_j), \ l = 1, \ldots, d, \tag{8}$$

with coefficients given by

$$\begin{pmatrix} \Sigma & D \\ D^T & 0 \end{pmatrix} \begin{pmatrix} B \\ A \end{pmatrix} = \begin{pmatrix} U \\ 0 \end{pmatrix}, \tag{9}$$

where

$$\Sigma_{ij} = \sigma(\mathbf{t}_i, \mathbf{t}_j),$$
$$A = (\mathbf{a}_1, \ldots, \mathbf{a}_d), \ \mathbf{a}_l = (a_1[l], \ldots, a_M[l])^T,$$
$$l = 1, \ldots, d,$$
$$B = (\mathbf{b}_1, \ldots, \mathbf{b}_d), \ \mathbf{b}_l = (b_1[l], \ldots, b_n[l])^T,$$
$$l = 1, \ldots, d,$$
$$U = (\mathbf{u}_1, \ldots, \mathbf{u}_d), \ \mathbf{u}_l = (u_1[l], \ldots, u_n[l])^T,$$
$$l = 1, \ldots, d,$$
$$D_{ij} = g_j(\mathbf{t}_i), \ i = 1, \ldots, n, \ j = 1, \ldots, M,$$
$$M = \begin{pmatrix} d + r \\ d \end{pmatrix} \tag{10}$$

As before we shall only be using a linear drift so we take $r = 1$ which gives $M = 3$ in two dimensions and $M = 4$ in three dimensions.

2.2. Inverse distance weighted interpolation

Methods using weights based on a distance measure have been used to solve the interpolation problem. The following is a method proposed by Shepard [19], it is a slightly modified version of this that we shall be using later. This method uses a weighted sum of the constraint values, where the weights are dependent on the distances from the observed point to the constraint sites.

Once again we have a set of n sites, $\mathbf{t}_i = (t_i[1], \ldots, t_i[d])^T$, at each of which we have a value, x_i, of our function. Let our transformation from $\mathbb{R}^d \to \mathbb{R}$ be given by,

$$f(\mathbf{t}) = \sum_{i=1}^{n} w_i(\mathbf{t}) x_i \tag{11}$$

where $f(\mathbf{t}_i) = x_i, \ i = 1, \ldots, n$ are our data constraints. In order that our constraints are satisfied we require a set of weights which have the following properties,

$$w_i(\mathbf{t}_i) = 1$$
$$\sum_{i=1}^{n} w_i(\mathbf{t}) = 1 \tag{12}$$
$$w_i(\mathbf{t}) \geq 0, \ i = 1, \ldots, n, \ \mathbf{t} \in \mathbb{R}^d$$

Shepard [19] put forward the following weight function,

$$w_i(\mathbf{t}) = \frac{q_i(\mathbf{t})}{\sum_{j=1}^{n} q_j(\mathbf{t})} \tag{13}$$

where

$$q_i(\mathbf{t}) = \frac{1}{s_i(\mathbf{t})^\mu}, \tag{14}$$

with $s_i(\mathbf{t})$ being the distance from $\mathbf{t}$ to site $\mathbf{t}_i$. The smoothness of this interpolation scheme is governed by the choice of μ. A value of $\mu > 1$ ensures that the first derivative is continuous.

A number, d, of these can be used in the same form as (7) to deform an image but this scheme is not ideal, see [18]. However, as we are not going to use these coefficients to perform the whole deformation these problems are not applicable.

2.3. Distance transforms

Distance transforms (DT) are algorithms developed to allow the distance, or an approximation of the distance, from any pixel to a predefined image feature to be easily obtained. They involve passing a mask over the image a number of times, generating an image in which each pixel contains a value that corresponds to the distance to the nearest feature pixel (see [7] for a detailed review). A commonly used DT is the 3-4 DT (see [12],[7]) and its mask is shown schematically in figure 1(a) alongside the two dimensional Euclidean distance transform mask (EDT), figure 1(b). The 3-4 DT is found by first segmenting the image into object and background and then passing, first the upper half of the mask (above the solid line) in figure 1(a) including 0 forwards over the image. The minimum of the current pixel value and the pixels which the masks covers plus their corresponding distance measure (either 3 or 4) is then assigned to the current pixel. Following this the lower portion of the mask, again including 0, is passed backwards over the image and again the minimum value is assigned to the current pixel.

The EDT is the most exact DT as it is two dimensional and if the 8 point sequential Euclidean distance mapping (8-SED), [9], is used then the chance of pixel misclassification is small. The EDT is found by passing portions of the mask shown in figure 1(b) over a segmented image a number of times in both the forward and backwards directions. The algorithm used is described in more detail in [9]. This results in a two dimensional vector for each pixel from which the distance to an object can be found by simply evaluating the length of the vector assigned to each pixel.

Figure 2 shows two distance transforms of a square, displayed using a cyclical grey scale colourmap. Figure 2(a) is the result of using a 3-4 DT and figure 2(b) is the result of using the 8-SED EDT and evaluating the lengths of the resulting vectors. It is clear that the 3-4 DT produces artifacts at the corners of the square. This is caused by the pixellation of the square and the approximate distance measurement of the 3-4 DT. If this transform were used for image deformation then artifacts would appear in the deformed image. Figure 2(b) is the EDT of the same square, it is clear that any artifacts due to the corners of the square are negligible. It is because of this that we have used the EDT in our deformation algorithm.

3. Deformations incorporating rigid structures

Our original problem is one where we wish to constrain parts of the image to be transformed subject to a pre-determined rigid body transformation, while using landmarks outside of the rigid bodies to define a deformation. Let us have n landmark sites given by $\mathbf{t}_i = (t_i[1], \ldots, t_i[d])^T$ which we wish to transform to new sites $\mathbf{u}_i = (u_i[1], \ldots, u_i[d])^T$ under the deformation. If we just have landmarks then we can form an interpolating deformation given by (5)-(10). We can rewrite (9) as follows

$$\Sigma B + DA = U \qquad (15)$$

we know Σ, D and U, and the matrix A represents the linear part of the transformation. Hence if we can control A we can control the linear part of the deformation and hence constrain parts of the image to have the required linear transformation at the objects. Further to that we need to ensure that the non-linear part of the transformation tends to zero as we move towards the objects, we can achieve this with careful selection of the function $\sigma(\mathbf{t}, \mathbf{t}_i)$.

First let us have n_o objects which we shall call O_i, $i = 1, \ldots, n_o$. Each O_i is the set of image pixels (or voxels) con-

tained in a segmented region. The objects may contain holes or even consist of two distinct image regions which form part of the same structure. We can then define an overall "object" set by $O_o = O_1 \cup O_2 \cup \ldots \cup O_{n_o}$. Each of the individual objects has an associated linear transformation which we shall denote by the matrices L_i, $i = 1, \ldots, n_o$. Each L_i is a $d \times M$ matrix of coefficients which when combined with the M basis functions $g_j(\mathbf{t})$, $j = 1, \ldots, M$ form a linear transformation. Each linear transformation is defined with respect to each individual objects centre of gravity.

We shall now evaluate $n_o + 1$ distance transforms, $\mathcal{D}_0(\mathbf{t}), \ldots, \mathcal{D}_{n_o}(\mathbf{t})$, in each element of which is a two dimensional vector. These consist of an overall distance transform, $\mathcal{D}_0(\mathbf{t})$, which represents the distance to the closest object, and n_o individual object distance transforms, $\mathcal{D}_i(\mathbf{t})$, $i = 1, \ldots, n_o$, which represent the distance from a point to object O_i, these are evaluated using [9].

In order to find a solution we now have to choose a kernel function which tends to zero as we move towards an object as well as a linear combination of the individual object transformations such that our object constraints are satisfied. We can define a basis function which tends to zero as we move towards any of the objects by weighting a valid basis function with the distance to the closest rigid body. For two points $\mathbf{t}$ and $\mathbf{t}_i$ this gives us,

$$\sigma'(\mathbf{t}, \mathbf{t}_i) = |\mathcal{D}_0(\mathbf{t})||\mathcal{D}_0(\mathbf{t}_i)|\sigma(\mathbf{t}, \mathbf{t}_i), \qquad (16)$$

this will tend to zero as the point $\mathbf{t}$ tends to any image object. Further if we form the matrix Σ' where $\Sigma'_{ij} = \sigma'(\mathbf{t}_i, \mathbf{t}_j)$ using (16) then we can decompose it in the following manner,

$$\Sigma' = K\Sigma K,$$

where

$$K_{ij} = \begin{cases} |\mathcal{D}_0(\mathbf{t}_i)| & i = j, \\ 0 & \text{otherwise} \end{cases} \quad \text{and } \Sigma_{ij} = \sigma(\mathbf{t}_i, \mathbf{t}_j)$$

as K is diagonal and $\mathcal{D}_0(\mathbf{t}_i) \neq 0$, as the landmarks are not on the objects, then K^{-1} exists. Further if $\sigma(\mathbf{t}, \mathbf{t}_i)$ is a valid basis function it follows that Σ is conditionally positive definite and hence Σ' is invertible and (16) is a valid basis function.

In order to define our linear term we have used a weighted sum of the individual object linear transformations. We shall use weights similar to (13) but with $s_i(\mathbf{t})$ replaced by $\mathcal{D}_i(\mathbf{t})$ giving,

$$w_i(\mathbf{t}) = \frac{q_i(\mathbf{t})}{\sum_{j=1}^{n_o} q_j(\mathbf{t})}$$

where

$$q_i(\mathbf{t}) = \frac{1}{\mathcal{D}_i(\mathbf{t})^\mu}.$$

So we have,

$$w_i(\mathbf{t}) = \begin{cases} 1 \text{ if } \mathbf{t} \in O_i \\ 0 \text{ if } \mathbf{t} \in O_j, \ j = 1, \ldots, n_o, \ j \neq i \end{cases} \qquad (17)$$

+4	+3	+4
+3	0	+3
+4	+3	+4

+(1,1)	+(0,1)	+(1,1)
+(1,0)	(0,0)	+(1,0)
+(1,1)	+(0,1)	+(1,1)

(a) (b)

Figure 1. Masks for two distance transforms, (a) the 3-4 distance transform mask, (b) the eight point sequential Euclidean distance transform mask.

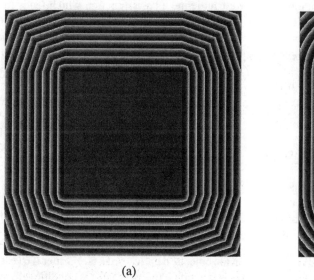
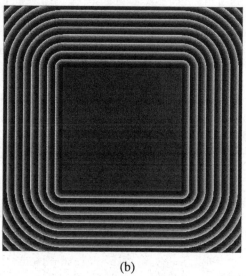

(a) (b)

Figure 2. Distance transforms for a square using two algorithms, displayed using a cyclical grey scale colourmap, (a) the 3-4 distance transform, (b) the eight point sequential Euclidean distance transform.

and

$$\sum_{i=1}^{n_o} w_i(\mathbf{t}) = 1. \qquad (18)$$

For any point $\mathbf{t}$ we define our linear transformation as

$$\mathcal{L}(\mathbf{t}) = \sum_{i=1}^{n_o} w_i(\mathbf{t})L_i, \qquad (19)$$

where (17) ensures the required linear transformation at the objects and (18) ensures the existence of the identity mapping.

Using (19) to define our linear transformation we can rewrite the coefficient equation (15) as

$$B = \Sigma'^{-1}(U - T), \qquad (20)$$

108

where

$$T = \begin{pmatrix} \mathbf{g}(\mathbf{t}_1)^T \mathcal{L}(\mathbf{t}_1)^T \\ \mathbf{g}(\mathbf{t}_2)^T \mathcal{L}(\mathbf{t}_2)^T \\ \vdots \\ \mathbf{g}(\mathbf{t}_n)^T \mathcal{L}(\mathbf{t}_n)^T \end{pmatrix} \qquad (21)$$

and

$$\mathbf{g}(\mathbf{t}_i) = (g_1(\mathbf{t}_i), \ldots, g_M(\mathbf{t}_i))^T. \qquad (22)$$

We can now write the interpolation solution for $\mathbb{R}^d \to \mathbb{R}^d$ in the following manner,

$$\mathbf{t} \to \mathbf{f}(\mathbf{t}) = \mathcal{L}(\mathbf{t})\mathbf{g}(\mathbf{t}) + \sum_{j=1}^{n} B_j^T \sigma'(\mathbf{t}, \mathbf{t}_j). \qquad (23)$$

where B_j is the jth row of B given by (20) and (10), $\sigma'(\mathbf{t}, \mathbf{t}_i)$ is given by (16) and $\mathcal{L}(\mathbf{t})$ by (19).

4. Results

In order to evaluate our deformations we must first choose a valid basis function. Ruprecht *et al.* [18] have experimented with a wide range of basis functions and have concluded that multiquadrics performed in a more satisfactory manner than other functions We shall now show some illustrative examples using a modified Hardy multiquadric [11] as our basis function, this is given by,

$$\sigma'(\mathbf{t}, \mathbf{t}_i) = |\mathcal{D}_o(\mathbf{t})||\mathcal{D}_o(\mathbf{t}_i)|(|\mathbf{t} - \mathbf{t}_i|^2 + R_i^2)^{\frac{\alpha}{2}}, \qquad (24)$$

and using (19)-(23) to form our deformation. The choices of α and R_i are subjective, we have used $\alpha = 1$, as proposed by [11], and taken R_i to be the distance from landmark $\mathbf{t}_i$ to the closest rigid body. The R_i's act as locality parameters, when R_i is small the deformation will be more elastic than when R_i is large.

Figure 3 shows the results of using both standard landmark based deformation and a deformation incorporating a rigid structure. The original image, with the square in grey and sixteen landmarks marked by black crosses, is plotted in figure 3(a). We shall assume that we know that the square is a rigid structure and we shall attempt to rotate it through 45°. Figure 3(b) shows the result of using eight of the sixteen landmarks, one at each corner of the image and one at each corner of the square. The four image corners have been fixed and the four corners of the square have been rotated through 45° with respect to the centre of the square. It is clear that if the square is known to be a rigid structure then we have a very unsatisfactory deformation. The image in the figure 3(c) shows the result of using all sixteen landmarks shown in 3(a), once again the image corners are fixed and the remaining landmarks rotated through 45° with respect to the centre of the square. The addition of extra landmarks has improved the transformation of the square but it is still

obviously deformed. We could carry on adding landmarks until the square takes a more rigid shape or, taking landmarks to their extreme, use a landmark at every pixel within the square. This is however not a satisfactory solution as the addition of these extra landmarks soon makes the computational cost of the deformation prohibitive. Figure 3(d) shows the result of using (19)-(24) with one rigid body, the square, and four landmarks, the four corners of the image. We have set L_1 to be the coefficients required for a 45° rotation. It is clear that we have achieved the desired rotation of of the square without any deformation of the object. This is a vast improvement over normal landmark based techniques as well as being quick to compute (quicker than computing 3(c)). It is possible to improve the landmark based approach by using derivative information such as edgels, see [6],[15]. This however becomes less useful as the shapes you wish to constrain become more complex.

The theory is valid for any number of rigid bodies and figure 4 shows two deformations of a simulated section of spine with five rigid bodies and four landmarks. The original image is figure 4(a) where the rigid bodies are the grey squares and we have a landmark at each of the four corners which we fix in position. Figure 4(b) shows a bending of the overall image, this is the sort of deformation one would expect in the spine where the squares could be thought of as the vertebrae. Here we have a smooth and reasonable deformation of the image surrounding the objects. In figure 4(c) we have moved the rigid bodies in a more random manner involving both translations and rotations. This image demonstrates the robustness of the algorithm to deformations which would not appear to be biologically reasonable. Deformations such as this may be difficult to model using a biomathematical model but could occur during a surgical procedure or due to a severe trauma.

Figure 5 shows the results of constructing a deformation incorporating rigid bodies for a sagittal MR image of the human spine. 5(a) and (b) show a sagittal slice through the head and neck of a volunteer with his neck in different positions. We are now going to match the images together. Figures 5(c) and (d) show segmentations of 5(a) and 5(b) respectively. These were achieved by drawing around the vertebrae and posterior of the skull by hand. We actually have nine rigid structures in this image, this is because the spinal processes, which appear to be separate from the spinal column are in fact attached to vertebrae. We have also used fifteen landmarks which are shown as white crosses in 5(a) and (b). Figure 5(e) shows the result of matching the fifteen landmarks and nine rigid bodies of 5(a) to those of 5(b). The linear transformations were found by first matching the centres of gravity of the rigid bodies and then rotating them to the correct position. These were evaluated automatically from the segmented images by matching the principal axes of the shapes. This is not an ideal solution as it is suscepti-

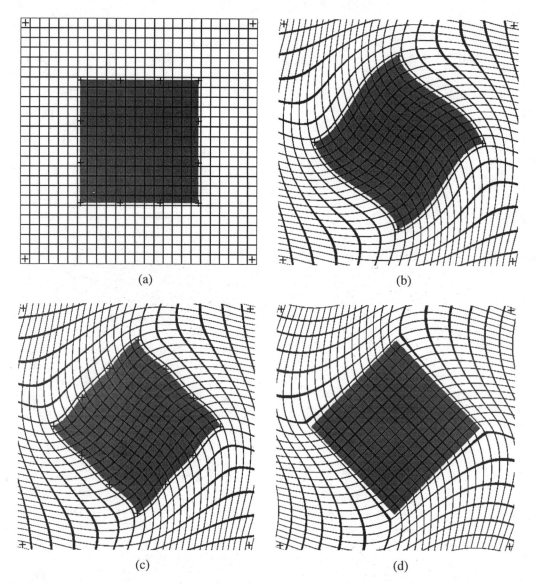

Figure 3. The rotation through 45° of a "rigid" square within an image while keeping the image corners fixed, (a) the original square, (b) a transformation using eight landmarks, (c) a transformation using sixteen landmarks, (d) the transformation using four landmarks and one rigid object, the square.

ble to noise in the segmentations, although it does work in this example. In the future we will investigate different rigid body matching methods including chamfer matching. Figure 5(f) shows a thresholded boundary of 5(e) overlaid onto 5(b). It is clear that we have achieved a high degree of accuracy for internal structures both at the rigid bodies and also in the surrounding deformable tissue, except at the skin surface which is not of clinical relevance.

5. Conclusions and discussion

We have provided an interpolating method of deformation which enables rigid structures within an image to be constrained as well as landmark information. The method moves user defined objects and landmarks exactly and provides a smooth interpolation elsewhere in the image. This method is valid in any number of dimensions.

We have chosen an interpolation approach with added constraints as a compromise between accuracy and speed of processing, all the figures in this paper took less than 6 min-

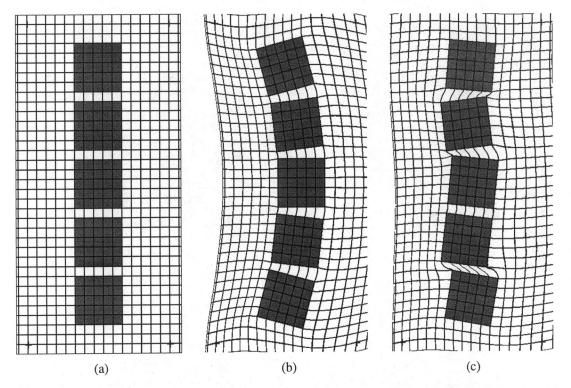

Figure 4. A simulated section of spine comprising five separate rigid squares (vertebrae), (a) in their original positions, and after two deformations (b) and (c), in both cases the squares move rigidly as the spine deforms.

utes on a SUN SPARC 20/61 to compute. Model based approaches can, if they are based on accurate image information, prove more accurate, but they are very computationally expensive. For interventional work we require a solution quickly (how quickly will depend on the interventional procedure) but not necessarily in real time as routinely there are periods of inactivity during a procedure. We intend to optimise the current code in order to significantly decrease the algorithm computation time.

Unlike rigid body registration where the result is predictable at all points in the image, incorporating deformations could lead to misleading or inaccurate results, especially far from landmarks or identified rigid bodies. The choice of basis function affects the interpolation solution, however in image deformation we do not know the "correct" interpolation scheme. In one deformation kriging may prove to be the best method, in another a thin-plate spline may be best, or a radial basis function solution may prove to be the best. There is no way of predicting which method will fit the data best away from the landmarks as we are only given information at certain points in the image. Validation of this approach is therefore an important issue especially as it is hoped that these methods will find applications in sur-

gical therapeutic interventions in order to improve the accuracy of image guidance. Validation will proceed by assessing the accuracy of transformation of structure boundaries and other features which have not been identified *a priori* as constraints. In certain circumstances it may also be possible to track structures such as surgical clips or other markers inserted during previous interventions. Detailed descriptions of our approaches to validation will be described in future submissions.

The use of derivative information can help to improve the accuracy of the transformation further, see [6],[15]. Our method can be extended to allow the use of derivative constraints at positions away from the rigid objects. Directional derivatives of the EDT's can be found numerically, μ in (14) can be chosen so that the weights are differentiable to the required order, and the basis function $\sigma(\mathbf{t}, \mathbf{t}_i)$ and the order r of the underlying drift can be chosen using the method laid down for kriging with derivatives in [14].

6. Acknowledgements

We are grateful for the financial support of Philips Medical Systems (EasyVision/ EasyGuide Advanced Develop-

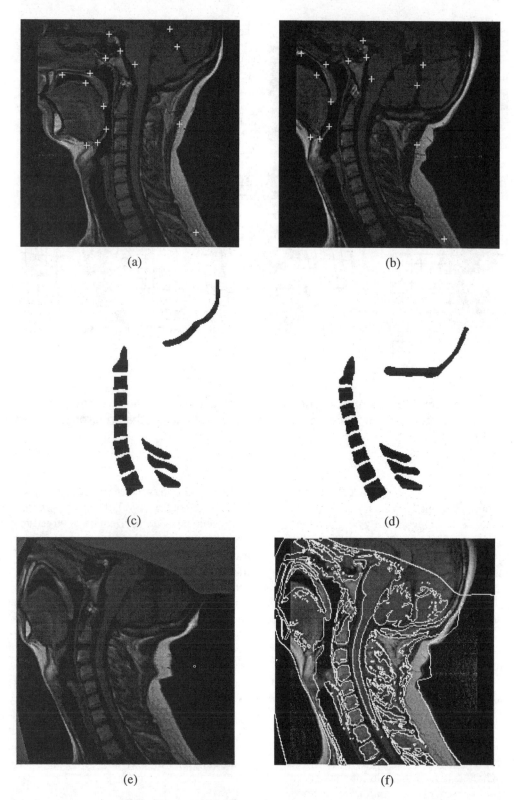

Figure 5. An image match incorporating rigid structures, (a) the original image with landmarks, (b) the destination image with corresponding landmarks, (c) the segmentation of (a), (d) the segmentation of (b), (e) the result of deforming (a) using the landmarks of (a) and (b) and matching the rigid bodies in (c) and (d), (f) a threshold overlay of (e) onto (b).

ment) (JAL) and the UK EPSRC (Grant No. GR/J90183) (DLGH, DJH). We would also like to thank Paul Summers for his help with the MR data acquisition and the assistance of other members of the Image Processing Group at Guy's Hospital. The support and encouragement of Prof. Andreas Adam and Dr. John Reidy is also greatly appreciated.

References

[1] N. Arad, N. Dyn, D. Reisfeld, and Y. Yeshurun. Image warping by radial basis functions: Application to facial expressions. *CVGIP: Graphical Models and Image Processing*, 56(2):161–172, Mar. 1994.

[2] N. Arad and D. Reisfeld. Image warping using few anchor points and radial functions. *Computer Graphics Forum*, 14(1):35–46, 1995.

[3] F. L. Bookstein. Principal warps: Thin-plate splines and the decomposition of deformations. *IEEE Trans. Patt. Anal. Mach. Intell.*, 11:567–585, 1989.

[4] F. L. Bookstein. *Morphometric Tools for Landmark Data.* Cambridge Univ. Press, Cambridge, 1991.

[5] F. L. Bookstein. Thin-plate splines and the atlas problem for biomedical images. In A. C. F. Colchester and D. J. Hawkes, editors, *Information Processing in Medical Imaging*, 1991.

[6] F. L. Bookstein and W. D. K. Green. A feature space for edgels in images with landmarks. *Jour. of Math. Imag. and Vis.*, 3:231–261, 1993.

[7] G. Borgefors. Distance transformations in digital images. *Computer Vision, Graphics and Image Processing*, 34:344–371, 1986.

[8] N. A. C. Cressie. *Statistics for Spatial Data.* Wiley, 2nd edition, 1993.

[9] P. Danielsson. Euclidian distance mapping. *Computer Graphics and Image Processing*, 14:227–248, 1980.

[10] P. J. Edwards, D. L. G. Hill, J. A. Little, V. A. S. Sahni, and D. J. Hawkes. Medical image registration incorporating deformations. In D. Pycock, editor, *British Machine Vision Conference*, pages 691–699, 1995.

[11] R. L. Hardy. Multiquadric equations of topography and other irregular surfaces. *Journal of Geophysical Research*, 76(8):1905–1915, 1971.

[12] D. L. G. Hill and D. J. Hawkes. Medical image registration using knowledge of adjacency of anatomical structures. *Image and Vision Computing*, 12:173–178, 1994.

[13] D. L. G. Hill, D. J. Hawkes, J. E. Crossman, M. J. Gleeson, T. C. S. Cox, E. E. C. M. L. Bracey, A. J. Strong, and P. Graves. Registration of MR and CT images for skull based surgery using point-like anatomical features. *The British Journal of Radiology*, 64:1030–1035, 1991.

[14] K. V. Mardia, J. T. Kent, C. R. Goodall, and J. A. Little. Kriging and splines with derivative information. *Biometrika*, 83(1):207–221, 1996.

[15] K. V. Mardia and J. A. Little. Image warping using derivative information. In F. L. Bookstein, J. S. Duncan, N. Lange, and D. C. Wilson, editors, *Mathematical Methods in Medical Imaging III, S.P.I.E. vol. 2099*, pages 16–31, San Diego, California, July 1994.

[16] C. A. Micchelli. Interpolation of scattered data: Distance matrices and conditionally positive definite functions. *Constructive Approximation*, 2:11–22, 1986.

[17] D. E. Myers. Kriging, cokriging, radial basis functions and the role of positive definiteness. *Computers Math. Applic.*, 24(12):139–148, 1992.

[18] D. Ruprecht, R. Nagel, and H. Müller. Spatial free-form deformation with scattered data interpolation methods. *Computers and Graphics*, 19(1):63–71, 1995.

[19] D. Shepard. A two-dimensional interpolation function for irregularly spaced data. In *Proc. 23rd Nat'l Conf. of the ACM*, pages 517–524, New York, 1968. ACM Press.

[20] C. Studholme, D. L. G. Hill, and D. J. Hawkes. Multi resolution voxel similarity measures for MR-PET registration. In Y. Bizais, B. C. di Paola, and R. di Paola, editors, *Information Processing in Medical Imaging*, Dordrecht, The Netherlands, in press, 1995. Kluwer Academic Publishers.

[21] G. Wahba. *Spline Models for Observational Data.* Philadelphia: Society for Industrial and Applied Mathematics, 1990.

[22] K. Waters. A physical model of facial tissue and muscle articulation derived from computer tomography data. In R. A. Robb, editor, *Visualization in Biomedical Computing*, pages 574–583, 1992.

[23] R. P. Woods, J. C. Mazziotta, and S. R. Cherry. MRI-PET registration with automated algorithm. *Journal of Computer Assisted Tomography*, 17(4):536–546, 1993.

Contour/Surface Registration Using a Physically Deformable Model

Jiang Qian, Theophano Mitsa
Department of Electrical and Computer Engineering
University of Iowa, Iowa City, IA 52242

Eric A. Hoffman
Department of Radiology, University of Iowa College of Medicine
University of Iowa, Iowa City, IA 52242
jqian@icaen.uiowa.edu

Abstract

This paper describes a new approach of surface/contour registration based on a physically deformable model. No prior knowledge about the types of geometric transformation is required for registration. Instead, our approach views the surface as made of elastic material that will change shape in response to the applied external force. The registration of two surfaces/contours is the deformation process of one shape towards the other governed by physical laws. Before the deformation, the two shapes are roughly registered with a global affine transformation. The physically deformable model is then applied to deform one shape to match the other. The point correspondences between the two shapes are established when one shape is finally deformed to the other. In the 2D case, the model is similar to the active contour model but registration is formulated as an equilibrium problem instead of minimization problem. The result is a set of decoupled linear system equations that are easy to solve. It is also shown that, because of physical constraints imposed, our model is an improved version of Burr's dynamic contour model. Experimental results are presented to demonstrate the performance of the model.

1 Introduction

Image registration is the process of determining a geometric transform that relates the contents of two images in a meaningful way and establishing the correspondence between the two images. The analysis of two or more digital images of the same scene taken from different places or at a different time often requires registration/matching of the images. The goal of image registration is to either expose differences of interest between the images or determine the parameters of the matching transformation that aligns the images.

Image registration is an important stage in many biomedical image analysis applications. Multimodality matching to register CT, MRI and PET integrates anatomical and functional information to study functional-structure relationships. Monomodality matching of images from the same object over a period of time assists the evaluation of changes that occurred in that period. Most registration methods assume that some type of geometric transformation is capable of aligning the images, then search over the domain of the transform to find the optimal transformation [4, 18]. However, when the knowledge of the transformation type is not available or when local variations among different regions are present, these methods are difficult to apply.

In this paper, we describe a new approach that registers images based on a physically deformable model. No prior knowledge about the types of geometric transformations is required. Instead, our approach simulates the manual registration process and models the registration as the deformation of an elastic material. Before registration, the contours of the images are extracted. The physically deformable model is applied to deform one contour, called the start contour, to match the other, the goal contour. The result is point correspondences between the contours. Then an intensity transformation is estimated from the matching points to warp one image to the other. The physically deformable model considers the contour as a set of vertices. Each has physical properties such as position, velocity, acceleration and mass. Each vertex is also being attached to its neighbor vertices by springs. When

114

Proceedings of MMBIA '96

an external force is acting on a vertex, it will change its position. In response neighboring vertices will generate internal elastic forces to resist the change. The contour is deformed until an equilibrium state between the internal and external forces is achieved.

Our physically deformable model is the unification of two existing contour models. The first model is for image segmentation(Active Contour Model[10, 19]), while the other is for contour registration(Burr's dynamic model[5, 6]). Our model can be easily extended to 3D surface registration. Active Contour Models (called snakes) are energy constraint deformable models for image segmentation. In [3], Bajscy uses a similar deformable model for registration purposes, but the registration problem is solved as a minimization problem with a cost functional that combines a deformable model and a similarity measure. In our registration method, using the deformable model, matching is formulated as an equilibrium problem. The motion of a vertex follows Newtonian mechanics–when a force is applied to a body, the body accelerates in the direction the force is acting. The body accelerates at a proportional rate to the size of the force. The equilibrium state is reached when the velocity and acceleration are zero for all vertices on the contour.

Our paper is organized as follows: In section 2, we provide a summary of related work. In section 3, we present a physically deformable model and the algorithm for contour/surface registration. Experimental results are presented in section 4 and a conclusion is provided in section 5.

2 Related Work

The most recent work in image registration has been the development of techniques which exploit deformable models. Unlike traditional approaches that assume some types of geometric transformation and find the optimal transformation among the admissible class of transformations, no assumptions about the types of geometric transformation are required. Instead, these approaches simulate the manual registration process and model the registration as the deformation of an elastic material. Imagine that we have two objects, one of them made from an elastic material, the other serving as a reference. By applying appropriate external forces we can change the shape of the elastic object so that it matches the reference. The Partial Differential Equation(PDE) that governs the deformation of the object through space can be written in Lagrange's form [17] as follows:

$$m\frac{\partial^2 \mathbf{p}}{\partial t^2} + \gamma\frac{\partial \mathbf{p}}{\partial t} + \frac{\delta\varepsilon(\mathbf{p})}{\delta\mathbf{p}} = \mathbf{f}(\mathbf{p}, t) \qquad (1)$$

where $\mathbf{p}(t)$ is the position of a finite element at time t. The first term on the left side of equation is the multiplication of mass density time acceleration and can be considered as the inertia force due to the model's distributed mass. The second term is proportional to the velocity and can be considered as the damping force due to dissipation. The third term is a variational derivative of the potential energy of the elastic deformation $\varepsilon(\mathbf{p})$ and can be considered as the internal elastic forces to resist the deformation. $\mathbf{f}(\mathbf{p})$ is the net external forces that drives the deformation of a object. Equation (1) can be rearranged to:

$$m\mathbf{a} = \mathbf{f}_{net} \qquad (2)$$

which is Newton's second law. $\mathbf{a} = \frac{\partial^2 \mathbf{p}}{\partial t^2}$ is acceleration and $\mathbf{f}_{net}$ is the force including damping force, internal elastic forces and external forces.

There are two types of models based on the PDE. One is the active contour model, the other one is Burr's dynamic contour model.

2.1 Active Contour Model

Kass, Witkin, and Terzopoulos presented their Active Contour Models in [10]. Snakes were originally used for segmentation or boundary extraction, however, if one contour is set as the initial guess for the extraction of the second contour, then snakes can be used for contour registration.

Snakes are a special case of deformable models because in snakes the governing PDE is the same as in equation 1 except that the term of damping force is set to zero. Using the variational method [9], the problem of solving the PDE is reformulated as the minimization problem of the derived functional. The derived functional represents the energy of the model and is expressed as:

$$\begin{aligned} E^*_{snake} &= \int_0^1 E_{snake}(\mathbf{v}(s))\,ds \\ &= \int_0^1 E_{int}(\mathbf{v}(s)) + P(\mathbf{v}(s))ds. \end{aligned} \qquad (3)$$

where $\mathbf{v}(s) = (x(s), y(s))$ represents a contour with the arc length, s, as parameter.

$P(\mathbf{v}(s))$ is the potential associated with the external forces. It is computed as a function of the image data. The internal energy E_{int} is written as:

$$E_{int} = (\alpha(s)|\mathbf{v}_s(s)|^2 + \beta(s)|\mathbf{v}_{ss}(s)|^2)/2. \qquad (4)$$

where α and β are weighting coefficients at each point to determine the extent to which the contour is allowed to stretch or bend at that point. The variables $\mathbf{v}_s(s)$ and $\mathbf{v}_{ss}(s)$ are the first and second derivative of $\mathbf{v}(s)$ respectively.

There is a number of different ways to discretize equations(3),(4) and implement the model. Amini [2] used dynamic programming to include hard constraints in the model. Cohen [7] modified the definition of external forces, derived from the gradient of the image, to obtain more stable results and introduced an extra pressure force which made the curve model behave like a balloon instead of snake. Bajscy [3] used multilevel(multigrid) techniques to perform deformations step-by-step in a coarse-to-fine strategy, increasing the local similarity and global coherence. Williams [19] proposed a fast algorithm for snakes which combines speed, flexibility, and simplicity compared to the original snake version. Lai [12, 11, 13] formulated generalized active contour models, or g-snakes, based on a stable and regenerative shape matrix, which is invariant and unique under rigid motions.

2.2 Dynamic Contour Model

Burr [5, 6] developed another model-based registration method by an iterative technique which depends on the local neighborhood whose size is progressively smaller with each iteration. The essence of the model is to determine a force field acting on one contour and try to distort it to be like the other one. In Burr's model two contours are defined by ordered lists of their vertices:

$$\mathbf{C1}(i) = \{(x1_i, y1_i)\}, 1 \leq i \leq \mathbf{N1}$$

and

$$\mathbf{C2}(j) = \{(x2_j, y2_j)\}, 1 \leq j \leq \mathbf{N2}$$

where $\mathbf{N}$ is the number of vertices in a contour and (x_i, y_i) are the $x-y$ coordinates of a vertex. A straight line segment is represented by its two end vertices (x_i, y_i) and (x_{i+1}, y_{i+1}). $\mathbf{C1}$(i) is the contour to be deformed, called start contour. $\mathbf{C2}$(j) serves as a reference and is called goal contour. An intermediate contour is generated at each iteration which progressively deforms to match the goal contour. There are three major steps at each iteration [15]:

1 Determine the displacement vector between a vertex in one contour and its nearest line segment in another contour.
Figure 1 shows the geometry of the displacement vectors. Displacement vectors in $\mathbf{D1}$ are the vectors from vertices in $\mathbf{C1}$ to their nearest line segment in $\mathbf{C2}$, similarly displacement vectors in $\mathbf{D2}$

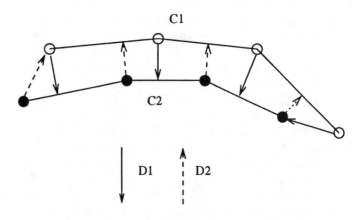

Figure 1. Geometry of displacement vectors.

are the vectors from vertices in $\mathbf{C2}$ to their nearest line segment in $\mathbf{C1}$. $\mathbf{D1}$ roughly represents the force pushing $\mathbf{C1}$ towards $\mathbf{C2}$, while negative $\mathbf{D2}$ represents the pulling force from $\mathbf{C2}$ to attract $\mathbf{C1}$ at those vertices.

2 Compose a force field for the whole image based on the displacement vectors of the two contours. A smoothed displacement vector at any point (x,y) is defined as a weighted average of neighboring displacement vectors. A Gaussian weight function is used to give more influence to near neighbors and less influence to far neighbors. The smoothed displacement field $\mathbf{DS}$(x,y) is a function of the pushing and pulling forces,

$$\mathbf{DS}(x,y) = \gamma^{-1}(\mathbf{DS}_{push} - \mathbf{DS}_{pull}) \quad (5)$$

where $\mathbf{DS}_{push}$ and $\mathbf{DS}_{pull}$ are:

$$\mathbf{DS}_{push} = \frac{\sum_{i=1}^{N1} G1_i \mathbf{D1}(i, J_i)}{\sum_{i=1}^{N1} G1_i}$$

$$\mathbf{DS}_{pull} = \frac{\sum_{j=1}^{N2} G2_j \mathbf{D2}(j, I_j)}{\sum_{j=1}^{N2} G2_j} \quad (6)$$

and G1 and G2 are Gaussian weights defined by

$$G1_i = exp\frac{-(x - x1_i)^2 - (y - y1_i)^2}{\sigma_k^2}$$

$$G2_j = exp\frac{-(x - x2_j - D2_x(j, I_j))^2}{\sigma_k^2} \cdot$$

$$exp\frac{-(y - y2_j - D2_y(j, I_j))^2}{\sigma_k^2} \quad (7)$$

J_i denotes the closest neighbor vertex in $\mathbf{C2}$ of vertex i in $\mathbf{C1}$. Similarly, I_j denotes the closest neighbor vertex in **C1** of vertex j in **C2**. The parameter σ_k is defined as

$$\sigma_k = \sigma_0 f^{-k} \qquad (8)$$

where f is a constant and $1 \leq f \leq 2$. Under this definition, σ_k will decrease gradually after each iteration, which effectively reduces the size of local neighborhood used to composite the displacement field.

3 Iterated Matching.

For the kth iteration, an intermediate contour $\mathbf{W}^k$ is generated from the previous contour $\mathbf{W}^{k-1}$ and the force field in step 2:

$$\mathbf{W}^k(i) = \mathbf{W}^{k-1}(i) + \mathbf{DS}^{k-1}(x_i^{k-1}, y_i^{k-1}) \quad (9)$$

$\mathbf{W}^0$ is defined as **C1**.

The iteration continues with $\mathbf{W}^{k-1}$ as **C1** in the kth iteration until the following stop condition is satisfied:

$$\frac{1}{N1} \sum_{i=1}^{N1} |\mathbf{DS}(x1_i, y1_i)| < \epsilon \qquad (10)$$

where ϵ is a predefined small number.

Burr's model focuses on the calculation of the external force that drives the matching of two contours. It will be demonstrated later in the discussion of our registration model that the intermediate result at each iteration is the numerical solution of the basic *PDE* without the term of internal forces. Moshfeghi [15] extended Burr's model to register 2D images from different modalities. He and his collaborators [16] recently extended their elastic matching method from 2D to 3D.

3 Methods

Figure 2 shows a diagram of the model-based image registration system. It consists of the following steps:

1. Preprocessing,

2. Initial Global Registration,

3. Model-based Contour/Surface Registration,

4. Image Registration.

In the preprocessing, images are segmented and features that are common to both images, which are the boundaries of the regions of interest, are extracted.

In initial global registration, we use a moment-based algorithm [1] to find a global affine transformation that roughly registers the two contours. A physically model-based contour registration is then applied to the two

globally aligned contours/surfaces to find the matching points on the contours. With the matching points between the two contours, a set of displacement vectors, required to register the vertices of the first object with the second, is obtained. These displacement vectors represent local nonlinear distortions of the contours. To warp the first image to the second one, a weighted interpolation of the displacement vectors is calculated to approximate distortions that deform the first image to the second [15]. The intensity of the deformed image is resampled using bilinear interpolation. As discussed later in the paper, our technique can be easily extended to 3D to perform surface registration.

In the following sections, the model-based contour/surface registration is discussed in detail.

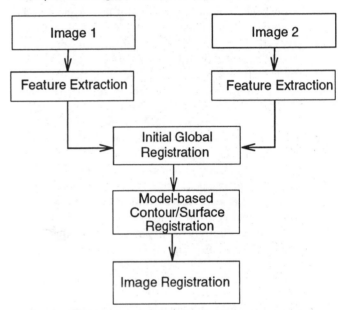

Figure 2. Block diagram of the physically model-based registration system.

3.1 Physically Model-based Registration

We first present 2D contour registration model then extend it to 3D surface registration.

In 2D contour registration model, the contours are presented by ordered lists of vertices. Each vertex's status is given by $\{\mathbf{p}, \mathbf{v}, \mathbf{a}, m\}$, where $\mathbf{p}$ is the position of the vertex; $\mathbf{v}$ is its velocity; $\mathbf{a}$ acceleration; m mass. The dynamic behavior of a vertex i is given by:

$$m_i \mathbf{a}_i = \mathbf{f}_i \qquad (11)$$

where $\mathbf{f}_i$ is the net force acting on vertex i. Three kinds of forces are included in the deformable model:

(1) an external force that drives the start contour to match the goal contour, (2) a damping force due to dissipation, (3) and internal spring force that resists the deformation.

The dynamic equation (1) is solved using numerical integration through time with the status of each vertex calculated at a sequence of discrete positions in time. From time t to time $t + \Delta t$, the deformation of a vertex i is described by [14]:

$$
\begin{aligned}
\mathbf{p}_i(t + \Delta t) &= \mathbf{p}_i(t) + \mathbf{v}_i(t)\Delta t \\
\mathbf{v}_i(t + \Delta t) &= \mathbf{v}_i(t) + \mathbf{a}_i(t)\Delta t \qquad (12) \\
\mathbf{a}_i(t + \Delta t) &= \frac{1}{m_i}\mathbf{f}_i(t + \Delta t)
\end{aligned}
$$

which means the new status of the vertex at time $t + \Delta t$ can be derived from the previous status at time t and the net force at the current time $t + \Delta t$.

Registration is an iterative deformation process. During each iteration, an intermediate contour, which is initially start contour, is deformed from the contour of the previous iteration. When the intermediate contour is finally deformed to be the goal contour, the vertices in the start contour are matched to points in the goal contour and point correspondences between the two contours are established.

There are two stages in one iteration. First the driving external force is calculated at each vertex based on the difference between the current intermediate contour and the goal contour. The external force $\mathbf{f}_{ext}$ acts on vertex i in a infinitely small time interval to set up the initial deformation velocity, i.e.

$$
\mathbf{v}_i(0) = \frac{\mathbf{f}_{ext,i}}{m_i} \qquad (13)
$$

The actual deformation happens at the second stage as described in equation (12) with initial velocity set by equation (13) and acceleration zero. During this stage, no external force, only damping and internal force are generated to resist the deformation. This is continued until a steady state is reached for all vertices, which results into a new intermediate contour that is more like the goal contour. The iteration repeats until the intermediate contour is deformed to be the goal contour or the difference is less then a predefined small number.

3.1.1 External force

The external force in the model is similar to the one defined by Burr [5] in his dynamic model for image registration (equation (5)). As Burr discussed, it is based on a simple estimation of the dissimilarity between two contours. The distance between each vertex in one contour and its nearest vertex in the second contour is determined. Similarly, these distances are found starting

with each vertex in the second contour. The contours are then pulled together by a composite of these displacements and their neighboring displacements which are weighted by their proximity. This composite vector is the major force that brings two contours together.

3.1.2 Internal and Damping Force

In the second stage of each iterative deformation, the total force $\mathbf{f}_i$ on vertex i is a summation of internal forces and damping force:

$$
\mathbf{f}_i = \mathbf{f}_{damp,i} + \mathbf{f}_{int,i} \qquad (14)
$$

The damping force is proportional to the vertex velocity, but negative in the direction.

$$
\mathbf{f}_{damp,i} = -w_{damp}\mathbf{v}_i \qquad (15)
$$

where w_{damp} is a damping coefficient.
The internal force at vertex i is

$$
\mathbf{f}_{int} = -\nabla E_{int} \qquad (16)
$$

where E_{int} is given in equation (4). Since E_{int} has two terms in (4), there are two corresponding internal elastic forces. The first internal force is due to the changes of the arc length s. Physically there are two springs that connect vertex i to i-1 and i+1. If d_i denotes the length between vertex i and i+1 and $\mathbf{f}_{spring,i}$ denotes the spring force along the spring, then, with an ideal Hookean spring:

$$
|\mathbf{f}_{spring,i}| = k(d_i(t) - d_i(t + \Delta t)) \qquad (17)
$$

where k is the spring constant. The internal spring force on vertex i is:

$$
\mathbf{f}_{int_1,i} = \mathbf{f}_{spring,i} - \mathbf{f}_{spring,i-1} \qquad (18)
$$

The second internal force is due to changes of curvature. Williams [19] summarized different methods to approximate the curvature. The formula we adopted for the estimation of the curvature at vertex i is:

$$
\mathbf{v}_{ss} \approx \frac{\mathbf{u}_i}{|\mathbf{u}_i|} - \frac{\mathbf{u}_{i+1}}{|\mathbf{u}_{i+1}|} \qquad (19)
$$

where $\mathbf{u}_i = \mathbf{p}_i - \mathbf{p}_{i-1}$
The second internal force, the curvature force, is thus given by:

$$
\mathbf{f}_{int_2,i} = \beta(\mathbf{v}_{ss}(t) - \mathbf{v}_{ss}(t + \Delta t)) \qquad (20)
$$

where β is a weighting coefficient for the curvature force.
The total internal force on vertex i is:

$$
\mathbf{f}_{int,i} = \mathbf{f}_{int_1,i} + \mathbf{f}_{int_2,i} \qquad (21)
$$

3.2 Comparison of our Model to Existing Models

Both our model and Terzopoulos's active contour model are based on the same *PDE* equation (equation (1)). However, our model has an additional term-the damping force. Also, a significant difference between the two models, is that matching is formulated as an equilibrium problem instead of minimization problem. As a consequence, the matching problem is converted into a set of decoupled linear equations which can be solved individually.

To see the relationship of our model and Burr's dynamic model, let us set the internal forces to zero and deform the start contour. At kth iteration, the external force sets the initial velocity and the deformation of vertex $\mathbf{p}$ is governed by:

$$
\begin{aligned}
m\ddot{\mathbf{p}}(t) &= -w_{damp}\dot{\mathbf{p}}(t) \\
\dot{\mathbf{p}}(0_+) &= \frac{\mathbf{f}_{burr}}{m} \\
\mathbf{p}(0_+) &= \mathbf{p}^{k-1}
\end{aligned}
\tag{22}
$$

The steady solution of this iteration, which is the vertex position at next iteration, is:

$$
\mathbf{p}^k = \mathbf{p}(\infty) = \mathbf{p}^{k-1} + \frac{\mathbf{f}_{burr}}{w_{damp}}
\tag{23}
$$

Comparing (23) with (9) we see they are identical if w_{damp} is one. Our model, therefore, is an improved version of Burr's dynamic model, in the sense that we are considering internal forces during the deformation.

3.2.1 Surface Registration

Extension of the above 2D contour registration model to 3D surface registration is quite straightforward and only a few modifications are required.

The first modification is the requirement of surface reconstruction from a set of 2D contours. This can be implemented using a tiling algorithm in [8]. A surface, $\mathbf{S}$, is then represented by its ordered vertex and triangle patch lists:

$$
\mathbf{S}(i,c) = \{(x_i, y_i, z_i), \Delta_c\}, 1 \le i \le \mathbf{N} \text{ and } 1 \le c \le \mathbf{T}
$$

where $\mathbf{N}$ is the number of vertices in a surface and (x_i, y_i, z_i) are the $x-y-z$ coordinates of vertex i; $\mathbf{T}$ is the number of triangle patches and Δ_c is triangle patch c.

The second modification is the extension of the external force. The procedure to determine the external force is similar to the procedure used to determine the force of Burr's model except that the displacement vector in step 1 of section 2.2 is now between a vertex and its nearest patch, instead of nearest line segment. The details of this procedure can be found in [16].

The last modification is in regards to the internal forces. The springs attached to a vertex are now not restricted to two neighboring vertices in the same contour. They also include springs from vertices in neighboring contours. Similarly, estimation of curvature in equation (19), using two neighboring vertices in the same contour, needs modification to include vertices in neighboring contours.

4 Registration Results

We have implemented the model-based registration in 2D. Figure 3 shows the deformation process of two synthetic contours. The parameters used in our model were:

1. $\sigma_0 = 110$

2. $\gamma = 1.3$

3. $f = 1.2$ for the external force

4. $w_{damp} = 0.8$ for the damping force

5. $k = 0.2$ for the spring constant and

6. $\beta = 0.5$ for the curvature force

Figure 3a shows the overlay of the start and goal contours where the outer contour is the start contour and inner one is the goal contour. Figure 3b shows the deformation after one iteration. The intermediate contour is between the start and goal contour. Figure 3c is the deformation at fifth iteration. Figure 3d is the final result after 21 iterations. The intermediate contour now is deformed to the goal contour. The arrows between the start contour and the goal contour show the displacement vectors and the point correspondences. We intentionally skipped the initial global matching to demonstrate the deformation process. As a result, the differences between the two contours are much larger than the differences after the global registration. Therefore, we need more iterations to register two contours (21 iterations in this example). Normally 5-10 iterations are sufficient when global registration is applied first.

To demonstrate the performance of our registration model, we generated a pair of contours with known matching points by applying a type of geometric transformation to the start contour to form the goal contour. The point matching results from our method can then be compared with the exact known matching points and the performance of our model can be evaluated.

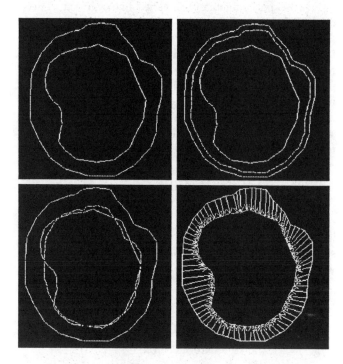

Figure 3. Contour registration results: (upper left) start and goal contour (upper right) first iteration with intermediate contour in the middle (bottom left) fifth iteration (bottom right) 21th iteration. The intermediate contour is deformed to the goal contour

	Exact parameter	Estimated parameter
Translation	(24, 17)	(21, 19.3)
Scale	(0.84, 0.84)	(0.79, 0.89)
Rotation	40°	37°

Table 1. Parameters of the exact transformation and the initial global matching.

The first example is an artificially generated goal contour from the start contour using a global affine transformation. Normally due to the noise in the sample data, there will be some error in the estimated transform parameters and in the matching result. Figure 4(left) shows the overlay of the start and goal contours. Figure 4(right) shows the two contours after initial global registration. The affine transformation parameters listed in table 1 are the exact and estimated parameters. After the initial global registration, the contours are further registered with our model. The matching results of the global registration and the model registration are compared with the known exact matching points. The mean error, maximum error, and error standard deviation with respect to the distance from the exact matching points are 7.75, 11.86 and 2.46 pixels respectively, using initial global matching. They were reduced to 1.62, 3.14, and 1.02 pixels respectively, when the model-based registration was applied.

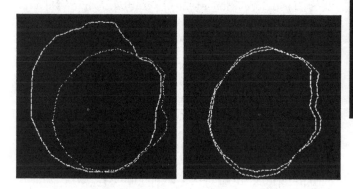

Figure 4. The overlay of the start and goal contours in the case of a global transformation: (left) before the global registration (right) after the global registration.

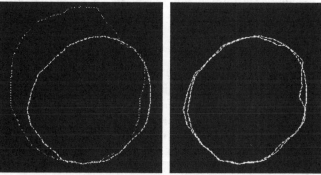

Figure 5. The overlay of the start and goal contours in the case of a polynomial transformation: (left) before the global registration. (right) after the global registration.

In the second example, we deformed the start contour with a second order polynomial transformation. Figure 5(left) is the overlay of the start and goal contours. Figure 5(right) is the overlay of the two contours after initial matching. The parameters for the deformation are same as in the first example. The mean error, maximum error, and error standard deviation with respect to the distance from the exact matching points are 5.21, 12.67, and 2.47 pixels respectively, using initial global matching. They were reduced to 3.06, 7.72 and 2.31 pixels respectively, when the model-based registration was applied with 10 iterations.

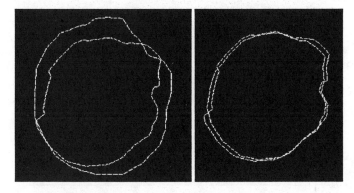

Figure 6. The overlay of the start and goal contours in the case of a piecewise linear transformation: (left) before the global registration (right) after the global registration.

In the next example, we deformed the start contour with piecewise local affine transformations. The start contour was divided into nine segments, where each segment was transformed by a different affine transformation with small random variation from each other. Figure 6(left) is the overlay of the two contours before initial matching, while Figure 6(right) is the overlay of the two contours after initial matching. Using the same parameters for the deformation model, the registration of the two contours is refined with 13 iterations. The mean error, maximum error, and error standard deviation with respect to the distance from the exact matching points are 5.0, 9.0, and 2.29 pixels respectively, using initial global matching. They became 1.75, 13.2 and 2.28 pixels using our model. Most parts of the two contours were well registered except for a few points near the boundary of two segments. The reason is that the above simulated deformation does not keep the continuity between two consecutive segments. That is why, in this example, our model gives better mean value but worse maximun error than the global matching.

5   Conclusion

A deformable model of surface/contour registration has been presented. The implementation of the model in 2D is described in detail while the extension to 3D is briefly mentioned. This model can be considered as the integration of Terzopoulos's active contour model and Burr's dynamic model. However, matching is formulated as an equilibrium problem instead of minimization problem. As a consequence, the problem is converted into a set of linear equations which reduces the algorithmic complexity. Another advantage over the original active contour model is that other hard constraints are easy to incorporate into this model, since the deformation is governed by *PDE* for each vertex individually. The introduction of Burr's external force is intuitive and can match two contours with small and local elastic deformations. The neighborhood size used to compose the force is reduced after each iteration, thus allowing for more "elastic" distortion until the two images have been matched as closely as desired. Experiment results simulating different deformation show good matching results even with some local deformations.

The initial global matching is necessary because: (1) It significantly reduces the number of iterations in the deformation process. (2) If not well globally registered, the dissimilarity of the two shapes may be too large for the deformation to be performed correctly. This is due to the assumption in the calculation of the driving external force of Burr's dynamic model.

The computation of the deformation at each iteration is proportional to the number of vertices and number of triangle patches of the two objects, not the size of the original data. So the computation cost can be controlled by the resolution of the surface/contour, hence is inversely proportional to the quality of the registration.

This model can be used in clinical applications, such as brain CT and lung CT image registration. If registration of two images is in the time domain, the intermediate results can be used for animation. One issue to be noted here is that, although the framework of this model is complete, the selection of the optimal parameters of the model under different situations is not studied in this paper and will be investigated in the future.

References

[1] N. M. Albert and J. F. K. D. The principal axes transformation-a method for image registration. *Journal of Nuclear Medicine*, 31(10):1717–1722, 1990.

[2] A. A. Amini, S. Tehrani, and T. E. Weymouth. Using dynamic programming for minimizing the energy of active contours in the presence of hard constraints. In *The Second International Conference on Computer Vision*, pages 95–99, 1988.

[3] R. Bajscy. Multiresolution elastic matching. *Computer Vision, Graphics, and Image Processing*, 46:1–21, 1989.

[4] L. G. Brown. A survey of image registration techniques. *ACM Computing Surveys*, 24(4):325–376, December 1992.

[5] D. J. Burr. A dynamic model for image registration. *Computer Graphics and Image Processing*, 15:102–112, 1981.

[6] D. J. Burr. Elastic matching of line drawings. *IEEE Trans. Pattern Analysis, and Machine Intelligence*, 3(6):708–713, 1981.

[7] L. D. Cohen. On active contour models and balloons. *CVGIP: Image Understanding*, 53(2):211–218, March 1991.

[8] S. Ganapathy and T. G. Dennehy. A new general triangulation method for planar contours. *Computer Graphics*, 16(3):69–75, July 1982.

[9] I. Gelfand and S. Fomin. *Calculus of Variations*. Prentice-Hall, NJ, 1963.

[10] M. Kass, A. Witkin, and D. Terzoppoulos. Snakes: Active contour models. *Int. J. Comput. Vision*, 1(4):321–331, 1988.

[11] K. F. Lai. *Deformable Contours: Modeling, Extraction, Detection and Classification*. PhD thesis, Electrical and Computer Engineering Department, University of Wisconsin - Madis on, August 1994.

[12] K. F. Lai and R. T. Chin. On regularization, formulation and initialization of active contour models (snakes). In *1st Asian Conf. on Computer Vision*, pages 542–545, 1993.

[13] K. F. Lai and R. T. Chin. Deformable contours: Modeling and extraction. In *Proc. Computer Vision and Pattern Recognition Conf.*, pages 601–608, IEEE Comp Soc Press, Los Alamitos, CA, 1994.

[14] S. Lobregt and M. A. Viergever. A discrete dynamic contour model. *IEEE Trans. Med. Imaging*, 14(1):12–24, March 1995.

[15] M. Moshfeghi. Elastic matching of multimodality medical images. *CVGIP: Graphical Models and Image Processing*, 53(3):271–282, May 1991.

[16] M. Moshfeghi, S. Ranganath, and K. Nawyn. Three-dimensional elastic matching of volumes. *IEEE Tran. on Image Processing*, 3(2):128–138, March 1994.

[17] D. Terzoppoulos, J. Platt, A. Barr, and K. Fleischer. Elastically deformable models. *Computer Graphics*, 21(4):205–214, July 1987.

[18] P. A. van den Elsen, E. D. Pol, and M. A. Viergever. Medical image matching–a review with classification. *IEEE Engineering in Medicine and Biology*, pages 26–39, March 1993.

[19] D. J. Williams and M. Shah. A fast algorithm for active contours and curvature estimation. *CVGIP: Image Understanding*, 55(1):14–26, January 1992.

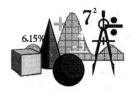

Session 4

Medial Axes

Marching Cores: A Method for Extracting Cores from 3D Medical Images

Jacob D. Furst and Stephen M. Pizer
Medical Image Display & Analysis Group
University of North Carolina
Chapel Hill, NC 27599-3175
furst@cs.unc.edu

David H. Eberly
SAS Institute
SAS Campus Drive
Cary, NC 27511

Abstract

We present an algorithm, called marching cores, that generates cores of 3D medical images and also generalizes to finding implicitly defined manifolds of codimension greater than one. As we march along the core, we use medialness kernels to generate new medialness values and then find ridges in the extended medial space using the geometric definition of height ridges and mathematical models of manifold intersections. Results from both a test image and a CT image illustrate the algorithm.

1. Introduction

Multiscale figural analysis of images has shown considerable potential in a variety of areas. Most of this work has been done with 2D images, but one wishes to be able to perform the same figural analysis on 3D images. One approach is to analyze a 3D image as a set of slices, applying 2D techniques to each slice and then combining the results in a 3D description. However, this is undesirable for the same reason that analyzing a 2D image by rows is undesirable: interslice information is added on after the initial analysis, rather than during this analysis. Thus, we will address the issue of applying 2D techniques in their full generality to 3D images. In either case, a multiscale analysis typically results in a space of one higher dimension than the image space. This has not presented an enormous problem for 2D images, since the resultant space is 3D, the space of everyday experience. (While the scale space is typically not a Euclidean space, many of the same concepts apply.) However, when the subject of analysis is a 3D image, the resulting scale space is 4D, and the rules must be altered. In particular, many of the algorithms designed for finding implicit surfaces in $\mathbf{R}^3$ do not apply in a $\mathbf{R}^3 \times \mathbf{R}^+$ scale space.

The particular application of this paper is to multiscale figural analysis by medial analysis: the core [14]. This analysis results from the intersection of multiscale analysis and the study of symmetry sets, most notably Blum's medial axis [2], [13] and has shown promise in a variety of medical image analysis tasks. First, one may use the core to approximate boundaries. These approximate boundaries provide a starting point for other techniques to converge to object boundaries. Second, the core may be used as a summary descriptor of figural shape. These summary descriptors may then be used to measure transformations and deformations. Third, in combination with other descriptors such as boundaries or figure hierarchies, the core can be used as a model for recognition, segmentation, and measurement. The success of the uses of figural analysis by cores is related to cores having the properties of rotational, translational, and zoom invariance, as well as insensitivities to noise, blurring, and certain changes in image intensity.

However, existing core extraction algorithms have been largely restricted to the calculation of 1D cores from 2D images (and thus from a 3D scale space). Some work has been done on the extraction of 1D cores from 3D images (and thus from a 4D scale space), but very little has been done on the more general problem of extracting 2D cores from 3D images. Further, the existing algorithms for extracting surfaces from 3D data sets turn out not to be extensible to finding surfaces in 4D data sets. We present a new algorithm, called *marching cores*, that generalizes existing surface-finding algorithms to the case of finding surfaces in $\mathbf{R}^4$. We will apply this algorithm to the particular problem of finding cores. The results of this algorithm can then be used in a variety of tasks, from image segmentation to registration to display.

After a brief description of the steps involved in multiscale medial analysis, we will describe related work and discuss some inadequacies of such work regarding our problem. Then we will describe the basic algorithm and improvements to the algorithm. Finally, we will show results of the algorithm on a test object and on a CT scan of a patient's head.

124

2. Multiscale medial analysis of medical images

The multiscale medial analysis of medical images typically involves three major stages [12]. The first two are typically combined algorithmically, although they are conceptually distinct. In this section, we will describe the analysis from a theoretical viewpoint; we will describe algorithm implementation and enhancements in later sections.

1. *Boundariness*
   The first step of analysis involves computing a measure of how like a boundary every point in the image is. Boundariness is a function of position, angle, and scale, and so the measurement of boundariness in 3D images requires 6 parameters: 3 of position, 2 of angle, and 1 of aperture. This is the multiscale extension of measuring the tangency of a sphere to a binary object's boundary. Instead of declaring that a point is or is not on the boundary of an object in a given direction, each point is given a graded measure of how much like a boundary it is, using each possible measurement aperture. When combined with a means of assuring that the scale is proportional to figural width, this is what provides much of the insensitivity of the core. Note also that each point is given such a measure at each possible measurement aperture, providing further insensitivities to image disturbances.

2. *Medialness*
   The second step of core finding (frequently combined with the first step) is to accumulate boundariness values along the surface of spheres. This is the multiscale analog of counting the number of tangencies of a sphere to a binary object's boundary. However, the measure is again graded, based on the integration of the graded boundariness values. The radius of the sphere of integration is proportional to the aperture at which boundariness was measured, and in the same direction in which boundariness was measured. Thus, medialness serves to collect boundariness values of like scale values which point to the same sphere center. It is a function of position and scale (having integrated boundariness across all orientations), and determines how like a medial axis each point in the scale space is. The proportionality between the aperture of the boundariness and the radius of the sphere results in zoom invariance of the medialness function.

The combination of the first two steps is typically performed by convolving the original image with a series of scale dependent medialness kernels. There are many such kernels available; they can be designed to do such things as reduce interfigural interference, reduce the influence of noise inside an object, and pre-

fer a particular orientation. Our algorithm currently uses the Morse medialness kernel [12].

3. *Ridge extraction*
   The final step in core generation requires extracting a meaningful locus from the medialness function. The locus we choose to use is the height ridge, or generalized maximum [4]. In particular, let $M(\vec{x}), \vec{x} \in \mathbf{R}^4$ be a function formed from the convolution of a 3D greyscale image with a range of scale dependent medialness kernels. Let ∇M be the vector of first order partial derivatives of M and let $H(M)$ be the matrix of second order partial derivatives of M. Finally, let $(\lambda_i, e_i), 1 \le i \le 4$ be the solutions to the eigensystem $He = \lambda e$, such that $\lambda_1 \le \lambda_2 \le \lambda_3 \le \lambda_4$. We call the vectors (e_1, e_2, e_3, e_4) the eigenframe of the Hessian matrix. The core is then defined implicitly by the two equations

$$P(\vec{x}) = e_1 \cdot \nabla M = 0$$
$$Q(\vec{x}) = e_2 \cdot \nabla M = 0$$

where, in addition, we require that $\lambda_1 < 0$ and $\lambda_2 < 0$. This last condition guarantees that e_1 and e_2 are the directions of greatest convexity while the first condition confirms that we are at a maximum along the e_1 and e_2 directions. Conceptually, the space defined by e_1 and e_2 is roughly equivalent to enlarging or reducing the radius of the medial kernel and moving the center of the medial kernel transverse to the projection of the core onto space.

The condition $P = 0$ defines a hypersurface, as does the condition $Q = 0$. Thus, finding the core can be thought of as finding the intersection of these two hypersurfaces.

This ridge of medialness is the core. Further, [3] and [10] have shown that this ridge is a manifold.

3. Related work

There already exist many computational algorithms for finding implicitly defined manifolds and they broadly divide into two categories. The first is a class of methods that samples the manifold directly, ignoring information about the containing space. The second is a class of methods that takes advantage of the coordinate grid of the containing space to determine where a surface lies.

Of the first class, there are generally two varieties. The first samples the manifold in a sequential fashion by first finding the manifold and then by restricting further sampling to the tangent space of the previous samples. The most well known of these algorithms is curve following. A curve has a 1D tangent space, so each step of the algorithm involves stepping along the tangent space and finding the curve in that neighborhood. The tangent space of the new sample is then calculated, and the process repeated. This process works less well even for surfaces, as the tangent space becomes 2D, and it is hard to ensure an adequate sampling of the surface. For higher dimensional manifolds, the problem becomes even worse. The second variety of sampling algorithms uses global repulsion functions and Lagrangian constraints to restrict a set of samples to the desired manifold [16]. Simpler versions of this method have a fixed size set of samples, while more advanced versions allow for the set of samples to change to sample the manifold more completely. Such algorithms have the great advantage of performing very well on dynamic surfaces as well as generalizing to arbitrary dimensional manifolds. However, they have no notion of manifold topology, and global repulsion (versus repulsion restricted to the surface) can cause insufficient sampling where the manifold is highly curved.

Of the second class, there are also two major varieties. The first assigns each 0D element (e.g., pixel or voxel) a boolean value based on the manifold intersecting that element or not [8]. The union of all such elements is then taken to be the manifold. Such a representation resembles a pile of n-dimensional sugar cubes. These representations are fairly easy to compute, and the regular nature of the spatial elements makes certain rendering tasks much easier. However, they typically rely on a thresholding technique to evaluate the predicate. Also, they throw away much of the information about the actual manifold in favor of their cuberille representation. The second variety, such as *marching cubes* [11] and *tracked partitioning* [1], assigns a graded values to each 0D element and traps 0's along the 1D elements (edges) connecting the 0D elements. These locations of the 0's along edges are then taken to be the samples of the surface. These methods enjoy the great advantage of being able to combine the samples with linear approximations, again immensely aiding the rendering process. However, this entire class of methods is best suited for finding hypersurfaces; that is, they are not immediately generalizable to other manifolds. *marching lines* [15] presents an extension of the *marching cubes* algorithm used for finding curves in 3D. It employs techniques similar to the ones we use.

There are other methods of finding manifolds, but most rely on having some representation of the manifold in terms of a set of its submanifolds (e.g., reconstructing a surface from a series of parallel curves on the surface [7]). That is, these methods already require some samples and reconstruct the manifold from these samples. Thus, they are generally not useful for finding manifolds for which no samples are available.

indent Our approach starts with the 0-trapping algorithms and works them into a general approach for finding arbitrary-dimensional manifolds in any space. We thus preserve many of the advantages of these methods in finding other manifolds.

4. Marching cores algorithm

The *marching cores* algorithm uses a breadth first traversal to locate the surface in the hypercubes of the 4D medialness space. Given a starting point near the surface (currently specified by the user), the algorithm will exhaustively search the space around the point until a surface point is found. This surface point then serves as the basis from which the core marches: each subsequent hypercube will either extend the search or stop it. When all extensions have been explored, the core has been found.

To locate the core surface in a hypercube, the algorithm determines where the surface intersects the hypercube. This is the first point of departure from existing algorithms. Current algorithms are able to mark each sample point of a cube, and use either a table lookup (marching cubes) or an edge traversal (tracked partitioning) to determine how the surface intersects the cube. This method is generally only applicable to hypersurfaces, which will always intersect at edges. However, by the theorems of manifold intersection based on dimension and codimension, our core surface will only intersect the hypercube on faces of the hypercube. There is no enumeration of samples, nor edge tracking method that we can use to find these intersections. We must adopt a different approach.

We first realize that any surface in 4D is really the intersection of two hypersurfaces. (These ideas do fully generalize to the problem of finding arbitrary manifolds in any space.) And we can use current algorithms to find these hypersurfaces. Then given the two hypersurfaces, we can intersect them to find the actual surface.

However, the two hypersurfaces that define the core are differential measurements on this medialness space and currently require principal frame fields at every vertex of the hypercube. Thus, the calculation of the core is considerably more complex than merely identifying a surface from given samples. In particular, we are required to match eigenframes between two samples, so that we can trap zeroes of measurements made in corresponding eigendirections.

Therefore, the first step of our algorithm is similar to existing ones: we calculate function values for each vertex of the hypercube. However, we must calculate four values for each vertex: P and Q and

$$R(\vec{x}) = e_3 \cdot \nabla M = 0$$

$$S(\vec{x}) = e_4 \cdot \nabla M = 0.$$

R and S are required to prevent errors in surface tracking caused by partial umbilics of $H(M)$. Since eigenvectors may swap at an umbilic, the P and Q functions may correspond to different eigenvectors at different samples. We calculate R and S so that we may trap zeroes of functions corresponding to the same eigen vectors. From these values, we find where the hypersurface intersects the hypercube. Note that the topology of the intersection is not of great interest because it will not aid in the intersection of the two surfaces; we are immediately interested in finding the actual location of the intersection. Figure 1 illustrates zero trapping along an edge of a hypercube.

hypersurfaces and the final surface with linear approximations. Figure 3 illustrates the final intersection of the core with an entire hypercube.

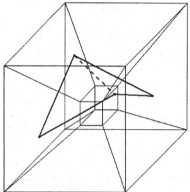

Figure 3. The intersection of the core and a hypercube.

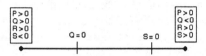

Figure 1. Finding zeroes of the directional derivatives.

Performing this step for all hypersurfaces produces up to four representations which we can then intersect. This is the surface which we are seeking. Figure 2 illustrates the intersections of three hypersurfaces and a face of the hypercube. We then check each intersection for the condition that $\lambda_1 < 0$ and $\lambda_2 < 0$. Points meeting that criterion are core points.

Then, each cube of the hypercube containing a segment of the core defines a new direction in which to search for the core. Figure 4 illustrates the indicated directions of search for the example core.

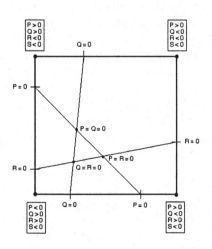

Figure 2. Finding core points.

As in existing algorithms, we choose to represent both

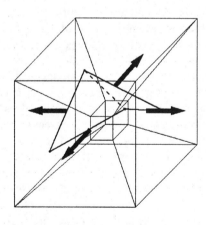

Figure 4. A marching core.

In summary, the marching cores algorithm finds core of 3D medical images by performing the following steps:

1. Read the 3D image into memory.

2. Solicit a starting point for the search from the user.

3. Calculate medialness values for all the vertices of the starting hypercube.

4. Calculate function values for both hypersurfaces at each vertex of the hypercube.

5. Using these function values, find the intersections of the hypersurface and edge via linear interpolation.

6. Represent each of the hypersurfaces with a linear approximation.

7. Intersect the two hypersurface representations.

8. Output the intersection.

9. Repeat from step 3 for each neighboring hypercube into which the core surface extends.

5. Enhancements

We have made modifications to the original *marching cores* algorithm that make it run faster and more stably.

5.1. Efficiency enhancements

The longest step in the algorithm is the medialness calculation. The simplest solution to avoid having to recompute any medialness values is to save each computed value in a table (the 4D medialness image.) However, the resultant use of memory is far from optimal. Given an image as small as $128 \times 128 \times 32$ examined at 16 different scales, the medialness table has 8M entries, most of which will never be used, since the ridges will generally be a sparse subset of the original image. At the other extreme, one can recalculate every medialness value, making optimum use of space, but requiring far more time. The compromise we have taken is a hash table, in which we save medialness values keyed by scale space coordinates. Given the high reuse of medialness values, hash table hit rates of 95% are fairly common, while the size of the table remains small. In addition, the breadth first nature of the marching provides a natural way of disposing of old medialness values should the table become too large.

The height ridge definition and the zero-trapping algorithm require that we be able to match eigenframes between two connected samples in the hypercubes. Such matching in inherently difficult, as the eigenspaces way swap smoothly, or rotate without smoothing in unpredictable ways. To reduce the complexity of this problem, we have adopted a slightly different approach to height ridges [6] in which we declare that one direction in which to search for maximal medialness is the scale direction. Once we have made this decision, we are left with the orthogonal image space in which to search for the other medialness maximum. While this still requires that we match eigenframe across edges, we have reduced the dimensionality of the problem, with an accompanying increase in stability.

Finally, we have used a a divided differences approach to calculating derivatives whenever we are at sample positions, rather than the more expensive spline approximations.

5.2. Functional enhancements

We have added capabilities that allow a user to search for multiple cores within an image, as well being able to change parameters of the program such as the interslice to interpixel distance, the ratio of radius to standard deviation, and the cut-off point for assuming that a Gaussian distribution is zero. Further, the user can choose from a number of methods of dealing with image boundaries.

6. Results

We have applied the *marching cores* algorithm to CT data as well as analytical functions. We present two case studies to illustrate the results of the algorithm. The surfaces and wireframes displayed in the following figures were generated using programs developed by [9].

6.1. Test object

The test object is defined by a central attenuated ellipsoid with two protruding attenuated half-ellipsoids, one emerging from the top of the center ellipsoid and one from the bottom. The two half-ellipsoids are oriented orthogonally to each other.

The attenuation of the ellipsoids is described by a parameter k_i for each coordinate axis x_i of the image:

$$\Sigma \frac{|x_i|^{k_i}}{c_i} = 1.$$

In this image, the k values chosen were 2, 2, (for the long axes) and 5 (for the short axis).

Figure 5 shows the core as a shaded surface, while the object is shown in wireframe. Note the cross-shape hole in the center of the core. Our research indicates that this is most likely due to the interference of the protruding ellipsoids. We have begun research to devise methods of avoiding this interfigural interference on core finding algorithms. Figure 6 shows the approximate boundary corresponding to the core (the boundary at the scale of the core, or BASOC) as a shaded surface, with the object again shown as wire frame. Note the correspondence between the BASOC and the surface of the object. This indicates that the width component of the core is accurately capturing object shape.

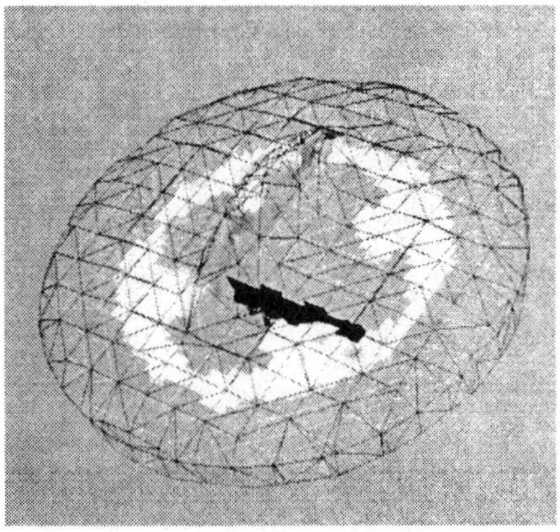

Figure 5. The core (tiled) and the test object (wireframe).

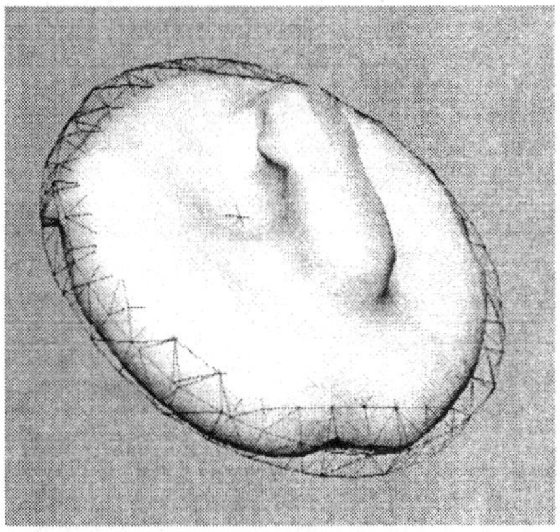

Figure 6. The BASOC (tiled) and the test object (wireframe).

6.2. CT skull

The second result was derived from a CT of a patient's head. We extracted the core of the skull, the surface inside the bone describing the middle between the inside of the skull and the outside of the skull. Figure 7 shows the core of the skull, with an intensity-contoured representation of the skull shown in wireframe. The core failed to extend throughout the entire skull, again most likely because of interobject interference in the original image. Figure 8 shows the boundary at the scale of the core as a shaded surface, with the skull contour again seen in wireframe. Again, the core has fairly accurately captured the shape of the skull.

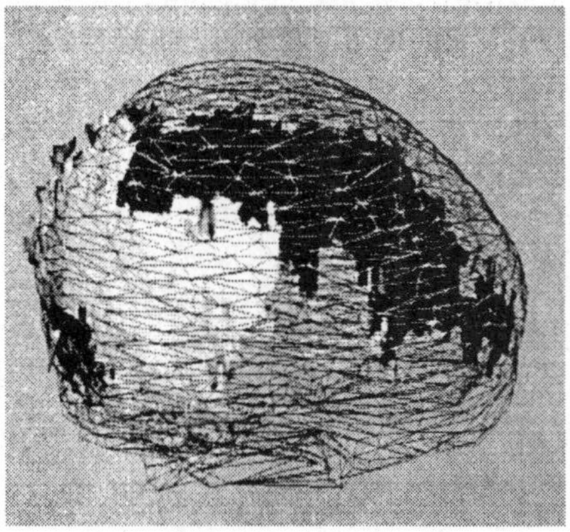

Figure 7. The core (tiled) and the CT skull (wireframe).

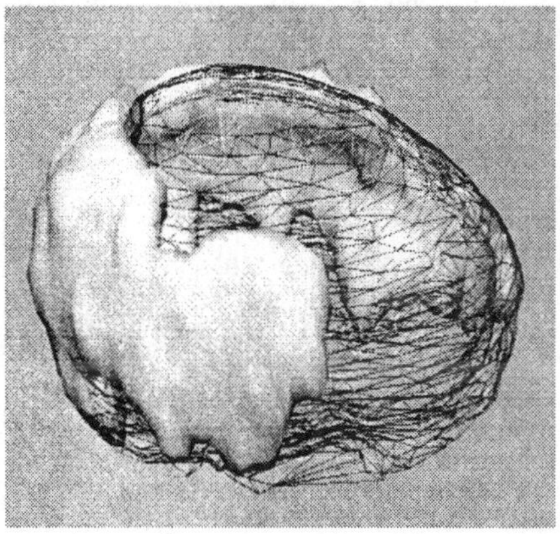

Figure 8. The BASOC (tiled) and the CT skull (wireframe).

7. Discussion

The *marching cores* algorithm presented here has been designed to find the 2D height ridge of a 4D medialness function. However, the same algorithm will also work to generate 2D height ridges of any 4D function. Further, the algorithm can be extended to find d-dimensional ridges of n-dimensional functions. Finally, note that this problem is an example of solving a system of d equations in n unknowns (d < n) in which the solution is known to be a manifold.

Regarding cores (and height ridges in general), the algorithm's greatest weakness is in the correspondence of eigenframes from sample to sample. Eberly [5] has produced alternative definitions for the height ridge that do not require the correspondence of eigenframes, although they have only been implemented for finding 1D cores. We are exploring other ways to avoid having to match eigenframes.

Finally, we are exploring the use of medialness functions other than those, like Morse medialness [12], that are unweighted for the relative orientation of boundaries. Initial study shows that such kernels are sensitive to interfigural interference. We are investigating the use of Gaussian weighting of the medialness kernels based on the relative orientation of a boundary pair and the direction of the core being extended to provide an improvement in interfigural interference.

8. Conclusions

Marching cores provides a method of finding cores of 3D medical images. These cores can then be used for medical image analysis. In addition, the algorithm provides a more general framework in which to find manifolds of arbitrary dimension in any space using the concept of intersecting hypersurfaces.

9. Acknowledgements

The authors wish to thank Chenwei Gu and Mitchel Soltys for providing programs allowing visualization of the core, as well as Stephen Aylward for helping with the interface between the *marching cores* program and the visualization programs. This work was supported partially by NIH grant PO1 CA47982.

References

[1] J. Bloomenthal. Polygonization of implicit surfaces. *Computer Aided Geometric Design*, pages 341–355, 1988.

[2] H. Blum and R. N. Nagel. Shape descriptions using weighted symmetric axis features. *Pattern Recognition*, 10:167–180, 1978.

[3] J. N. Damon. Properties of ridges and cores for two dimensional images. Preliminary version.

[4] D. Eberly. *Geometric Methods for Analysis of Ridges in N-Dimensional Images*. PhD thesis, The University of North Carolina at Chapel Hill, January 1994.

[5] D. H. Eberly, 1995. Personal communication.

[6] D. S. Fritsch. *Registration of Radiotherapy Images using Multiscale Medial Descriptions of Image Structure*. PhD thesis, The University of North Carolina at Chapel Hill, 1993.

[7] H. Fuchs, Z. M. Kedem, and S. P. Uselton. Optimal surface reconstruction from planar contours. *Communications of the ACM 20*, 10:693–702, October 1977.

[8] G. T. Herman and J. K. Udupa. Display of 3d digital images: Computational foundations and medical applications. *IEEE COmputer Graphics and Applications 3*, 5:39–46, August 1983.

[9] H. Hoppe, T. DeRose, T. Duchamp, J. McDonald, and W. Stuetzle. Surface reconstruction from unorganized points. In *Computer Graphics Proceedings*, Annual Conference Series, pages 71–78. ACM SIGGRAPH, July 1992.

[10] R. S. Keller. Summary of results for 1- and 2-dimensional ridges (cores) in 3+1 space. Preliminary version.

[11] W. E. Lorenson and H. E. Cline. Marching cubes: a high resolution 3d surface construction algorithm. *Computer Graphics*, 21(4):163–169, July 1987.

[12] B. S. Morse. *Computation of Object Cores from Grey-level Images*. PhD thesis, The University of North Carolina at Chapel Hill, 1994.

[13] L. R. Nackman and S. M. Pizer. Three-dimensional shape description using the symmetric axis transform, i: Theory. *IEEE Transactions of Pattern Analysis and Machine Intelligence*, 6(2):187–202, 1985.

[14] S. M. Pizer, D. H. Eberly, D. S. Fritsch, and B. S. Morse. Zoom invariant vision of figural shape: the mathematics of cores. Submitted for publication.

[15] J.-P. Thirion and A. Gourdon. The marching lines algorithm: new results and proofs. Technical Report 1881-2, Institut National de Recherche en Informatique et en Automatique, April 1993.

[16] A. P. Witkin and P. S. Heckbert. Using particles to sample and control implicit surfaces. In *Computer Graphics Proceedings*, Annual Conference Series, pages 269–277. ACM SIGGRAPH, July 1994.

Intensity Ridge and Widths
for Tubular Object Segmentation and Description

Stephen Aylward[1]
Elizabeth Bullitt[2]
[1]Dept. of Computer Science
Medical Image Display and Analysis Group
University of North Carolina
Chapel Hill, 27599-3175
aylward@cs.unc.edu
bullitt@med.unc.edu

Stephen Pizer[1]
David Eberly[1]
[2]Dept. of Surgery, Division of Neurosurgery
Medical Image Display and Analysis Group
University of North Carolina
Chapel Hill, 27599-7060
smp@cs.unc.edu
eberly@cs.unc.edu

Abstract

This paper introduces a technique for the automated description of tubular objects in 3D medical images. The goal of automated 3D object description is to extract a representation which consistently details the location, size, and structure of objects in 3D images using minimal user interaction. Such a representation provides a means by which objects can be classified, quantifiably evaluated, and registered. It also serves as a region of interest specification for visualization processes.

The technique presented in this paper is suited for generating representations of 3D objects with nearly circular cross sections which have, possibly as a result of a global operation (e.g., blurring), intensity extrema near their centers. Such tubular objects commonly occur within human anatomy (e.g., vessels and selected bones). The medial axis of each of these objects is well approximated by its intensity ridge. The scales of the local maxima in medialness at all points along the ridge can be mapped to local width estimates. Together these measures capture the location, size, and structure of tubular objects.

This paper covers the mathematical basis, the implementation issues, and the application of this technique to the extraction of vessels from 3D magnetic resonance angiographic images and bones from 3D X-ray computed tomographic images.

1. Introduction

Three-dimensional (3D) medical images can be acquired as a whole (e.g., 3D magnetic resonance images (MRI) or 3D ultrasound images) or generated via the stacking of slices (e.g., stacked 2D MRI or stacked X-ray computed tomography). The goal of automated 3D object description is to extract a representation which consistently details the location, size, and structure of objects of interest in 3D images using minimal user interaction. Such a representation can be used for a variety of classification, quantitative evaluation, and registration tasks. It can also be used to define a region of interest for visualization processes. Existing technologies for these tasks include intensity, landmark, boundary, and medial methods.

Intensity methods include pixel labeling [1, 17] and stochastic registration [7, 15] techniques. Although highly automated, these techniques fail to summarize the geometry (i.e., structure and size) of the objects. Additionally, these processes usually only consider small scale image information which reduces the range of applications for which they can produce sufficient results.

Landmark-based methods [2, 16] have been demonstrated to be appropriate for a wide range of tasks, however they require the existence, specification, and accurate and consistent identification of localized landmark. Landmarks also usually only exist at sparse, discrete locations, thus they do not explicitly capture the intervening characteristics of continuous objects.

Boundary methods include active contour techniques [8, 14]. They too have been shown to be applicable to numerous problems. Recent work [14] has the potential to reduce the otherwise significant user interaction required for their initialization. However, boundary methods are, in general, sensitive to small scale image and boundary noise. Most boundary methods also fail to summarize the geometric information of an object beyond providing an outline.

Medial methods include cores [11] and steered filters [13]. Core methods have been proven to be invariant to a wide range of image noise and object disturbances [10]. They capture the multilocal information of an object and have been demonstrated to be appropriate for classification, quantitative evaluation, registration and visualization tasks. Core representations require near minimal user-interaction to initiate. Steered filters are less computationally expensive than cores but are not as invariant to object disturbances and image noise.

131

Many objects in medical images have circular cross sections with, possibly as a result of a global process (e.g., blurring), intensity extrema near their center (e.g., vessels in MRAs and selected bones in CT). For each such tubular objects, their intensity ridge and an estimate of the object width at points on that ridge can be quickly generated from a single mouse click and an initial width estimate. While the ridge is generated using information only at a single scale, the width estimates use multiscale information and thus are invariant to small scale boundary disturbances. Thus, for tubular objects, capturing their intensity ridges and widths results in a fast and accurate representation.

In situations for which the tubular constraints no longer hold and a general object description is still desired, core methods should probably be used. The technique presented in this paper is based on the methods of cores. Cores represent the loci in scale and space of the generalized maxima in medialness of objects. They are generalized maxima in that they are maximal in a subset of directions (e.g., 1D cores in 3D or 2D cores in 3D). They will not necessarily be maximal in the direction of their locus. For a tubular object, the spatial location of its 1D core is well approximated by its intensity ridge. The generalized maxima in medialness at points on that ridge thus approximate the scale component of the core. While intensity ridges and widths can be easily initiated and rapidly calculated, they are not invariant to as wide a range of image noise and object disturbances as 1D cores are. Additionally, 2D cores must be used to accurately describe objects of arbitrary shape in 3D images.

This representation, as with cores, can be combined with the other representations. By using the ridge and width to locate and characterize landmark points (e.g., branching points or points of maximum object curvature), the landmark identification process can include multiscale geometric information. If a small scale boundary representation is still desired, the ridge and width representation can serve as the starting point for the

boundary generation process. The width estimate also suggests an appropriate aperture with which boundary measures should be made.

Section 2 details the process of intensity ridge and width extraction. Section 3 demonstrates its application to vessel extraction from stacked 2D magnetic resonance angiographic (3D MRA) images and to the extraction of bones from stacked X-ray computed tomography (3D CT) images. Section 4 contains the conclusion and a description of the future work.

2. Intensity ridges and widths extraction

As mentioned in Section 1, the process presented in this paper finds the approximate 1D loci of the maxima in medialness (i.e., a 1D core) for tubular objects. An intensity ridge, measured using a single aperture and defined using 1D height ridge criterion, is used to approximate the spatial component (Section 2.1). The loci of the maxima through scale at points on that ridge approximate the scale component (Section 2.2).

For each application, a single aperture size was used to extract all of the ridges. This intensity ridge aperture was empirically selected so as to ensure the existence of intensity critical points near the centers of the cross sections of the objects of interest. Dependent on image noise and the shape and content of the cross sections, additional processing (e.g., morphological operations or convolutions) may be needed to create central cross section intensity extrema or to improve contrast for the width estimation. For the extraction of the assortment of vessels and bones demonstrated in this paper, however, such preprocessing was not necessary.

2.1. Intensity ridges

By mapping image intensity to height, a 3D image can be viewed as a 3D surface in 4D. A similar mapping can be performed for a 2D image as demonstrated in Figures 1

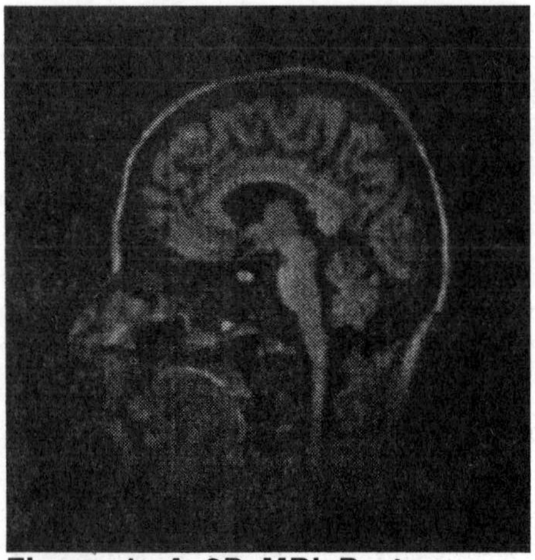

Figure 1. A 2D MRI Proton Density slice.

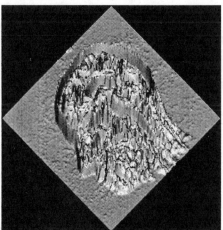

Figure 2. Associated 2D intensity height surface in 3D.

and 2. Height ridge definitions can be applied to such surfaces in order to extract intensity ridges. [5]

The following gives the conditions for a 1D height ridge on a 3D surface, $\mathbf{F}$, above a point $\mathbf{x} \in \Re^3$,

Define

α, β, and γ as ascending-ordered eigenvalues of the Hessian of $\mathbf{F}$ at $\mathbf{x}$

$\mathbf{u}$, $\mathbf{v}$, and $\mathbf{w}$ as the corresponding eigenvectors of the Hessian

and the directional derivatives:

$$\mathbf{P} = \mathbf{u} \cdot \nabla \mathbf{F} \qquad \mathbf{Q} = \mathbf{v} \cdot \nabla \mathbf{F} \qquad \mathbf{R} = \mathbf{w} \cdot \nabla \mathbf{F}$$

Then the following conditions must hold at $\mathbf{x}$:

$$\alpha \leq \beta < 0 < \gamma \qquad \mathbf{P} = 0 \text{ and } \mathbf{Q} = 0$$

The conditions of equality to zero are conveniently tested by formulating the function $\mathbf{J} = \mathbf{P}^2 + \mathbf{Q}^2$ and testing $\mathbf{J} < \text{Tolerance}$ (e.g., 1.0e-4).

For both the ridge and widths calculations, sub-voxel surface height and first and second derivatives need to be calculated. Interpolating cubic splines can be fit to the surface to provide the sub-voxel values. The necessary derivatives can then be calculated via the derivatives of the splines. Cubic splines assure C^0 continuity of the second derivatives which is important for some of the minimization algorithms employed.

2.1.1. Flowing to a ridge point

Given an initial starting point (e.g., user mouse click), its associated intensity ridge can be found using a conjugate directions search with respect to the Hessian so as to minimize $\mathbf{J}$. Two conjugate direction searches are usually sufficient. Thus, a line search is performed from $\mathbf{x}$ in the direction $\mathbf{u}$ to find the local minimum of $\mathbf{J}$, and then, if necessary, the direction $\mathbf{v}$ is searched from that minimum. If the resulting minimum of $\mathbf{J}$ is not within tolerance, a new stimulation point is required. For the examples in this paper, the bisection method [12] was used to perform the line searches.

2.1.2. Traversing the ridge

Once a ridge point is found, two methods exist for traversing the ridge: 1) the tangent to the ridge can be explicitly calculated and used to perform each step or 2) a step can be taken in the approximate direction of the tangent and then a flow to the ridge can be performed if the resulting point is too far off the actual ridge (i.e., $\mathbf{J}$ is larger than its tolerance). [5]

The calculation of the tangent requires the calculation of third derivative information. The method is detailed in [11]. To maintain C^0 continuity of the third derivative information, quardic interpolating splines are needed. Thus, the approximate tangent method is used so as to reduce computational complexity.

By stepping in the approximately tangent direction $\mathbf{w}$ (or -$\mathbf{w}$ when traversing the ridge in the opposite direction) and using the flow algorithm if $\mathbf{J}$ becomes large, the ridge

can be traversed using only the eigenvalues and eigenvectors of the Hessian. This technique also circumvents many of the difficulties associated with the discontinuities in the eigenvector field of an image. In fact, it is sufficient to test and correct for the swapping of $\mathbf{u}$ and $\mathbf{v}$ between consecutive ridge points to handle the remaining discontinuities. [5]

For the examples presented in this paper, the traversal step size was 0.1 voxel units. Termination of ridge traversal occurs when the ridge criterion are no longer upheld. Section 2.3 introduces some implementation specific termination criterion.

2.2. Estimating an object's local width

Given the intensity ridge as an approximation to the central skeleton (i.e., medial axis) of the tubular object, the scales of the maxima in medialness at all points along that ridge need to be calculated to complete the representation. It was empirically determined that the identity function provides an accurate mapping from scale to width.

Evaluating points on the ridge in the order they were extracted, the user-supplied initial width estimate, σ_0, is used to find the scale of the local maximum in medialness, σ_1, at the first ridge point, $\mathbf{x}_1$, using a medialness function, $\mathbf{M}(\mathbf{x};\sigma)$. Each subsequent local maximum in scale, σ_t, is found with respect to the previously found local maximum in scale, σ_{t-1}.

$$\underset{\sigma_t}{\arg \text{ local-max}}\{\mathbf{M}(\mathbf{x}_t;\sigma_t) \mid \sigma_{t-1}\}$$

One form of medialness is the response from convolution with the normalized Laplacian of a Gaussian (LOG) at a given spatial location and scale [11]. Figure 3 depicts a 1D LOG at a fixed σ.

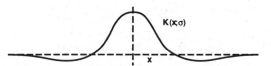

Figure 3. 1D normalized Laplacian of a Gaussian, $K(x;\sigma)$, at a fixed σ

For a 3D image, the LOG kernel is

$$K(\mathbf{x};\sigma) = -\sigma^2 \nabla^2 G(\mathbf{x};\sigma)$$

where $G(\mathbf{x};\sigma)$ is the equation of a 3D Gaussian

$$G(\mathbf{x};\sigma) = \frac{1}{(2\pi)^{3/2}\sigma^3} e^{-\frac{|\mathbf{x}|^2}{2\sigma^2}}$$

Thus, the medialness value at a point, $\mathbf{x}_t$, on the intensity ridge, and at a scale, σ, for an image, I, is

$$\mathbf{M}(\mathbf{x}_t;\sigma) = K(\mathbf{x}_t;\sigma) * I(\mathbf{x}_t) \qquad * = \text{convolution}$$

Any line search technique can be applied to localize the maximum in medialness through scale at a ridge point. For the work presented in this paper, the maximum is initially bracketed using a fixed step size of 1. The bisection method is then used to determine the scale of the maximum within 1.0e-3 tolerance. Due to the slowly varying width of the objects being considered, determining the maxima in medialness at voxel spacing along the ridge is sufficient.

2.3. Implementation issues

To integrate the algorithms given in Sections 2.1 and 2.2 into a usable software package, two ridge termination criterion and a medialness constraint need to be added. They are as follows

- No intensity ridge can enter the area covered by previous ridges and their widths. This prevents the formation of redundant representations of object segments. Thus, for example, a single representation of a branch point is formed.

- Intensity ridges are only allowed to make steps at an angle less than $\pi/8$ compared to the previous step direction. Intensity ridges can often pass branches. However, the intensities can be such that the ridge instead follows those branches. Terminating when this limit is exceeded halts the integration of interfering objects in most situations and only rarely interferes with normal object traversal.

- Near branching points, the proximity of the neighboring branch interferes with the medialness calculations and causes a rapid increase in the local width estimates (see Figure 4). By monitoring the rate of change in width, these biased widths can be automatically replaced by interpolating the surrounding widths. For the applications detailed in this paper, linear interpolation is used. If the interpolation segment length is beyond a threshold (e.g., 10 voxels), it is assumed that a truly wide object segment has been encountered (i.e., an aneurysm) and no interpolation is performed.

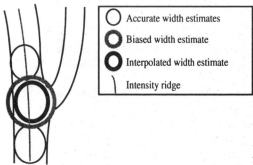

Figure 4. At branches and crossings, medialness estimates undergo rapid changes.

Additionally, having automatically identified potential branching points by monitoring for rapid changes in width, the object boundary about those points can be checked for traversing intensity ridges, and, if found, the objects associated with those ridges can be automatically included. This technique has been implemented for core methods [6]. Work is underway to integrate this automatic branch traversal technique with this software.

3. Applications

Three-dimensional images are usually visualized using volume or surface rendering techniques. These visualization techniques require the selection of a number of parameters including clipping plane orientation, view point selection, and opacity functions or surface generation criterion.

Even for modest sized 3D images, the real time manipulation of these parameters usually requires expensive, specialized hardware, and the selection of appropriate parameters can be difficult. The parameter selection process is often confounded by the fact that multiple objects can have overlapping intensity ranges (e.g., vessels and bones in CTA, or extraneous vessels versus surgically relevant vessels within an MRA) and by the fact that image noise can introduce object boundary disturbances which may vary as a function of these parameters.

By defining regions of interest using ridges and widths, not only can the speed of visualization be increased due to data reduction, but the parameter selection process can be greatly simplified by the removal of interfering objects and the localization of parameter effects. Significant research using core representations in this regard has been performed by David Chen at UNC.

3.1. Vessel and aneurysm definition from MRA

The 3D image for this test set was generated via time-of-flight MRA in a Siemens 10mT/m Magnetom SP4000 unit with a quadrature head coil. Off resonance (1500 Hz) magnetization transfer suppression (75 Hz) was used to further suppress background stationary tissue. Images were acquired as a 4.8 cm stack using 48 1 mm contiguous partitions. The following parameters were used: TR = 38 msec, TE = 7 msec, FOV = 200 mm, flip angle = 20°, signal averages = 1, and a 192x256 matrix with superior venous presaturation pulse.

The resulting 3D MRA image is a stack of 48 slices each 256x256 pixels. Figure 6 shows slice 38 in which the M1 segment of the middle cerebral artery and the A1 segment of the anterior cerebral artery are clearly visible. The coarse hand segmentation along the skull was performed for other purposes and has no bearing on the results of these experiments. Figure 7 shows a maximum intensity projection volume visualization of the entire (i.e., without a limiting region of interest) MRA image. The parameters were chosen so as to maximally differentiate between the vessels and the background. Other researchers (e.g., [9]) have developed MRA data processing techniques which improve the resulting

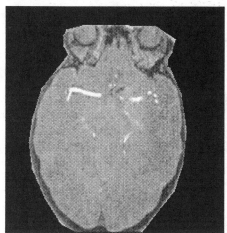

Figure 6. One slice of the 3D MRA image.

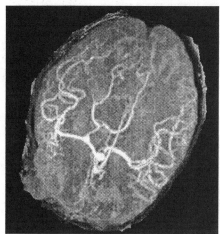

Figure 7. Maximum intensity projection volume visualization of the entire 3D MRA image

visualizations, but such methods do not extract quantitative representations of the vessels and therefore were not considered.

From a **single** mouse click in slice 38 on the M1 segment and an initial local width estimate of 0.32 cm, an

intensity ridge at the inner scale of the image (i.e., without blurring) traversing approximately 250 voxels is extracted, and its local widths determined. This process takes approximately 12 seconds on a HP 715/100. Figure 8 shows slices 36-38 of the 3D MRA with the

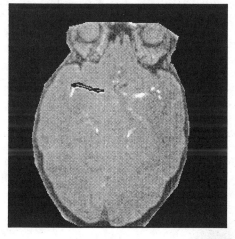

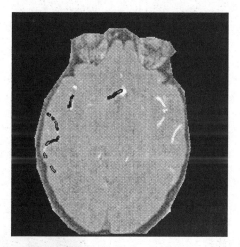

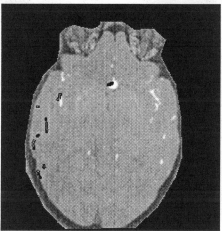

Figure 8. Consecutive slices through a vessel defined from a single mouse click

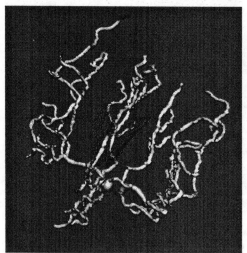

Figure 9. Vessel tree defined from 105 mouse clicks

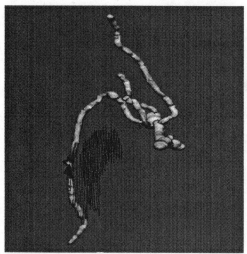

Figure 10. Visualization of relevant vessels and the aneurysm viewed from the optimal surgical approach

intensity ridge indicated in medium gray within the area contained by the local width estimates which is shown in dark gray. Note how the local width is accurately estimated for the wide M1, across vessel branches, and throughout its narrowing until its termination.

In approximately 20 minutes, 105 vessel definitions can be extracted from the MRA data. Figure 9 is a visualization of those definitions. It was made using surface rendering software developed at UNC by Mitch Soltys. By viewing these definitions as opposed to directly viewing the MRA data (Figure 7), noise is eliminated. Note also the smooth and regular vessel boundaries generated from the estimated widths in this rendering compared to the boundary irregularities depicted in the maximum intensity projection (Figure 7). The location and approximate width of the neck of the anterior communicating artery aneurysm can be clearly distinguished. A hand contouring of the ventricles is (easily) included in the rendering for reference.

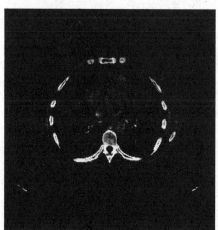

Figure 11. Slice 49 from the CT image

Additionally, a variety of post processing techniques can be applied to these representations.

Post processing software developed by Elizabeth Bullitt enables the elimination of extraneous vessel definitions from view so that one can, for example, visualize only those vessels likely to be seen from a particular surgical approach (see Figure 10 which also includes the hand contour of the ventricles for reference). Post processing techniques can also be used to perform quantitative evaluations (i.e., identification of a possible stenosis), classifications (e.g., vessel segment, branch point, etc.), registrations, and multimodal integration (vessels not appearing in an MRA due to flow patterns can be defined in X-ray angiograms and inserted into a common visualization). [3, 4] detail many of these techniques and demonstrate their application to surgical planning.

3.2. Bone definition from 3D CT

The 3D image for this test set contains 78 256x256 slices. Intra-slice pixel spacing is 0.169492 cm. Inter-slice spacing is 0.4 cm.

Figure 11 shows one slice of the CT data. Several ribs, the sternum, and the spinal column are clearly visible. Figure 12 contains two volume visualizations of the entire 3D CT image.

Clicking within each rib, the spinal cord, and the sternum allows the data associated with these bones to be extracted. The ridge calculations are performed with a Gaussian aperture of 0.24 cm. This gives the ribs an approximately Gaussian cross section. For the spinal column and sternum, the intensity valley associated with the spinal cord and the bone marrow, respectively, are used to approximate the medial axis. Valley extraction is accomplished by simply inverting the pixel intensities for the ridge flow and traversal algorithms. All width

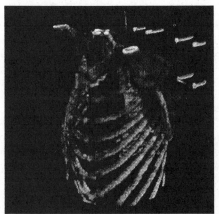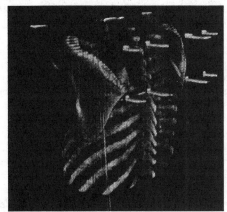

Figure 12. Two volume visualization of the entire 3D CT image

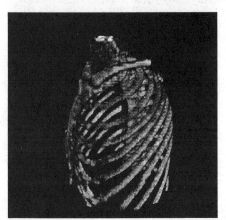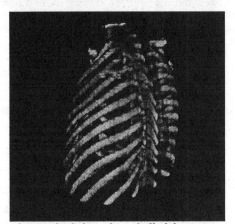

Figure 13. Two volume visualizations of the data bounded by the definitions extracted from the 3D CT image

calculations are performed without modification. An initial width estimate of 6.4 cm is used to extract a definition of the spinal column. An initial width estimate of 1.6 cm is used during the extraction of the ribs. Figure 13 is a volume visualization of the data bounded by the extracted definitions whose widths are twice the computed widths in the definitions. It is important to note that all other visualization parameters are the same for Figures 12 and 13.

4. Conclusion

This paper introduces a technique for the automated description of tubular objects in 3D images. This technique enhances the visualization of and enables the quantitative evaluation, classification, and registration of tubular objects in 3D images. Tubular objects are defined as having nearly circular cross sections of relatively uniform content. Such objects are common in human anatomy, and their representation using intensity ridges and widths has been demonstrated to be sufficiently accurate for several applications.

Current work is focusing on the integration of automated branch traversal techniques into the representation extraction process. Subsequent work will concentrate on the integration of boundary evolution processes so that the boundaries estimated by the ridges and widths can be refined as needed. Each of these tasks has already been applied to core methods [6] and this work will rely heavily that research.

This work was supported in part by NCI-NIH grant P01 CA47982.

References

[1] Aylward, S.R. and Coggins, J.M., "Spatially Invariant Classification of Tissues in MR Images." *Visualization in Biomedical Computing*, Rochester, MN, 1994

[2] Bookstein, F. and Green, W., "A Thin-Plate Spline for Deformations with Specified Derivatives." *Mathematical Methods in Medical Imaging II*, SPIE, vol. 2035, 1993 p. 14-44

[3] Bullitt, E., Aylward, S., Soltys, M., Boxwala, A., Rosenman, J. and Pizer, S., "Intracerebral Vessel Display I. Core-based Extraction of Vessels from

Magnetic Resonance Angiograms." *American Journal of Neuroradiology*, vol. Submitted, 1996

[4] Bullitt, E., Liu, A. and Pizer, S.M., "Intracerebral Vessel Display II. Three-Dimensional Reconstruction of Aneurysms from Angiographic Images." *American Journal of Neuroradiology*, vol. Submitted, 1996

[5] Eberly, D., Gardner, R.B., Morse, B.S., Pizer, S.M. and Scharlach, C., "Ridges for Image Analysis." *Journal of Mathematical Imaging and Vision*, vol. 4, 1994 p. 351-371

[6] Fritsch, D.S., Eberly, D., Pizer, S.M. and McAuliffe, M.J., "Stimulated Cores and their Applications in Medical Imaging." *IPMI 1995: Information Processing in Medical Imaging*, Kluwer Series in Computational Imaging and Vision, 1995 p. 385-368

[7] Hill, D.L.G., Studholme, C. and Hawkes, D.J., "Voxel Similarity Measures for Automated Image Registration." *Visualization in Biomedical Computing*, SPIE, Rochester, MN, vol. 2359, 1994 p. 205-216

[8] Kass, M., Witkin, A. and Terzopoulos, D., "Snakes: Active Contour Models." *International Journal of Computer Vision*, vol. 1, no. 4. 1988 p. 321-331

[9] Michiels, J., Bosmans, H., Nuttin, M., Knauth, M., Verbeeck, R., Vandermeulen, D., Wilms, G., Marchal, G., Suetens, P. and Gybels, J., "The use of Magnetic Resonance Angiography in Stereotactic Neurosurgery." *Journal of Neurosurgery*, vol. 82, 1995 p. 982-987

[10] Morse, B.S., Pizer, S.M., Puff, D.T. and Gu, C., "Zoom-Invariant Vision of Figural Shape: Effects on Cores of Image Disturbances." *Computer Vision and Image Understanding*, vol. Submitted, 1996

[11] Pizer, S.M., Eberly, D., Morse, B.S. and Fritsch, D.S., "Zoom-invariant Vision of Figural Shape: the Mathematics of Cores." *Computer Vision and Image Understanding*, vol. Submitted, 1996

[12] Press, W.H., Flannery, B.P., Teukolsky, S.A. and Vetterling, W.T., Numerical Recipes in C. Cambridge University Press, Cambridge, 1990

[13] Szekely, G., Koller, T., Kikinis, R. and Gerig, G., "Structural Description and Combined 3D Display for Superior Analysis of Cerebral Vascularity from MRA." *SPIE P*, 1994 p. 272-281

[14] Tek, H. and Kimia, B.B., "Volumetric Segmentation of Medical Images by Three-Dimensional Bubbles." *Workshop on Physics-Based Modeling*, IEEE Press, 1995 p. 9-16

[15] van den Elsen, P.A., Pol, E.-J.D., Sumanaweera, T.S., Hemler, P.F., Napel, S. and Adler, J.R., "Grey Value Correlation Techniques used for Automatic Matching of CT and MR Brain and Spine Images." *Visualization in Biomedical Computing*, SPIE, Rochester, MN, vol. 2359, 1994 p. 227-237

[16] Vignaud, J., Rabischong, P., Yver, J.P., Pardo, P. and Thurel, C., "Multidirectional Reconstruction of Angiograms by Stereogrammetry and Computer. Application to Computed Tomography." *Neuroradiology*, vol. 18, 1979 p. 1-7

[17] Wells, W.M., Grimson, W.E.L., Kikinis, R. and Jolesz, F.A., "Statistical Gain Correction and Segmentation of MRI Data." *Visualization in Biomedical Computing*, SPIE, Rochester, MN, vol. 2359, 1994

Characterization and Recognition of 3D Organ Shape in Medical Image Analysis Using Skeletonization

M. Näf[a], O. Kübler[a], R. Kikinis[b], M.E. Shenton[c] and G. Székely[a]

[a] Communication Technology Laboratory, Swiss Federal Institute of Technology ETH,
Gloriastr. 35, CH-8092 Zurich, Switzerland
[b] Department of Radiology, MRI Division, Brigham & Women's Hospital
Harvard Medical School, 75 Francis Street, Boston MA 02115, USA
[c] Department of Psychiatry 116A, Harvard Medical School and Brockton VACM
090 Belmont Street, Brockton, MA 02401, USA

Abstract

The paper describes a procedure for the generation of the Blum skeleton (Medial Axis) of large, complex, digitized 3D objects. The proposed algorithm is a 3D generalization of the Voronoi Skeleton concept, which is already in routine use for 2D shapes. A specific algorithm for the generation of 3D Voronoi Diagrams of very large point sets (containing several 100'000 generating points) is described. The pitfalls and drawbacks of pruning procedures are discussed, and a topologically correct regularization algorithm is given for the necessary regularization of the resulting Voronoi diagram. The performance of the developed procedures is illustrated on synthetic objects, as well as on large, complex anatomical data, e.g. the segmented white matter of a human brain extracted from MR data.

Keywords: *Multidimensional Volume Models, shape analysis, skeletonization*

1. Introduction

Analysis of organs in 3D radiological data calls for shape description methods which are capable of dealing with the variability and complexity of the human anatomy including organs of extremely complex shapes like the human brain. Our investigations will concentrate on the following two different aspects of organ shape analysis:

- Recognition of organs of the human anatomy in 3D radiological data. We want to concentrate especially on the aspect of finding robust methods for matching generic anatomical knowledge coded in anatomical atlases with individual anatomy found in acquired radiological data. The basic problem of such inter-individual anatomical matching is, that while brains are very similar in their overall shapes, the surface of individual brains (i.e. the structure of sulci and gyri) is fingerprint-like, no two brains are the same. This makes classical, surface-based methods fairly useless and we have to search for methods which are able to separate the general global brain shape from the individual variations in a well controlled and robust way.

- Analysis and characterization of the morphological structure of the cortex. This problem is complementary to the first one in the sense, that here we do not care about generic shape characteristics but want to analyze the unique individual variations.

One has to realize that the requirements for the shape descriptor to be used are actually complementary for these two cases.

- In the first case we regard the different objects as samples of a population. An ideal object shape descriptor would allow us to search for the common properties of the object class without being much disturbed by the individual variations of the single entities. In other words we are looking for methods capable of describing *global*, general shape.

- in the second case we want to investigate, how the individuum differs from other members of its class. We want to characterize its unique, distinctive features. For this purpose we need a shape descriptor which can code and handle *local*, specific details efficiently.

The concept of local symmetry, originating from the pioneering work of Blum [2] has the potential of unifying these requirements for the description of biological objects. The shape descriptor resulting from a skeletonization process consists of hierarchically organized local symmetry axes, allowing task-dependent differentiation between global ob-

Proceedings of MMBIA '96

ject shape and local individual features. We will also investigate, how serious limitations of the skeletal representation can be potentially eliminated by generalizing the concepts of Blum to a collection of all local symmetries of a scene and how skeletons and the Multi-scale Medial Axis concept of Pizer et.al. [12] can be possibly combined to a powerful tool for object recognition in complex anatomical scenes.

2. Voronoi Skeletons in 2D

During the last two decades skeletonization has been an important research area for image processing and computer vision, concentrating primarily on the basic problem of how the MAT concept could be implemented on the digital image raster. As rotational invariance is essential for reliable shape description, an Euclidean metric (or a reasonable approximation of it) has to be reconciled with the raster-type connectivity during the skeleton generation procedure.

An elegant way to generate topologically, as well as geometrically correct skeletons is the reformulation of Blum's concept in a semi-continuous way. Objects on the raster plane can be faithfully represented by their discrete boundary points, providing the densest possible sampling of their (unknown) continuous outline [16, 4, 19, 14]. The Voronoi Diagram of these boundary points is a superset of the MAT [4] and can be generated very efficiently [14]. The Voronoi Diagram (VD) is a fundamental structure in computational geometry. It is defined on a set S of n points in d-dimensional Euclidean space E^d. The points of S are called sites (sometimes other basic elements, e.g. polygons, are used as sites). The VD of S splits E^d into regions with one region for each site, so that the points in the region for site $s \in S$ are closer to s than to any other site in S. The Delaunay triangulation (DT) of S is the dual of the VD. It decomposes the convex hull of S into a number of convex cells having elements of S as vertices. Each cell has the property that its vertices lie on a d-dimensional circumscribing ball and that there are no other sites lying inside this ball. More details on VD's and DT's can be found in [15]

Several regularization procedures have been proposed to reduce the resulting 2D VD to its stable, essential parts (pruning). They can most easily be understood by referring to the straight line dual of the VD, the DT. The object can be envisaged as being composed of Delaunay triangles. The goal of regularization is to identify those peripheral Delaunay triangles which are irrelevant for representing the object at coarser scales, and to suppress the corresponding parts of the VD in order to obtain the desired Voronoi skeleton.

Several procedures have been proposed to measure the relevance of the different branches of the VD:

- Brandt and Algazi [4] use the maximal distance between the original outline segment of the object and

the Delaunay-edge it is replaced by,

- Ogniewicz [14] calculates the difference in length between the original outline segment and the Delaunay edge and

- Meyer [11], Talbot and Vincent [19] as well as Attali and Montanvert [1] propose to use the angle between the fire-fronts which meet at the selected skeleton branch. It can be easily shown, that the 'pointedness' of the appropriate Delaunay triangles provides the same measure.

While it has been shown that the inner VD of the boundary points is homotopically equivalent to the skeleton of the object [16], simply thresholding the branches will not necessarily preserve the topology of the VD, that is the topology of the original object. In order to be sure that no homotopical changes happen, another regularization approach must be taken. The deletion of Delaunay triangles can be made in a recursive manner by deleting only those triangles on the border (i.e. those having two sides on the actual outline of the object, and one side through the object) which ensures that the graph topology remains unaltered.

Recursive regularization algorithms also need a measure which decides where the consecutive deletion of triangles has to stop. All kinds of measures (such as the previously discussed ones) can be used for this purpose. The recursive deletion ensures that no topological changes occur. Note, however, that the first two of the proposed measures change monotonically during the successive deletion procedure, therefore simple thresholding will also guarantee the preservation of homotopy. This is not the case for the third ('pointedness') measure, which means that it must be combined with a recursive deletion algorithm. In this case, however, small pointed triangles on the object boundary can block the regularization process, in effect making irrelevant branches of the VD undeletable. This is a general problem of non-monotonic regularization measures.

In the following we will study the 3D generalization of the skeleton. In contrast to the 2D case, only few studies have been published [18, 1, 3, 13], consequently many theoretical and implementational problems remain unsolved. While the generation of the 3D VD of very large point sets poses 'only' technical difficulties, no satisfactory procedure for 3D pruning has been proposed. We discuss the 3D generalization of some 2D regularization measures and show preliminary results.

3. 3D Voronoi Skeletons

3.1. Skeletons in 3D

The analysis of real 3D image scenes requires methods capable of dealing with the shape of truly 3D objects. Such scenes arise e.g. in medical image analysis, where current radiological image acquisition techniques deliver high-resolution true 3D images of the individual patient anatomy. Traditional slice-by-slice methods are generally misleading and especially troublesome if dealing with object shape. Computer representation and handling of biological objects calls for 3D shape analysis methods dealing with the complexity and variability of the anatomy. Such techniques may find broad application in image analysis (e.g. for computer representation and manipulation of anatomical knowledge) as well as in computer graphics (e.g. for efficient manipulation and deformation of 3D objects). Skeletonization (originally emerging from the analysis of the morphology of biological objects) appears to be one of the few promising techniques to achieve these goals.

The MAT concept of Blum can be generalized straightforwardly to 3D. Usually, the fire-fronts initiated at the boundary of an object meet on surfaces, resulting in a skeleton consisting of branched 2D manifolds. However, in degenerate cases (as e.g. perfectly cylindrical objects) the quenching procedure will produce curves instead of surfaces. As we do not want to make any a priori restrictions on the shape of the object investigated, the skeletonization algorithm should be able to generate 3D skeletons that contain both surface (2D) and lineal (1D) parts.

The basic theoretical results behind the 2D Voronoi skeleton generation procedures [16, 4] can also be generalized to 3D. The strategy to be followed is then analogous to 2D: the boundary of the object to be analyzed is sampled, the VD of the sample points is generated and finally the irrelevant branches have to be pruned to get the 3D Voronoi skeleton which is a reasonably good approximation of the continuous skeleton. It has to be noted, that the proven theorems require a maximally dense sampling, i.e. sampling the boundary at voxel level. Due to the enormous algorithmic difficulties caused by the huge amount of boundary points in a maximally dense sampling, some proposals have been made for sparse boundary sampling. It seems to be intuitive to generate less dense sampling on surface patches with low local curvature. Such approximations, however, are only admissible if the object is approximated by polygons , in which case entirely different algorithms for the generation of the skeleton of continuous objects have to be found [10]. Otherwise, in addition to large distortions in the skeleton algorithmically disturbing side-effects have to be expected as e.g. parts of the inner skeleton may become disconnected.

3.2. 3D Voronoi diagram generation

Maximal sampling of the boundary of 3D objects on a 256^3 image raster usually results in several 100'000 generating points. Unfortunately, the extremely efficient 2D VD generation algorithm has no direct generalization to 3D because it takes advantage of the explicit ordering of the edges incident in a vertex which is given in 2D but not in 3D.

In computational geometry many algorithms for 3D VD generation have been proposed and some implementations are available. Most of them, however, run into serious problems when faced with such a large number of generating points. In addition, they are usually unable to handle degenerate cases caused by more than four cospherical points; a situation that is unavoidable among point samples located on a regular image raster. Handling cospherical points calls for more flexible data structures to represent a DT consisting not only of tetrahedra but of general convex polyhedra.

In our implementation we extended an existing algorithm [5] adapting it to deal with cospherical input points and supplying it with a uniform grid for fast point location, a technique which is well known from computer graphics applications. The algorithm actually computes the DT of a point set which is the dual representation of the VD. It is based on the divide & conquer (D&C) paradigm, which basically consists of recursively applying two phases: a subdivision of the problem into subproblems and a merging of the subproblems' solutions. The efficiency of the D&C algorithm depends on an efficient merging of the local DT's computed in the previous phase. The merging requires a number of local modifications on both DT's which is an expensive task. This can be avoided if instead of merging partial results in a second step, the merging part of the DT is built first and then the independent parts of the DT are computed on subsets of the input points.

We have chosen to follow Cignoni's algorithm both for its time characteristics (it can be parallelized and has been proved to be optimal in 2D both in terms of mean and worst time complexity) and its memory requirements: the Delaunay polyhedra can be stored to disk immediately when they are generated and only a relatively small list of Delaunay faces have to be retained in memory.

The local DT's are generated by successively constructing new Delaunay polyhedra from already computed Delaunay faces. For that a new vertex must be searched in the input point-set so that together with the Delaunay face it forms a new Delaunay polyhedron. This operation can be speeded up considerably if one uses the fact that in most cases one has to search the missing vertex only among a limited number of points when choosing an appropriate scanning of the space. In fact the missing vertex must lie on the other side of the Delaunay face and within a sphere of unknown radius which passes through the corner vertices of the Delaunay face. Hence a sequence of such spheres with increasing radius can be generated and the space inside of them scanned until the missing vertex is found. The uniform grid, in our case a regular, non-hierarchical partitioning of the 3D space in cubic grid cells, is used as an indexing scheme for fast selection of points contained in a given sphere. To avoid sphere to cell conversion the search is performed in the smallest circumscribed cube of the sphere.

The VD can be directly obtained from the DT by the following substitutions. Each Delaunay polyhedron becomes a Voronoi vertex located at the center of the polyhedron's circumsphere. Each Delaunay face becomes a Voronoi edge joining the circumsphere centers of the two Delaunay polyhedra which are in touch over that face. Finally each Delaunay edge becomes a Voronoi face made up of all the Voronoi vertices representing the Delaunay polyhedra which meet at that edge.

With our implementation we have been able to generate 3D VD's of large medical objects with over 250'000 boundary points.

3.3. The Delaunay Triangulation as a cell complex

Cell complexes are used to define topological properties of finite sets. They have been proposed to image processing by Kovalevsky [9]. We will introduce here just a few basic definitions.

A **cell complex** $\mathcal{C}(C, B, \dim)$ is a set C of abstract elements provided with an antisymmetric, irreflexive and transitive binary relation $B \subset C \times C$ called the bounding relation and with a dimension function $\dim : C \mapsto I$ from C into the set I of the non-negative integers such that $\dim(c') < \dim(c'')$ for all pairs $(c', c'') \in B$.

In our case the DT of an object can be described as a cell complex $\mathcal{D}(D, B, \dim)$ where D is the set of vertices, edges and faces of the DT. The bounding relation B is a partial order in D. It indicates the ordered pairs (e', e'') of elements such that e' is said to bound e'', which is denoted by $e' \prec e''$. A cell is said to bound a cell of higher dimension if it is part of its boundary. For $\mathcal{D}$ we choose the bounding relation in such a way that an edge is bounded by two vertices and a face by some edges together with the vertices of those edges and so on. The dimension function dim assigns 0 to vertices, 1 to edges, 2 to faces and 3 to polyhedra.

A **subcomplex** $\mathcal{S}(S, B_S, \dim_S)$ of a given complex $\mathcal{C}(C, B, \dim)$ is a complex whose set S is a subset of C and the relation B_S is the intersection of B with $S \times S$. The dimension function remains unchanged for all elements in the subset. Hence to define a subcomplex it is sufficient to define a subset S of elements. This is important because it allows us to use the common formulae of set theory to define intersections, unions and complements of subcomplexes. A subcomplex $\mathcal{S} \subset \mathcal{C}$ is called **open** if for every element e' of the set S all elements of C which are bounded by e' are also contained in S.

A **topological space** $(X, \mathcal{T})$ consists of a set X of elements and a system $\mathcal{T} = \{S_1, \ldots, S_i, \ldots\}$ of subsets S_i of X. These subsets are called the open subsets of the space and must fulfill 3 fundamental axioms:

A1 $X \in \mathcal{T}$ and $\emptyset \in \mathcal{T}$

A2 the union of an arbitrary number of sets in $\mathcal{T}$ must be contained in $\mathcal{T}$

A3 the intersection of a finite number of sets in $\mathcal{T}$ must be contained in $\mathcal{T}$

It is easy to see that the open subcomplexes in $\mathcal{C}$ as defined above satisfy these axioms. Hence cell complexes are topological spaces and provide us a mean to describe consistently topological properties of a DT.

Every open subcomplex $\mathcal{S} \subset \mathcal{C}$ is called an open **neighborhood** of its elements $e \in S$. We denote it by $N(e)$. Since $\mathcal{C}$ is finite an element e can have only a finite number of open neighborhoods. Hence the intersection of all of them is according to axiom A3 again an open neighborhood. We call it the smallest open neighborhood of e and denote it by $N_0(e)$.

Then the **boundary** $\partial(\mathcal{S})$ of a subcomplex $\mathcal{S} \subset \mathcal{C}$ is the set of elements which contain in their smallest neighborhood at least one element of both the subcomplex $\mathcal{S}$ and its complement $\mathcal{C} \setminus \mathcal{S}$.

We already mentioned in the 2D case that the VD and the DT are dual representations. The duality of two cell complexes can be defined as follows:

Two n-dimensional cell complexes $\mathcal{C}(C, B, \dim)$ and $\mathcal{C}'(C', B', \dim')$ are called **dual** if there exists a one-to-one mapping $\alpha : C \mapsto C'$ with the following properties: if $\alpha(e_1) = e_1'$ and $\alpha(e_2) = e_2'$ then

(a) $e_1 \prec e_2 \Leftrightarrow e_1' \prec e_2'$
(b) $\dim'(e_1') = n - \dim(e_1)$ and $\dim'(e_2') = n - \dim(e_2)$

Hence the 3D VD generation of a point-set $\{v_i\}$ which describes the boundary of an object will yield two dual cell complexes as a result; the DT $\mathcal{D}$ and the VD $\mathcal{V}$ which are related by the mapping α as defined at the end of section 3.2. Then in a first step we define a subcomplex $\mathcal{V}_0 \subset \mathcal{V}$ which represents the 'inner' VD and contains only those elements strictly lying inside the object. By duality a subcomplex $\mathcal{D}_0 \subset \mathcal{D}$ with $D_0 = \alpha(V_0)$ is defined on which the regularization will take place. It can be seen that $\mathcal{D}_0$ is an open subcomplex.

3.4. Regularization

As discussed in the 2D case, the regularization needs:

- a measure expressing the significance of a Voronoi branch.
- a deletion sequence ensuring topology preservation.

The inner VD of the generating boundary points has a special structure in 2D. For a simply connected object without holes it is an acyclic graph representing a tree. Hence every Voronoi edge connects exactly two parts of the graph.

This enforces a hierarchy between branches, defining a natural deletion sequence when progressing from the outmost branches to the inside of the graph. Equivalently every Delaunay edge (the dual counterpart of a Voronoi edge in 2D) cuts the object into two disjoint parts. This allows easy definition of significance measures based on 2D form considerations, expressing the importance of the removed subpart for the overall appearance of the object. These nice properties lead to the definition of different significance measures in 2D, making simple regularization techniques as discussed in the previous section applicable. Note that the situation for an object with holes is similar since the cycles that will show up in the Voronoi graph reflect the object's topology and therefore must be preserved anyway.

In 3D however the Voronoi graph rather resembles a net containing many cycles, and thus lacks the hierarchical organization which has been proved so useful in 2D. This means that there is no natural deletion sequence, uniquely defined by the topology of the cell complex. It can be shown, that apart from trivial degenerate cases, there are always many substantially different deletion sequences of the Voronoi faces equally respecting the topology of the object. As no theoretical results are known about the effect of the deletion sequence to the resulting skeleton, the uniqueness of the resulting skeleton may be questioned. There is of course no difficulty in defining arbitrarily a partial ordering e.g. on Voronoi faces but in general it is hard to find an ordering which ensures the invariance of the skeleton after pruning.

During the recursive regularization procedure the DT or equivalently the VD is stepwise reduced by deleting single Delaunay polyhedra when operating on the DT or Voronoi faces when operating on the VD. In both cases the dual representation is updated, i.e. the deletion of a polyhedron on the DT implies the deletion of its corresponding vertex on the VD. The sequence in which those elements are removed is called the deletion sequence. The deletion sequence must ensure that after each step the remaining part of the DT is again an open subcomplex of $\mathcal{D}$ and is homotopically equivalent to $\mathcal{D}_0$. For this purpose different checks for topological equivalence have to be implemented. In the following, the topological check for Delaunay polyhedra will be described.

The regularization process produces a sequence of subcomplexes $(\mathcal{D}_i)$ by removing a subcomplex $\mathcal{S}_i$:

$$\mathcal{D}_{i+1} = \mathcal{D}_i \setminus \mathcal{S}_i$$

$\mathcal{S}_i$ must be a closed cell complex so that $\mathcal{D}_{i+1}$ is again an open subcomplex. These are homotopically equivalent if their boundaries are homotopically equivalent. Hence if we want to remove a single polyhedron p_i in the i-th step we must also remove the cells which bound p_i. So the (i+1)-th

subcomplex can be described as:

$$\mathcal{D}_{i+1} = \mathcal{D}_i \setminus \{p_i, \partial(p_i)\}$$

To ensure homotopical equivalence between $\mathcal{D}_i$ and $\mathcal{D}_{i+1}$ one must ensure that at each step the boundary of the newly generated subcomplex is homotopically equivalent (denoted by $\cong$) to the previous one: $\partial(\mathcal{D}_i) \cong \partial(\mathcal{D}_{i+1})$. The deletion of p_i changes the boundary of $\mathcal{D}_i$ only locally, namely at the bounding elements of p_i. This means that the homotopical equivalence of $\mathcal{D}_i$ and $\mathcal{D}_{i+1}$ can be decided locally by the following deletability criterion:

Consider the bounding elements of p_i. They can be grouped into two categories according to whether they belong to the boundary of $\mathcal{D}_i$ or not. The elements which belong to the boundary are called outside elements, the others inside elements. We can group them into connected components containing only inside or only outside elements using the bounding relation B. Then the deletability criterion is defined by two conditions:

1. there is exactly one inside and one outside component.
2. the boundary between the two components is a non self-intersecting, closed line.

In a practical implementation we only need to consider the outside components and the boundaries between inside and outside components. A component can have dimensionality 0,1 or 2 according to the maximal dimensionality of the elements contained in it.

From the fact that all vertices lie on the object's boundary we directly conclude that all vertices are outside elements and hence must belong to one single outside component. In other words if several 1D outside components (isolated vertices) exist the criterion is not fulfilled.

The existence of 1D outside components again makes p_i not deletable as the boundary of a 1D component is not a closed line.

The boundary of 2D components consists of vertices and edges. We don't consider the vertices since they are all outside elements. Three types of outside edges can be distinguished: those bounding 2 outside faces, those bounding 2 inside faces and those bounding both an inside and an outside face. The first ones are lying in the inner of the component and do not belong to the component's boundary. The second ones do belong to the component's boundary which is self-intersecting at this edge, and thus p_i is not deletable. Then we determine whether the third ones make up exactly one closed line which does not self-intersect in a vertex. If this is true p_i is deletable.

In listing 1 the deletability criterion is given in pseudocode. The function takes a polyhedron p_i as input and returns a boolean value depending on whether p_i is deletable or not. Let us step through the algorithm:

```
function is_deletable(p_i)

1.  oi_edgs = make_list()
    oo_edgs = make_list()
    boundary = make_list()
2.  FOR each outside face f_i ∈ p_i DO
        FOR each edge e_i ∈ f_i DO
3.          IF member(e_i,oi_edgs)
                remove(e_i,oi_edgs)
                insert(e_i,oo_edgs)
            ELSE
                insert(e_i,oi_edgs)
4.  FOR each inside face f_i ∈ p_i DO
        FOR each outside edge e_i ∈ f_i DO
5.          IF not member(e_i,oi_edgs) and
                not member(e_i,oo_edgs)
                RETURN not deletable
6.  IF size(oi_edgs) > 0
7.      e_0 = get_edg(oi_edgs)
        v_0 = start_vrt(e_0)
        v_i = end_vrt(e_0)
8.      insert(v_0,boundary)
9.      WHILE (e_i=get_edg(oi_edgs,v_i))>0 DO
10.         IF member(v_i,boundary)
                RETURN not deletable
11.         insert(v_i,boundary)
12.         IF start_vrt(e_i) == v_i
                v_i=end_vrt(e_i)
            ELSE
                v_i=start_vrt(e_i)
13. IF size(oi_edgs) > 0
        RETURN not deletable
14. o_vrts = make_list(boundary)
15. FOR all e_i ∈ oo_edgs DO
        insert(start_vrt(e_i),o_vrts)
        insert(end_vrt(e_i),o_vrts)
16. IF size(o_vrts) == nr_of_vrts(p_i)
        RETURN deletable
    ELSE
        RETURN not deletable
```

Figure 1. Pseudocode of the deletability criterion

lines 1–3 Two lists of outside edges are filled. The list oo_edgs holds the edges bounding two outside faces, the list oi_edgs those bounding an inside and an outside face.

lines 4–5 Then outside edges bounding two inside faces are detected. If such edges are found the function can immediately return with a negative answer. Notably this addresses not only the case of 1-dimensional but also 2-dimensional components with a boundary that is self-intersecting along an edge.

lines 6–12 One of possibly several component boundaries is constructed as follows. An arbitrary edge is taken from the list oi_edgs (function get_edg()), one of its vertices (v_0)is added to the list boundary and the other (v_i) used to retrieve the next edge (e_i) starting at v_i with the function get_edg(). After a test whether the vertex v_i of the new edge is already part of the component's boundary, and therefore the boundary would be self-intersecting (line 10), v_i is added to the list boundary (line 11). This is done repeatedly until the component's boundary is complete.

line 13 At this point the list oi_edgs should be void, otherwise there are more than one outside components.

lines 14–16 The last check is whether all vertices make part of the single outside component we found. This is done by collecting all vertices belonging to outside edges in the inner of the component and the vertices of the component's boundary in the list o_vrts. If o_vrts contains all vertices, p_i is deletable otherwise it is not.

The function is_deletable() is used to define a deletion sequence for the Delaunay polyhedra which corresponds to a peeling of the object. First the layer with all boundary polyhedra is selected. Then polyhedra of this layer are removed from the object one at a time as long as two requirements are fulfilled:

- they are still deletable.
- their significance (determined by a significance measure as described below) is less than a chosen threshold.

This generates a new layer of boundary polyhedra on which the peeling proceeds until no more polyhedra satisfying the above conditions can be found.

The Generalization of some significance measures from 2D to 3D is not straightforward. In 3D a Delaunay face generally doesn't cut the object into two parts, making the definition of measures based on part-subpart comparisons more complicated than in 2D. A possible solution is to use a cutting surface composed of faces from *several* Delaunay polyhedra that have already been removed instead. Such a cutting surface cannot, however, be defined uniquely based solely on the topology of the cell complex, as already discussed above. In addition, the resulting cutting surface can become fairly complex and the question arises whether the substitution of the original outline with that cutting surface is really a simplification of the object. On the other side, the "pointedness measure" based on the angularity criterion

144

can be easily generalized to 3D by measuring 3D angles of the Delaunay tetrahedra [1]. For general convex polyhedra, however, it is not evident how to generalize the angular criterion. Therefore we propose an alternative measure based on distance ridges, related to the angular criterion.

According to the definition of the MAT by the centers of all maximal inscribing spheres the skeleton of an object is equivalent to the ridges of its distance map (DM). Euclidean DM's can be generated very efficiently following e.g. a sequential algorithm proposed by Danielsson in 1980 [6]. In the past it has already been tried to extract ridges directly from DM's, but the connectivity of the resulting skeleton is not guaranteed. Hence several approaches tried to join the separated portions of the skeleton in a post-processing step, which turns out to be a very difficult task already in 2D.

The strength of the ridges in the DM, however, can well be used for the characterization of the significance of single Voronoi faces. The detection of the ridge strength is a much easier problem, as the Voronoi faces specify the exact position of the ridge to be investigated, and even define the orthogonal direction to it.

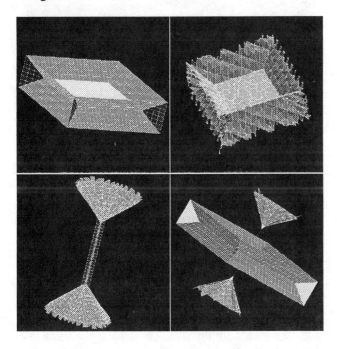

Figure 2. 3D Voronoi Skeletons of artificial objects. Upper left: skeleton of a cuboid. Upper right: the same cuboid rotated by $\phi = 15°$, $\theta = 65°$. Lower left: elongated cylinder. Lower right: cylinder and cuboid combined.

The ridge-strength measure turns out to be a combination of the information at hand from the VD (i.e. exact location and orientation of possible skeletal faces) and the information derived from the DM (how well a candidate face

represents a ridge in the DM). The quality of a ridge can be described at every point of a candidate face by the local curvature found in the DM in direction of the face's normal. One has to note here that in general ridges will not always be faces; the skeleton will converge to lines where the object's shape shows radial symmetry. An analysis of the Hessian matrix of the DM can be used to determine the type of the local object symmetry. The number of its eigenvalues that are almost zero corresponds to the dimensionality of the ridge. This way the dimensionality of the skeleton can be determined locally without any prior decision about the expected object shape.

We used the above procedure to generate skeletons of different artificial test objects. Some results, cuboids, cylinders and their composition are shown in figure 2.

4. Skeleton based object recognition

We have illustrated that skeletal description of 3D objects offers a solution to cope with problems of description and analysis of complex shapes. Application of this methodology is, however, impeded by the following major problems:

- The calculation of the hierarchical skeleton will be, even after solving the open problems discussed in this paper, computationally expensive and algorithmically complex. This means that skeletal description has to be restricted to cases where approximation techniques are feasible, or where the additional information provided by the skeletal description (basically the hierarchical organization of the shape) is really necessary, justifying the large additional costs against simpler methods.

- The methods discussed for skeletonization require a binary object for the analysis, which necessitates prior segmentation of the scene. In some cases, however, segmentation can be difficult, making the routine application of skeletal analysis illusory.

- The idea of skeletonization only produces a (small) part of the full symmetry set. Large parts of the general symmetry information about the object are suppressed by the procedure. This can be easily seen in the case of a rectangle, where the formation of the symmetry axes of the two smaller sides is blocked by the 'quicker' burning up between the longer sides. This feature is essential for the skeletal description and is mainly responsible for the branching topography which is the basis of the skeleton hierarchy. On the other hand, changes in the object which deeply influence the burning pattern will result in basic reorganization of the skeletal branches. The notorious sensitivity of skeletons to topological noise is a well known consequence of this, and we expect this situation to be even worse in three dimensions. The mutual position of objects (e.g. objects embedded one in another or touching one another) in a complex scene will lead to similar changes in the object's skeleton. This problem can only be avoided if the objects are segmented and isolated before skeletonization. A requirement which makes skeletons nearly useless for the recognition of objects in complex scenes.

Calculation of symmetry transforms of images using mixed wave/diffusion processes [17] or the Multi-scale Medial Axis (MMA) transformation [12] offers an appealing way to cope with many of the above mentioned problems. The basic idea of this general symmetry transformation is the propagation of edge information into the object, creating local symmetry or medialness information where evidence generated by opposite object boundaries accumulates without terminating front propagation at quenching points. These methods can process directly gray-valued images and also allow the boundary points to participate in any number of symmetry relations. This way one gets the complete symmetry set without the suppression effect observed in the MAT transformation.

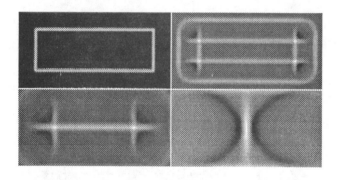

Figure 3. Medialness measure of a rectangle on different scales.

Figure 3 shows the 3D medialness field of a binary rectangle, as generated by the MMA transformation. The single images illustrate the medialness information on different scales. The images demonstrate that both symmetry axes between the long and the short sides survive, providing complete information about the symmetry of the original object.

The different symmetry axes can be found as 1D ridges in the 3D medialness space (note, that the medialness field has an extra dimension in addition to the spatial one, the scale). Figure 4 shows the result of ridge extraction in the 3D medialness field and a projection to the plane of the spatial coordinates. One can clearly see the classical skeleton as part of the symmetry structure, while the remaining symmetries have been constructed, too.

The mixed application of the MAT and this general symmetry transformation opens a promising way for using skeletons in object recognition and matching. In many applications (as e.g. anatomical atlas matching) it is reasonable to create a model of the objects under investigation. As the model is created only once, the amount of work required for its generation is not critical. The MAT of such a model can be produced by the methods discussed in the previous section, creating a structured description of the object. For an object to be recognized in a complex scene the MMA transformation of the whole scene can be generated, and we can try to fit our skeletal model elastically onto the resulting ridges the same way, as we identify the skeleton of the rectangle in the medialness field. Generalizations of the well known snakes [7] offer a possible way to perform this kind of matching.

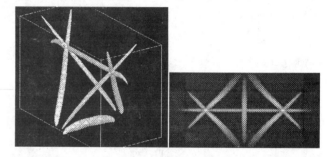

Figure 4. Ridges in the 3D medialness field of a rectangle. In the right figure the detected ridges have been projected to the subspace of the spatial coordinates.

5. Skeletal characterization of organs based on 3D radiological data

We would like to illustrate the power of skeletal representation on two prototypical medical applications. In the first case bone thickness in the acetabulum has to be investigated for optimal prosthesis placement in hip joint replacement operations. In the second example the generation of skeletons of a human brain extracted from 3D MRI data will be demonstrated.

5.1. Bone thickness characterization using skeletonization

Optimal placement of hip joint replacement prosthesis requires general knowledge about the thickness of the surrounding bone structures. Such knowledge can be extracted from the analysis of the anatomical variation in a selected training population. Quantitative evaluation, however, is not possible without adequate representation of the innominate bone. Skeletal description provides a natural basis for this analysis and proved to be useful for the characterization and visualization of the thickness of the hip bone around the acetabulum.

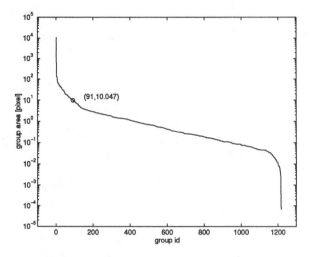

Figure 5. Overall area of the face groups making up the hip bone skeleton after the first regularization step.

Figure 7 shows a 3D rendering of an innominate bone to be analyzed. The dataset contained 49'733 boundary points, which produced 65'073 Delaunay polyhedra and 102'447 elementary Voronoi faces. After a first regularization step using the ridge strength as significance measure 29'928 elementary Voronoi faces were left. The remaining faces can be sewn together at edges where only two of them meet. This aggregation of individual faces into groups representing unbranched skeletal parts produced 1'218 face groups. An analysis of these groups shows that many of them represent insignificantly small skeletal parts (cf. figure 5). Hence a second regularization step acting on these face groups and using the overall area of the group as significance measure has been done to clean up the skeleton. All groups with an overall area of less than 10 pixels have been removed if homotopical equivalence could be guaranteed. Thereafter 28'196 faces were left. Obviously this produced an additional number of edges joining only two elementary Voronoi faces. Hence the aggregation procedure has been repeated which lead to 179 face groups. Figure 8 shows the resulting skeleton after the two regularization steps as a fusible stereo pair.

For the visualization of the skeleton the use of elementary Voronoi faces is acceptable. However for the representation and analysis of the 3D shape of the organ, the face groups which represent global medial surfaces are used.

Figure 6 shows the single medial surface that has been produced by the aggregation procedure and represents the acetabulum. It is shaded according to the local thickness. Areas representing thick bone structures capable of supporting hip joint replacement prosthesis are well visible.

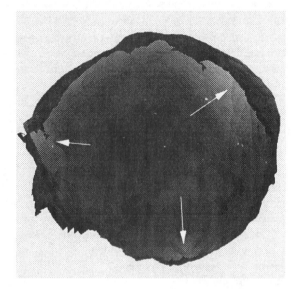

Figure 6. The medial surface representing the acetabulum of the hip bone colored by the local bone thickness (from black to white). The arrows indicate optimal areas for prosthesis support.

5.2. Analysis of the cortical structure of the brain

Neuroanatomical and histological findings from post-mortem brains, as well as in vivo findings from MRI studies suggest the presence at morphological temporal lobe abnormalities in schizophrenia. To determine, whether or not sulco-gyral pattern abnormalities in the temporal lobe could be detected in vivo, computerized surface rendering techniques for MR data have been developed in order to make qualitative and quantitative analysis of three-dimensional reconstruction of the temporal and frontal cortex. 3D renderings of the brain surface have been used to determine characteristics of the sulco-gyral patterns correlating with clinical findings [8].

One of the basic problems of this analysis was, that the structural description of the brain surface has been derived from a single 2D view of the rendered data. This is a basically 2D approach which cannot completely catch the complex 3D structure of the cortical surface.

Skeletal representation offers a promising way to generate more precise descriptors of the sulco-gyral foldings. In our analysis the white brain matter extracted from an MR acquisition was processed by the skeletonization software. The dataset contained 205'848 boundary points, which produced 300'563 Delaunay polyhedra and 488'504 elementary Voronoi faces. After regularization 87'205 elementary Voronoi faces were left. The original data and the resulting elementary Voronoi faces of the skeleton are shown as fusible stereo pair in figure 9. In this case the Voronoi faces are colored according to the importance measure (ridge-strength of the DM) used in the regularization process. The structure of the cortical surface is now coded in the branching of the individual skeletal sheets, clearly visible on the image. An extension of the face aggregation procedure used in the previous example is in progress, allowing the representation of the sulco-gyral structure using the branching lines on the skeletal surface.

6. Conclusions

We presented an overview about the conceptual, algorithmic and practical aspects of the generation of 3D hierarchical skeletons, and showed that, while the basic ideas of Voronoi skeleton generation can be extended to 3D, several theoretical and algorithmic implementation problems arise. While the technical aspects of the 3D VD generation have been solved, regularization remains an open problem. This is basically due to the lack of a hierarchical organization of the Delaunay cells, providing no clue about a reasonable sequence for the deletion of the Delaunay polyhedra.

While the 3D hierarchical skeleton promises to be a possible tool for handling complex shapes of the human anatomy, some drawbacks limit its applicability. However, combination of the Blum skeleton concept of binary objects with the recently proposed concept of the MMA applicable for gray-scale images opens a wide range of possible applications for skeletal description.

Two prototypical applications in medical image analysis have been presented demonstrating the power of skeletal representation in organ shape analysis problems. The complex branching structure of skeletal sheets provides an appropriate representation of the underlying organ shape and can carry the information necessary for subsequent quantitative shape analysis.

The presented work provides only a first step in the direction of skeleton based shape analysis. Further development is in progress allowing the generation of the complete skeletal hierarchy of the skeletons of anatomical objects. This hierarchy will allow us to concentrate selectively on the parts of the skeleton which are relevant to a specific application.

References

[1] Attali D. and Montanvert A. Semicontinuous Skeletons of 2D and 3D Shapes. In *Proc. 2nd Int. Workshop on Visual Form*, pages 32–41. World Scientific, 1994.

[2] Blum H. A Transformation for Extracting New Descriptors of Shape. In W. Walthen-Dunn, editor, *Models for the Perception of Speech and Visual Form*. MIT Press, 1967.

[3] Brandt J.W. Describing a solid with the three-dimensional skeleton. In *Proc. SPIE Conf. Curves and Surfaces in Comp. Vision and Graphics III*, volume 1830, pages 258–269, Boston, 1992.

[4] Brandt J.W. and Algazi V.R. Continuous Skeleton Computation by Voronoi Diagram. *CVGIP:IU*, 55(3):329–338, 1992.

[5] Cignoni P., Montani C. and Scopigno R. A merge-first divide & conquer algorithm for E^d triangulations. Technical Report 92-16, Istituto CNUCE-C.N.R., Pisa, Italy, 1992.

[6] P. Danielsson. Euclidean distance mapping. *Computer Vision, Graphics, and Image Processing*, 14:227–248, 1980.

[7] M. Kass, A. Witkin, and D. Terzopoulos. Snakes: Active contour models. *International Conference on Computer Vision*, pages 259–268, June 1987.

[8] Kikinis R., Shenton M.E., Gerig G., Hokama H., Haimson J., O'Donnel B.F., Wible C.G., McCarley R.W., Jolesz F.A. Temporal lobe sulco-gyral pattern anomalies in schizophrenia: an mr three-dimensional surface rendering study. *Neuroscience Letters*, 182:7–12, 1994.

[9] V. Kovalevsky. Finite topology as applied to image analysis. *Computer Vision, Graphics, and Image Processing*, 46:141–161, 1989.

[10] Lee D.T. Medial Axis Transformation of a Planar Shape. *IEEE PAMI*, 4(4):363–369, 1982.

[11] Meyer F. Skeletons and Perceptual graphs. *Signal Processing*, 16:335–363, 1989.

[12] Morse B.S., Pizer S.M. and Burbeck C.A. General Shape and Specific Detail: Context-dependent Use of Scale in Determining Visual Form. In *Proc. 2nd Int. Workshop on Visual Form*, pages 374–383. World Scientific, 1994.

[13] Nackman L.R. and Pizer S.M. Three-Dimensional Shape Description Using the Symmetric Axis Transformation I: Theory. *IEEE PAMI*, 7(2):187–202, 1985.

[14] Ogniewicz R.L. and Ilg M. Voronoi Skeletons: Theory and Applications. In *IEEE CVPR*, pages 63–69. IEEE Computer Society Press, 1992.

[15] Preparata F.P., Shamos M.I. *Computational Geometry.* Springer-Verlag, New York, 1985.

[16] Schmitt M. Some Examples of Algorithms Analysis in Computational Geometry by Means of Mathematical Morphological Techniques. In *Lecture Notes in Computer Science: Geometry and robotics*, volume 391, pages 225–246. Springer-Verlag, 1989.

[17] Scott G.L., Turner S.C. and Zisserman A. Using a mixed wave/diffusion process to elicit the symmetry set. *Image and Vision Computing*, 7(1):63–70, 1989.

[18] Székely G., Brechbühler Ch., Kübler O., Ogniewicz R.L. and Budinger T. Mapping the human cerebral cortex using 3D medial manifolds. In *Proc. VBC*, volume 1808, pages 130–144, Chapel Hill, October 1994. SPIE.

[19] Talbot H. and Vincent L. Euclidean Skeletons and Conditional Bisectors. In *Proc. SPIE Conf. Medical Imaging V: Image Processing*, volume 1818, pages 862–876, 1992.

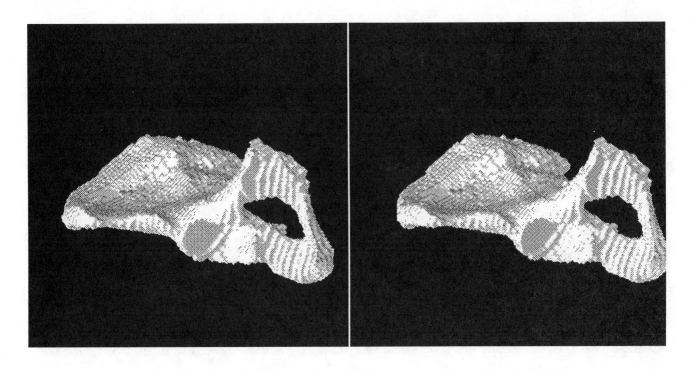

Figure 7. Fusible stereo pair of the 3D rendered hip bone under study.

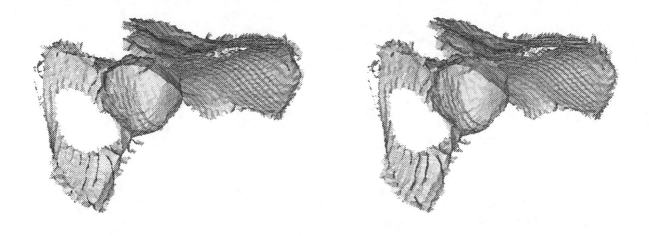

Figure 8. Fusible stereo pair of the 3D rendered hip bone skeleton.

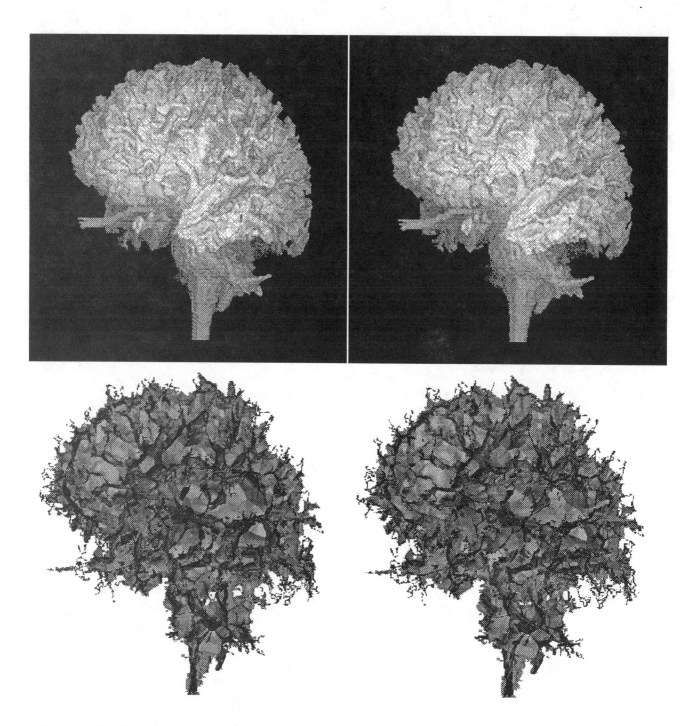

Figure 9. Original object and 3D Voronoi Skeleton of a human brain's white matter, shown as fusible stereo pairs. The skeletal faces are colored according to the importance measure (ridge-strength of the DM) used in the regularization process.

Finding 3D Parametric Representations of the Deep Cortical Folds

Marc Vaillant, Christos Davatzikos* and R. Nick Bryan
Neuroimaging Laboratory
Department of Radiology
Johns Hopkins School of Medicine
600 N. Wolfe street, Baltimore MD 21287
WWW: http://ditzel.rad.jhu.edu

Abstract

Parametric representations of anatomical structures provide useful mathematical descriptions for many medical imaging applications, including morphological analysis of the brain. In this paper, we develop a methodology for obtaining a parametric representation of the deep cortical folds of the brain utilizing characteristics of the cortical shape. We first find a mathematical representation of the outer cortical surface using a deformable surface algorithm. Using the principal curvatures of the resulting surface, we then identify the edges on the sulci on it, and we initialize active contours along them. An external force field guides an active contour to the deep edge of a sulcus, along the medial surface of a cortical fold. A parametric description of a sulcal surface is obtained as the active contour traverses the sulcus, sweeping a surface resembling a convoluted ribbon embedded in 3D. In this paper we present results using magnetic resonance images.

1. Introduction

The representation of the shape of complex anatomical forms, such as the cortex of the human brain, has been a challenging problem for the medical imaging community. The focus of our work is the development of an automated methodology for finding parametric representations of the deep cortical folds. Studying the morphology of these folds, which are often the location of important functional areas of the brain, extends our understanding of the structure and function of the human brain.

The region between two juxtaposed sides of a cortical fold, called a *sulcus*, is a thin convoluted ribbon embedded

---

* Address correspondence to C. Davatzikos in the address above. E-mail: marc@jhu.edu, hristos@welchlink.welch.jhu.edu, rnbryan@rad.jhu.edu

in 3D. Cross-sections of various sulci are shown in Fig. 1 superimposed on magnetic resonance images of the brain. The cerebral sulci are important brain structures, since they are believed to be associated with functionally distinct cortical regions. In particular, during the development of the brain in the embryo connections between specific cortical regions and connections between cortical regions and subcortical structures are believed to induce the sharp inward folding of the cortex, resulting in the formation of the sulci. Moreover, the roots of the sulci often demarcate the boundaries between functionally and structurally different cortical regions [14, 15]. Most notably, the central sulcus is the boundary between its posteriorly located primary somatosensory cortex and its anteriorly located primary motor cortex. Along the central sulcus is a fairly consistent somatotopic distribution of functional regions of the cortex, known as Penfield's homunculus.

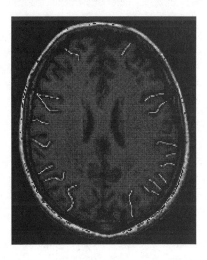

Figure 1. A sample magnetic resonance image with several sulci outlined.

In order to study the cerebral sulci and the distribution

Proceedings of MMBIA '96

of the function along their associated cortical folds, we first need to establish a quantitative methodology for describing the shape of these ribbon-like structures. In this paper we present steps toward the development of a methodology for finding parametric representations of the sulcal ribbons.

Related to our work is the work in [15], which studies the cortical topography by determining a graph of the sulci. Also, related is the work in [19, 18], which determines the medial axis of arbitrary shapes at multiple scales. Both of these approaches yield important information about the overall topography of the cortex. Our work focuses on quantitatively analyzing the geometry of individual sulci and on determining a coordinate system suitable to the shape of the sulci.

The method we propose in this paper is a physically-based algorithm utilizing the particular characteristics of the cortical shape. Specifically, our algorithm uses the outer cortical surface as a starting point, and it identifies the outer edges of the sulcal ribbons, which lie on the outer cortical surface, using the principal curvatures [7]. By placing active contours [13, 8] along these edges, which are then let free to move inward following the cortical gyrations, our method obtains a parametric representation of the sulcal ribbons. These representations can be used to calculate geometric cortical features (e.g. curvature) suitable for shape analysis. Moreover, they can serve as the basis for finding average shapes and for quantifying anatomical differences between the normal and the abnormal brain.

The primary application of this work is the morphological analysis of the cortex. However, our methodology can potentially find application in two other medical imaging problems. The first one is image-guided surgery, in which a key issue is to find minimally invasive surgical paths. Certain sulcal and gyral regions are optimal routes for approaching deeply located targets. These natural pathways are better utilized in surgical planning if functional data (fMRI, EEG, MEG) and structural data (MRI, MR angiograms and venograms, atlases adapted to the shape of the patient's brain) can be projected on a reference system located on the sulcal ribbons. An optimal route in this reference system can then be found as the curve optimizing some kind of risk measure derived from these data.

Finally, another application of our algorithm is in the spatial normalization and registration of brain images, in which a key issue is often obtaining a parametric representation of distinct surfaces which can then be matched based on their geometric characteristics [9, 21]. The sulcal ribbons of distinct cortical folds can be used for this purpose in shape transformation methodologies [6, 16, 5, 12, 1].

2. Methods

2.1. Overview

The proposed algorithm utilizes two specific characteristics of the cortex:

1. The cortical folds tend to branch off the outer cortex in a direction nearly perpendicular to it. This direction can change considerably toward the deep parts of the folds.

2. The cortex has a fairly uniform thickness. Moreover, the two juxtaposed sides of a cortical fold are nearly in contact. Therefore, the effective thickness of the cortex at its sharp inward folds is twice the actual cortical thickness (see Fig. 2). We observe that the points that lie on the medial surface of a sulcus coincide with the center of the cortical mass included in a neighborhood around them (see Fig. 2); the same is not true for points not it.

We use these two cortical features to derive a force field which guides an active contour, initially placed along the outer cortical surface, to the deepest part of a sulcus. This force field is comprised of two components. The first component, denoted by $\mathbf{F}_1$, restricts the motion of the active contour to be along the medial surface of a sulcus. The second force, denoted by $\mathbf{F}_2$, resembles a gravitational force and is responsible for the inward motion of the active contour deep into the cortical folds (see Fig. 3). The collection of the deformed configurations of the active contour defines a surface, which resembles a convoluted ribbon embedded in 3D and has the shape of the medial sulcal surface.

2.2. Initialization of the Active Contour

The active contour is initialized along the outer edge of a sulcus, i.e. its edge that lies on the outer cortical surface. In order to find such an edge, we first obtain a parametric representation of the outer cortical surface using a deformable surface algorithm described elsewhere [7]. A deformable surface, initially having a spherical configuration surrounding the brain, deforms like a contracting elastic membrane attracted by the outer cortical boundary. We determine the outer cortical boundary through a sequence of three operations: a morphological erosion which detaches the brain tissue from the nearby skull and bone marrow, a seeded region growing which extracts the brain tissue, and a conditional morphological dilation which recaptures the brain tissue lost in the erosion step.

Resulting from the deformable surface algorithm is a parametric representation of the outer cortical surface, denoted by $\mathbf{b}(u, v)$, where (u, v) takes values in a planar domain in which the deformable surface is parameterized. The intersections of this surface with the sulcal ribbons are the outer edges of the sulci, and are identified along the outer cortical surface using the minimum (principal) curvature [17] of $\mathbf{b}(u, v)$, which has high value along them [7]. On these high curvature curves we then initialize active contours having evenly spaced points. The initial configuration of an active contour will be denoted by $\mathbf{x}(s, 0) = \mathbf{x}(s, t)|_{t=0}$. Here, the parameter t denotes time. As $s \in [0, 1]$ sweeps the unit interval, $\mathbf{x}(s, t)$ runs along the active contour at its configuration at time t. Equivalently, $\mathbf{x}(s, t)$ and $\mathbf{x}(s, t + \Delta t)$ are two consecutive deformed configurations of the active contour.

2.3. Active Contour Deformation

After its initial placement along the outer edge of a sulcus, the active contour slides along the medial surface of the sulcus under the influence of its internal elastic forces and two external force fields which are described next.

Restoring Force. The first force field, $\mathbf{F}_1$, acting on the active contour restricts its motion to be on the sulcal medial surface. This force is based on the observation that the points lying on the medial surface of a sulcus satisfy the following condition (see Fig. 2):

$$\mathbf{X} = \mathbf{c}(\mathbf{X}), \qquad (1)$$

where $\mathbf{c}(\mathbf{X})$ is the center of the cortical mass included in a spherical neighborhood, $\mathcal{N}(\mathbf{X})$, centered on $\mathbf{X}$ [1]. Accordingly, we define the force acting on a point located at $\mathbf{X}$ as

$$\mathbf{F}_1(\mathbf{X}) = \frac{\mathbf{c}(\mathbf{X}) - \mathbf{X}}{\rho(\mathbf{X})}, \qquad (2)$$

where $\rho(\mathbf{X})$ is the radius of $\mathcal{N}(\mathbf{X})$ and is spatially varying, as described below.

If the cortex had exactly uniform thickness throughout its extent, and if the two juxtaposed sides of the cortical folds were always in contact with each other, then ρ in (2) would be fixed to a value equal to the cortical thickness. In that case, $\mathbf{F}_1$ would be exactly zero on the sulci. However, this is often not the case. In order to account for variations in the cortical and sulcal thickness, we allow $\rho(\mathbf{X})$ to vary throughout the cortex; at each point $\mathbf{X}$, $\mathcal{N}(\mathbf{X})$ adapts its size to encompass the cortical gray matter in its full width. In particular, at each point $\mathbf{X}$, $\rho(\mathbf{X})$ is defined as the radius of the smallest spherical neighborhood intersecting the cortical boundaries on both sides of a cortical fold.

Now consider an active contour point located at $\mathbf{X}$. If $\mathbf{X}$ is exactly on the medial axis of the sulcus then $\mathbf{F}_1(\mathbf{X}) = 0$;

---

[1] In the experiments herein, the cortical mass is the indicator function of the cortex, and is obtained at a pre-segmentation step.

in this case $\mathbf{F}_1$ does not effect this point. Otherwise, $\mathbf{F}_1$ moves the point towards the sulcal medial axis (see Fig. 2). After a sequence of incremental movements, the point balances at a position satisfying (1) (within some preset tolerance factor) where $\mathbf{F}_1$ vanishes. It is important to note that $\rho(\cdot)$ adapts continuously to the cortical thickness during this restoring motion. At equilibrium, the spherical neighborhood balances between the two opposite boundaries of the cortical fold.

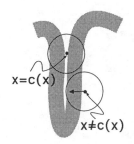

Figure 2. Schematic diagram of the cross-section of a sulcus and its surrounding cortex. The effective thickness of the cortex around a sulcus is twice its actual thickness, illustrating that the center of mass of a circular neighborhood represents the location of the medial surface of a sulcus. The force $\mathbf{c}(\mathbf{X}) - \mathbf{X}$ moves a point towards this axis.

Inward Force.

The second force field, $\mathbf{F}_2$, acting on the active contour is responsible for its inward motion toward the deepest edge of a sulcus. At the active contour's initial configuration $\mathbf{x}(s, 0)$, $\mathbf{F}_2$ at each contour point is in the direction of the inward normal to the outer cortical surface, which is denoted by $\mathbf{F}_N[\mathbf{x}(s, 0)]$. As mentioned earlier, the orientation of the sulci tend to deviate from this normal direction at positions deep in the brain. Accordingly, we adapt $\mathbf{F}_2$ as the active contour moves inward. If $\mathbf{x}(s, t)$ is the position of an active contour point at time t, then $\mathbf{x}_t(s, t)$, and $\mathbf{x}_{tt}(s, t)$ respectively represent speed and acceleration components of the active contour's dynamics. These terms effectively provide a directional estimation of the active contour's motion. We now define $\mathbf{F}_2(s, 0)$ as

$$\mathbf{F}_2(s, t) = \alpha \mathbf{x}_t + \beta \mathbf{x}_{tt} + \gamma \mathbf{F}_N[\mathbf{x}(s, 0)], \qquad (3)$$

where subscripts denote partial derivatives.

The first two terms in (3) give rise to damping and inertial influences which have the effect of averaging the previously traveled direction of the active contour with the initial inward direction. This actively adapts the inward force to the shape of the sulcus.

Under the influence of the two force fields, $\mathbf{F}_1$ and $\mathbf{F}_2$, the active contour deforms elastically, sliding along the medial surface of a sulcus towards its deepest edge. The inward trajectory of each active contour point is terminated when the magnitude of the total force acting on it becomes less than a threshold $\zeta \in [0,1]$. This typically occurs at the bottom parts of the cortical folds where $\mathbf{F}_1$ and $\mathbf{F}_2$ have almost opposite directions (see Fig. 3).

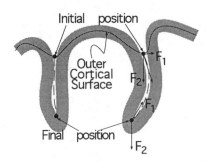

Figure 3. A 2D schematic diagram of the force field acting on the active contour. $\mathbf{F}_1$ attracts an active contour point along the medial axis of a sulcus. $\mathbf{F}_2$ guides and active contour point inward to the deep edge of the sulcus. The outer cortical contour, (solid curve) represents a cross-section of the outer cortical surface. The dashed curves represent the trajectories of points belonging to two different active contours, (one for each sulcus) oriented perpendicularly to the image plane.

2.4. Refinement of the Sulcal Surface

The collection of the deformed configurations of the active contour constitute a surface, parameterized by $\mathbf{x}(s,t)$. This surface tends to be smooth along one family of isoparametric curves, the one obtained by fixing t, because of the internal elastic forces of the active contour which are along these curves. However, it is not necessarily smooth along the other family of isoparametric curves, the one obtained by fixing s, which are oriented along the direction of the inward motion. In order to obtain a smooth surface, $\mathbf{y}(s,t)$, from $\mathbf{x}(s,t)$ we solve the following regularization problem:

$$\text{Minimize} \iint \|\mathbf{y}(s,t) - \mathbf{x}(s,t)\|^2 ds dt$$
$$+ K \iint \left(\|\mathbf{y}_s(s,t)\|^2 + \|\mathbf{y}_t(s,t)\|^2 \right) ds dt, \quad (4)$$

where subscripts denote partial derivatives.

In (4), the surface $\mathbf{y}(s,t)$ is an elastic membrane which adapts to the shape of the sulcal surface $\mathbf{x}(s,t)$, while maintaining a certain degree of smoothness determined by the elasticity parameter K. Equation (4) is discretized and solved iteratively, resulting in a smoother surface parameterized by $\mathbf{y}(s,t)$.

2.5. The Sulcal Coordinate System

The way in which the sulcal ribbons fold in 3D varies considerably across individuals. However, the distribution of function along the surrounding cortex is believed to be more consistent[2]. This suggests that it may be beneficial to perform the analysis of structural and functional data pertaining to the cortical folds in a coordinate system that is independent from the way in which the sulci fold in 3D, rather than a standard three-dimensional cartesian coordinate system. Our parameterization readily provides a map from a sulcus to the planar domain $\mathcal{D} = [0,1] \times [0,1]$. The analysis of shape properties of the sulci in this domain is independent from their embedding in 3D.

In order to obtain a map from a sulcus to $\mathcal{D}$ we resample the s-isoparametric curves and the t-isoparametric curves of $\mathbf{y}(s,t)$ by the same number of points. An iterative procedure [7] is finally used to find a nearly homothetic map. Having mapped a particular sulcus from a population onto $\mathcal{D}$, we can then analyze the shape of the sulcus in that population in a common framework. In particular, if N subjects have sulcal parameterizations $\mathbf{p}_1(u,v), \mathbf{p}_2(u,v), \cdots, \mathbf{p}_N(u,v)$, $(u,v) \in \mathcal{D}$, we can define an average sulcus as,

$$\bar{\mathbf{p}}(u,v) = \frac{1}{N} \sum_{i=1}^{N} \mathbf{p}_i(u,v). \quad (5)$$

More elaborate shape averaging schemes, such as the Procrustes algorithm [4], can also be applied.

Functional data can also be mapped to the sulcal domain, allowing for the analysis of the distribution of function along the surrounding cortex. The statistical analysis of functional images in stereotactic spaces has been shown to considerably reduce the undesirable effects of low sensitivity and resolution of functional images such as PET and fMRI[11, 10].

3. Experiments

2D Results. A 2D version of the algorithm was first tested on a synthetic image of the brain consisting of three gray level values representing CSF, gray matter and white matter. An active contour algorithm was used to obtain a parameterization of the boundary denoted by $\mathbf{b}(s)$, the 2D analog of $\mathbf{b}(u,v)$. The result is shown in Fig. 4a superimposed on the synthetic image. We then initialized a set of *probe points*, the 2D analog of active contours, which move independently, at high points of curvature along the contour and applied our algorithm. The resulting probe trajectories are shown in Fig. 4b and are nearly identical to the truth. Fig. 4d shows the resulting probe trajectories after applying

---

[2] A notable example is the somatotopic projection of sensory and motor function along the central sulcus.

the algorithm to a synthetic image corrupted by noise of standard deviation $\sigma = 30$. The same parameters were used as in the previous experiment and it is clear that the noise did not alter the performance of the algorithm significantly.

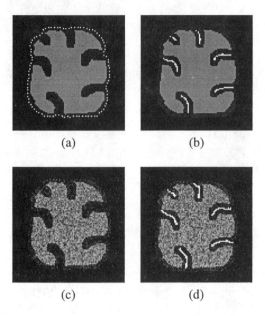

Figure 4. Experiments with a synthetic image. (a) Initial outer contour points superimposed on the image. (b) Resulting trajectories of the probes found by the algorithm. (c) Synthetic image corrupted by noise, $\sigma = 30$. (d) Resulting trajectories.

In order to obtain quantitative error measurements in this example, we manually traced the medial axes of the sulci. Error measurements were obtained by recording the maximum distance in pixels between manually generated sulci and the trajectories generated by our algorithm. We obtained a maximum and average error for each trajectory as well as a maximum and average over all trajectories in the image. This error measure, however, does not reflect probe trajectories which did not reach the end of the sulcus. Specifically, each point in such a trajectory is close to some manually traced sulcal point. However, there are parts of the manually traced sulci which were not reached by any probe. In order to account for such errors, we also obtained a second error measure. This measure is similar to the one described above except that it measures the distance between each *manually* traced sulcus and its nearest probe trajectory. The traced trajectories were not parameterized and therefore, for the second error measure we could not localize the error to individual trajectories and could only compute a maximum and average error over all trajectory points in the image. We ran the algorithm for several variations of the parameters and found that the average error for a single trajectory, using the first error measurement, was

between 0 and 2 pixels and the maximum error was between 3 to 5 pixels. The average error for each image was less than one pixel. The average error for each image, using the second error measurement, was between 1 to 5 pixels and the maximum error was between 5 to 9 pixels. The larger error observed from the second error measure can be attributed to probes which stopped before reaching the end of the sulcus due to poor selection of the parameters. The selection of the appropriate parameter values alleviated this problem; therefore it is apparent that the success of the algorithm is somewhat dependent on the choice of these parameters. Developing methodologies for automatic parameter selection is a future direction of research.

The algorithm was next tested on a transaxial slice from a 3D MR brain data set. The resulting trajectories of the probes, which were initially placed on selected local extrema of the curvature of the outer cortical boundary, are shown in Fig. 5. Specific sulci in the slice were selected based on their close resemblance to the path which would be traversed by the algorithm in 3D. In particular those sulci which were oriented orthogonal to the cross-sectional slice were chosen. This figure shows that, in general, the probe trajectories adapted to the sulcal shape. The main errors occurred when a probe's neighborhood encompassed cortical mass from branching or neighboring sulci, offsetting the center of mass function.

Some probes terminated their search early as a result of cortical folds greatly deviating from an orientation normal to the outer cortical contour. The major variability in orientation occurs deep within the brain and work is being investigated to automatically adapt the parameters to modify $\mathbf{F}_2$ as the probes proceed. Experiments have shown that initiating the trajectory with a large γ (see equation (3)) and allowing the parameter to relax as the probes proceed may provide a more robust adaptation of $\mathbf{F}_2$ because $\mathbf{F}_N$ provides a less accurate representation of the orientation of the folds as the probes penetrate deep into the brain.

3D Results. A deformable surface algorithm was first run on a 3D volume data set to parameterize the outer cortical surface [7]. From this parameterization, the curvature and the inward normals on the surface were calculated. A flattened representation of the curvature map of the top of the brain, which has high values at the cerebral sulci, was used to manually outline the central sulcus and a linear interpolation was used to equally space the outlined points(see Fig. 6). The active contour was initialized at these points and the algorithm was applied next. The sulcal ribbon generated from the resultant trajectories is shown in Fig. 7. Cross-sections of the same sulcal ribbon are shown in Fig. 8 superimposed on the corresponding MR images. Figures 7 and 8 show that the ribbon obtained by the algorithm lies along the medial surface of the sulcus. A grid highlighting the active contour and the trajectories of its points at regular

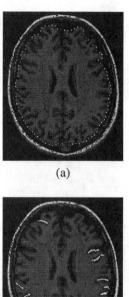

(a)

(b)

Figure 5. 2D Trans-axial MR slice: (a) initial outer contour points superimposed, (b) resulting central axes of selected sulci superimposed.

intervals is superimposed on the sulcus in Fig. 7b to illustrate the smooth uniform spacing along the $t-$isoparametric and $s-$isoparametric curves. Fig. 7c is a top view clearly showing the gyrations of the sulcus along its long axis.

We applied this procedure to the central sulcus of five subjects. The resulting sulcal surfaces and their average are shown in Fig 9. Our experiments have shown that the results remained stable over a varying range of parameter values. The central sulcus of these five subjects appear to have a fairly consistent folding pattern. Moreover, the average sulcus reveals two fairly prominent folds, which further suggest a consistency in the folding pattern of the central sulcus in these five subjects.

4. Discussion

We have developed a method for finding and parameterizing the medial surfaces of sulci utilizing particular characteristics of the cortical folds. A force field guides a set of active contour points along the medial surfaces of sulci, thereby parameterizing the sulcal "ribbons". This technique was tested in 2D and 3D on synthetic and real data.

The advantage of our method is that a parameterized representation of the cortical folds is automatically obtained. The limitation of previous methods for medial axis finding

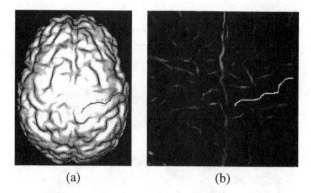

(a)   (b)

Figure 6. (a) Outer cortical surface with the initial active contour superimposed. (b) Flattened outer cortical map of the minimum (principal) curvature with the initial active contour superimposed.

is the difficulty in parameterization of the result. Traditional axis-width descriptors as described in [2, 3] often generate noisy medial axes with spurious gaps, making parameterization and subsequent shape analysis very difficult. Moreover, axes in the whole image are extracted, most of which do not correspond the sulci and therefore must be manually removed at a post-processing step. The Multiscale Medial Axis method described in [19, 18] separates small scale detail from larger scale shape properties; again, specific axes such as those representing the sulci must be manually selected and parameterized.

Several extensions of this basic approach are possible. In particular, a current limitation of our algorithm is the requirement for the manual initialization of the active contour. The automation of this procedure is a very difficult task, primarily because of the complexity of the cortical structure. Specifically, although sulcal edges can be identified from the peaks of the absolute value of the minimum curvature of the outer cortical surface [7, 22, 20], the differentiation between the sulci eventually requires a higher level model. Our current and future work in this direction focuses on the use of prior probability distributions which reflect our expectation for finding a particular sulcal edge at a given coordinate (u, v) of the outer cortical surface $\mathbf{b}(u, v)$. These priors, together with geometric properties of the outer cortex, such as curvatures, can potentially lead to the automatic identification of specific sulci, and the initial placement of the active contour along them.

Another possible extension of our algorithm is in the refinement procedure of Section 2.4. In particular, one could constrain the surface $\mathbf{y}(s, t)$ to the center of mass of the sulcus rather than $\mathbf{x}(s, t)$, therefore allowing it to freely slide along the medial surface rather than "being tied" to $\mathbf{x}(s, t)$. For example, the first term in equation (4) could be replaced by, $\iint \|\mathbf{y}(s, t) - \mathbf{c}(s, t)\|^2 ds dt$ where $\mathbf{c}(s, t)$ is the center of mass of a neighborhood at $\mathbf{y}(s, t)$. As well, an elastic warping of the sulci based on matching curvature can help to achieve a better map between subjects[9].

Currently, we are performing experiments over a wide parameter range for further validation of the performance of our algorithm. We also plan to apply our methodology to a large set of subjects in order to perform meaningful statistical analysis, utilizing more elaborate averaging techniques such as the Procustes algorithm for shape averaging, to help eliminate averaging error resulting from differences in the overall orientation of the sulci.

References

[1] R. Bajcsy and S. Kovacic. Multiresolution elastic matching. *Comp. Vision, Graphics, and Image Proc.*, 46:1–21, 1989.

[2] H. Blum. A transformation for extracting new descriptors of shape. In W. Wathen-Dunn, editor, *Models for the Perception of Speech and Visual Form*, pages 363–380. MIT Press, Cambridge, MA, 1967.

[3] H. Blum and R. Nagel. Shape description using weighted symmetric axis features. *Patt. Recog.*, 10:167–180, 1978.

[4] F. Bookstein. Thin-plate splines and the atlas problem for biomedical images. *Proc. of the 12th Int. Conf. on Inf. Proc. in Med. Imaging*, pages 326–342, 1991.

[5] G. Christensen, R. Rabbitt, and M. Miller. 3D brain mapping using a deformable neuroanatomy. *Phys. Med. Biol.*, 39:609–618, 1994.

[6] C. Davatzikos. Spatial normalization of 3D images using deformable models. *J. Comp. Assist. Tomogr.*, 1996. To appear May/June 1996.

[7] C. Davatzikos and R. Bryan. Using a deformable surface model to obtain a mathematical representation of the cortex. *Proc. of the IEEE Comp. Vision Symp.*, pages 212–217, Nov. 1995.

[8] C. Davatzikos and J. Prince. An active contour model for mapping the cortex. *IEEE Trans. on Medical Imaging*, 14:65–80, 1995.

[9] C. Davatzikos, J. Prince, and R. Bryan. Image registration based on boundary mapping. *IEEE Trans. on Med. Imaging*, Feb. 1996.

[10] P. Fox, M. Mintum, E. Reiman, and M. Reichle. Enhanced detection of focal brain responses using inter-subject averaging and distribution analysis of subtracted PET images. *J. Cerebral Flow and Metabolism*, 8:642–653, 1988.

[11] K. Friston, J. Ashburner, C. Frith, J. Poline, J. Heather, and R. Frackowiak. Spatial registration and normalization of images. *Human Brain Mapping*, 1995.

[12] J. Gee, M. Reivich, and R. Bajcsy. Elastically deforming 3D atlas to match anatomical brain images. *J. Comp. Assist. Tomogr.*, 17:225–236, 1993.

[13] M. Kass, A. Witkin, and D. Terzopoulos. Snakes: Active contour models. *International Journal of Computer Vision*, 1:321–331, 1988.

[14] A. Luria. *Higher Cortical Functions In Man*. Basic Books, Inc. and Consultants Bureau Enterprises, Inc., 1966.

[15] J.-F. Mangin, J. Regis, I. Bloch, V. Frouin, Y. Samson, and J. López-Krahe. A MRF based random graph modelling the human cortical topography. In *Proc. First Int. Conf., CVRMed*, pages 177–183, Nice, France, 1995.

[16] M. Miller, G. Christensen, Y. Amit, and U. Grenander. Mathematical textbook of deformable neuroanatomies. *Proc. of the National Academy of Sciences*, 90:11944–11948, 1993.

[17] R. Millman and G. Parker. *Elements of Differential Geometry*. Prentice Hall, 1977.

[18] B. Morse, S. Pizer, and A. Liu. Multiscale medial analysis of medical images. *Image and Vision Computing*, 12(6):327–338, July/August 1994.

[19] S. Pizer, J. Coggins, C. Burbeck, B. Morse, and D. Fritsch. Object shape before boundary shape: Scale-space medial axes. *Journal of Mathematical Imaging and Vision*, 4:303–313, 1994.

[20] G. Subsol, J. Thirion, and N. Ayache. First steps towards automatic building of anatomical atlases. *INRIA, Technical Report N° 2216*, 1994.

[21] G. Subsol, J. Thirion, and N. Ayache. A general scheme for automatically building 3D morphometric anatomical atlases: application to a skull atlas. *INRIA Technical Report N° 2586*, 1995.

[22] J. Thirion, O. Monga, S. Benayoun, A. Gueziec, and N. Ayache. Automatic registration of 3-D images using surface curvature. *SPIE Proc., Mathematical Methods in Medical Imaging*, 1768:206–216, 1992.

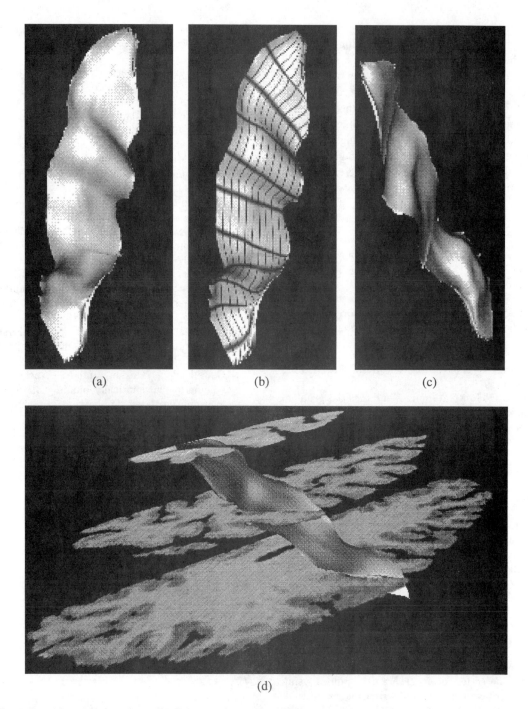

(a)   (b)   (c)

(d)

Figure 7. (a) Resulting sulcal surface. (b) Sulcal surface with grid lines superimposed. The thinner and longer grid lines indicate the configuration of the active contour at various times. The thicker and shorter lines indicate the trajectory of selected points of the active contour. (c) Top view orientation of the sulcal surface illustrating gyrations along the long axis. (d) Cross-sections of the MR volumetric image, (left hemisphere) intersected by the sulcal surface.

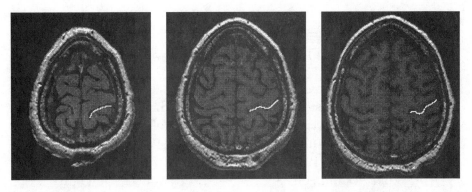

Figure 8. Cross-sections of the resulting sulcal surface superimposed on the corresponding MR slices.

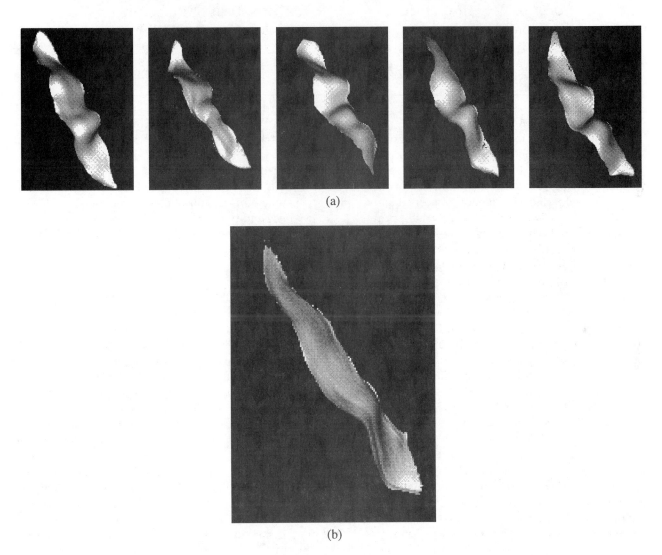

(a)

(b)

Figure 9. (a) The resulting central sulcus of five subjects and (b), the average central sulcus.

Tracking 3-D Pulmonary Tree Structures

Chandrasekhar Pisupati
Dept of Computer Science
The Johns Hopkins University
Baltimore, MD-21218
{pcsekhar@cs.jhu.edu}

Lawrence Wolff
Dept of Computer Science
The Johns Hopkins University
Baltimore, MD-21218
{wolff@cs.jhu.edu}

Wayne Mitzner
Dept of Env. Health Sci.
The Johns Hopkins Medical Institutions
Baltimore, MD-21205
{wmitz@welchlink.welch.jhu.edu}

Elias Zerhouni
Dept of Radiology
The Johns Hopkins Medical Institutions
Baltimore, MD-21205
{zerhouni@mri.jhu.edu}

Abstract

Physiological measurements like branch angles, branch lengths, branch diameters and branch cross-sectional area of the 3-D pulmonary tree structures are clinically essential in evaluating the function of normal and diseased lung and during the breathing process. In order to facilitate these measurements and study relative structural changes, the 3-D lung tree volumes are reduced to a **3-D Euclidean straight line central axis tree**. The central axis tree captures the branch topology and geometric features of the tree volume. Since matching 3-D tree volumes is complex, as they change in branch topology and geometry, we accomplish it by designing an efficient algorithm that matches their corresponding central axis trees.

The algorithm takes two binary central axis trees $T_1 = (V_1, E_1, W_1)$ and $T_2 = (V_2, E_2, W_2)$, where W_1 and W_2 are set of tuples containing geometric attributes corresponding to the nodes in T_1 and T_2, as inputs and returns the **one-to-one** matching function $\mathbf{f}$ of nodes in T_1 to T_2 that preserves the tree topology and closely matches the geometric attributes of these trees i.e. branch points, branch lengths, and branch angles between mapped nodes of T_1 and T_2. Since the topology match alone could result in many choices of the mapping function $\mathbf{f}$, we prune these choices by incorporating constraints on the geometric attributes of nodes in T_1 and T_2. We design a **linear time** algorithm that matches the branch topology and geometric features of T_1 and T_2. Our algorithm produced accurate matchings on various airway data sets of a dog lung obtained from Computed Tomography under simulated breathing conditions. T_1 and T_2 are obtained by running a two-pass *central axis algorithm* on the tree volumes.

1. Introduction

The lung contains a complex system of branching trees that conduct air and blood down to the small gas exchanging regions. The physiological function of the lung is based on the structural geometry of the various trees present in the lung. Hence, the ability to accurately measure the geometric parameters of these trees is essential not only in evaluating the function of the normal lungs, but also in diagnosing diseased lungs. Some of the geometric parameters of clinical interest are the branch angles, branch cross-sectional area, branch lengths and branch points. Inhalation and exhalation of air cause changes in these geometric parameters. Breathing can be viewed as dynamic motion of the lung tree structures as a function of time. Not only is it important to measure these parameters accurately, but in order to compare these parameters between a normal and diseased lung (in a clinical setting) or to study the relative change in tree structure during various phases of breathing, one needs to **correspond/match** these tree volumes.

160

We provide a brief overview of lung physiology [5]. Each lobe of a lung has an *airway tree* which contains the air we breath, and *vascular trees* which contain blood. The airway tree is surrounded throughout by an airway wall which, in turn, is blood filled. There are two types of blood filled vascular trees (or vessels) : Pulmonary Arterial (PA) and Pulmonary Venous (PV) tree. The PA tree has similar branching structure as the airway tree. It aligns adjacent to the airway tree throughout, with the airway wall separating them. Using High Resolution Computed Tomography (HRCT), one can obtain multislice lung data sets. In this paper, we assume that the three tree structures are already segmented [3] from the lung volume.

There are three types of lung tree volume correspondences possible :
(1) match tree volumes of the same type under different breathing conditions i.e. airways with airways, PA tree with PA tree, and PV tree with PV tree.
(2) match tree volumes of one type with the other at the same breath-hold.
(3) match tree volumes of same type obtained from different lung specimens.
The second type of matching could be used to better segment the airway tree using the knowledge of the PA tree. The third type occurs in a purely clinical setting. The proposed matching algorithm, though in principle, can be used for any of these types, we show our results on airway trees obtained from HRCT under different static pressures, thereby simulating normal breathing process.

The *Central Axis Tree* (CAT) of a 3-D tree volume can be informally defined as a connected union of *straight line spine segments* wherein each spine segment best approximates the axis of the branch. They are binary in nature, since lung trees have binary branching. The nodes of the CAT contain as attributes 3-D branch points which act as **anatomical tracking points**, and the three direction vectors corresponding to branch axes at each bifurcation. The edges of the CAT are obtained by joining the nodes using the branching information of the 3-D tree volume. The *branch length* is defined as the Euclidean distance between two successive branch points of the CAT. The *branch angle* is defined as the angle between the two direction vectors (originating from the branch point) which best approximate the branch axes.

The lung trees expand and contract as we breath-in and breath-out air during the breathing process. This process is experimentally simulated by varying the air pressure on the static lung. The image sequences of the lung at varying pressures is obtained using HRCT. In case of airways, due to low intensity gradient between small airway branches and the airway wall, these airways are not captured by HRCT, at lower pressures. But, by increasing the pressure, these smaller branches which are otherwise missing become more pronounced due to the increase in branch diameter, and are hence captured by the HRCT. This results in more branches in the airways at higher pressure. This, in turn, corresponds to more edges in the CAT of the tree volume at higher pressure, thus complicating the matching process of these CATs. These extra branches provide the **rationale for mapping edges** of the CAT (say, T_1) corresponding to tree volume at lower pressure **to edge-disjoint paths** of the CAT (say, T_2) corresponding to tree volume at higher pressure (See Fig. 1).

Previous work on pulmonary tree volume correspondence [7] involved manual processing in order to compare their central axis tree representations. In [7], the tree volume was reduced to a CAT. Starting from the root, the edges of the CAT were appended with binary values (0 or 1) based on the cross-sectional area of the corresponding branch. This results in a binary string sequence corresponding to each edge of the CAT. String sequences which are identical in two different CAT representations obtained at different breathing conditions (i.e. different pressures) may not map onto the same branch, due to the appearance of new branches corresponding to the tree volume at higher pressure when compared to the one at lower pressure. This arises due to the limitations in the resolution of HRCT or due to improper segmentation of these new branches in the smaller tree volume. Hence, the CAT correspondences were done manually [7].

We provide an algorithm to **correspond** dynamically varying 3-D tree volumes by matching their tree topology and geometry. Our approach involves matching CATs corresponding to these tree volumes. The CAT is computed from the 3-D tree volume using a robust central axis algorithm [4].

We illustrate some of the difficulties involved in matching CATs (refer Fig. 1). The dotted arrows in Fig. 1 correspond to the mapping of nodes from T_1 to T_2. The circles at each node in T_1 correspond to spheres of different radii $(r_1, r_2, \ldots)$ by which the nodes of T_1 displace to become nodes in T_2, due to the breathing process. We want a one-to-one mapping of nodes of T_1 to T_2 which involves mapping the edges in T_1 to disjoint paths in T_2 such that the **parent-child relationship** is preserved i.e. if node v_i of T_1 is mapped to v_i' of T_2, then the two children of v_i should map to descendant nodes which lie on the edge disjoint paths starting from v_i' in T_2 (Fig. 1). In Fig. 1, node P of T_1 may have two choices to map onto P' or P'' in T_2. Similarly, R has

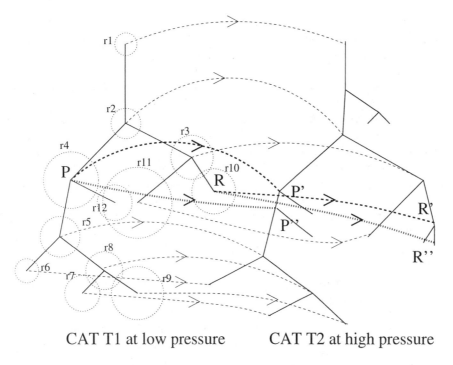

CAT T1 at low pressure   CAT T2 at high pressure

Figure 1. Matching two 3-D central axis trees at different pressures

two choices in R' or R''. We break the tie by using the geometric attributes at each candidate node and pick the node which best matches the geometric features.

Related work on pattern matching used 2-D and 3-D Euclidean point sets without considering topology/connectivity information. Pattern matching under Euclidean motion (rotation and translation) was done in 2-D [2] and in 3-D [1] but our problem involves matching patterns which are *non-uniform scaled* versions of one another with the additional constraint of tree topology and maintaining parent-child relationship. There are two components associated with matching the CAT's : (1) Topology match (2) geometric feature match. If we try to match the topology alone, we have too many ways of mapping edges of T_1 to paths of T_2 and hence we cannot decide which mapping "best" matches the geometric features, unless we enumerate all possible mappings and compare the geometric features. In terms of the geometric features, displacement of nodes in T_1 around spheres of different radii to nodes in T_2, result in changes in branch lengths, branch angles and branch points.

If we use the proximity of 3-D branch points in T_1 and T_2 as the *minimization* criteria, the Hausdorff distance metric [6] results in a *many-to-one* matching of nodes in T_1 to T_2, but, we require a *one-to-one* matching. On the other hand, though bipartite matching

corresponding to 3-D branch points in T_1 and T_2 produces a one-to-one mapping of the nodes in T_1 and T_2, it does not guarantee the parent-child relationship and tree topology. An example of this is shown in Fig. 2, where the leaf node $a1$ of T_1 gets mapped to node $b2$ of T_2 instead of node $a2$ of T_2, if we use the Euclidean proximity criteria. The basic problem with Hausdorff and bipartite matching is that they do not incorporate tree topology. One could perhaps do better if one can estimate the varying displacement of each of the branch points in T_1 to obtain T_2, but we have no knowledge of the relative displacements. Our algorithm relies on one-to-one matching of nodes in T_1 and T_2 based not only on topology but also on the "proximity" of branch points, and "similarity" in branch angles, branch lengths and branch diameters. Though, one cannot exactly quantify the amount of variation in each of the geometric parameters, as they vary across each node of T_1, we assign maximum relaxation bounds on these parameters. Since, very few candidate nodes satisfy the geometric constraints imposed by these relaxation bounds, our algorithms work well in our application domain.

The organization of the paper is as follows: In section 2, we provide an overview of the central axis algorithm to compute the central axis tree from 3-D tree volume. The interested reader is referred to [4] for

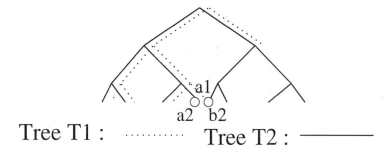

Tree T1 : ··········· Tree T2 : ──────

Figure 2. Node a1 in $T1$ is mapped to node b2 (instead of a2) in $T2$

more details. In section 3, we provide a **linear time algorithm** that matches two central axis trees and in section 4 we provide the results of the matching algorithm on airway data sets of a dog lung obtained from HRCT at different pressures. We conclude in section 5 looking at applying these algorithms for better segmentation of airways.

2. Central Axis Algorithm (CAA)

The central axis algorithm [4] uses a two-pass region growing of the tree volume and obtains branch points by solving a non-linear optimization formulation. By connecting the branch points using the tree topology, we obtain the central axis tree.

In the **first phase**, we use a recursive region growing procedure to go down the tree volume. As we traverse the tree volume, we obtain the branching information by constructing the topological tree T. The nodes in T correspond to branches of the lung tree volume and the edges in T correspond to adjacent branches. At each stage of the region growth, we check to see if the current set S' is a *single connected component* or not. If S' contains two disjoint voxel sets, this implies that the parent branch is branching to two daughter branches and hence we update T by adding two new nodes to the current node of T. We continue region growth recursively by expanding on the two disjoint voxel sets, updating T along the way. T reflects the branching structure of the bronchial tree. In each of the nodes of T, we maintain *centroid* (first order moments) information of current voxel sets as we go down that branch. We use T to guide the second phase of our algorithm.

The **second phase** involves traversing the tree volume bottom-up from the leaves of the lung tree. Note that, in the first phase, the region growth can occur oblique to the axis of the branch thereby providing few centroid points for the nodes of T. The objective of the second phase is to direct the region growth along

the axis of the branch, so as to facilitate more centroid points corresponding to each branch, than the first phase. More importantly, this phase tries to avoid the region growth at branch junctions thereby providing good centroid points, for branch point computation.

After the completion of second phase, at each bifurcation, the branch point and the three direction vectors along the branches are computed, by formulating it as a $3-cluster$ problem (described below) that minimizes the **least square error** of the centroid points corresponding to that branch.

Let $M_1, M_2, \ldots, M_k$ be the number of points in each of the k clusters respectively. Let p_i^j correspond to the ith point in the jth cluster. In the case of pulmonary trees, k equals three (Fig. 3) as there are three branches at each bifurcation. Moreover, the points in each cluster correspond to the centroid points obtained during the second phase of region growing of that branch in the tree volume. We define the $k-cluster$ or $k-star$ problem as follows:

Given a group of k disjoint clusters with $M_1, M_2, \ldots, M_k$ Euclidean points in R^3, find a center point C and k unit direction vectors $u_1, u_2, \ldots, u_k$ emanating from C such that the Euclidean perpendicular distance from the M_i points in cluster i to its direction vector u_i is *minimized* **and this is summed over all clusters $i = 1, 2, \ldots, k$.**

We formulate it as the following non-linear program : ($\bullet$ denotes dot product)

$$Minimize \sum_{j=1}^{k} \sum_{i=1}^{M_j} \|(p_i^j - C) - ((p_i^j - C) \bullet u_j)u_j\|^2$$

$$subj. \ to \ \|u_j\|^2 - 1 = 0 \quad \forall j = 1, \ldots, k$$

We run the $3-cluster$ subroutine at each of the branch bifurcations in order to obtain branch points. By con-

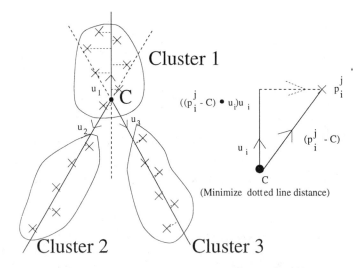

Figure 3. 3-Cluster problem at a branch junction (X represents centroid point)

necting the appropriate branch points with straight lines using the topological tree T, we obtain a **straight line central axis tree**.

3. Tree Volume Correspondence

The central axis trees obtained from the central axis algorithm are 3-D Euclidean trees, with different number of nodes and edges corresponding to lung volumes at various pressures. Note that each node of the CAT contains the 3-D Euclidean coordinates of the branch point, three direction vectors that best fit the branch axes at a bifurcation, three branch lengths and three branch diameters corresponding to the branches, as geometric attributes. The branch diameter is the average diameter over the entire branch. Tracking dynamically moving branch points of two central axis trees is crucial in corresponding tree volumes, since displacement in branch points result in relative change in other geometric attributes like branch lengths, and branch angles.

In what follows, we shall use the central axis tree representation where we consider just the 3-D branch point as the geometric attribute of each node of the CAT.

Let $T_1 = (V_1, E_1, W_1)$ where $\mid V_1 \mid = n$ and $T_2 = (V_2, E_2, W_2)$ where $\mid V_2 \mid = m$ where $W_i : V_i \to R^3, i = 1, 2$ be the two central axis trees generated by CAA. Let $V_1 = \{v_1, v_2, \ldots, v_n\}$ and $V_2 = \{v_1, v_2, \ldots, v_m\}$ be the vertices of T_1 and T_2. W_1 and W_2 correspond to the 3-D branch points on lung trees which act as anatomical landmarks. T_1 and T_2 are the central axis trees corresponding to lung volumes at lower and higher pressures respectively. The additional nodes in T_2 correspond

to missing branches not captured in T_1 either by the HRCT imaging modality or due to poor segmentation.

We need to track each of the nodes $v_1, v_2, \ldots, v_n$ in T_1 displaced within spheres of different radii (i.e. $\epsilon_1, \epsilon_2, \ldots, \epsilon_n$) to the nodes $v_1', v_2', \ldots, v_n'$ of T_2. Hence, it is difficult to solve the tree matching problem as one needs to exactly estimate the displacements ϵ_i 's of the branch points in order to produce accurate matchings. Since, we have no a priori knowledge of the values of ϵ_i's, we simplify the problem to the following minimization problem of the Euclidean distance between the mapped branch points of T_1 and T_2. This version of the matching problem has the drawback that it does not allow any relaxation in terms of the branch point movement.

INPUT 1:
Two geometric binary trees $T_1 = (V_1, E_1, W_1)$ and $T_2 = (V_2, E_2, W_2)$ where $W_i : V_i \to R^3, i = 1, 2$.

PROBLEM:
Is there a one-to-one matching function $\mathbf{f}$ of nodes in T_1 to T_2 such that the two edges emanating from a node v_1 in T_1 map to edge-disjoint paths starting from $\mathbf{f}(v_1)$ in T_2? If so, amongst all such maps $\mathbf{f}$, compute an $\mathbf{f}$ that minimizes the function:

$$\sum_{v_i \in V_1} \|(\mid W_1(v_i) - W_2(\mathbf{f}(v_i))\mid)\|_2^2.$$

Note that we map **edges** in T_1 **to edge-disjoint paths** in T_2 due to the extra branches and twigs which appear in the tree volume corresponding to T_2. One approach to solve the above problem is to consider just the topology and enumerate all possible **f**'s, and then compute the Euclidean difference between the branch points of T_1 and T_2 for each of the **f**'s, to obtain the minimum displacement of nodes in T_1 to T_2.

INPUT 2:
Two *rooted binary* trees $T_1 = (V_1, E_1)$ and $T_2 = (V_2, E_2)$ (W's not considered)

PROBLEM:
How many distinct mappings of **f** are possible such that the edges in T_1 map to edge-disjoint paths in T_2?

In the case of **complete binary trees**, there can be an **exponential** number of distinct mapping functions between nodes in T_1 and T_2. Let $P(n, k)$ denote the number of distinct mappings(n $= \|V_2\|$ and k $= \|V_1\|$ n $= 2^m - 1$ and k $= 2^l - 1$ and $l < m$). We formulate the following recurrence equation :

$$P(n, k) = 0 \ if \ n < k, \ P(n, n) = 1$$

$$P(n, 1) = n, \ P(n, 0) = 0$$

$$P(n, k) = 2 * P((n-1)/2, k) + \{P((n-1)/2, (k-1)/2)\}^2$$

The root of T_1 is : (i) mapped to root of T_2
(ii) not mapped to root of T_2.
In the first case, we have $P((n-1)/2, (k-1)/2)$ ways to map the left subtree of T_1, $P((n-1)/2, (k-1)/2)$ ways to map the right subtree of T_1, and since both these are independent, hence the product. In the second case, we have $2 * P((n-1)/2, k)$ ways of mapping T_1 to T_2. We shall prove the following result on the exponential nature of $P(n, k)$.

THEOREM : For any fixed n, $P(n, k)$ monotonically increases as k increases where $k = 1, 3, 7, \ldots, (n-1)/2$

Proof : By induction on k.

Basis : For k $= 3$, we show $P(n, 3) > P(n, 1)$, since

$$P(n, 3) = 2 * P((n-1)/2, 3) + \{P((n-1)/2, 1)\}^2$$
$$P(n, 3) = 2 + (n-1)/2)^2 > P(n, 1) = n$$

The above equation holds when $n \geq 5$ which is true since $k = 3 \leq (n-1)/2$. Also, observe that $\{P(n, 3) - P(n, 1)\} > 2$.

Inductive Hypothesis : P(n,k) is monotonically increasing for all values of $k = 1, 3, 7, 2^l - 1$. Moreover, $\{P(n, k) - P(n, (k-1)/2)\} > 2$, $\{P(n, (k-1)/2) - P(n, (k-3)/4)\} > 2$ and so on. For all $k \leq 2^l - 1$, the following holds:

$$P(n, k) > P(n, (k-1)/2) > \ldots > P(n, 1)$$

Inductive Step : For $k = 2^{l+1} - 1$ and $n \geq (2 * k + 1)$, we need to show $P(n, k) > P(n, (k-1)/2)$.

$$P(n, k) = 2 * P((n-1)/2, k) + \{P((n-1)/2, (k-1)/2)\}^2$$
$$\geq 2 + \{P((n-1)/2, (k-1)/2)\}^2$$
$$P(n, (k-1)/2) =$$
$$2 * P((n-1)/2, (k-1)/2) + \{P((n-1)/2k, (k-3)/4)\}^2$$

Therefore, we need to show that

$$2 + \{P((n-1)/2, (k-1)/2)\}^2 >$$
$$2 * P((n-1)/2, (k-1)/2) + \{P((n-1)/2, (k-3)/4)\}^2$$
$$\implies \{P((n-1)/2, (k-1)/2) - 1\}^2 >$$
$$\{P((n-1)/2, (k-3)/4) - 1\}\{P((n-1)/2, (k-3)/4) + 1\}$$

which hold true since

$$\{P((n-1)/2, (k-1)/2) - 1\} >$$
$$\{P((n-1)/2, (k-3)/4) - 1\}$$
by Ind. Hypothesis
$$\{P((n-1)/2, (k-1)/2) - 1\} \geq$$
$$\{P((n-1)/2, (k-3)/4) + 1\}$$
by Ind. Hypothesis and the fact
$$\{P((n-1)/2, (k-1)/2) - P((n-1)/2, (k-3)/4)\} > 2$$
holds true for $k \leq 2^l - 1$

From the above theorem, we know that the largest P(n,k) occurs when k $= (n-1)/2$ and this implies $P(n, (n-1)/2) = P(3, 1)^{2^{log(n)-2}} = O(3^n)$. Due to the exponential number of possible mappings, we cannot enumerate all of them and compute the "best" possible match. Therefore, we resort to a *linear time greedy algorithm* that matches T_1 to T_2 and takes into account the geometric constraints imposed by the movement of branch points between T_1 and T_2.

3.1. Tree Matching Algorithm

The **matching algorithm** starts by mapping a common reference node i.e. the roots of T_1 and T_2. Then it performs a **breadth-first** traversal on T_1 mapping nodes in T_1 to nodes in T_2. We use a *linear time recursive algorithm* to match the nodes of T_1 to T_2 and this algorithm does not perform any backtracking.

Let $L(p, q)$ denote the Euclidean distance between 3-D branch points corresponding to the nodes p and q present in the same CAT or two different CATs. Let $N(p)$ be the total number of nodes in the subtree rooted at p and $H(p)$ be the **height** of the node p in a CAT. Let BD_bound, BL_bound, BP_bound, BA_bound be the maximum relaxation bounds on the branch diameters, branch lengths, branch points and branch angles respectively.

Inductively, we assume that all nodes of T_1 at a particular **depth** d are mapped to nodes in T_2. Let us assume node v_1 at depth d in T_1 is matched with node v_1' in T_2 (Fig. 4). The crucial step then is to **match** the two children of v_i i.e. c_1 and c_2 (at depth $d + 1$) with

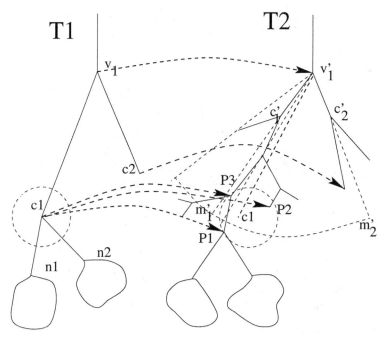

Edge (v1,c1) of T1 mapped to path (v'1, *) of T2 and
Edge (v1,c2) of T1 mapped to path (v'1, *) of T2
(* indicates potential nodes)

Figure 4. Matching children of v_1 in T_1 to descendants of v_1' in T_2

the descendants of v_1'. Let c_1' and c_2' be the two children of v_1'. Note that both c_1 and c_2 should map to nodes which lie on the edge-disjoint paths emanating from v_1' in T_2. If c_1 is mapped to some descendant node k_1' of v_1' in T_2, then it is the *best possible candidate node* that satisfies the following topological and geometric criteria which are **weighted equally**. The same criteria hold true for mapping c_2 of T_1 to a descendant node of v_1' in T_2. The first two criteria based on tree topology **must** be satisfied and all other geometric criteria may or may not be satisfied.

(i) $N(k_1') \geq N(c_1)$.

(ii) $H(c_1) \leq H(k_1')$

iii) The difference in branch diameters should be within the BD_bound i.e. the diameter of the branch corresponding to the edge (v_1, c_1) in T_1 must be similar to the diameter of the branches all along the path starting from v_1' to k_1' in T_2.

iv) The path from v_1' to k_1' must not be too curved (Fig. 5). The rationale being that an edge in T_1 should map to an almost straight path in T_2 since the new smaller branches in T_2 hardly deviate the straight path. In Fig. 4, candidate nodes $P1$ and $P3$ are preferred as a match for c_1 over $P2$ due to this reason (note that

all of them are within the sphere of influence of c_1).

v) The Euclidean difference in distance between branch point corresponding to c_1 and k_1' should not exceed the BP_bound i.e. $L(c_1, k_1') \leq$ BP_bound.

vi) $L(v_1', k_1') \leq L(v_1, c_1) +$ BL_bound. Moreover, the two vectors $(v_1 - c_1)$ and $(v_1' - k_1')$ should not differ significantly in only one of the X, Y, and Z components.

vii) The three angles (2 angles due to parent-child, one due to child-child) should be within the BA_bound of their corresponding counterparts in T_1.

In order to **identify candidate nodes** that are descendants of v_1' in T_2 that can be mapped to the node c_1 of T_1, we march from v_1' along a downward path every time pruning one subtree component. The nodes along the path are candidates for matching with c_1 in T_1. Pruning the subtree component is done by extending the length of both the edge segments (v_1', c_1') and (v_1', c_2') until they equal $L(v_1, c_1) +$ BL_bound. Let the end points of the extended segments be m_1' and m_2' respectively. If m_1' is closer to c_1 than m_2' in terms of the Euclidean distance, then the subtree rooted at c_2' in T_2 is pruned (provided $L(m_2', c_1) >$ BP_bound) and its descendant nodes are not considered as candidate nodes. If both $L(m_1', c_1) <$ BP_bound and $L(m_2', c_1) <$

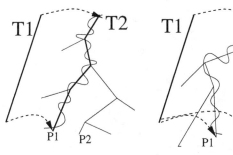

Edge in T1 mapped to an
almost straight path in T2

Bad case for matching algorithm
as edge in T1 is forced to map
to one of the curved paths in T2

Figure 5. Two scenerios to map an edge in T_1 to paths in T_2

BP_bound, then we use the above geometric criteria to decide as to which subtree needs to be pruned. Assuming that the subtree rooted at c_2' is pruned, we iterate the above process at the children of c_1' in T_2, every time pruning one of the subtree component. All the nodes along the path from v_1' are candidate nodes provided, the absolute difference in Euclidean distance between them and c_1 in T_1 is less than the BP_bound. We apply the above seven geometric criteria weighted equally to these candidate nodes and pick the node with the **best score** as the matched node of c_1 of T_1. We use the same procedure to match the node c_2 of T_1.

In order to decide at which node along the path from v_1' in T_2 the pruning needs to stop, we assume that we have two ways in which the absolute difference in Euclidean distance between c_1 and the candidate nodes on the path from v_1' varies : (i) decreases and then continues to increase or (ii) keeps increasing. We stop traversing the path to identify candidate nodes as soon as the absolute difference in distance between c_1 and the candidate node increases beyond the BP_bound. At this point, we evaluate the seven criteria for all candidate nodes. In Fig. 4, $P2$ may not be identified as a potential match node for c_1 in T_1 because, though m_2' lies within the BP_bound, the path from v_1' to $P2$ is more curved than the path to either $P3$ or $P1$.

After having mapped the children c_1 and c_2 of v_1 in T_1 to nodes in T_2 which lie on edge disjoint paths starting from v_1', we process the children of c_1 and c_2 which are at depth $d + 2$. In this manner, we map all the nodes in T_1 to nodes in T_2. The **time complexity** of the algorithm is $O(|V_2|)$ since we visit each node of T_2 constant number of times, and check for various criteria at each node of T_2.

4. Results

The dog lung data was obtained using HRCT at different static pressures of 3cm, 10cm and 20 cm of water. The images had an in-plane pixel resolution of 0.5mm on each side with a 1mm interslice spacing and a slice thickness of 2mm. Linear interpolation was used to obtain cubic voxel data. Each image stack contained around 170 images each of which is a 256x128 8-bit grayscale image (reduced from 16 bit HRCT data). We segmented the airway trees and ran the central axis algorithm [4] on them. The central axis tree obtained by joining the 3-D branch points is superimposed in Fig. 6 for the airway volume at 20cm of H_2O pressure.

We ran the central axis algorithm on airway volumes at all three pressures. For the sake of brevity, we show the results of the matching algorithm on the central axis trees at 3cm and 20cm pressures (Fig. 7). Note the reduction in number of branches as the static pressure is decreased. The matching algorithm performed quite well in corresponding nodes when comparing CATs at 20cm and 10cm, 10cm and 3cm , and at 20cm and 3cm pressure. This could be due to relatively little movement of branch points between airway volumes at successive pressures. In the case of matching CATs at 20cm and 3cm, the branch points moved significantly when compared to matching CATs at successive pressures, as expected. A *fixed* relaxation bound parameter BP_bound was set at a high value in order to allow for more candidate nodes, for all CAT match pairings. The matching algorithm is quite robust, since gradually evolving tree volumes were compared in which the branch points moved relatively less. We hope to run the matching algorithms on human airway data sets in a clinical setting which could provide more branch point motion due to actual breathing conditions.

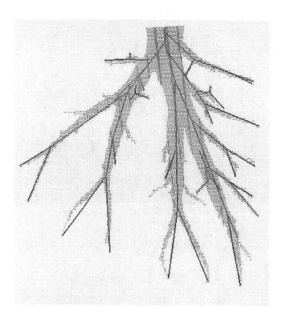

Figure 6. Airway volume at 20 cm H_2O pressure and the superimposed central axis tree

5. Conclusions

We designed a matching algorithm to match the central axis trees of 3-D tree structures which incorporates both tree topology and geometry. Our methods are simple and work well on real data sets. We are currently generating complex data sets of the central axis trees to incorporate bad situations (Fig. 5) which make the matching algorithm fail. This, in turn, helps develop new and more robust *heuristics*. It turns out that the PA trees are easier to segment than the airway trees [7] and since both airway and PA tree run in parallel all along the lung with similar branching structure, one can use the information provided by the extra edges in the CAT of the PA tree to identify missing airway branches. By corresponding the CATs of airway and PA tree using the proposed matching algorithms, one can enhance the airway segmentation algorithm by locating missing airway branches.

6. Acknowledgements

We thank Kumar Ramaiyer and Dr. Ramana Motakuri for useful discussions on matching algorithms.

7. References

[1] M.T. Goodrich, J.S. Mitchell and M.W. Orletsky, "Practical Methods for Approximate Geometric Pattern Matching under Rigid Motion," *Proc. 10th Annu. ACM Sympos. Comput. Geom*, pp. 103-112, 1994.

[2] P. Chew, M.T. Goodrich et al, "Geometric pattern matching under Euclidean Motion," *Proc. 5th Canadian conf. Comput. Geom*, pp. 151-156, 1993.

[3] C. Pisupati, L. Wolff et al, "Segmentation of 3-D Pulmonary Trees using Mathematical Morphology," *International Symposium on Mathematical Morphology*, Atlanta, GA, May 1996.

[4] C. Pisupati, L. Wolff et al, "A Central Axis Algorithm for 3D Bronchial Tree Structures," *IEEE International Symp. on Computer Vision*, Miami, FL, pp. 259-264, 1995.

[5] E.R. Weibel, "Lung Morphometry and Models in Respiratory Physiology," *Respiratory Physiology - An analytical Approach* Editors : Chang, Paiva.

[6] F.P. Preparata and M.I. Shamos, "*Computational Geometry: An Introduction*," Springer-Verlag, New York, 1985.

[7] S. Wood, E.A. Zerhouni et al, "Measurement of of three-dimensional lung tree structures by using Computed Tomography," *Journal of Applied Physiology*, Vol. 79(5), pp. 1687-1697, 1995.

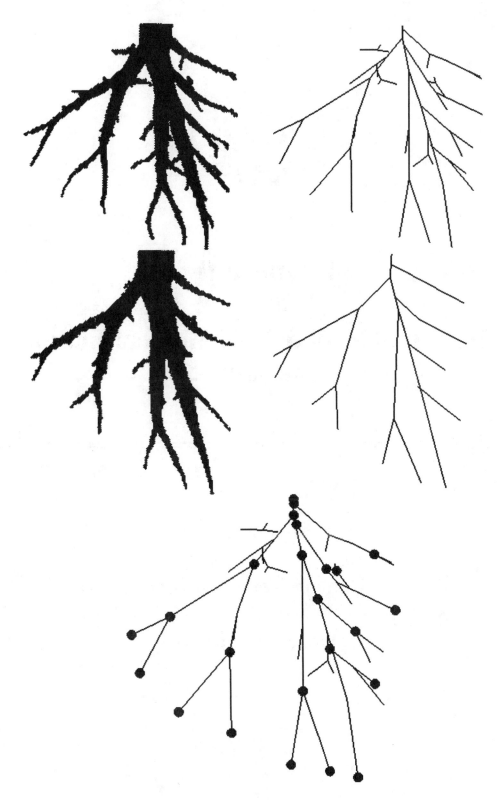

Figure 7. Airways and Central Axis Trees (CATs) at 20cm and 3cm pressure. Also, the matched nodes of the CAT at 20cm pressure with CAT at 3cm pressure displayed as spheres

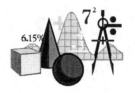

Keynote II

"Deformable Models in Medical Image Analysis"

Speakers

Demetri Terzopoulos
and
Tim McInerney

Deformable Models in Medical Image Analysis[1]

Tim McInerney and Demetri Terzopoulos

Department of Computer Science, University of Toronto, Toronto, ON M5S 3H5, Canada

Abstract

This article surveys deformable models, a promising and vigorously researched computer-assisted medical image analysis technique. Among model-based techniques, deformable models offer a unique and powerful approach to image analysis that combines geometry, physics, and approximation theory. They have proven to be effective in segmenting, matching, and tracking anatomic structures by exploiting (bottom-up) constraints derived from the image data together with (top-down) a priori knowledge about the location, size, and shape of these structures. Deformable models are capable of accommodating the significant variability of biological structures over time and across different individuals. Furthermore, they support highly intuitive interaction mechanisms that, when necessary, allow medical scientists and practitioners to bring their expertise to bear on the model-based image interpretation task. This article reviews the rapidly expanding body of work on the development and application of deformable models to problems of fundamental importance in medical image analysis, including segmentation, shape representation, matching, and motion tracking.

1 Introduction

The rapid development and proliferation of medical imaging technologies is revolutionizing medicine. Medical imaging allows scientists and physicians to glean potentially life-saving information by peering noninvasively into the human body. The role of medical imaging has expanded beyond the simple visualization and inspection of anatomic structures. It has become a tool for surgical planning and simulation, intra-operative navigation, radiotherapy planning, and for tracking the progress of disease. For example, ascertaining the detailed shape and organization of anatomic structures enables a surgeon preoperatively to plan an optimal approach to some target structure. In radiotherapy, medical imaging allows the delivery of a necrotic dose of radiation to a tumor with minimal collateral damage to healthy tissue.

With medical imaging playing an increasingly prominent role in the diagnosis and treatment of disease, the medical image analysis community has become preoccupied with the challenging problem of extracting, with the assistance of computers, clinically useful information about anatomic structures imaged through CT, MR, PET, and other modalities [94, 85, 5, 13, 6]. Although modern imaging devices provide exceptional views of internal anatomy, the use of computers to quantify and analyze the embedded structures with accuracy and efficiency is limited. Accurate, repeatable, quantitative data must be efficiently extracted in order to support the spectrum of biomedical investigations and clinical activities from diagnosis, to radiotherapy, to surgery.

Segmenting structures from medical images and reconstructing a compact geometric representation of these structures is difficult due to the sheer size of the datasets and the complexity and variability of the anatomic shapes of interest. Furthermore, the shortcomings typical of sampled data, such as sampling artifacts, spatial aliasing, and noise, may cause the boundaries of structures to be indistinct and disconnected. The challenge is to extract boundary elements belonging to the same structure and integrate these elements into a coherent and consistent model of the structure. Traditional low-level image processing techniques which consider only local information can make incorrect assumptions during this integration process and generate infeasible object boundaries. As a result, these model-free techniques usually require considerable amounts of expert intervention. Furthermore, the subsequent analysis and interpretation of the segmented objects is hindered by the pixel- or voxel-level structure representations generated by most image processing operations.

This article surveys deformable models, a promising and vigorously researched model-based approach to computer-assisted medical image analysis. The widely recognized potency of deformable models stems from their ability to segment, match, and track images of anatomic structures by exploiting (bottom-up) constraints derived from the image data together with (top-down) *a priori* knowledge about the location, size, and shape of these structures. Deformable models are capable of accommodating the often significant variability of biological structures over time and across different individuals. Furthermore, deformable models support highly intuitive interaction mechanisms that allow medical scientists and practitioners to bring their expertise to bear on the model-based image interpretation task when necessary. We will review the basic formulation of deformable models and survey their application to fundamental medical image analysis problems, including segmentation, shape

---

[1] An extended version of this paper appears as reference [72].

171

representation, matching, and motion tracking.

2 Mathematical Foundations

The mathematical foundations of deformable models represent the confluence of geometry, physics, and approximation theory. Geometry serves to represent object shape, physics imposes constraints on how the shape may vary over space and time, and optimal approximation theory provides the formal underpinnings of mechanisms for fitting the models to measured data.

Deformable model geometry usually permits broad shape coverage by employing geometric representations that involve many degrees of freedom, such as splines. The model remains manageable, however, because the degrees of freedom are generally not permitted to evolve independently, but are governed by physical principles that bestow intuitively meaningful behavior upon the geometric substrate. The name "deformable models" stems primarily from the use of elasticity theory at the physical level, generally within a Lagrangian dynamics setting. The physical interpretation views deformable models as elastic bodies which respond naturally to applied forces and constraints. Typically, deformation energy functions defined in terms of the geometric degrees of freedom are associated with the deformable model. The energy grows monotonically as the model deforms away from a specified natural or "rest shape" and often includes terms that constrain the smoothness or symmetry of the model. In the Lagrangian setting, the deformation energy gives rise to elastic forces internal to the model. Taking a physics-based view of classical optimal approximation, external potential energy functions are defined in terms of the data of interest to which the model is to be fitted. These potential energies give rise to external forces which deform the model such that it fits the data.

Deformable curve, surface, and solid models gained popularity after they were proposed for use in computer vision [103] and computer graphics [101] in the mid 1980's. Terzopoulos introduced the theory of continuous (multidimensional) deformable models in a Lagrangian dynamics setting [99], based on deformation energies in the form of (controlled-continuity) generalized splines [100]. Ancestors of the deformable models now in common use include Fischler and Elshlager's spring-loaded templates [41] and Widrow's rubber mask technique [109]. The deformable model that has attracted the most attention to date is popularly known as "snakes" [56]. Snakes or "deformable contour models" represent a special case of the general multidimensional deformable model theory [99].

An extended version of this paper [72] reviews the basic mathematical machinery of deformable models.

3 Medical Image Analysis with Deformable Models

Although originally developed for application to problems in computer vision and computer graphics, the potential of deformable models for use in medical image analysis has been quickly realized. They have been applied to images generated by imaging modalities as varied as X-ray, computed tomography (CT), angiography, magnetic resonance (MR), and ultrasound. Two dimensional and three dimensional deformable models have been used to segment, visualize, track, and quantify a variety of anatomic structures ranging in scale from the macroscopic to the microscopic. These include the brain, heart, face, cerebral, coronary and retinal arteries, kidney, lungs, stomach, liver, skull, vertebra, objects such as brain tumors, a fetus, and even cellular structures such as neurons and chromosomes. Deformable models have been used to track the nonrigid motion of the heart, the growing tip of a neurite, and the motion of erythrocytes. They have been used to locate structures in the brain, and to register images of the retina, vertebra and neuronal tissue.

In the following sections, we review and discuss the application of deformable models to medical image interpretation tasks including segmentation, matching, and motion analysis.

3.1 Image Segmentation with Deformable Curves

The segmentation of anatomic structures—the partitioning of the original set of image points into subsets corresponding to the structures—is an essential first stage of most medical image analysis tasks, such as registration, labeling, and motion tracking. These tasks require anatomic structures in the original image to be reduced to a compact, analytic representation of their shapes. Performing this segmentation manually is extremely labor intensive and time-consuming. A primary example is the segmentation of the heart, especially the left ventricle (LV), from cardiac imagery. Segmentation of the left ventricle is a prerequisite for computing diagnostic information such as ejection-fraction ratio, ventricular volume ratio, heart output, and for wall motion analysis which provides information on wall thickening, etc. [90].

Most clinical segmentation is currently performed using manual slice editing. In this scenario, a skilled operator, using a computer mouse or trackball, manually traces the region of interest on each slice of an image volume. Manual slice editing suffers from several drawbacks. These include the difficulty in achieving reproducible results, operator bias, forcing the operator to view each 2D slice separately to deduce and measure the shape and volume of 3D structures, and operator fatigue.

Segmentation using traditional low-level image processing techniques, such as region growing, edge detection, and mathematical morphology operations, also requires considerable amounts of expert interactive guidance. Furthermore, automating these model-free approaches is difficult because of the shape complexity and variability within and across individuals. In general, the underconstrained nature of the segmentation problem limits the efficacy of approaches that consider local information only. Noise and other image artifacts can cause incorrect regions or boundary discontinuities

172

in objects recovered by these methods.

A deformable model based segmentation scheme, used in concert with image pre-processing, can overcome many of the limitations of manual slice editing and traditional image processing techniques. These connected and continuous geometric models consider an object boundary as a whole and can make use of *a priori* knowledge of object shape to constrain the segmentation problem. The inherent continuity and smoothness of the models can compensate for noise, gaps and other irregularities in object boundaries. Furthermore, the parametric representations of the models provide a compact, analytical description of object shape. These properties lead to a robust and elegant technique for linking sparse or noisy local image features into a coherent and consistent model of the object.

Among the first and primary uses of deformable models in medical image analysis was the application of deformable contour models, such as snakes [56], to segment structures in 2D images [12, 28, 105, 87, 29, 61, 18, 48, 66, 33]. Typically users initialized a deformable model near the object of interest and allowed it to deform into place. Users could then use the interactive capabilities of these models and manually fine-tune them. Furthermore, once the user is satisfied with the result on an initial image slice, the fitted contour model may then be used as the initial boundary approximation for neighboring slices. These models are then deformed into place and again propagated until all slices have been processed. The resulting sequence of 2D contours can then be connected to form a continuous 3D surface model [64, 23, 28, 29].

The application of snakes and other similar deformable contour models to extract regions of interest is, however, not without limitations. For example, snakes were designed as interactive models. In non-interactive applications, they must be initialized close to the structure of interest to guarantee good performance. The internal energy constraints of snakes can limit their geometric flexibility and prevent a snake from representing long tube-like shapes or shapes with significant protrusions or bifurcations. Furthermore, the topology of the structure of interest must be known in advance since classical deformable contour models are parametric and are incapable of topological transformations without additional machinery.

Various methods have been proposed to improve and further automate the deformable contour segmentation process. Cohen and Cohen [29] used an internal "inflation" force to expand a snakes model past spurious edges towards the real edges of the structure, making the snake less sensitive to initial conditions (inflation forces were also employed in [103]). Amini *et al.* [3] use dynamic programming to carry out a more extensive search for global minima. Poon *et al.* [84] and Grzeszczuk and Levin [46] minimize the energy of active contour models using simulated annealing which is known to give global solutions and allows the incorporation of non-differentiable constraints.

Poon *et al.* [84] also use a discriminant function to incorporate region based image features into the image forces of their active contour model. The discriminant function allows the inclusion of additional image features in the segmentation and serves as a constraint for global segmentation consistency (i.e. every image pixel contributes to the discriminant function). The result is a more robust energy functional and a much better tolerance to deviation of the initial guess from the true boundaries. Others researchers [86, 22, 21, 52, 42, 68] have also integrated region-based information into deformable contour models in an attempt to decrease sensitivity to insignificant edges and initial model placement.

Recently, several researchers [60, 19, 67, 108, 20, 71, 89] have been developing topology independent shape modeling schemes that allow a deformable contour or surface model to not only represent long tube-like shapes or shapes with bifurcations, but also to dynamically sense and change its topology.

3.2 Volume Image Segmentation with Deformable Surfaces

Segmenting 3D image volumes slice by slice, either manually or by applying 2D contour models, is a laborious process and requires a post-processing step to connect the sequence of 2D contours into a continuous surface. Furthermore, the resulting surface reconstruction can contain inconsistencies or show rings or bands. The use of a true 3D deformable surface model on the other hand, can result in a faster, more robust segmentation technique which ensures a globally smooth and coherent surface between image slices. Deformable surface models in 3D were first used in computer vision [103]. Many researchers have since explored the use of deformable surface models for segmenting structures in medical image volumes. Miller [74] constructs a polygonal approximation to a sphere and geometrically deforms this "balloon" model until the balloon surface conforms to the object surface in 3D CT data. The segmentation process is formulated as the minimization of a cost function where the desired behavior of the balloon model is determined by a local cost function associated with each model vertex. The cost function is a weighted sum of three terms: a deformation potential that "expands" the model vertices towards the object boundary, an image term that identifies features such as edges and opposes the balloon expansion, and a term that maintains the topology of the model by constraining each vertex to remain close to the centroid of its neighbors.

Cohen and Cohen [27, 29] and McInerney and Terzopoulos [70] use finite element and physics-based techniques to implement an elastically deformable cylinder and sphere, respectively. The models are used to segment the inner wall of the left ventricle of the heart from MR or CT image volumes. These deformable surfaces are based on a thin-plate under tension surface spline, which controls and constrains the stretching and bending of the surface. The models are fitted to data dynamically by integrating Lagrangian equations of motion through time in order to adjust the deformational degrees of freedom. Furthermore, the finite element method is used to represent the models as a continuous surface in the form of weighted sums of local polynomial basis functions. Unlike Miller's [74] polygonal model, the finite element method provides an analytic surface representation and the use of high-order polynomials means that fewer elements are required to accurately represent an object. Pentland and Sclaroff [83] and Nastar and Ayache [78] also develop physics-based models but use a reduced modal basis for the finite elements (see Section 3.5).

Staib and Duncan [93] describe a 3D surface model used for geometric surface matching to 3D medical image data. The model uses a Fourier parameterization which decomposes the surface into a weighted sum of sinusoidal basis functions. Several different surface types are developed such as tori, open surfaces, closed surfaces and tubes. Surface finding is formulated as an optimization problem using gradient ascent which attracts the surface to strong image gradients in the vicinity of the model. An advantage of the Fourier parameterization is that it allows a wide variety of smooth surfaces to be described with a small number of parameters. That is, a Fourier representation expresses a function in terms of an orthonormal basis and higher indexed basis functions in the sum represent higher spatial variation. Therefore, the series can be truncated and still represent relatively smooth objects accurately.

In a different approach, Szeliski et al. [97] use a dynamic, self-organizing oriented particle system to model surfaces of objects. The oriented particles, which can be visualized as small, flat disks, evolve according to Newtonian mechanics and interact through external and interparticle forces. The external forces attract the particles to the data while interparticle forces attempt to group the particles into a coherent surface. The particles can reconstruct objects with complex shapes and topologies by "flowing" over the data, extracting and conforming to meaningful surfaces. A triangulation is then performed which connects the particles into a continuous global model that is consistent with the inferred object surface.

Other notable work involving 3D deformable surface models and medical image applications can be found in [37, 108, 98, 32] as well as several models described in the following sections.

3.3 Incorporating A Priori Knowledge

In medical images, the general shape, location and orientation of objects is known and this knowledge may be incorporated into the deformable model in the form of initial conditions, data constraints, constraints on the model shape parameters, or into the model fitting procedure. The use of implicit or explicit anatomical knowledge to guide shape recovery is especially important for robust automatic interpretation of medical images. For automatic interpretation, it is essential to have a model that not only describes the size, shape, location and orientation of the target object but that also permits expected variations in these characteristics. Automatic interpretation of medical images can relieve clinicians from the labor intensive aspects of their work while increasing the accuracy, consistency, and reproducibility of the interpretations.

A number of researchers have incorporated knowledge of object shape into deformable models by using deformable shape templates. These models usually use "hand-crafted" global shape parameters to embody a priori knowledge of expected shape and shape variation of the structures and have been used successfully for many applications of automatic image interpretation. The idea of deformable templates can be traced back to the early work on spring loaded templates by Fischler and Elshlager [41]. An excellent example in computer vision is the work of Yuille et al. [114] who construct deformable templates for detecting and describing features of faces, such as the eye. In medical image analysis, Lipson et al. [65] note that axial cross sectional images of the spine yield approximately elliptical vertebral contours and consequently extract the contours using a deformable ellipsoidal template.

Deformable models based on superquadrics are another example of deformable shape templates that are gaining in popularity in medical image research. Superquadrics contain a small number of intuitive global shape parameters that can be tailored to the average shape of a target anatomic structure. Furthermore, the global parameters can often be coupled with local shape parameters such as splines resulting in a powerful shape representation scheme. For example, Metaxas and Terzopoulos [73] employ a dynamic deformable superquadric model [102] to reconstruct and track human limbs from 3D biokinetic data. Their models can deform both locally and globally by incorporating the global shape parameters of a superellipsoid with the local degrees of freedom of a membrane spline in a Lagrangian dynamics formulation. The global parameters efficiently capture the gross shape features of the data, while the local deformation parameters reconstruct the fine details of complex shapes. Using Kalman filtering theory, they develop and demonstrate a biokinetic motion tracker based on their deformable superquadric model.

Vemuri and Radisavljevic [107, 106] construct a deformable superquadric model in an orthonormal wavelet basis. This multi-resolution basis provides the model with the ability to continuously transform from local to global shape deformations thereby allowing a continuum of shape models to be created and to be represented with relatively few parameters. They apply the model to segment and reconstruct anatomical structures in the human brain from MRI data.

As a final example, Bardinet et al. [9, 11, 10] fit a deformable superquadric to segmented 3D cardiac images and then refine the superquadric fit using a volumetric deformation technique known as free form deformations (FFDs). FFDs are defined by tensor product trivariate splines and can be visualized as a rubber-like box in which the object to be deformed (in this case the superquadric) is embedded. Deformations of the box are automatically transmitted to embedded objects. This volumetric aspect of FFDs allows two superquadric surface models to be simultaneously deformed in order to reconstruct the inner and outer surfaces of the left ventricle of the heart and the volume in between these surfaces. Further examples of deformable superquadrics can be found in [82, 24] (see Section 3.5).

Several researchers cast the deformable model fitting process in a probabilistic framework and include prior knowledge of object shape by incorporating prior probability distributions on the shape variables to be estimated [106, 92, 110]. For example, Staib and Duncan [92] use a deformable contour model on 2D echocardiograms and MR images to extract the LV of the heart and the corpus callosum of the brain, respectively. This closed contour model is parameterized using an elliptic Fourier decomposition and *a priori* shape information is included as a spatial probability expressed through the likelihood of each model parameter. The model parameter probability distributions are derived from a set of example object boundaries and serve to bias the contour model towards expected or more likely shapes.

Szekely *et al.* [96] have also developed Fourier parameterized models. Furthermore, they have added elasticity to their models to create "Fourier snakes" in 2D and elastically deformable Fourier surface models in 3D. By using the Fourier parameterization followed by a statistical analysis of a training set, they define mean organ models and their eigen-deformations. An elastic fit of the mean model in the subspace of eigenmodes restricts possible deformations and finds an optimal match between the model surface and boundary candidates.

Cootes *et al.* [30] and Hill *et al.* [53] present a statistically based technique for building deformable shape templates and use these models to segment various organs from 2D and 3D medical images. The statistical parameterization provides global shape constraints and allows the model to deform only in ways implied by the training set. The shape models represent objects by sets of landmark points which are placed in the same way on an object boundary in each input image. For example, to extract the LV from echocardiograms, they choose points around the ventricle boundary, the nearby edge of the right ventricle, and the top of the left atrium. The points can be connected to form a deformable contour. By examining the statistics of training sets of hand-labeled medical images, and using principal component analysis, a shape model is derived that describes the average positions and the major modes of variation of the object points. New shapes are generated using the mean shape and a weighted sum of the major modes of variation. Object boundaries are then segmented using this "point distribution model" by examining a region around each model point to calculate the displacement required to move it towards the boundary. These displacements are then used to update the shape parameter weights.

3.4 Matching

Matching of regions in images can be performed between the representation of a region and a model (labeling) or between the representation of two distinct regions (registration). Registration of 2D and 3D medical images is necessary in order to study the evolution of a pathology in an individual, or to take full advantage of the complementary information coming from multimodality imagery. Recent exam-

ples of the use of deformable models to perform medical image registration are found in [76, 77, 47, 40, 14, 50, 59, 104]. These techniques primarily consist of constructing highly structured descriptions for matching. This operation is usually carried out by extracting regions of interest with an edge detection algorithm, followed by the extraction of landmark points or characteristic contours (or curves on extracted boundary surfaces in the case of 3D data). In 3D, these curves usually describe differential structures such as ridges, or topological singularities. An elastic matching algorithm can then be applied between corresponding pairs of curves or contours where the "start" contour is iteratively deformed to the "goal" contour using forces derived from local pattern matches with the goal contour [76].

An example of matching where the use of explicit *a priori* knowledge has been embedded into deformable models is the extraction and labeling of anatomic structures in the brain, primarily from MR images. The anatomical knowledge is made explicit in the form of a 3D brain atlas. The atlas is modeled as a physical object and is given elastic properties. After an initial global alignment, the atlas deforms and matches itself onto corresponding regions in the brain image volume in response to forces derived from image features. The assumption underlying this approach is that at some representational level, normal brains have the same topological structure and differ only in shape details. The idea of modeling the atlas as an elastic object was originated by Broit [17], who formulated the matching process as a minimization of a cost function. Subsequently, Bajcsy and Kovacic [8] implemented a multiresolution version of Broit's system where the deformation of the atlas proceeds step-by-step in a coarse to fine strategy, increasing the local similarity and global coherence. The elastically deformable atlas technique has since become a very active area of research and is being explored by several researchers [39, 43, 88, 25, 15, 16, 35, 69, 36, 95, 34, 91].

There are several problems with the deformable atlas approach. The technique is sensitive to initial positioning of the atlas—if the initial rigid alignment is off by too much, then the elastic match may perform poorly. The presence of neighboring features may also cause matching problems—the atlas may warp to an incorrect boundary. Finally, without user interaction, the atlas can have difficulty converging to complicated object boundaries. One solution to these problems is to use image preprocessing in conjunction with the deformable atlas. Sandor and Leahy [88] use this approach to automatically label regions of the cortical surface that appear in 3D MR images of human brains. They automatically match a labeled deformable atlas model to preprocessed brain images, where preprocessing consists of 3D edge detection and morphological operations. These filtering operations automatically extract the brain and sulci (deep grooves in the cortical surface) from an MR image and provide a smoothed representation of the brain surface to which their 3D B-spline deformable surface model can rapidly converge.

3.5 Motion Tracking and Analysis

The idea of tracking objects in time-varying images using deformable models was originally proposed in the context of computer vision [56, 103]. Deformable models have been used to track nonrigid microscopic and macroscopic structures in motion, such as blood cells [63] and neurite growth cones [49] in cine-microscopy, as well as coronary arteries in cine-angiography [62]. However, the primary use of deformable models for tracking in medical image analysis is to measure the dynamic behavior of the human heart, especially the left ventricle. Regional characterization of the heart wall motion is necessary to isolate the severity and extent of diseases such as ischemia. Magnetic resonance and other imaging technologies can now provide time varying three dimensional images of the heart with excellent spatial resolution and reasonable temporal resolutions. Deformable models are well suited for this image analysis task.

In the simplest approach, a 2D deformable contour model is used to segment the LV boundary in each slice of an initial image volume. These contours are then used as the initial approximation of the LV boundaries in corresponding slices of the image volume at the next time instant and are then deformed to extract the new set of LV boundaries [90, 105, 7, 51, 44]. This temporal propagation of the deformable contours dramatically decreases the time taken to segment the LV from a sequence of image volumes over a cardiac cycle. Singh *et al.* [90] report a time of 15 minutes to perform the segmentation, considerably less than the 1.5-2 hours that a human expert takes for manual segmentation. McInerney and Terzopoulos [70] have applied the temporal propagation approach in 3D using a 3D dynamic deformable "balloon" model to track the LV.

In a more involved approach, Amini and Duncan [2] use bending energy and surface curvature to track and analyze LV motion. For each time instant, two sparse subsets of surface points are created by choosing geometrically significant landmark points, one for the endocardial surface, and the other for the epicardial surface of the LV. Surface patches surrounding these points are then modeled as thin, flexible plates. Making the assumption that each surface patch deforms only slightly and locally within a small time interval, for each sampled point on the first surface they construct a search area on the LV surface in the image volume at the next time instant. The best matched (i.e. minimum bending energy) point within the search window on the second surface is taken to correspond to the point on the first surface. This matching process yields a set of initial motion vectors for pairs of LV surfaces derived from a 3D image sequence. A smoothing procedure is then performed using the initial motion vectors to generate a dense motion vector field over the LV surfaces.

Cohen *et al.* [26] also employ a bending energy technique in 2D and attempt to improve on this method by adding a term to the bending energy function that tends to preserve the matching of high curvature points. Goldgof *et al.* [45, 55, 54, 75] have also been pursuing surface shape matching ideas primarily based on changes in Gaussian cur-

vature and assume a conformal motion model (i.e. motion which preserves angles between curves on a surface but not distances).

An alternative approach is that of Chen *et al.* [24], who use a hierarchical motion model of the LV constructed by combining a globally deformable superquadric with a locally deformable surface using spherical harmonic shape modeling primitives. Using this model, they estimate the LV motion from angiographic data and produce a hierarchical decomposition that characterizes the LV motion in a coarse-to-fine fashion.

Pentland and Horowitz [82] and Nastar and Ayache [78, 79] are also able to produce a coarse-to-fine characterization of the LV motion. They use dynamic deformable models to track and recover the LV motion and make use of modal analysis, a well-known mechanical engineering technique, to parameterize their models. This parameterization is obtained from the eigenvectors of a finite element formulation of the models. These eigenvectors are often referred to as the "free vibration" modes and variable detail of LV motion representation results from varying the number of modes used.

The heart is a relatively smooth organ and consequently there are few reliable landmark points. The heart also undergoes complex nonrigid motion that includes a twisting (tangential) component as well as the normal component of motion. The motion recovery methods described above are, in general, not able to capture this tangential motion without additional information. Recently, magnetic resonance techniques, based on magnetic tagging [4] have been developed to track material points on the myocardium in a non-invasive way. The temporal correspondence of material points that these techniques provide allow for quantitative measurement of tissue motion and deformation including the twisting component of the LV motion. Several researchers have applied deformable models to image sequences of MR tagged data [112, 113, 81, 38, 58, 57, 1]. For example, Amini *et. al* [1] and Kumar and Goldgof [58] use a 2D deformable grid to localize and track SPAMM (Spatial Modulation of Magnetization) tag points on the LV tissue. Park *et al.* [80, 81] fit a volumetric physics-based deformable model to MRI-SPAMM data of the LV. The parameters of the model are functions which can can capture regional shape variations of the LV such as bending, twisting, and contraction. Based on this model, the authors quantitatively compare normal hearts and hearts with hypertrophic cardiomyopathy.

Another problem with most of the methods described above is that they model the endocardial and epicardial surfaces of the LV separately. In reality the heart is a thick-walled structure. Duncan *et al.* [38] and Park *et al.* [80, 81] develop models which consider the volumetric nature of the heart wall. These models use the shape properties of the endocardial and epicardial surfaces and incorporate mid-wall displacement information of tagged MR images. By constructing 3D finite element models of the LV with nodes in the mid-wall region as well as nodes on the endocardial and epicardial surfaces, more accurate measurements of the LV motion can be obtained. Young and Axel [111, 113], and

Creswell [31] and have also constructed 3D finite element models from the boundary representations of the endocardial and epicardial surfaces.

4 Conclusion

The increasingly important role of medical imaging in the diagnosis and treatment of disease has opened an array of challenging problems centered on the computation of accurate geometric models of anatomic structures from medical images. Deformable models offer an attractive approach to tackling such problems, because these models are able to represent the complex shapes and broad shape variability of anatomical structures. Deformable models overcome many of the limitations of traditional low-level image processing techniques, by providing compact and analytical representations of object shape, by incorporating anatomic knowledge, and by providing interactive capabilities. The continued development and refinement of deformable models should remain an important area of research into the foreseeable future. An extended version of this paper [72] includes a discussion of the key issues in this regard and indicates some promising research directions.

Acknowledgements

We would like to thank the following individuals for providing citation information that improved the completeness of the bibliography: Amir Amini, Nicholas Ayache, Ingrid Carlbom, Chang Wen Chen, James Duncan, Dmitry Goldgof, Thomas Huang, Stephane Lavallee, Francois Leitner, Gerard Medioni, Dimitri Metaxas, Alex Pentland, Stan Sclaroff, Ajit Singh, Richard Szeliski, Baba Vemuri, Alistair Young, and Alan Yuille. TM is grateful for the financial support of an NSERC postgraduate scholarship. DT is a fellow of the Canadian Institute for Advanced Research. This work was made possible by the financial support of the Information Technologies Research Center of Ontario.

References

[1] A. Amini, R. Curwen, A. Klein, T. Egglin, J. Pollak, F. Lee, and J. Gore. Physics based snakes, Kalman snakes, and snake grids for feature localization and tracking in medical images. In Bizais et al. [13], pages 363–364.

[2] A. Amini and J. Duncan. Bending and stretching models for LV wall motion analysis from curves and surfaces. *Image and Vision Computing*, 10(6):418–430, July 1992.

[3] A. Amini, T. Weymouth, and R. Jain. Using dynamic programming for solving variational problems in vision. *IEEE Trans. on Pattern Analysis and Machine Intelligence*, 12(9):855–867, 1990.

[4] L. Axel and L. Dougherty. Heart wall motion: Improved method of spatial modulation of magnetization for MR imaging. *Radiology*, 172:349–350, 1989.

[5] N. Ayache. Medical computer vision, virtual reality and robotics. *Image and Vision Computing*, 13(4):295–313, 1995.

[6] N. Ayache, editor. *Proc. First International Conf. on Computer Vision, Virtual Reality and Robotics in Medicine (CVRMed'95), Nice, France, April, 1995*, volume 905 of *Lectures Notes in Computer Science*, Berlin, Germany, 1995. Springer–Verlag.

[7] N. Ayache, I. Cohen, and I. Herlin. Medical image tracking. In A. Blake and A. Yuille, editors, *Active Vision*, chapter 17. MIT Press, Cambridge, MA, 1992.

[8] R. Bajcsy and S. Kovacic. Multiresolution elastic matching. *Computer Vision, Graphics, and Image Processing*, 46:1–21, 1989.

[9] E. Bardinet, L. Cohen, and N. Ayache. Superquadrics and free-form deformations: A global model to fit and track 3D medical data. In Ayache [6], pages 319–326.

[10] E. Bardinet, L. Cohen, and N. Ayache. Analyzing the deformation of the left ventricle of the heart with a parametric deformable model. Research report 2797, INRIA, Sophia-Antipolis, France, Feb. 1996.

[11] E. Bardinet, L. Cohen, and N. Ayache. A parametric deformable model to fit unstructured 3D data. *Computer Vision and Image Understanding*, 1996. In press. Also research report 2617, INRIA, Sophia-Antipolis, France.

[12] M. Berger. Snake growing. In O. Faugeras, editor, *Computer Vision – Proc. First European Conf. on Computer Vision (ECCV'90), Antibes, France, April, 1990*, Lectures Notes in Computer Science, pages 570–572. Springer–Verlag, 1990.

[13] Y. Bizais, C. Barillot, and R. D. Paola, editors. *Information Processing in Medical Imaging: Proc. 14th Int. Conf. (IPMI'95), Ile de Berder, France, June, 1995*, volume 3 of *Computational Imaging and Vision*, Dordrecht, The Netherlands, 1995. Kluwer Academic.

[14] F. Bookstein. Principal warps: Thin-plate splines and the decomposition of deformations. *IEEE Trans. on Pattern Analysis and Machine Intelligence*, 11(6):567–585, June 1989.

[15] F. Bookstein. Thin-plate splines and the atlas problem for biomedical images. In H. Barret and A. Gmitro, editors, *Information Processing in Medical Imaging: Proc. 12th Int. Conf. (IPMI'91), Wye, UK, July, 1991*, Lectures Notes in Computer Science, pages 326–342. Springer–Verlag, 1991.

[16] I. Bozma and J. Duncan. A modular system for image analysis using a game theoretic framework. *Image and Vision Computing*, 10(6):431–443, July 1992.

[17] C. Broit. *Optimal Registration of Deformed Images*. PhD thesis, Computer and Information Science Dept., University of Pennsylvania, Philadelphia, PA, 1981.

[18] I. Carlbom, D. Terzopoulos, and K. Harris. Computer-assisted registration, segmentation, and 3D reconstruction from images of neuronal tissue sections. *IEEE Trans. on Medical Imaging*, 13(2):351–362, 1994.

[19] V. Caselles, F. Catte, T. Coll, and F. Dibos. A geometric model for active contours. *Numerische Mathematik*, 66, 1993.

[20] V. Caselles, R. Kimmel, and G. Sapiro. Geodesic active contours. In *Proc. Fifth International Conf. on Computer Vision (ICCV'95), Cambridge, MA, June, 1995*, pages 694–699, Los Alamitos, CA, 1995. IEEE Computer Society Press.

[21] A. Chakraborty and J. Duncan. Integration of boundary finding and region-based segmentation using game theory. In Bizais et al. [13], pages 189–200.

[22] A. Chakraborty, L. Staib, and J. Duncan. Deformable boundary finding influenced by region homogeneity. In *Proc. Conf. Computer Vision and Pattern Recognition (CVPR'94), Seattle, WA, June, 1994*, pages 624–627, Los Alamitos, CA, 1994. IEEE Computer Society Press.

[23] L. Chang, H. Chen, and J. Ho. Reconstruction of 3D medical images: A nonlinear interpolation technique for reconstruction of 3D medical images. *Computer Vision, Graphics, and Image Processing*, 53(4):382–391, July 1991.

[24] C. Chen, T. Huang, and M. Arrott. Modeling, analysis and visualization of left ventricle shape and motion by hierarchical decomposition. *IEEE Trans. on Pattern Analysis and Machine Intelligence*, 16:342–356, April 1994.

[25] G. Christensen, R. Rabbitt, M. Miller, S. Joshi, U. Grenander, T. Coogan, and D. van Essen. Topological properties of smooth anatomic maps. In Bizais et al. [13], pages 101–112.

[26] I. Cohen, N. Ayache, and P. Sulger. Tracking points on deformable objects using curvature information. In G. Sandini, editor, *Computer Vision – Proc. Second European Conf. on Computer Vision (ECCV'92), Santa Margherita Ligure, Italy, May, 1992*, Lectures Notes in Computer Science, pages 458–466. Springer–Verlag, 1992.

[27] I. Cohen, L. Cohen, and N. Ayache. Using deformable surfaces to segment 3D images and infer differential structures. *CVGIP: Image Understanding*, 56(2):242–263, 1992.

[28] L. Cohen. On active contour models and balloons. *CVGIP: Image Understanding*, 53(2):211–218, March 1991.

[29] L. Cohen and I. Cohen. Finite element methods for active contour models and balloons for 2D and 3D images. *IEEE Trans. on Pattern Analysis and Machine Intelligence*, 15(11):1131–1147, November 1993.

[30] T. Cootes, A. Hill, C. Taylor, and J. Haslam. The use of active shape models for locating structures in medical images. *Image and Vision Computing*, 12(6):355–366, July 1994.

[31] L. Creswell, S. Wyers, J. Pirolo, W. Perman, M. Vannier, and M. Pasque. Mathematical modelling of the heart using magnetic resonance imaging. *IEEE Trans. on Medical Imaging*, 11(4):581–589, Dec. 1992.

[32] C. Davatzikos and R. Bryan. Using a deformable surface model to obtain a mathematical representation of the cortex. In *International Symp. on Computer Vision, Coral Gables, FL, November, 1995*, pages 212–217, Los Alamitos, CA, 1995. IEEE Computer Society Press.

[33] C. Davatzikos and J. Prince. An active contour model for mapping the cortex. *IEEE Trans. on Medical Imaging*, 14(1):65–80, March 1995.

[34] C. Davatzikos, J. Prince, and R. Bryan. Image registration based on boundary mapping. *IEEE Trans. on Medical Imaging*, 15(1):112–115, Feb. 1996.

[35] J. Declerck, G. Subsol, J. Thirion, and N. Ayache. Automatic retrieval of anatomic structures in 3D medical images. In Ayache [6], pages 153–162.

[36] K. Delibasis and P. Undrill. Anatomical object recognition using deformable geometric models. *Image and Vision Computing*, 12(7):423–433, Sept. 1994.

[37] H. Delingette, M. Hebert, and K. Ikeuchi. Shape representation and image segmentation using deformable surfaces. *Image and Vision Computing*, 10(3):132–144, April 1992.

[38] J. Duncan, P. Shi, A. Amini, R. Constable, L. Staib, D. Dione, Q. Shi, E. Heller, M. Singer, A. Chakraborty, G. Robinson, J. Gore, and A. Sinusas. Towards reliable, noninvasive measurement of myocardial function from 4D

images. In *Medical Imaging 1994: Physiology and Function from Multidimensional Medical Images*, volume 2168 of *SPIE Proc.*, pages 149–161, Bellingham, WA, Feb 1994. SPIE.

[39] A. Evans, W. Dai, L. Collins, P. Neelin, and S. Marrett. Warping of a computerized 3D atlas to match brain image volumes for quantitative neuroanatomical and functional analysis. In *Medical Imaging V: Image Processing*, volume 1445 of *SPIE Proc.*, pages 236–246, Bellingham, WA, 1991. SPIE.

[40] J. Feldmar and N. Ayache. Locally affine registration of free-form surfaces. In *Proc. Conf. Computer Vision and Pattern Recognition (CVPR'94), Seattle, WA, June, 1994*, pages 496–501, Los Alamitos, CA, 1994. IEEE Computer Society Press.

[41] M. Fischler and R. Elschlager. The representation and matching of pictorial structures. *IEEE Trans. on Computers*, 22(1):67–92, 1973.

[42] J. Gauch, H. Pien, and J. Shah. Hybrid boundary-based and region-based deformable models for biomedical image segmentation. In *Mathematical Methods in Medical Imaging III*, volume 2299 of *SPIE Proc.*, pages 72–83, San Diego, CA, 1994. SPIE.

[43] J. Gee, M. Reivich, and R. Bajcsy. Elastically deforming 3D atlas to match anatomical brain images. *Journal of Computer Assisted Tomography*, 17(2):225–236, March-April 1993.

[44] D. Geiger, A. Gupta, L. Costa, and J. Vlontzos. Dynamic programming for detecting, tracking and matching deformable contours. *IEEE Trans. on Pattern Analysis and Machine Intelligence*, 17(3):294–302, March 1995.

[45] D. Goldgof, H. Lee, and T. Huang. Motion analysis of nonrigid surfaces. In *Proc. Conf. Computer Vision and Pattern Recognition (CVPR'88), Ann Arbor, MI, June, 1988*, pages 375–380, Los Alamitos, CA, 1988. IEEE Computer Society Press.

[46] R. Grzeszczuk and D. Levin. Brownian strings: Segmenting images with stochastically deformable contours. In Robb [85], pages 72–89.

[47] A. Gueziec and N. Ayache. Smoothing and matching of 3D space curves. *International Journal of Computer Vision*, 12(1):79–104, February 1994.

[48] A. Gupta, T. O'Donnell, and A. Singh. Segmentation and tracking of cine cardiac MR and CT images using a 3-D deformable model. In *Proc. IEEE Conf. on Computers in Cardiology, September, 1994*, 1994.

[49] S. Gwydir, H. Buettner, and S. Dunn. Non-rigid motion analysis and feature labelling of the growth cone. In *IEEE Workshop on Biomedical Image Analysis, Seattle, WA, June, 1994*, pages 80–87, Los Alamitos, CA, 1994. IEEE Computer Society Press.

[50] A. Hamadeh, S. Lavallee, R. Szeliski, P. Cinquin, and O. Peria. Anatomy-based registration for computer-integrated surgery. In Ayache [6], pages 212–218.

[51] I. Herlin and N. Ayache. Features extraction and analysis methods for sequences of ultrasound images. *Image and Vision Computing*, 10(10):673–682, December 1992.

[52] I. Herlin, C. Nguyen, and C. Graffigne. A deformable region model using stochastic processes applied to echocardiographic images. In *Proc. Conf. Computer Vision and Pattern Recognition (CVPR'92), Urbana, IL, June, 1992*, pages 534–539, Los Alamitos, CA, 1992. IEEE Computer Society Press.

[53] A. Hill, A. Thornham, and C. Taylor. Model-based interpretation of 3D medical images. In *Proc. 4th British Machine Vision Conf. (BMVC'93), Surrey, UK, September, 1993*, pages 339–348. BMVA Press, 1993.

[54] W. Huang and D. Goldgof. Adaptive-size meshes for rigid and nonrigid shape analysis and synthesis. *IEEE Trans. on Pattern Analysis and Machine Intelligence*, 15(3), March 1993.

[55] C. Kambhamettu and D. Goldgof. Point correspondence recovery in nonrigid motion. *CVGIP: Image Understanding*, 60(1):26–43, July 1994.

[56] M. Kass, A. Witkin, and D. Terzopoulos. Snakes: Active contour models. *International Journal of Computer Vision*, 1(4):321–331, 1988.

[57] D. Kraitchman, A. Young, C. Chang, and L. Axel. Semiautomatic tracking of myocardial motion in MR tagged images. *IEEE Trans. on Medical Imaging*, 14(3):422–432, Sept. 1995.

[58] S. Kumar and D. Goldgof. Automatic tracking of SPAMM grid and the estimation of deformation parameters from cardiac MR images. *IEEE Trans. on Medical Imaging*, 13(1):122–132, March 1994.

[59] S. Lavallée and R. Szeliski. Recovering the position and orientation of free-form objects from image contours using 3D distance maps. *IEEE Trans. on Pattern Analysis and Machine Intelligence*, 17(4):378–390, 1995.

[60] F. Leitner and P. Cinquin. Complex topology 3D objects segmentation. In *Model-Based Vision Development and Tools*, volume 1609 of *SPIE Proc.*, pages 16–26, Bellingham, WA, 1991. SPIE.

[61] F. Leitner and P. Cinquin. From splines and snakes to Snakes Splines. In C. Laugier, editor, *Geometric Reasoning: From Perception to Action*, volume 708 of *Lectures Notes in Computer Science*, pages 264–281. Springer–Verlag, 1993.

[62] J. Lengyel, D. Greenberg, and R. Popp. Time-dependent three-dimensional intravascular ultrasound. In *Proc. SIGGRAPH'95, Los Angeles, CA, August, 1995, in Computer Graphics Proc., Annual Conf. Series 1995*, pages 457–464, New York, NY, 1995. ACM SIGGRAPH.

[63] F. Leymarie and M. Levine. Tracking deformable objects in the plane using an active contour model. *IEEE Trans. on Pattern Analysis and Machine Intelligence*, 15(6):635–646, 1993.

[64] W. Lin and S. Chen. A new surface interpolation technique for reconstructing 3D objects from serial cross-sections. *Computer Vision, Graphics, and Image Processing*, 48:124–143, Oct. 1989.

[65] P. Lipson, A. Yuille, D. O'Keefe, J. Cavanaugh, J. Taaffe, and D. Rosenthal. Deformable templates for feature extraction from medical images. In O. Faugeras, editor, *Computer Vision – Proc. First European Conf. on Computer Vision (ECCV'90), Antibes, France, April, 1990*, Lectures Notes in Computer Science, pages 477–484. Springer–Verlag, 1990.

[66] S. Lobregt and M. Viergever. A discrete dynamic contour model. *IEEE Trans. on Medical Imaging*, 14(1):12–24, March 1995.

[67] R. Malladi, J. Sethian, and B. Vemuri. Shape modeling with front propagation: A level set approach. *IEEE Trans. on Pattern Analysis and Machine Intelligence*, 17(2):158–175, Feb. 1995.

[68] J. Mangin, F. Tupin, V. Frouin, I. Bloch, R. Rougetet, J. Regis, and J. Lopez-Krahe. Deformable topological models for segmentation of 3D medical images. In Bizais et al. [13], pages 153–164.

[69] D. McDonald, D. Avis, and A. Evans. Multiple surface identification and matching in magnetic resonance images. In Robb [85], pages 160–169.

[70] T. McInerney and D. Terzopoulos. A dynamic finite element surface model for segmentation and tracking in multidimensional medical images with application to cardiac 4D image analysis. *Computerized Medical Imaging and Graphics*, 19(1):69–83, January 1995.

[71] T. McInerney and D. Terzopoulos. Topologically adaptable snakes. In *Proc. Fifth International Conf. on Computer Vision (ICCV'95), Cambridge, MA, June, 1995*, pages 840–845, Los Alamitos, CA, 1995. IEEE Computer Society Press.

[72] T. McInerney and D. Terzopoulos. Deformable models in medical image analysis: A survey. *Medical Image Analysis*, 1(2), 1996.

[73] D. Metaxas and D. Terzopoulos. Shape and nonrigid motion estimation through physics-based synthesis. *IEEE Trans. on Pattern Analysis and Machine Intelligence*, 15(6):580–591, 1993.

[74] J. Miller, D. Breen, W. Lorensen, R. O'Bara, and M. Wozny. Geometrically deformed models: A method for extracting closed geometric models from volume data. In *Computer Graphics (Proc. SIGGRAPH'91 Conf., Las Vegas, NV, July, 1991)*, volume 25(4), pages 217–226, July 1991.

[75] S. Mishra, D. Goldgof, and T. Huang. Non-rigid motion analysis and epicardial deformation estimation from angiography data. In *Proc. Conf. Computer Vision and Pattern Recognition (CVPR'91), Maui, HI, June, 1991*, pages 331–336, Los Alamitos, CA, 1991. IEEE Computer Society Press.

[76] M. Moshfeghi. Elastic matching of multimodality medical images. *CVGIP: Graphical Models and Image Processing*, 53:271–282, 1991.

[77] M. Moshfeghi, S. Ranganath, and K. Nawyn. Three-dimensional elastic matching of volumes. *IEEE Trans. on Image Processing*, 3:128–138, 1994.

[78] C. Nastar and N. Ayache. Fast segmentation, tracking, and analysis of deformable objects. In *Proc. Fourth International Conf. on Computer Vision (ICCV'93), Berlin, Germany, May, 1993*, pages 275–279, Los Alamitos, CA, 1993. IEEE Computer Society Press.

[79] C. Nastar and N. Ayache. Non-rigid motion analysis in medical images: A physically based approach. In A. Colchester and D. Hawkes, editors, *Information Processing in Medical Imaging: Proc. 13th Int. Conf. (IPMI'93), Flagstaff, AZ, June, 1993*, Lectures Notes in Computer Science, pages 17–32. Springer–Verlag, 1993.

[80] J. Park, D. Metaxas, and L. Axel. Volumetric deformable models with parameter functions: A new approach to the 3D motion analysis of the LV from MRI–SPAMM. In *Proc. Fifth International Conf. on Computer Vision (ICCV'95), Cambridge, MA, June, 1995*, pages 700–705, Los Alamitos, CA, 1995. IEEE Computer Society Press.

[81] J. Park, D. Metaxas, and L. Axel. Analysis of left ventricular wall motion based on volumetric deformable models and MRI–SPAMM. *Medical Image Analysis*, 1(1), 1996.

[82] A. Pentland and B. Horowitz. Recovery of nonrigid motion and structure. *IEEE Trans. on Pattern Analysis and Machine Intelligence*, 13(7):730–742, July 1991.

[83] A. Pentland and S. Sclaroff. Closed-form solutions for physically based shape modelling and recognition. *IEEE Trans. on Pattern Analysis and Machine Intelligence*, 13(7):715–729, July 1991.

[84] C. S. Poon, M. Braun, R. Fahrig, A. Ginige, and A. Dorrell. Segmentation of medical images using an active contour model incorporating region-based images features. In Robb [85], pages 90–97.

[85] R. Robb, editor. *Proc. Third Conf. on Visualization in Biomedical Computing (VBC'94), Rochester, MN, October, 1994*, volume 2359 of *SPIE Proc.*, Bellingham, WA, 1994. SPIE.

[86] N. Rougon and F. Prêteux. Deformable markers: Mathematical morphology for active contour models control. In *Image Algebra and Morphological Image Processing II*, volume 1568 of *SPIE Proc.*, pages 78–89, Bellingham, WA, 1991. SPIE.

[87] N. Rougon and F. Prêteux. Directional adaptive deformable models for segmentation with application to 2D and 3D medical images. In *Medical Imaging 93: Image Processing*, volume 1898 of *SPIE Proc.*, pages 193–207, Bellingham, WA, 1993. SPIE.

[88] S. Sandor and R. Leahy. Towards automatic labelling of the cerebral cortex using a deformable atlas model. In Bizais et al. [13], pages 127–138.

[89] G. Sapiro, R. Kimmel, and V. Caselles. Object detection and measurements in medical images via geodesic deformable contours. In *Vision Geometry IV*, volume 2573 of *SPIE Proc.*, pages 366–378, Bellingham, WA, 1995. SPIE.

[90] A. Singh, L. von Kurowski, and M. Chiu. Cardiac MR image segmentation using deformable models. In *Biomedical Image Processing and Biomedical Visualization*, volume 1905 of *SPIE Proc.*, pages 8–28, Bellingham, WA, 1993. SPIE.

[91] J. Snell, M. Merickel, J. Ortega, J. Goble, J. Brookeman, and N. Kassell. Model-based boundary estimation of complex objects using hierarchical active surface templates. *Pattern Recognition*, 28(10):1599–1609, 1995.

[92] L. Staib and J. Duncan. Boundary finding with parametrically deformable models. *IEEE Trans. on Pattern Analysis and Machine Intelligence*, 14(11):1061–1075, November 1992.

[93] L. Staib and J. Duncan. Deformable Fourier models for surface finding in 3D images. In R. Robb, editor, *Proc. Second Conf. on Visualization in Biomedical Computing (VBC'92), Chapel Hill, NC, October, 1992*, volume 1808 of *SPIE Proc.*, pages 90–104, Bellingham, WA, 1992. SPIE.

[94] M. Stytz, G. Frieder, and O. Frieder. Three–dimensional medical imaging: Algorithms and computer systems. *ACM Computing Surveys*, 23(4):421–499, December 1991.

[95] G. Subsol, J. Thirion, and N. Ayache. A general scheme for automatically building 3D morphometric anatomical atlases: Application to a skull atlas. In *Proc. Second International Symp. on Medical Robotics and Computer Assisted Surgery (MRCAS'95), Baltimore, MD, November, 1995*, pages 226–233, 1995.

[96] G. Székely, A. Kelemen, C. Brechbuhler, and G. Gerig. Segmentation of 2-D and 3-D objects from MRI volume data using constrained elastic deformations of flexible Fourier surface models. *Medical Image Analysis*, 1(1), 1996.

[97] R. Szeliski, D. Tonnesen, and D. Terzopoulos. Modeling surfaces of arbitrary topology with dynamic particles. In *Proc. Conf. Computer Vision and Pattern Recognition (CVPR'93), New York, NY, June, 1993*, pages 82–87, Los Alamitos, CA, 1993. IEEE Computer Society Press.

[98] H. Tek and B. Kimia. Shock-based reaction-diffusion bubbles for image segmentation. In Ayache [6], pages 434–438.

[99] D. Terzopoulos. On matching deformable models to images. Technical Report 60, Schlumberger Palo Alto Research, 1986. Reprinted in *Topical Meeting on Machine Vision,* Technical Digest Series, Vol. 12 (Optical Society of America, Washington, DC) 1987, 160-167.

[100] D. Terzopoulos. Regularization of inverse visual problems involving discontinuities. *IEEE Trans. on Pattern Analysis and Machine Intelligence*, 8(4):413–424, 1986.

[101] D. Terzopoulos and K. Fleischer. Deformable models. *The Visual Computer*, 4(6):306–331, 1988.

[102] D. Terzopoulos and D. Metaxas. Dynamic 3D models with local and global deformations: Deformable superquadrics. *IEEE Trans. on Pattern Analysis and Machine Intelligence*, 13(7):703–714, July 1991.

[103] D. Terzopoulos, A. Witkin, and M. Kass. Constraints on deformable models: Recovering 3D shape and nonrigid motion. *Artificial Intelligence*, 36(1):91–123, 1988.

[104] J. Thirion. Extremal points: Definition and application to 3D image registration. In *Proc. Conf. Computer Vision and Pattern Recognition (CVPR'94), Seattle, WA, June, 1994*, pages 587–592, Los Alamitos, CA, 1994. IEEE Computer Society Press.

[105] N. Ueda and K. Mase. Tracking moving contours using energy-minimizing elastic contour models. In G. Sandini, editor, *Computer Vision – Proc. Second European Conf. on Computer Vision (ECCV'92), Santa Margherita Ligure, Italy, May, 1992*, Lectures Notes in Computer Science, pages 453–457. Springer–Verlag, 1992.

[106] B. Vemuri and A. Radisavljevic. Multiresolution stochastic hybrid shape models with fractal priors. *ACM Trans. on Graphics*, 13(2):177–207, April 1994.

[107] B. Vemuri, A. Radisavljevic, and C. Leonard. Multiresolution 3D stochastic shape models for image segmentation. In A. Colchester and D. Hawkes, editors, *Information Processing in Medical Imaging: Proc. 13th Int. Conf. (IPMI'93), Flagstaff, AZ, June, 1993*, Lectures Notes in Computer Science, pages 62–76. Springer–Verlag, 1993.

[108] R. Whitaker. Volumetric deformable models. In Robb [85].

[109] B. Widrow. The rubber mask technique, part I. *Pattern Recognition*, 5(3):175–211, 1973.

[110] M. Worring, A. Smeulders, L. Staib, and J. Duncan. Parameterized feasible boundaries in gradient vector fields. In A. Colchester and D. Hawkes, editors, *Information Processing in Medical Imaging: Proc. 13th Int. Conf. (IPMI'93), Flagstaff, AZ, June, 1993*, Lectures Notes in Computer Science, pages 48–61. Springer–Verlag, 1993.

[111] A. Young and L. Axel. Non-rigid wall motion using MR tagging. In *Proc. Conf. Computer Vision and Pattern Recognition (CVPR'92), Urbana, IL, June, 1992*, pages 399–404, Los Alamitos, CA, 1992. IEEE Computer Society Press.

[112] A. Young, L. Axel, L. Dougherty, D. Bogen, and C. Parenteau. Validation of tagging with MR imaging to estimate material deformation. *Radiology*, 188:101–108, 1993.

[113] A. Young, D. Kraitchman, L. Dougherty, and L. Axel. Tracking and finite element analysis of stripe deformation in magnetic resonance tagging. *IEEE Trans. on Medical Imaging*, 14(3):413–421, Sept. 1995.

[114] A. Yuille, P. Hallinan, and D. Cohen. Feature extraction from faces using deformable templates. *International Journal of Computer Vision*, 8:99–111, 1992.

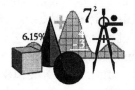

Session 5

Deformable Models I

Cardiac Motion Simulator for Tagged MRI

Edo Waks*, Jerry L. Prince*, and Andrew S. Douglas[†]
* Department of Electrical and Computer Engineering
[†] Department of Mechanical Engineering
Johns Hopkins University
Baltimore, MD 21218
E-mail: prince@jhu.edu

Abstract

This paper describes a computational simulator for use in cardiac imaging using tagged magnetic resonance imaging. The simulator incorporates a 13-parameter model of left-ventricular motion due to Arts et al. (1992) and applies it to a confocal prolate spherical shell, resembling the shape of the left ventricle. Using parameters determined in other work, our model can be made to assume a configuration representing one of 60 phases in the cardiac cycle. In this paper, we determine the inverse motion map analytically, allowing pointwise correspondences to be made between two points at any two times. Using this mathematical relationship, we simulate the (tagged) magnetic resonance imaging process using a standard (tagged) spin-echo imaging equation. Image sequences can be synthesized at arbitrary orientations at any phase. We currently synthesize a SPAMM tag pattern with arbitrary spatial frequency, but other patterns can be readily incorporated. To accommodate two-dimensional motion estimation algorithms, we have created a two-dimensional simulator which restricts the three-dimensional motion to two dimensions. In either two or three dimensions, a true motion is output so that motion estimation algorithms can be compared against the truth. We conclude with a simple demonstration of the performance of the simulator.

Keywords — motion analysis of biomedical images, cardiac magnetic resonance imaging, representation and description of multidimensional shape.

1 Introduction

Tagged MR imaging [8] can provide important information about the motion of the left ventricle (LV) of the heart. In this technique, a pattern of spatially varying magnetism is embedded in the LV using a special tagging pulse sequence. This intensity deforms along with the LV wall during the heart cycle, and is imaged by standard MRI techniques. Motion estimation methods attempt to determine the motion of the heart from the deformation of the tag pattern within an image sequence [2] [6] [4] [7] [3].

In order to test the effectiveness of a motion estimation algorithm it is highly desirable to obtain a set of images representing a known motion. Ideally, a deformable phantom would be used for this purpose. But such phantoms are difficult to build and control, and *a priori* knowledge of the motion they generate is often not available. Furthermore, such phantoms are usually restricted to simple deformations such as compressions and rotations. Computer simulation is an alternative which does not suffer from many of the problems encountered by phantoms. In this approach, a computer is used to generate a series of synthetic images which display some form of motion. The underlying mathematical transformation responsible for the motion displayed by these images is known, making this a good control experiment. But care must be taken to ensure that these simulations are representative of a true medical imaging experiment.

In this research, our goal was to develop an accurate simulator that could generate a control experiment for motion estimation from tagged cardiac MR images. In order to develop a representative simulation, we first selected a shape that is both similar to the LV, and also easy to work with. Our model is based on a prolate spheroidal geometry, and we implement a mechanical model for LV motion developed by Arts et al. [1]. We generate realistic tag patterns using a tagged MR imaging equation described by Prince and McVeigh [6]. These mathematical models have been used to form an accurate simulator capable of generating complex motion as well as perfectly calculable displacement fields.

This research was supported by NIH grant R29-HL47405, and NSF grant MIP-9350336. Correspond to prince@jhu.edu.

2 Background

2.1 Model Shape

In our approach we begin with a three-dimensional volume, and then take two-dimensional slices in order to simulate the MR imaging process. The basis of our geometric model is the prolate sphere, which is a three-dimensional ellipse-like object, as shown in Figure 1.

A prolate sphere is defined to have a constant radius λ which determines its size. Points which lie on this surface can be identified by the parameter λ, along with the elevation angle η and the azimuthal angle ϕ, shown in Figure 1. A point (λ, η, ϕ) in prolate spheroidal coordinates has the following Cartesian coordinates:

$$
\begin{aligned}
x &= \delta \sinh \lambda \sin \eta \cos \phi \,, \\
y &= \delta \sinh \lambda \sin \eta \sin \phi \,, \\
z &= \delta \cosh \lambda \cos \eta \,.
\end{aligned} \tag{1}
$$

The fixed parameter δ is the focal radius (the distance from the origin to either focus). A point (x, y, z) in Cartesian coordinates has the following prolate spheroidal coordinates:

$$
\begin{aligned}
r_1 &= \sqrt{x^2 + y^2 + (z + \delta)^2} \,, \\
r_2 &= \sqrt{x^2 + y^2 + (z - \delta)^2} \,, \\
\lambda &= \cosh^{-1} \frac{r_1 + r_2}{2\delta} & \lambda > 0 \,, \\
\eta &= \cos^{-1} \frac{r_1 - r_2}{2\delta} & 0 \le \eta \le 180 \,, \\
\phi &= \tan^{-1} \frac{y}{x} & 0 \le \phi < 360 \,.
\end{aligned} \tag{2}
$$

where r_1 and r_2 are the distances between (x, y, z) and each focus.

The LV itself can be modeled by defining it to lie between a pair of confocal prolate spheres with radii λ_i and λ_o such that $\lambda_i < \lambda_o$, as shown in Figure 2 (note that coordinate axes have been rotated for display purposes). The top of this volume is cut off by restricting η to the range $0 \le \eta \le 120^o$ in order to better approximate the shape of the LV. Thus, a point (x, y, z) is defined to lie inside the *model LV* if its prolate spheroidal coordinates satisfy $\lambda_i \le \lambda \le \lambda_o$ and $0 \le \eta \le 120^o$. This model LV defines the material points for the motion, described next.

2.2 Motion Model

Having selected a geometric model of the LV, it is now necessary to model the motion of the LV. We have chosen to implement the motion model designed by Arts et al. [1] because of the wide variety of intricate motions it can provide. Complex motion is achieved in this model by applying a series of thirteen three-dimensional transformations controlled by thirteen motion parameters, k_1 through k_{13}.

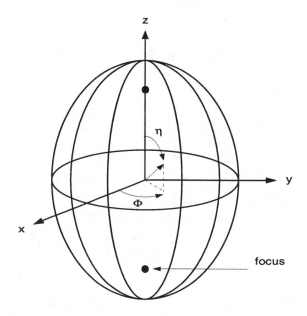

Figure 1. A prolate sphere, centered at the origin and aligned along the z-axis..

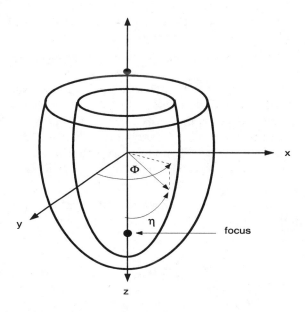

Figure 2. Prolate spheroidal model for the left ventricular myocardium.

Table 1. Description of the thirteen k-parameters.

k_1	Radially dependent compression
k_2	Left ventricular torsion
k_3	Ellipticallization in long axis planes
k_4	Ellipticallization in short axis planes
k_5	Shear in x direction
k_6	Shear in y direction
k_7	Shear in z direction
k_8	Rotation about x-axis
k_9	Rotation about y-axis
k_{10}	Rotation about z-axis
k_{11}	Translation in x direction
k_{12}	Translation in y direction
k_{13}	Translation in z direction

Table 1 lists these parameters, referred to as k-parameters, and the transformations to which they correspond.

All transformations listed in Table 1 are three-dimensional, but we have introduced a fourth dimension which allows us to express the overall transformation as a single matrix map. The fourth dimension is incorporated in order to allow translations to be expressed as matrix transformations. This technique improves computational efficiency and simplifies the overall algorithm. It does not present any theoretical improvement on the motion model itself, but is merely a mathematical convenience.

Motion in the left ventricle is specified through a transformation which maps a *material point* to a corresponding *spatial point* at time t. A material point is a specific location defined on the model LV, and the spatial point is its location in space at a certain time instant. As the LV deforms, the spatial coordinates of each material point change. We express this mathematically as $\mathbf{r} = r(\mathbf{p}, t)$, where the material point $\mathbf{p}$ moves to the spatial point $\mathbf{r}$ at time t. The *reference map* is the inverse transformation $\mathbf{p} = p(\mathbf{r}, t)$.

The overall matrix equation that transforms point $\mathbf{p} = (p_x, p_y, p_z, 1)$, a point inside the model LV, into $\mathbf{r} = (r_x, r_y, r_z, 1)$ is:

$$\mathbf{r} = F_a F_6 F_5 F_4 F_3 F_2 F_1 F_0 \mathbf{p}, \qquad (3)$$

where

$$F_0 = \begin{bmatrix} a^{1/3} & 0 & 0 & 0 \\ 0 & a^{1/3} & 0 & 0 \\ 0 & 0 & a^{-2/3} & 0 \\ 0 & 0 & 0 & 1 \end{bmatrix}$$

$$F_1 = \begin{bmatrix} \epsilon & 0 & 0 & 0 \\ 0 & \epsilon & 0 & 0 \\ 0 & 0 & \epsilon & 0 \\ 0 & 0 & 0 & 1 \end{bmatrix},$$

$$\epsilon = \sqrt[3]{1 + \frac{3 k_1 V_w}{4\pi |F_0 \mathbf{p}|^3}}$$

$$F_2 = \begin{bmatrix} \cos ak_2 z_1/|\mathbf{r}_1| & -\sin ak_2 z_1/|\mathbf{r}_1| & 0 & 0 \\ \sin ak_2 z_1/|\mathbf{r}_1| & \cos ak_2 z_1/|\mathbf{r}_1| & 0 & 0 \\ 0 & 0 & 1 & 0 \\ 0 & 0 & 0 & 1 \end{bmatrix}$$

$$\mathbf{r}_1 = F_1 F_0 \mathbf{p} = \begin{bmatrix} x_1 \\ y_1 \\ z_1 \\ 1 \end{bmatrix}$$

$$F_3 = \begin{bmatrix} a^{-1/3} e^{k_4 - (k_3/2)} & 0 & 0 & 0 \\ 0 & a^{-1/3} e^{-k_4 - (k_3/2)} & 0 & 0 \\ 0 & 0 & a^{2/3} e^{k_3} & 0 \\ 0 & 0 & 0 & 1 \end{bmatrix}$$

$$F_4 = \begin{bmatrix} 1 & k_5 & 0 & 0 \\ k_5 & 1 + k_5{}^2 & 0 & 0 \\ 0 & 0 & 1 & 0 \\ 0 & 0 & 0 & 1 \end{bmatrix}$$

$$F_5 = \begin{bmatrix} 1 & 0 & k_6 & 0 \\ 0 & 1 & 0 & 0 \\ k_6 & 0 & 1 + k_6{}^2 & 0 \\ 0 & 0 & 0 & 1 \end{bmatrix}$$

$$F_6 = \begin{bmatrix} 1 & 0 & 0 & 0 \\ 0 & 1 & k_7 & 0 \\ 0 & k_7 & 1 + k_7{}^2 & 0 \\ 0 & 0 & 0 & 1 \end{bmatrix}$$

$$F_a = A_4 A_3 A_2 A_1$$

$$A_1 = \begin{bmatrix} 1 & 0 & 0 & 0 \\ 0 & \cos k_8 & -\sin k_8 & 0 \\ 0 & \sin k_8 & \cos k_8 & 0 \\ 0 & 0 & 0 & 1 \end{bmatrix}$$

$$A_2 = \begin{bmatrix} \cos k_9 & 0 & \sin k_9 & 0 \\ 0 & 1 & 0 & 0 \\ -\sin k_9 & 0 & \cos k_9 & 0 \\ 0 & 0 & 0 & 1 \end{bmatrix}$$

$$A_3 = \begin{bmatrix} \cos k_{10} & -\sin k_{10} & 0 & 0 \\ \sin k_{10} & \cos k_{10} & 0 & 0 \\ 0 & 0 & 1 & 0 \\ 0 & 0 & 0 & 1 \end{bmatrix}$$

$$A_4 = \begin{bmatrix} 1 & 0 & 0 & k_{11} \\ 0 & 1 & 0 & k_{12} \\ 0 & 0 & 1 & k_{13} \\ 0 & 0 & 0 & 1 \end{bmatrix}$$

It is possible to deduce what each transformation does by using Table 1, and referring to Reference [1].

Aside from the k-parameters, there are two constants in this model: a and V_w. V_w is the wall volume of the model LV. The constant a is a correctional parameter present in matrix F_0. F_0 transforms a prolate spheroidal shell into a more spherical shape in anticipation of the next transformation, which is a radially dependent compression in spherical coordinates. Ideally, we want all points on the surface of the prolate sphere to compress uniformly, but points in the model LV can have different spherical radii, in general, and nonuniform compression will result. By converting the model LV to a more spherical shape we reduce this undesirable distortion. The effect of F_0 is undone in matrix F_3.

In order for the motion model to be useful one needs the ability to generate realistic cardiac motion. Since a medical imaging sequence involves a discrete set of time frames, the thirteen k-parameters must be determined for each of these frames. This can be characterized as a parameter estimation problem, where the k-parameters are estimated so that the model LV is transformed as close as possible to the actual state of the LV for each time frame. One approach to this problem was presented by Arts et al. [1], where a least squares criterion is minimized using the Levenberg-Marquardt method.

3 A Computational Model

3.1 Overview

The computational model that we have developed first generates a three-dimensional LV model and applies a motion. Next, an imaging plane is selected to intersect the (deformed) LV. An image is generated by selecting points on the imaging plane and assigning them a value which depends on whether they lie inside or outside the LV volume. If they lie outside, they are assigned a value of 0, otherwise they are assigned a value determined by a spatial intensity pattern and an MR imaging equation. Motion estimation algorithms can then be applied to these images.

Testing the effectiveness of a motion estimation algorithm requires two additional pieces of information which must be generated by our computational model: a segmentation, which determines which pixels are inside the LV wall; and a displacement field, which represents the true displacement of the model. The displacement field can be compared with that generated by the motion estimation algorithm, and statistics such as mean square error can then be calculated.

Development of the computational model roughly parallels the steps of generating an actual series of MR images, providing a realistic three-dimensional simulation. But some motion estimation algorithms deal only with two-dimensional motion within the image plane. A three-dimensional simulation would be inappropriate for these algorithms because the LV is moving through the plane, generating an additional displacement component which cannot be accounted for in two-dimensional algorithms. The displacement fields generated by these two methods cannot be compared. Therefore, adjustments have to be made to the simulator in order to create a feasible two-dimensional control experiment. We will first discuss the three-dimensional model, and then outline the adjustments necessary to implement a two-dimensional motion simulator.

3.2 Additional Computations

Several issues have to be resolved before we can begin to develop the computational model. The first issue involves what values to assign the constants V_w and a. A closed form equation for V_w was obtained by integrating in prolate spheroidal coordinates over the boundary $\lambda_i \leq \lambda \leq \lambda_o$, $0 \leq \eta \leq 120, 0 \leq \phi \leq 360$. The result is:

$$V_w = \frac{\pi \delta^3}{4}$$
$$\times \left(3(\cosh \lambda_o - \cosh \lambda_i) + 4(\cosh^3 \lambda_o - \cosh^3 \lambda_i)\right).$$
$$(4)$$

Assigning a value for a is slightly more complicated. For a point with prolate spheroidal coordinates (λ, η, ϕ) the ideal value for a can be determined to be:

$$a = \frac{\cosh \lambda}{\sinh \lambda}. \qquad (5)$$

This value transforms a prolate sphere with radius λ into a sphere. But a dilemma arises when deforming a point inside confocal prolate spheres. Points within this volume have λ values between λ_i and λ_o; therefore, the exact value of a changes within the LV. Our solution is to find the appropriate value of a for the inner and outer shells, and take an average, so that it is approximately correct for all shells within the volume. There may be more accurate methods to select a, but this technique has proven to be quite effective experimentally.

A third issue that needs to be addressed is the calculation of the reference map. When dealing with nonlinear transformations it is often difficult to find the reference map, and one must settle for an approximation using iterative methods or other techniques. In this case, however, an explicit expression can be derived; it is given by

$$\mathbf{p} = R_0 R_1 R_2 R_L \mathbf{r}, \qquad (6)$$

where

$$\begin{aligned}
R_0 &= F_0^{-1}, \\
R_1 &= F_1^{-1}, \\
R_2 &= F_2^{-1}, \\
R_L &= [F_a F_6 F_5 F_4 F_3]^{-1}.
\end{aligned}$$

Determining R_0 and R_L is straightforward, because these are inverses of constant-valued, non-singular, matrices, and can be calculated numerically. The matrices F_1 and F_2 represent nonlinear transformations, however, so their inverses are a little more difficult to calculate. To find the matrix R_2 it is necessary to notice that the operation of F_2 is a rotation around the z-axis. We define $\mathbf{r}_1$ and $\mathbf{r}_2$ as follows:

$$\begin{aligned} \mathbf{r}_1 &= F_1 F_0 \mathbf{p}, \\ \mathbf{r}_2 &= F_2 F_1 F_0 \mathbf{p}. \end{aligned}$$

Since these two vectors differ only by a rotation around the z-axis, it follows that $z_1/|\mathbf{r}_1| = z_2/|\mathbf{r}_2|$, where z_1 and z_2 are the z-components of $\mathbf{r}_1$ and $\mathbf{r}_2$ respectively. Therefore,

$$R_2 = \begin{bmatrix} \cos a k_2 z_2/|\mathbf{r}_2| & \sin a k_2 z_2/|\mathbf{r}_2| & 0 & 0 \\ -\sin a k_2 z_2/|\mathbf{r}_2| & \cos a k_2 z_2/|\mathbf{r}_2| & 0 & 0 \\ 0 & 0 & 1 & 0 \\ 0 & 0 & 0 & 1 \end{bmatrix}. \tag{7}$$

Now we define $\mathbf{r}_0$:

$$\mathbf{r}_0 = F_0 \mathbf{p}.$$

Since $\mathbf{r}_0$ and $\mathbf{r}_1$ differ only by a scalar multiple in three dimensions, only the magnitudes of the vectors change. We can express this change of magnitude as follows:

$$|\mathbf{r}_1| = |\mathbf{r}_0| \sqrt[3]{1 + \frac{3k_1 V_w}{4\pi |\mathbf{r}_0|^3}}.$$

which can be rearranged to get:

$$|\mathbf{r}_0| = |\mathbf{r}_1| \sqrt[3]{1 - \frac{3k_1 V_w}{4\pi |\mathbf{r}_1|^3}}.$$

Thus, we can express the matrix R_1 as follows:

$$R_1 = \begin{bmatrix} \hat{\epsilon} & 0 & 0 & 0 \\ 0 & \hat{\epsilon} & 0 & 0 \\ 0 & 0 & \hat{\epsilon} & 0 \\ 0 & 0 & 0 & 1 \end{bmatrix}, \tag{8}$$

where

$$\hat{\epsilon} = \sqrt[3]{1 - \frac{3k_1 V_w}{4\pi |\mathbf{r}_1|^3}}.$$

3.3 3-D Simulation

We begin with the three-dimensional simulator because it is simpler than the two-dimensional model. A regular grid of points is first selected on the imaging plane which, ideally, encompasses the intersection of LV with the imaging plane. Next, we define a set of time instants $t_0 < t_1 < \ldots < t_n$. Time t_0 is referred to as the *tag*

reference time, and is the time when the tag pattern is initially applied (usually end-diastole). Next, given a spatial point $\mathbf{r}_i$ at time t_i, we must define the following function:

$$\mu = \Upsilon(\mathbf{r}_i, t_i) \tag{9}$$

where μ is the intensity value corresponding to point $\mathbf{r}_i$ at time t_i.

The value of μ depends on whether $\mathbf{r}_i$ is inside or outside the LV. The procedure for determining this is referred to as *segmentation*. The spatial point $\mathbf{r}_i$ is inside the LV if its corresponding material point $\mathbf{p}_i = p(\mathbf{r}_i, t_i)$ is inside the model LV. That is, if $\mathbf{p}_i = (\lambda, \eta, \phi)$ where $\lambda_i \leq \lambda \leq \lambda_o$ and $0 \leq \eta \leq 120$, then $\mathbf{r}_i$ is inside the LV. If $\mathbf{r}_i$ is outside the LV, then $\mu = 0$.

In order to determine μ when $\mathbf{r}_i$ is inside the LV, we must know where it came from at time t_0. This relationship is given by

$$\mathbf{r}_0 = r(p(\mathbf{r}_i, t_i), t_0) \tag{10}$$

The value of μ is given by the following tagged spin-echo MR imaging equation [6]

$$\mu = D_0 e^{-T_E/T_2}$$
$$\times \left\{ 1 + \left[\left(1 - e^{-(T_R - T_d)/T_1} \right) \xi(\mathbf{r}_0) - 1 \right] e^{-T_d/T_1} \right\}, \tag{11}$$

although other equations are readily incorporated. Here, $T_d = t_i - t_0$, and the constants D_0, T_1, and T_2 (the spin density, longitudinal relaxation time, and transverse relaxation time) are determined by the material properties of the LV being modeled and must be specified. The imaging parameters T_E and T_R (the echo time and the pulse repetition time) must also be specified. The function $\xi(\mathbf{r}_0)$ is the applied spatial tag pattern. In our simulation we used a two-dimensional SPAMM (spatial modulation of magnetization) tag pattern, characterized by the following equation [6]

$$\xi(\mathbf{r}) = \left(\cos^2 \theta - \sin^2 \theta \cos k_x r_x \right)$$
$$\times \left(\cos^2 \theta - \sin^2 \theta \cos k_y r_y \right). \tag{12}$$

Here, k_x and k_y are radial spatial frequencies in the x and y directions respectively, and θ is the tag pattern tip angle. Other tag patterns can be easily substituted into the simulation.

Having developed the mathematics to synthesize the images, our next step is to generate a truth displacement field; that is, a a vector field indicating the motion from one frame to the next. Given a point $\mathbf{r}_i$ at time t_i, we want to find the point $\mathbf{r}_{i+1}$ to which point $\mathbf{r}_i$ moves at time t_{i+1}. The expression for this is

$$\mathbf{r}_{i+1} = r(p(\mathbf{r}_i, t_i), t_{i+1}). \tag{13}$$

The displacement field is defined as $d_i(\mathbf{r}_i, t_i) = \mathbf{r}_{i+1} - \mathbf{r}_i$.

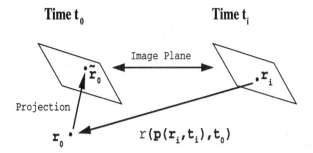

Figure 3. Pattern application in synthetic MR image.

3.4 2-D Model

Using the procedure just outlined, one can generate a full image sequence comprising both short-axis images and long-axis images, and test any three-dimensional motion estimation algorithm. But many algorithms only work in a two-dimensional setting using one imaging plane. These require a control experiment in which the simulated motion is two-dimensional. In other words, we want to generate a two-dimensional object and deform it so that each point on the object remains in the plane.

Again, we must define the value for μ in Equation 9 for all r_i at all times t_i. If r_i is outside the LV then $\mu = 0$ still holds. But the procedure for finding μ when r_i is in the LV must be modified. In the three-dimensional case we found the point r_0, and used it to find the proper intensity using a tag pattern and MR imaging equation. But in general, r_0 will not be located on the imaging plane. Therefore, we replace it with the point $\tilde{r}_0$, the projection of r_0 onto the imaging plane; Figure 3 illustrates this procedure. Instead of using r_0 in Equation (11), we use $\tilde{r}_0$, thereby forcing the motion to be two-dimensional.

The segmentation method must also be modified. In the three-dimensional case, we said that r_i is in the LV if its corresponding material point p_i is in the model LV. Here, we define r_i to be in the LV if $\tilde{r}_0$ is in the LV, which is equivalent to asking whether $\tilde{p}_0 = p(\tilde{r}_0, t_0)$ is in the model LV.

The biggest mathematical challenge in this 2-D simulation is in defining the displacement. Given a spatial point r_i at one time t_i, where does it move to at time t_{i+1}? Chances are that the actual material point corresponding to our spatial point moves off the plane. But we are no longer interested in the actual material point. Any point which, when shifted back to t_0 and projected to the imaging plane, lands on $\tilde{r}_0$ will carry the exact same intensity as that of r_{i+1}. There are an infinite number of points which project onto $\tilde{r}_0$, and they all lie on a line which is perpendicular to the

imaging plane and passing through point r_0. If we assume that our motion is not pathological, then exactly one of these points will intersect the imaging plane at each time instant. We find this point computationally by doing a line search using the Golden Section Search [5], using r_0 as an initial guess. Our minimization criterion is the magnitude of the distance vector from the estimated $\tilde{r}_{i+1}$ to the image plane. The resulting 2-D displacement field is given by $d_i(r_i, t_i) = \tilde{r}_{i+1} - r_i$.

4 Simulation Results

The k-parameters underlying our simulation were derived from a bead experiment on a dog heart [1]. They are shown for 60 different times within a single cardiac cycle in Figure 4. This figure shows the k-parameters as a function of the frame number 1 through 60. In a 1 second cardiac cycle, the time frames are equally spaced in steps of 0.017 seconds. All k-parameters are unitless except for the rotational parameters k_8 through k_{10}, which are in units of radians, and the translational parameters k_{11} through k_{13}, which are in units of centimeters. The six columns labeled (a)–(f) indicate key times at which we will show results below. Column (a) is approximately at end-diastole and is also the tag reference frame, while column (e) approximately represents end-systole. Table 2 lists the other key constants used in our simulation and their values.

Figure 5 shows the three-dimensional model at six phases of cardiac deformation. The image plane is also shown. The images generated along this imaging plane are shown in Figure 6. These images are generated for two-dimensional simulation. The tag patterns are seen to clearly deform as time progresses, and the effect of tag fading is also apparent (images get brighter overall).

Finally, the 2-D displacement fields for these times are shown in Figure 7. Each arrow represents the direction of displacement, and the size of the arrow corresponds to the magnitude of the displacements. The arrow lengths have been rescaled for visual enhancement, and do not actually point to the spatial location to which the points move. A larger arrow does however mean that a greater displacement has taken place. As can be seen, the simulator is capable of generating a relatively continuous and intricate displacement field.

5 Discussion

We have presented a LV motion simulator capable of generating tagged MR image studies used in motion estimation. This simulator effectively works in two modes, a three-dimensional and a two-dimensional mode. The mode of operation depends on the type of motion estimation algorithm being tested.

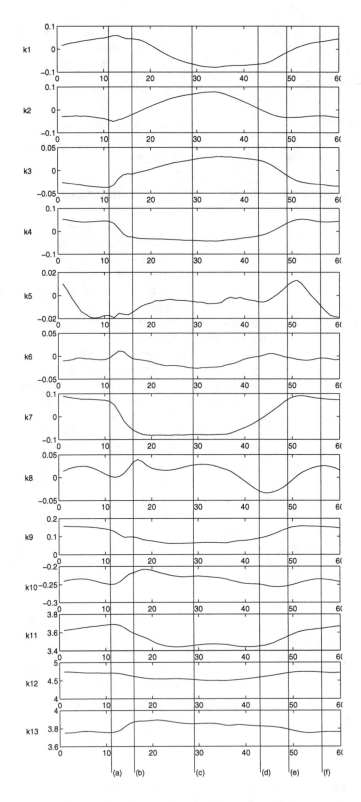

Figure 4. Estimated k-parameters. Vertical lines indicate the time instants used in future plots. Column (a) represents end-diastole and is also the tag reference frame, and column (e) is end-systole.

188

Table 2. Constant values

Constant	Description	value	units
λ_i	inner radius	0.35	none
λ_0	outer radius	0.55	none
δ	focal radius	4.00	cm
D_0	spin density	300.0	AU *
T_E	echo time	0.03	sec
T_R	pulse repetition time	10.0	sec
T_1	longitudinal relaxation time	0.60	sec
T_2	transverse relaxation time	0.10	sec
k_x	frequency in radial x	8.00	rad/cm
k_y	frequency in radial y	8.00	rad/cm
θ	tip angle of tag pattern	45.0	degrees

* Arbitrary units.

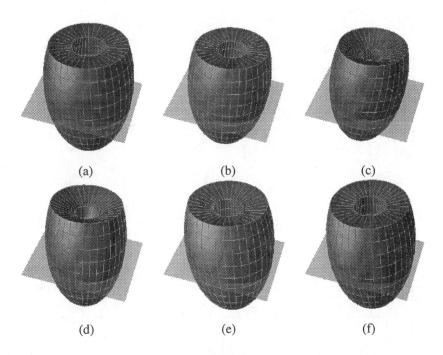

(a)　　　　　　(b)　　　　　　(c)

(d)　　　　　　(e)　　　　　　(f)

Figure 5. Three dimensional model and imaging plane shown at the time instants depicted in Figure 4

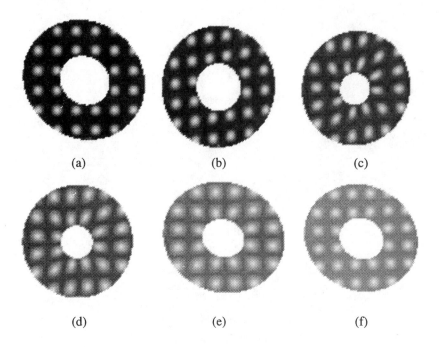

(a)   (b)   (c)

(d)   (e)   (f)

Figure 6. Synthesized MR images for the time instants depicted in Figure 4. The background is shown as white for clarity.

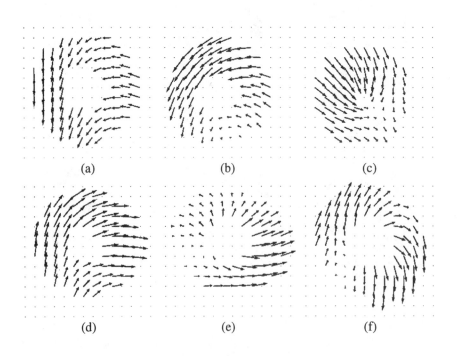

(a)   (b)   (c)

(d)   (e)   (f)

Figure 7. Displacement fields for the different time instants depicted in Figure 4.

Although the simulator functions well in its current stage, several issues remain to be addressed. The issue of parameter estimation has still not been completely resolved. As stated earlier, the simulation parameters were obtained from bead data of a dog heart. It would be very useful to be able to estimate these parameters from cardiac MR images. This approach is non-invasive and would allow us to work with human heart data. One of our next steps will be to try to develop a parameter estimation method using this kind of data.

There are also several additions to the simulator which would improve the overall realism of the output. These include adding a background, noise model, as well as a point spread function. Furthermore, there are countless imaginative improvements which would help generate more representative experiments. With a little ingenuity, we are confident that this simulator can be modified to generate data which can be used to test a wide variety of cardiac motion estimation algorithms.

References

[1] T. Arts, W. Hunter, A. Douglas, A. Muijtjens, and R. Reneman. Description of the deformation of the left ventricle by a kinematic model. *J. Biomechanics*, 25(10):1119–1127, 1992.

[2] T. S. Denney and J. L. Prince. Reconstruction of 3-d left ventricular motion from planar tagged cardiac MR images: An estimation theoretic approach. *IEEE Trans. Med. Imag.*, 14(4):625–635, December 1996.

[3] F. G. Meyer, R. T. Constable, A. G. Sinusas, and J. Duncan. Tracking myocardial deformation using spatially constrained velocities. In Y. Bizais, C. Barillot, and R. D. Paola, editors, *Information Processing in Medical Imaging*. Kluwer, 1995.

[4] W. G. O'Dell, C. C. Moore, W. Hunter, E. A. Zerhouni, and E. R. McVeigh. Displacement field fitting for calculating 3-d myocardial deformations from tagged MR images. *Radiology*, 1995. submitted.

[5] W. Press, B. Flannery, S. Teukolsky, and W. Vetterling. *Numerical Recipes in C*. Cambridge University Press, 1988.

[6] J. Prince and E. McVeigh. Motion estimation from tagged MR image sequences. *IEEE Transactions on Medical Imaging*, 11(2):238–249, June 1992.

[7] A. A. Young, D. L. Kraitchman, L. Dougherty, and L. Axel. Tracking and finite element analysis of stripe deformation in magnetic resonance tagging. *IEEE Trans. Med. Imag.*, 14(3):413–421, 1995.

[8] E. A. Zerhouni, D. M. Parish, W. J. Rogers, A. Yangand, and E. P. Shapiro. Human heart: tagging with MR imaging — a method for noninvasive assessment of myocardial motion. *Radiology*, 169:59–63, 1988.

Deformable B-Solids and Implicit Snakes for Localization and Tracking of SPAMM MRI-Data

Petia Radeva, Amir Amini*,†, Jiantao Huang† and Enric Martí
CVC, Departament d'Informatica,
Universitat Autonoma de Barcelona, 08193 Bellaterra (Barcelona), SPAIN
petia,enric@upisun1.uab.es

Departments of †Electrical Engineering and *Diagnostic Radiology,
Yale University, New Haven, CT 06520, USA
e-mail: amini,wangjz@minerva.cis.yale.edu

Abstract

To date, MRI-SPAMM data from different image slices have been analyzed independently. In this paper, we propose an approach for 3D tag localization and tracking of SPAMM data by a novel deformable B-solid. The solid is defined in terms of a 3D tensor product B-spline. The iso-parametric curves of the B-spline solid have special importance. These are termed implicit snakes as they deform under image forces from tag lines in different image slices. The localization and tracking of tag lines is performed under constraints of continuity and smoothness of the B-solid. The framework unifies the problems of localization, and displacement fitting and interpolation into the same procedure utilizing B-spline bases for interpolation. To track motion from boundaries and restrict image forces to the myocardium, a volumetric model is employed as a pair of coupled endocardial and epicardial B-spline surfaces. To recover deformations in the LV an energy-minimization problem is posed where both tag and LV boundary data are used. The framework has been implemented on tag data from Short Axis (SA) cardiac images, as well as SA left ventricle (LV) boundaries, and is currently being extended to include Long Axis (LA) data.

1. Introduction

Tagged MRI is an excellent technique for measuring non-rigid tissue motion. SPAMM[3] produces a grid pattern of signal voids on the tissue - two perpendicular sets of tag planes, each perpendicular to the imaging planes (see Fig. 5). The resulting pattern defines a time-varying curvilinear coordinate system on the tissue.

Accurate detection of tags is crucial to measurement of deformations and understanding of myocardial function. In [2, 6, 9] detection of tag stripes is performed by graph search and tag profile fitting. In order to determine the tag locations, tag profiles are simulated as a function of time using physics of MRI. The profile fitting approach has been improved by utilizing a template matching procedure in [1, 2]. In [1, 10, 18], authors have adopted a 2D snake technique for different image slices to recover within slice tag motion. Their approach aims to minimize an external energy which is the sum of intensities for each slice, together with an internal energy which provides smoothness. As pointed out in [10], detection of tag data with varying contrast needs spatially varying parameters for snakes, making automated localization non-trivial.

Our goal in this work is to develop a model for detection of local deformations of the LV based on tag and contour data. We extend to 3D the previous approach of detecting locally deforming tag stripes using 2D deformable grids [1, 2, 18]. We employ a planar surface description for the tag planes in the form of deformable iso-parametric surfaces of a B-solid, and provide the necessary smoothness constraints required in robust localization of tag information. Such an extension is justified by the fact that different slices represent parts of the same continuous body. In particular, tag lines appearing in different slices belong to continuous tag planes and thus should satisfy across and within slice smoothness constraints. For this purpose tag lines in different slices are detected by a set of implicit snakes that are part of the B-solid model. As an additional point, inhomogeneities in T_1 of myocardial tissue leads to different tag points being visible up to different times. Propagation of information across slices helps with such data analysis issues.

The B-solid is implemented as a 3D tensor product B-

192

Proceedings of MMBIA '96

spline model. This is a compact model, yet it is flexible enough to follow the movement of the LV with high accuracy. Its compactness results from the B-solid being completely defined by a set of control points much smaller in number than the number of voxels in the volume. In the deformable B-solid, two sets of iso-parametric surfaces are aligned with parallel lines of tag grids from the sequence of SA images. A set of twice iso-parametric curves links the tag intersections from different slices. We refer to the curves which are formed from intersection of iso-parametric surfaces with image slices as implicit snakes. Implicit snakes are attracted to tag data and deform the B-solid.

Detection and estimation of three-dimensional local tag deformation were previously considered as two separate procedures [12, 13, 18]. Usually, the second step corresponds to constructing a volumetric heart model using information from tags and contours. All of these perform a global fit with the heart contours and deform in accordance with the tag data displacements. In the B-solid approach, as a byproduct of representing the tags by implicit snakes, localization and displacement fitting and interpolation of tag information are performed in a single procedure (interpolation is performed with B-spline bases). Appropriate external forces of the B-solid attract these curves to tag data, adjusting the B-solid, and hence tracking the local deformation of the tissue. In this paper, we consider only SA image slices, and as such consider external forces from the image planes which alter the position of the implicit snakes within image slices. Though external forces thus far come from image slices, internal forces are applied in 3D to the B-solid.

A common feature of most heart motion reconstruction schemes is that they only use tag intersections [13, 18] or intersections between tags and myocardial contours to detect the local deformation of the heart tissue. Analysis with such sparse tag data neglect valuable information contained at other locations along tag lines [2]. The B-solid also uses all the information contained in tag displacements. Furthermore, the B-solid has no parameters to adjust except the parameters of elasticity of the implicit snakes.

Improvements are also proposed here, for snake analysis of tag data. In particular, the usual internal forces are modified to preserve characteristics of an ideal B-solid. As a consequence, the shrinking problem of the snakes is bypassed. To provide a contrast-independent detector for dark tag bands, we construct directional potential fields from principal curvature features of tagged images. The directional sensitivity of the potentials has the advantage that implicit snakes are attracted only by tag lines with similar orientations.

In addition to the deformable B-solid, we consider a B-spline representation for the LV boundaries [8] attached to the B-solid. The deformable B-spline LV model possesses local control, allowing the representation to better adjust to

the data and interpolate the contours providing an accurate representation for the heart. In contrast, most of the available models [13, 18] are designed to perform a global fit to the heart contours, and hence can at best roughly approximate the contours.

The rest of the paper is organized as follows: section 2 introduces the deformable B-solid, section 3 discusses energies associated with the B-solid, sections 4 and 5 define the localization by the B-solid and heart model, and section 6 considers the tracking problem for the B-solid. In section 7 an extension of the B-solid approach to SA and LA images analysis is outlined and finally, conclusions are given.

2. Deformable B-Solid

In this section, we discuss implicit snakes and the B-solid. As will be described, implicit snakes track the deformations resulting from the tag data. A heart model will be described which is designed to track the endocardial and epicardial boundaries, and is attached to the B-solid. The use of two models is necessary to achieve high precision in representing both tag and contour structures.

2.1. Definition of Deformable B-Solid

We define the B-solid as a 3D tensor product B-spline with iso-parametric surfaces corresponding to the tagging and imaging planes (see Fig. 1). The B-solid has all the attractive properties of B-splines: (1) B-splines provide local control of shape, allowing for exactly fitting the deformed tag planes. In addition, individual movement of control points only affect the solid's shape locally. (2) Cubic B-splines possess second order continuity everywhere. Moreover, due to parametric continuity, representing tag lines with B-splines allows for sub-pixel localization of tag features. (3) The degree of blending polynomials is independent of the number of control points, and furthermore the solid is completely specified by few control points.

We define the B-solid as a 3D tensor product B-spline,

$$Q(u, v, w) = \sum_{i=0}^{I} \sum_{j=0}^{J} \sum_{k=0}^{K} S_{kji} B_i(u) B_j(v) B_k(w),$$

where $B_i(u)$, $B_j(v)$ and $B_k(w)$ are the B-spline blending functions and $S_{kji}, k = 0, ...K, j = 0, ...J, i = 0, ...I$, are the control points of the B-solid. Cubic B-splines have an optimal approximation property, namely, that among all interpolants they minimize the norm of the second derivative. As we will consider thin-plate energy of the B-solid in our energy-based formulation, it is also reasonable to construct the deformable model with a cubic degree.

In a SA acquisition, the u and v iso-parametric surfaces are aligned with tag planes, and the $u - v$ iso-parametric

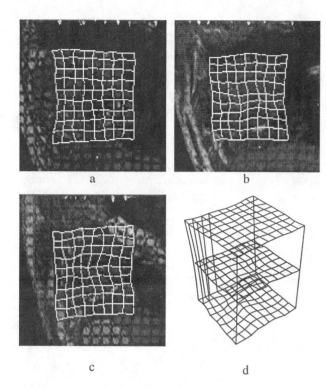

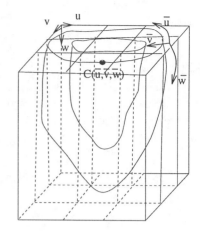

Figure 1. Tag grids detected by implicit snakes of the B-solid on different image slices (a,b,c) determine a B-solid (d)

Figure 2. Coordinate systems of B-solid $(u - v - w)$ and heart model $(\overline{u} - \overline{v} - \overline{w})$ (see text)

curves link tag intersections from different slices (see Fig. 1 and Fig. 2). Thus, u and v iso-parametric planes deform with tag planes and w - with SA imaging planes.

2.2. Heart Model

Given the epicardial and endocardial surfaces of the heart, we can represent this information as a pair of coupled boundary surfaces of the endocardium and epicardium using tensor product B-splines:

$$H(x,y,z) = \sum_{o=0}^{O} \sum_{p=0}^{P} \sum_{q=0}^{Q} H_{qpo} B_o(\overline{u}) B_p(\overline{v}) B_q(\overline{w})$$

where H_{qpo} are the control points and $(\overline{u}, \overline{v}, \overline{w})$ are the coordinates of the LV model. The $\overline{u}$ iso-parametric curves coincide with the inner and outer contours from each slice and, due to the closed curves, the corresponding blending functions are periodic. The $\overline{v}$-iso-parametric curves link the epicardial and endocardial contour from each slice, and the $\overline{w}$-iso-parametric curves go through the contours from the different slices (see Fig. 2). Their corresponding classes of blending functions are non-periodic. To consider the complete shape from apex to base, we place multiple knots at apex, hence creating the oval shape of the LV.

Non-linear blending functions of the parameters $\overline{u}$ and $\overline{w}$ give a realistic shape to the heart. As for the parameter $\overline{v}$, we have used linear spline functions because our heart model is a coupled boundaries model containing information only from the epicardial and endocardial surfaces. In Fig. 3 heart contours and LV's surfaces are shown. A volumetric heart model and its LA intersection can be seen in Fig. 4.

2.3. Relation between Tag and Heart Models

In this section we show how the coordinates of points of the heart model can be expressed as functions of the parameters of the B-solid model. This will be a required step in integrating the tags and contours in the same framework. Let the point $C(\overline{u}, \overline{v}, \overline{w}) = (x, y, z)$ be a control point in the heart model (see Fig. 2). We need to find the parameters (u, v, w) from the B-solid so that $C = \sum_{i=0}^{I} \sum_{j=0}^{J} \sum_{k=0}^{K} S_{kji} B_i(u) B_j(v) B_k(w)$, where S_{kji} are the control vertices of the tag model.

To solve, we consider a two step procedure [14]: The first step consists of finding a linear approximation (u_0, v_0, w_0) of the parameters by solving the system,

$$C = \sum_{i=0}^{I} \sum_{j=0}^{J} \sum_{k=0}^{K} S_{kji} B_i^1(u) B_j^1(v) B_k^1(w) \quad (1)$$

where B^1 are linear spline blending functions of the parameters and S_{kji} are the control vertices of the B-solid. The parameters (u_0, v_0, w_0) determine a point $C_0 = (x_0, y_0, z_0)$ in the cubic tag model,[1] so that: $(x_0, y_0, z_0) = \sum_{i=0}^{I} \sum_{j=0}^{J} \sum_{k=0}^{K} S_{kji} B_i(u_0) B_j(v_0) B_k(w_0)$.

---

[1] Here the blending functions are cubic according to the tag model

194

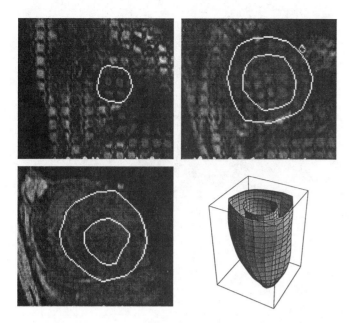

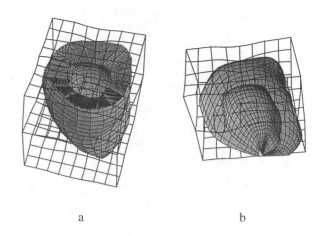

a b

Figure 4. Heart volumetric model located in a B-solid (a) and its LA (b) intersection

Figure 3. Heart contours and constructed endocardial and epicardial boundaries

Using a Taylor series expansion on (1) but with cubic blending functions and after simplifications, we obtain the following iterative procedure for the parameters (u, v, w),

$$
\begin{aligned}
x - x_l = (u_{l+1} - u_l) \sum_{i=0}^{I}\sum_{j=0}^{J}\sum_{k=0}^{K} X_{kji} B_i'(u_l) B_j(v_l) B_k(w_l) + \\
(v_{l+1} - v_l) \sum_{i=0}^{I}\sum_{j=0}^{J}\sum_{k=0}^{K} X_{kji} B_i(u_l) B_j'(v_l) B_k(w_l) + \\
(w_{l+1} - w_l) \sum_{i=0}^{I}\sum_{j=0}^{J}\sum_{k=0}^{K} X_{kji} B_i(u_l) B_j(v_l) B_k'(w_l) \\
y - y_l = (u_{l+1} - u_l) \sum_{i=0}^{I}\sum_{j=0}^{J}\sum_{k=0}^{K} Y_{kji} B_i'(u_l) B_j(v_l) B_k(w_l) + \\
(v_{l+1} - v_l) \sum_{i=0}^{I}\sum_{j=0}^{J}\sum_{k=0}^{K} Y_{kji} B_i(u_l) B_j'(v_l) B_k(w_l) + \\
(w_{l+1} - w_l) \sum_{i=0}^{I}\sum_{j=0}^{J}\sum_{k=0}^{K} Y_{kji} B_i(u_l) B_j(v_l) B_k'(w_l) \\
z - z_l = (u_{l+1} - u_l) \sum_{i=0}^{I}\sum_{j=0}^{J}\sum_{k=0}^{K} Z_{kji} B_i'(u_l) B_j(v_l) B_k(w_l) + \\
(v_{l+1} - v_l) \sum_{i=0}^{I}\sum_{j=0}^{J}\sum_{k=0}^{K} Z_{kji} B_i(u_l) B_j'(v_l) B_k(w_l) + \\
(w_{l+1} - w_l) \sum_{i=0}^{I}\sum_{j=0}^{J}\sum_{k=0}^{K} Z_{kji} B_i(u_l) B_j(v_l) B_k'(w_l)
\end{aligned}
$$

where $l = 0, 1, \ldots$. It can be shown using the Weierstrass theorem that $\{(x_l, y_l, z_l)\}$ converges to the point (x, y, z). The procedure described here is applied to all control points of the LV model individually.

2.4. Tensor Product Representation of B-Solids

Considering the large amount of data in a 3D volume, the compact representation of a model and its computational complexity become of great importance. Gueziec in [5], working on the problem of surface reconstruction from 3D edge data, introduced surface representation with deformable splines by means of a 2D tensor product. There, a surface $Q(x, y, z) = \sum_{i=0}^{I}\sum_{j=0}^{J} S_{ji} B_i(u) B_j(v)$, in terms of a tensor product B-spline with $I \times J$ control points, is presented in a compact way: for all points of the surface, a matrix notation is employed: $Q = B_v^T S B_u$, where S is the control points matrix of dimensions $J \times I$, whose elements are the control vertices $S_{ji} \in R^3$. B_u (B_v) has dimensions $I \times I$ ($J \times J$) gathering all spline evaluations in the blending functions $B_i(u), i = 0, ..., I$ ($B_j(v), j = 0, ..., J$),

$$
B_u = \begin{bmatrix}
B_0(u_0) & 0 & 0 & \ldots \\
B_1(u_0) & B_1(u_1) & 0 & \ldots \\
B_2(u_0) & B_2(u_1) & B_2(u_2) & \ldots \\
B_3(u_0) & B_3(u_1) & B_3(u_2) & \ldots \\
0 & B_4(u_1) & B_4(u_2) & \ldots \\
\cdot & \cdot & \cdot & \cdot
\end{bmatrix} \quad (2)
$$

Generalizing this notation to the solid, the control points form a 3D tensor. Using square brackets to distinguish the tensor from the matrix notation, we can write: $[Q] = [S]_{kji} \otimes_i B_u \otimes_j B_v \otimes_k B_w$, where $[Q]$ is a 3D tensor of 3-vectors representing all the sampled points of the B-solid. B_u, B_v and B_w are matrices of the form in (2), corresponding to the 3 classes of blending functions with respect to the parameters u, v and w. $[S]_{kji} =$

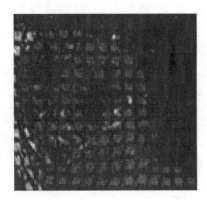

Figure 5. Original SPAMM image

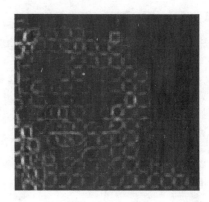

Figure 6. Map of principal curvatures

$\{S_{kji}\}_{i=0,\ldots I, j=0,\ldots J, k=0,\ldots K}$ is a 3D tensor, whose elements are the 3-vectors of control points. In particular, the elements of $[S]_{kji}$ are ordered in such a way that fixing k and j, we obtain the control points of all u iso-parametric curves, by fixing k and i we obtain the control points of the v iso-parametric curves, etc. Each matrix of the tensor $[S_{kji}]$ formed by fixing the index k contains the control points S_{kji}, belonging to the $k-$ plane (i.e. to the w iso-parametric surface of the B-spline model), and fixing the parameters j and i we obtain the $v-$ and $u-$iso-parametric planes of the B-solid, respectively.

The operation $\otimes_l$, where l denotes an index of a tensor (e.g. $l \in \{i, j, k\}$), is defined as follows,

$$[S]_{kji} \otimes_i B_{im} = [\sum_{i=0}^{I} S_{kji} B_{im}]_{kjm}, [S]_{kji} \otimes_j B_{jm} =$$

$$[\sum_{j=0}^{J} S_{kji} B_{jm}]_{kmi}, [S]_{kji} \otimes_k B_{km} = [\sum_{k=0}^{K} S_{kji} B_{km}]_{mji}.$$

The operation $\otimes_l$ is considered in more details in [14].

Because of the similarity of the multiplication $\otimes_l$ to multiplication of matrices and for sake of simplicity we shall omit the operator $\otimes_l$ accepting the following notations,

$$[S]_{kji} B_u := [S]_{kji} \otimes_i B_{im}(u)$$
$$[S]_{kji} B_v := [S]_{kji} \otimes_j B_{jm}(v)$$
$$[S]_{kji} B_w := [S]_{kji} \otimes_k B_{km}(w)$$

3. Energy of the Deformable B-Solid

The B-solid is a deformable body with an associated energy composed of internal and external energies,

$$E_{solid} = E_{int} + E_{ext} \qquad (3)$$

External forces attract the B-solid towards the tag data by minimizing its external energy E_{ext}, whereas internal forces try to preserve an ideal shape of the solid by minimizing the internal energy, E_{int}.

3.1. Tag External Energy of the Deformable B-Solid

In this paper, we propose to detect tag lines by applying a valley detector based on Haralick's facet model [7] as a more robust and invariant technique to variations in image contrast than by searching for dark regions in the image, as previously proposed. With the facet model, a pixel neighborhood is approximated by a continuous surface. All subsequent analysis is performed on the analytical representation of the facet. By observing that locations of interest in the image are dark ridges, we create a potential field whose valleys correspond to pixels with maximal principal curvature of the intensity surface, $C_{max} = \frac{1}{2}(T_{xx} + T_{yy}) + \sqrt{(T_{xx} - T_{yy})^2 + 4T_{xy}^2}$, where T denotes the surface facet (see Fig. 5 and Fig. 6).

In SPAMM-images, two sets of tag lines with approximate perpendicular orientations are present. When an implicit snake is not exactly aligned with its corresponding tag line, an attraction force from tags of perpendicular orientation acts on it which may lead the snake to settle in a wrong valley. To surmount this problem, we create two directional potential fields by filtering by a directional Gaussian the map of principal curvatures. The effect is that for the horizontal potential field, the influence of vertical features in horizontal potential field is diminished. An analogous situation holds for the vertical potential field. Thereafter, LV contours (which will be discussed later) are used to provide constant potential outside of LV myocardium. As a result implicit snakes are attracted by external forces only within the myocardium. The potential energy for each point q of an implicit snake from the deformable model Q is given by its height in the potential surface P^{tag}, $E_{ext}^{tag}(q) = P^{tag}(q)$, $q \in Q$. In each step of the iterative procedure, the implicit snake is pushed by the external forces towards tag lines of same orientation.

196

3.2. Contour External Energy of the Heart Model

Without attempting to have any *a priori* boundary point correspondences, we consider two classes of external forces: first external force is associated with tag data, as was discussed in the last section, and the second is associated with LV boundaries.

We construct contour potentials for each image slice from successive frames using a distance map. A continuous surface with valleys corresponding to the contours is obtained by an optimization procedure described in [8]. Locating a model Q on the contour potential field, P^{cont} the potential energy of a point q is given by its height in the contour potential field $E_{ext}^{cont}(q) = P^{cont}(q),\ q \in Q$.

3.3. Internal Energy of the Deformable B-Solid

The internal energy of the classical B-snakes [11] defined in terms of derivatives up to second order preserves its continuous and smooth shape. However, minimizing the derivatives result in undesired shrinking effects. To avoid this problem, some authors minimize the difference in the membrane and thin-plate energies for the snake from an ideal model [15, 17]. In our case, we are interested in small deformations of our three dimensional solid using as a reference an ideal rectangular three dimensional model, $Q(x,y,z) = \sum_{i=0}^{I} \sum_{j=0}^{J} \sum_{k=0}^{K} S_{kji}^{0} B_u B_v B_w$. We define the internal energy as follows,

$$
\begin{aligned}
E_{int} = \tfrac{1}{2}\Big\{ &\sum_{r,s,t=1}^{2} \sum_{\overline{u},\overline{v},\overline{w}\in U,\ \overline{u}\neq\overline{v}\neq\overline{w}} \alpha_{\frac{u}{u}}^{2-r}\alpha_{\frac{v}{v}}^{2-s}\alpha_{\frac{w}{w}}^{2-t}\beta_{\frac{u}{u}}^{r-1}\beta_{\frac{v}{v}}^{s-1}\beta_{\frac{w}{w}}^{t-1} \\
&\quad \|SB_{\overline{u}}^{(r)}B_{\overline{v}}^{(s)}B_{\overline{w}}^{(t)} - S^0 B_{\overline{u}}^{(r)}B_{\overline{v}}^{(s)}B_{\overline{w}}^{(t)}\|^2 + \\
\sum_{r,s=1}^{2} \sum_{\overline{u},\overline{v}\in U,\ \overline{u}\neq\overline{v}} &\alpha_{\frac{u}{u}}^{2-r}\alpha_{\frac{v}{v}}^{2-s}\beta_{\frac{u}{u}}^{r-1}\beta_{\frac{v}{v}}^{s-1} \|SB_{\overline{u}}^{(r)}B_{\overline{v}}^{(s)} - S^0 B_{\overline{u}}^{(r)}B_{\overline{v}}^{(s)}\|^2 \\
+ \sum_{r=1}^{2} \sum_{\overline{u}\in U} &\alpha_{\frac{u}{u}}^{2-r}\beta_{\frac{u}{u}}^{r-1}\|SB_{\overline{u}}^{(r)} - S^0 B_{\overline{u}}^{(r)}\|^2 \Big\}
\end{aligned}
$$

where superscripts in parantheses denote derivatives, U is the set of parameters $\{u,v,w\}$, $B_{\overline{u}}^{(r)}, B_{\overline{u}}^{(s)}, \ldots$ are matrices formed by the r,s,t-derivatives of the blending functions with respect to the parameter $\overline{u}$ as shown in (2) and α and β are parameters of elasticity that determine the relative weight between the internal and external energies. Note that the notation: $\sum_{r=1}^{2} \sum_{\overline{u}\in U} \ldots B_{\overline{u}}^{(r)}$ in fact expresses all first and second derivatives of blending functions with respect to each parameter (u,v,w). In our case, we have empirically obtained that $\alpha = 0.4$ and $\beta = 10$ provide good weights for different energies. Defined in this way the internal energy of the B-solid tries to minimize the distance between the deformable body and the model.

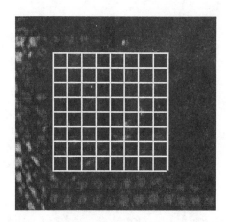

Figure 7. An intersection of the initial B-solid

4. Non-Rigid Registration of B-Solid to Tag Data

The problem of localization of tag data by a B-solid is an energy-minimizing problem. The B-solid is placed around data, and the implicit snakes are attracted by the image data. Since they determine the iso-parametric curves of the B-solid, deforming the implicit snakes deforms the solid. The local minimum of the energy that is found in image slices in the first volumetric temporal frame solves the localization problem. The resulting B-solid from each frame is then used as the initial solid in the subsequent frame in order to track the deformations.

4.1. Initialization of the B-Solid

We consider a B-solid initialization, where we do not put constraints on necessarily good approximation of the data by the implicit snakes. Instead, we consider appropriate internal forces that cope with the inexact initial positions of the deformable B-solid. The user only delimits the region of interest in one or each slices of images from the initial temporal frame and gives the initial distance between the u and v iso-parametric planes. The distance between the w-iso-parametric planes is determined by the slice separation in volumetric SA SPAMM images. The initial B-solid is defined as the minimum three-dimensional rectangular grid which contains the region(s) of interest (see Fig. 7). Since the internal force takes charge of local displacements [15], rotation and displacement of the implicit snakes between subsequent images is limited to half of the tag line inter-distances.

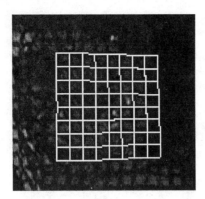

Figure 8. Tags localization by B-solid

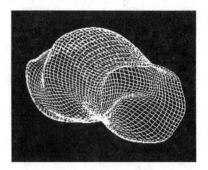

Figure 9. Endocardial B-spline approximation

4.2. Energy-Minimization Procedure

Let us consider equation (3). We are looking for a solid S that gives a minimum of the energy, E_{solid},

$$\frac{\partial E_{solid}}{\partial S} = \frac{\partial E_{int}}{\partial S} + \frac{\partial E_{ext}^{tag}}{\partial S} = 0 \qquad (4)$$

A solution can be viewed as one which achieves an equilibrium between the internal and external forces in the energy equation. The solid is under the control of internal forces that impose regularity on the B-solid, whereas external forces attract the B-solid towards the data. Finding a global minimum of the considered problem is too complicated to be treatable for the B-solid. Therefore, it is important to define the external and internal forces, reflecting the need for tag localization as well as boundary tracking so that the found local minimum is a good solution for the localization problem.

To provide dynamics for the deformable body, the associated evolution equation is considered,

$$-\frac{\partial S}{\partial t} = \frac{\partial E_{int}}{\partial S} + \frac{\partial E_{ext}^{tag}}{\partial S} \qquad (5)$$

A solution to the static problem (4) is achieved when the solution $S(t)$ of (5) stabilizes.

Substituting the derivatives of both energy in (5) and reducing the expression [14], we get,

$$S^{l+1} = (S^l + F_{init}(S^0) - F^{tag} B_u B_v B_w) \\ (K_u + I)^{-1}(K_v + I)^{-1}(K_w + I)^{-1} \qquad (6)$$

where $K_t := \alpha_t A_t' + \beta_t A_t''$, $A_t^{(r)} := B_t^{(r)} B_t^{(r)T}$, t is one of $\{u, v, w\}$, $F_{init}(S^0) = S^0(K_u + I)(K_v + I)(K_w + I) - S^0$, I denotes the identity matrix and $r = 1, 2$ denotes derivative. F_{init} can be thought of as a force that always tries to push the deformable body towards the model S^0. The combination of external force and F_{init} force allows for some displacement for the deformable body and thus less dependence on initial position. In Fig. 8 a result of the localization procedure can be seen.

The linear system (6) contains three independent linear equations for (X, Y, Z) coordinates of the control vertices. Similar to the case of 1D and 2D deformable models, the three stiffness matrices regarding the three parameters $(K_u + I)$, $(K_v + I)$ and $(K_w + I)$ are diagonal, symmetric, and positive definite. Given that the parameters of elasticity are constant over time, the factorization of the matrices is done only once. This in fact, is very important for handling the 3D model fitting to the 3D data, as well as for speeding up the computational process. It is worthwhile to emphasize that in (6) the smoothing operator is presented by decoupled operators with respect to the parameters. Thus, the smoothing effect of each of them can be estimated.

5. B-Spline Approximation to Endocardium and Epicardium

The problem of localization of the LV is considered here in order to construct a LV model using the endocardial and epicardial contours in image slices in the first temporal volumetric frame. For this purpose we need approximations to endocardium and epicardium of the LV by B-spline surfaces [8]. To fit the complexity of the heart shape we have used a cubic-quadric partially closed surface with 6 slices of control points and 16 control points in each slice. We assume the heart ventricle contour points are first determined by a low-level process from tagged images or are specified on the images by the user. A potential function is defined as a distance map of the contour points and the surface model is optimized by conjugate gradient descent. This potential tolerates large deviations of the initial model to the object because even when there are some false contour points. Smoothness was enforced by applying second order derivative penalties at all points along the surface. The heart boundaries approximation allows us to construct the heart model expressed by means of the control points of the B-spline surfaces (see Fig. 9 and Fig. 10).

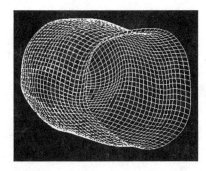

Figure 10. Epicardial B-spline approximation

6. Tracking of Heart Motion by B-Solid

The tracking procedure is analogous to the localization procedure with the only difference that tag and heart models contribute to the energy of the B-solid.

6.1. Integrated Tag Grid and Heart Boundaries Tracking

Both tag and heart models are interdependent since they are part of the same tissue. Hence, the energy minimization is done affecting only the B-solid model. The tracking problem is an energy minimizing process where the energy of the B-solid is defined by its internal, tag external and contour external energies,

$$E_{solid} = E_{int} + \omega_{tag}E_{ext}^{tag} + \omega_{cont}E_{ext}^{cont}$$

To assign equal importance to both external energies we have used equal weights $\omega_{tag} = \omega_{cont} = 1$. The contour external energy at point (x, y, z) of the solid is,

$$E_{ext}^{cont} = ||S/_H(x,y,z) - C(x,y,z)||^2 = \sum_{r=0}^{R}\sum_{s=0}^{S}\sum_{t=0}^{T}$$
$$|| \sum_{o=0}^{O}\sum_{p=0}^{P}\sum_{q=0}^{Q} H_{qpo}B_o(\overline{u}_r)B_p(\overline{v}_s)B_q(\overline{w}_t) - C(x,y,z)||^2$$

where H_{qpo} denotes the control vertices of number $O \times P \times Q$ of the heart boundaries and $(\overline{u}_r, \overline{v}_s, \overline{w}_t), r = 0, ..., R, s = 0, ..., S, t = 0, ..., T$ are the knots[2].

In order to find the control points S_{kji} of the B-solid associated with the control vertices H_{qpo} in the contour external energy, we apply the procedure that defines the relation between the tag and heart model given in section 2.3. Following the same energy-minimization procedure as in the tracking problem, we obtain the following iterative procedure for integrated tracking of tag and contour data,

$$S^{l+1} = (S^l + F_{init}(S^0) - F^{tag}B_uB_vB_w - F^{cont}) (K_u + I)^{-1}(K_v + I)^{-1}(K_w + I)^{-1} \quad (7)$$

---

[2] Since we only have endocardial and epicardial surfaces available, $P = S = 1$ and B_p is linear.

where $F_{kji}^{cont} = 2\sum_{o=0}^{O}\sum_{p=0}^{P}\sum_{q=0}^{Q}\sum_{r=0}^{R}\sum_{s=0}^{S}\sum_{t=0}^{T} B_o(\overline{u}_r) B_p(\overline{v}_s) B_q(\overline{w}_t)B_i(u_0)B_j(v_0)B_k(w_0)$.

In Fig. 11 and Fig. 12 an example of two frames considered in the tracking process is shown. At the base of the heart the grid is not deformed because the external force is applied only to the heart tissue. In Fig. 12 (c) and (d) a slice of the tracked heart located in the B-solid can be seen.

Note that no correspondence of points between nodes of the model and tag intersections is necessary. In addition, the interpolation of forces to nodes of the model is implicit.

6.2. Numerical Complexity

In the usual way of treating high-dimensional deformable models problem [17], the data are presented in a vector and the resulting linear systems (6) and (7) will be of size $((IJK) \times (IJK))$. In addition, the matrices are sparse but not diagonal [17, 18]. In the case of B-solid from (6) and (7), it can be seen that the numerical complexity of each iteration of the energy-mimizing procedure is $O(I \times J \times K)$ and the 3 stiffness matrices are diagonal. This fact is very important so as to make the procedure practical and in dealing with real 3D image analysis problems. The B-solid algorithm is implemented in C on a SUN Sparc station and takes about 6 minutes for each temporal frame to localize or track a B-solid with 600 control points.

7. Extension of the Approach to the Analysis of SA and LA Images

In case of SA images since the external forces of the implicit snakes belong to the imaging planes, the deformation of the B-solid caused by the tag and contour data is mainly in the plane $(x - y)$. The internal forces are three-dimensional yet this is not sufficient to provide out-of-plane movement of the material points of the heart. To solve this problem, authors have combined images of short and long axes views.

Here we describe how to obtain three-dimensional tissue movement by treating SA images with two-dimensional tags and LA images with one-dimensional tags; i.e., we assume that in the SA views there are two sets of perpendicular tag planes, whereas in the LA images there is only one set of horizontal tag planes. Let us consider SA view images where the imaging planes are parallel to the $(x-y)$ plane. From the fact that tagging planes are orthogonal to the imaging planes, it follows that the tagging planes are parallel to the planes $(x - z)$ and $(y - z)$ initially. Without loss of generality, we can consider that in the LA view the imaging planes are parallel to the plane $(x-z)$ and the tagging planes are parallel to the planes $(x-y)$ (see Fig. 13 and 14). Since a main source of information about the tissue movement is given by the deformation of the tag planes, we define the B-solid so that the

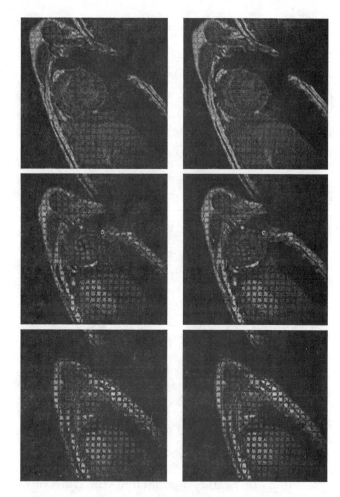

Figure 11. Tracking of deformation: different slices of images from two consecutive frames given in the first and second column

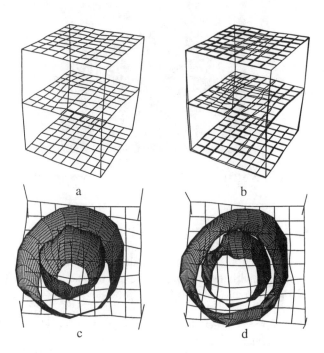

a   b

c   d

Figure 12. B-solids from first (a) and two consequetive frames (b) and slices of heart boundaries from both temporal frames (c) and (d).

iso-parametric planes correspond to the tagging planes. In particular, u and v iso-parametric planes are aligned with tag planes from the SA images and w iso-parametric planes are aligned with the tag planes from the LA images.

By definition the external forces of the B-solid are applied to the control vertices. The external forces of the B-solid are obtained by running patches on the iso-parametric curve and assigning the overall external force to the control vertices. In the case of B-solids constructed by SA view images, the u and v iso-parametric curves belong to the imaging planes. Since the potential field is constructed by considering the features (principal curvatures) of the imaging planes, the external forces are defined for each point of the imaging plane, in particular for the points of the iso-parametric curves.

In case of B-solid constructed by SA and LA view images, the iso-parametric curves do not belong to the imaging planes. The iso-parametric curves (e.g. the curve SP in

Fig. 13) intersect the imaging planes in tag lines (e.g. curves PU and PV). We estimate the external force on the control points considering the tag lines analogous to the case of implicit snakes in B-solid constructed from SA images [14]. Once we have determined the external forces on the implicit snakes, we apply the energy-minimization procedure to localize the tag and contour data and track the heart motion.

8. Conclusions

In conclusion, a novel three-dimensional B-solid deformable model is proposed for locating, and tracking the LV deformations in a time sequence of 3D volumetric SPAMM images with implicit snakes. B-spline bases provide local control of shape, compact representation, and parametric smoothness. The B-solid proposed in the paper deforms in space, adjusting to tag and contour data from different slices reflecting the natural continuity and smoothness of the three-dimensional tissue deformations. As a consequence of the approach, localization, displacement fitting and interpolation of tag and contour information are performed in a single procedure making use of B-spline bases. A LV volumetric model was also constructed to incorporate data from endocardial and epicardial boundaries and restricts the image

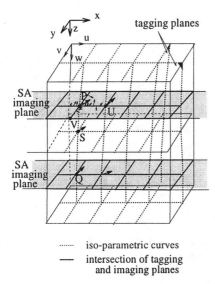

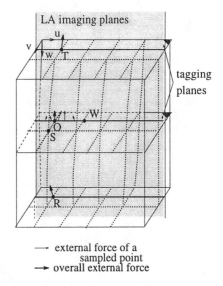

iso-parametric curves
— *intersection of tagging and imaging planes*

Figure 13. B-solid intersection with a SA image

— *external force of a sampled point*
→ *overall external force*

Figure 14. B-solid intersection with a LA image

forces to the heart tissue.

In applying the B-solid to tagged images, information from data in different slices are used, making the approach robust and precise against noise. Although the deformable B-solid presented here was created from tensor product of non-periodic B-splines in the cartesian coordinate frame, it is also possible to create B-solids adaptable to analysis of star-burst tagged MR images.

The B-solid defined here detects local heart's deformations. Our future work includes extraction of 3D motion of LV's material points with B-solids as discussed in section 7.

Acknowledgements

This work has been supported by a grant TIC91-0430 from MEC of Spain and grants from NSF and The Whitaker Biomedical Engineering Foundation.

References

[1] A. Amini. *Energy Minimizing Deformable Grids for Tracking Tagged MR Cardiac Images*. Proc. of CiC, 1992.

[2] A. Amini, R. Curwen, and J. Gore. *Snakes and Splines for Tracking Non-Rigid Heart Motion*. ECCV, UK, 1996.

[3] L. Axel and L. Dougherty. MR imaging of motion with spatial modulation of magnetization. *Radiology*, 171(3), 1989.

[4] R. Bartels, J. Beatty, and B. Barsky. *An Introduction to Splines for Use in Computer Graphics and Image Modelling*. Morgan Kauffmann, 1987.

[5] A. Gueziec. Surface representation with deformable splines: Using decoupled variables. *IEEE Comp. Sci. and Engineering*, 1995.

[6] M. A. Guttman, J. L. Prince, and E. R. McVeigh. Tag and contour detection in tagged MR images of the left ventricle. *Trans. on Med. Imaging*, 1994.

[7] R. M. Haralick and L. G. Shapiro. *The Facet Model*. Computer and Robot Vision, Addison-Wesley, 1992.

[8] J. Huang and A. Amini. *Deformable B-Spline Surfaces for Localization of Tubular Structures in 3D Medical Images*. Tech. Report, Yale University, New Haven, USA, 1996.

[9] D. L. Kraitchman, A. A. Young, C.-N. Chang, and L. Axel. Semi-automatic tracking of myocardial motion in mr tagged images. *IEEE Trans. Med. Imaging*, 14(3):422–433, 1995.

[10] S. Kumar and D. Goldgof. Automatic tracking of spamm grid and the estimation of deformation parameters from cardiac mr images. *IEEE Trans. Med. Imaging*, 13(1), 1994.

[11] S. Menet, P. Saint-Marc, and G. Medioni. *B-Snakes: Implementation and Application to Stereo*. Proc. DARPA Image Understanding Workshop, Pittsburgh, 1990.

[12] W. G. O'Dell, C. C. Moore, W. C. Hunter, E. A. Zerhouni, and E. R. McVeigh. Three-dimensional myocardial deformations: Calculation with displacement field fitting to tagged MR images. *Radiology*, 195, 1995.

[13] J. Park, D. Metaxas, and L. Axel. *Volumetric Deformable Models with Parameter Functions: A New Approach to the 3D Motion Analysis of the LV from MRI-SPAMM*. Proc. of ICCV, MIT, 1995.

[14] P. Radeva, A. Amini, J. Huang, and E. Martí. *Deformable B-Solid: Application to Tracking of MRI-SPAMM Data*. Tech. Report, UPIIA, UAB, 1996.

[15] P. Radeva, J. Serrat, and E. Martí. *A Snake for Model-Based Segmentation*. Proc. of ICCV, Cambridge, 1995.

[16] K. R. Symon. *Mecanica*. Aguilar, Madrid, 1970.

[17] D. Terzopoulos, J. Platt, A. Barr, and K. Fleisher. Elastically deformable models. *Computer Graphics*, 21(4), 1987.

[18] A. A. Young, D. L. Kraitchman, L. Dougherty, and L. Axel. Tracking and finite element analysis of stripe deformation in magnetic resonance tagging. *IEEE Trans. on Med. Imaging*, 14(3):413–421, 1995.

Fusion of Short-Axis and Long-Axis Cardiac MR Images

A. Ardeshir Goshtasby, Ph.D.
Computer Science and Engineering
303 Russ Engineering Ctr
Dayton, OH 45435
ardeshir@cs.wright.edu

David A. Turner, M.D.
Diagnostic Radiology and Nuclear Medicine
Rush-Presbyterian-St. Luke's Med Ctr
Chicago, IL 60612
dturner@rad.rpslmc.edu

Abstract

A method is introduced for fusing the short-axis and long-axis cardiac MR images into an isotropic volume image. A volume image obtained by this method contains the left ventricular (LV) cavity in one piece, facilitating measurement of its shape and volume. The main goal in this image fusion is to reconstruct the LV cavity in volume form and in high resolution. The accuracy of the method is measured using a synthetic image. Examples of image fusion using real images are also presented.

1. Introduction

The accurate measurement of cardiac function requires that the volume and shape of the left ventricular (LV) cavity be accurately determined at different phases of the cardiac cycle [2] [7] [13] [18] [20] [22]. In the past, long-axis [5] [22] and short-axis [2] [7] [18] [20] [21] images have been used separately to measure the LV volume. Short-axis images provide high-resolution information about the shape of the LV at several cross-sections normal to the LV major axis while providing poor resolution along the axis. On the other hand, long-axis images provide high-resolution information at a few cross-sections parallel to the LV major axis while providing poor resolution normal to the axis. The objective in this work is to combine the long-axis and the short-axis images obtained under the same MR coordinate system and produce an image that provides high resolution information both along and normal to the LV major axis.

Reconstructing the LV cavity at a higher resolution enables the LV volume and shape to be measured more accurately. In the past, the ellipsoid has been used as a model to represent the LV cavity and estimate LV regions that are missing from given image slices. By fusing the long-axis and short axis images, we would like to reconstruct the entire LV cavity in high-resolution and measure its shape and volume without using a model. The shape of the LV cavity deviates considerably from an ellipsoid at some phases of the cardiac cycle. We will determine the shape of the LV cavity at a cardiac phase by segmenting the volumetric image obtained from the fusion of the long-axis and short-axis images at that phase.

To reconstruct the entire LV cavity at a particular cardiac phase, we map the long-axis and short-axis images obtained in that phase back into the "MR viewing window" (an orthogonal volume encompassing the imaged volume). This mapping determines some entries of the 3-D image, which represents the MR window. Other entries of the 3-D image are estimated by approximation. Once an isotropic volume image of the heart is obtained, the entire LV cavity will be extracted by segmentation.

In the following, first the existing methods that measure the LV volume using either the long-axis or the short-axis MR images are reviewed. Then, a method is introduced that measures the LV volume using both the long-axis and short-axis MR images. Finally, experimental results are given and evaluated using synthetic and real images.

2. Background

The left ventricular ejection fraction, a measure of cardiac function, is determined by measuring the LV volume at the end-systolic and end-diastolic phases of the cardiac cycle. Past methods have used either the short-axis or the long-axis images to determine the LV volume. Methods that are based on the long-axis images use a single image of the cross-section of the LV cavity that contains the LV major axis [22]. Assuming that the LV cavity is an ellipsoid, its cross-section with a plane that contains its major axis is an ellipse.

Proceedings of MMBIA '96

By fitting an ellipse to an obtained LV boundary, the parameters of the ellipsoid are determined. LV volume obtained by the estimated ellipsoid is then adjusted using experimental results [5]. Attempts to automate this method have been made by delineating LV boundaries using a computer program. Lilly *et al.* [15] developed a model-based approach to LV boundary extraction, while Duncan *et al.* [6] developed a method that was based on an energy-minimizing criterion.

Methods that are based on the short-axis images try to reconstruct the LV cavity first and then measure its volume [2] [7]. The challenge here is to acquire images that contain the entire LV cavity at the end-systolic and end-diastolic phases of the cardiac cycle, and also to accurately delineate the LV boundary. To determine the short-axis LV boundaries, Wang *et al.* [24] and Fleagle *et al.* [9] used interactive methods while Cohen [4] used an automatic method based on an energy minimizing process. Suh *et al.* [23] and Faber *et al.* [8] developed model-based methods for extraction of LV cross-sections.

An attempt has also been made to combine cardiac MR images obtained at transverse, coronal, and sagittal cross-sections. Kuwahara and Eiho [17] first manually traced ventricular boundaries in two transverse, two coronal, and two sagittal cross-sections of the heart, and then combined the images to reconstruct the LV cavity in 3-D. In contrast to the method of Kuwahara and Eiho, which combines LV boundary contours obtained at three orthogonal cross-sections of the heart, we combine the original short-axis and long-axis images (not their boundary contours) to construct a volumetric image of the LV cavity and the surrounding tissues. In addition, our method is automatic and does not require any manual tracing. The proposed method maps the long-axis and short-axis image slices back into 3-D. For each known pixel intensity in the image slices, it determines the corresponding voxel intensity in the 3-D image. It then estimates 3-D image intensities that are not obtained by this mapping through approximation. The details of the method are discussed below.

3. Method

Figure 1 shows a sequence of eight short-axis MR images of the heart, while Figure 2 shows a sequence of four long-axis images. These images represent cinematic (cine) MR images acquired with a 1.5-Telsa device (Signa: GE Medical Systems, Milwakee). Imaging sections were $1cm$ thick and contiguous; the matrix size was 256×256, and the field of view was $31cm \times 31cm$. The cine MR images were acquired with software pro-

vided by the manufacturer [10]. Blood that flows into the imaged volume during the acquisition of images with this technique emits signals of higher intensity than tissue that remains in the volume during the entire acquisition (e.g., ventricular myocardium), a phenomenon known as "flow enhancement." Thus the blood pools appear brighter than other tissues in an acquired image. Figure 3a depicts the locations of the 2-D image slices of Figures 1 and 2 in the 3-D MR window. Figure 3b shows the 2-D images as they appear after being mapped into the window. This mapping partially determines the intensity of voxels in the 3-D image. It is possible that a pixel in a short-axis slice and a pixel in a long-axis slice map to the same voxel in 3-D. In such a situation, we let the intensity at the voxel equal the average of the two pixel intensities.

The equation describing the location of each MR slice in 3-D can be determined from the information provided in the header of the slice. By reading the 3-D coordinates of the upper-left, upper-right, and lower-left corners of each image slice from its header, the equation of the plane in 3-D from which the image was scanned can be determined. Assuming the coordinates of points in an image slice are represented by (x, y) and the coordinates of the same points in 3-D are represented by (X, Y, Z), the relation between the coordinates of corresponding points in 2-D and 3-D can then be written as:

$$X = a_1x + a_2y + a_3 \qquad (1)$$

$$Y = a_4x + a_5y + a_6 \qquad (2)$$

$$Z = a_7x + a_8y + a_9 \qquad (3)$$

A 2-D image is obtained by translating, rotating, and scaling a cross-section of the 3-D window. This transformation is linear and can be represented by relations (1)-(3). There are nine unknown parameters in this transformation, (a_1-a_9), which can be determined by substituting the coordinates of the upper-left, upper-right, and lower-left corners of an image slice in 2-D and their correspondences in 3-D into equations (1)-(3). The obtained system of equations can then be solved. Note that each image corner has three coordinates. When the coordinates of three corners are substituted into equations (1)-(3), nine equations will be obtained from which the nine unknowns are determined.

Once the unknown parameters of equations (1)-(3) are determined, and the coordinates (x, y) of a pixel in an image slice are substituted into equations (1)-(3), the corresponding voxel position in the 3-D image can be computed. Relations (1)-(3) thus establish correspondence between pixels in a sequence of image slices and the corresponding voxels in the 3-D image. By mapping the image slices to 3-D in this manner, we obtain the image shown in Figure 3b. The planes in the MR window corresponding to the long-axis and short-axis slices are shown in Figure 3a. Only a small portion of image 3b, as shown in Figure 4b, contains the LV cavity. We concentrate on the subwindow, which contains the LV cavity and discard the rest. The stripes in Figure 4b occur because the MR window was quantized into a 3-D array whose cross-section was slightly larger than its corresponding 2-D image slice. For voxels falling on the narrower stripes, no corresponding image pixels existed in the provided image slices. Figure 4a more clearly shows voxels where image intensities did not exist in the given image slices. We approximate the intensities of these voxels as well as the intensities of voxels that lie in between the image slices.

Suppose $\mathbf{P} = (X, Y, Z)$ is an image voxel whose intensity is not known. In the following, we estimate the intensity at $\mathbf{P}$ using intensities of N voxels closest to it whose values are known. Let's suppose $\{\mathbf{P}_i : i = 1, \ldots, N\}$ are the coordinates and $\{I_i : 1, \ldots, N\}$ are the intensities of the N voxels. We approximate the intensity I at voxel $\mathbf{P}$ using a weighted sum of intensities at the N voxels:

$$I(\mathbf{P}) = \frac{\sum_1^N I_i \, D_i(\mathbf{P})}{\sum_1^N D_i(\mathbf{P})} \qquad (4)$$

where

$$D_i(\mathbf{P}) = \left[(X - X_i)^2 + (Y - Y_i)^2 + (Z - Z_i)^2\right]^{-1}. \quad (5)$$

$D_i(\mathbf{P})$ represents the inverse squared distance between voxels $\mathbf{P}$ and $\mathbf{P}_i$. The farther voxel $\mathbf{P}_i$ is from voxel $\mathbf{P}$, the smaller the contribution of its intensity to the estimated intensity at $\mathbf{P}$. And conversely, the closer voxel $\mathbf{P}_i$ is to $\mathbf{P}$, the larger is its influence on the estimated intensity at $\mathbf{P}$. The square-root of formula (5) has been widely used as the basis function of *multiquadrics* in approximation theory [3] [12] [14] [19]. The basis functions in multiquadrics, however, decrease gradually from a center point and are not suitable for our purposes. In our formulations, we use the square distances, which decrease more rapidly from a center point and are computationally faster also. We introduce a smoothness parameter r^2 into equation (5) as is done in the basis functions of multiquadrics, to obtain:

$$D_i(\mathbf{P}) = \left[(X - X_i)^2 + (Y - Y_i)^2 + (Z - Z_i)^2 + r^2\right]^{-1} \quad (6)$$

As parameter r^2 is increased the contribution from farther voxels on an estimated intensity increases, thus producing a smoother approximation. However, as r^2 is decreased, the contributions increase from the immediate neighbors of the voxel whose intensity is being estimated. Thus a more detailed approximation is produced.

Although N can represent the total number of voxels whose intensities are known in a 3-D image, in practice however, the estimated intensity at voxel $\mathbf{P}$ depends mainly on the intensities of a small number of voxels neighboring $\mathbf{P}$. As one of these voxels moves away from $\mathbf{P}$, the effect of the image voxels on the estimated intensity vanishes rapidly. The neighborhood size to be used in this approximation depends on the distance between the given image slices and also on parameter r^2. As the distance between image slices increases, larger neighborhoods should be used to allow a sufficiently large number of voxels to participate in the approximation. Also, as r^2 increases, the basis function used in the approximation becomes wider, covering a larger portion of the image and requiring a larger neighborhood for the approximation. For the interslice distance of d pixels, we have found that the windows of size $w \times w \times w$, where $w = (2dr^2 - 1)$, must be used to achieve an approximation error less than half a pixel. For instance, when $r^2 = 1$ and $d = 8$, we need windows of size $15 \times 15 \times 15$, when $r^2 = 2$ and $d = 8$, we need windows of size $31 \times 31 \times 31$, and so on. Voxels falling outside of these windows have no effect on an estimated intensity with digital accuracy.

Applying the approximation of formulas (4) and (6) to the data of Figure 4b, we obtain the image shown in Figure 4c (only cross-sections of the volumetric image with its bounding planes are depicted). In the computations, we used $r^2 = 1$. Oblique cross-sections of this image are shown in Figure 5 (here also only the cross-sections of the volumetric image with its bounding planes are shown). In the following, we determine the accuracy of the approximation by reconstructing a synthetic volume image whose geometry is known, from its cross-sections.

4. Evaluation

In this section to determine the accuracy of a reconstructed volume image from given short-axis and long-axis image slices, we use an image that contains an object whose geometry is known. A $128 \times 128 \times 128$ synthetic image containing an object composed of a cylinder, a cube, a cone, and a sphere was generated. The intensity of voxels belonging to the object was 200 while that of the background was 100. Figure 6a depicts the obtained object after thresholding the synthetic image at 150. The synthetic image was partitioned into $128 \times 128 \times 8$ subimages, and each subimage was reduced to a 128×128 image by averaging the eight voxels along the Z-axis into a pixel value in the 2-D image. Next, the 3-D image was partitioned into $128 \times 8 \times 128$ subimages, and each subimage was reduced to a 128×128 image in the same fashion.

Assuming that the obtained 2-D images represented MR slices obtained at two orthogonal scan directions, we then fused them together using the method described in the preceding section. The reconstructed image is shown in Figure 6b. Parameter r^2 was equal to 0.5 in this approximation. On increasing r^2 to 1.0 and 2.0, we obtained the results shown in Figures 6c and 6d, respectively. As parameter r^2 is increased, the approximation neighborhood becomes larger, producing a smoother approximation. These figures show the surfaces obtained after thresholding the reconstructed images at 150.

The root-mean-squared difference between intensities of Figure 6a and intensities of Figures 6b-d were 7.45, 6.50, and 8.64, respectively. As parameter r^2 is increased, intensities in large gaps are determined more accurately. As r^2 is decreased, intensities near known voxels become more accurate. Among these three cases, average error was the smallest when $r^2 = 1.0$.

As interslice distance decreases, a denser distribution of voxels whose intensities are known becomes available. In such a situation, a smaller r^2 should be used so the details in the image are not smoothed out. As interslice distance increases, a larger r^2 should be used to allow a sufficiently large number of voxels to participate in estimating the intensities of large gaps.

Figure 7 shows the blood pools of Figure 4c obtained by the *marching cubes* algorithm [16]. The threshold value used in the algorithm was determined by interactively varying the intensity in one of the image slices until the best LV boundary was obtained by a radiologist's judgement. Then, the same threshold value was used in the marching cubes algorithm to determine the blood pools. More elaborate segmentation techniques [1] [4] [8] [11] may also be used to extract the blood pools once the volume image is constructed.

Parameter r^2 was equal to 0.5 in Figures 7a-b. On increasing r^2 to 1.0 and 2.0, we obtained the images shown in Figures 7c-d and 7e-f, respectively. As parameter r^2 is increased, a smoother approximation is obtained. A smoother approximation reduces image noise. At the same time, however, image details are also smoothed out. As can be observed in Figure 7, as r^2 is increased, details on extracted ventricular surfaces reduce. A second example is shown in Figure 8 using the same parameters as in Figure 7. We see that in Figures 7 and 8 the entire LV cavity and the left atrium have been extracted. Most parts of the right ventricular cavity has also been extracted. The short-axis and long-axis images used in these experiments did not contain the right atrium and, therefore, the right atrium was not obtained in the reconstructed images. The important point to note in these images is that the fusion process produces images that contain the entire LV cavity in high resolution. The process may be repeated on images from different phases of the cardiac cycle to extract the LV cavity in its entirety, thus enabling measurement of dynamic shape and volume of the LV cavity.

5. Summary and Conclusions

Measurement of volume-based indices of cardiac function requires measurement of the LV volume and shape at different phases of the cardiac cycle. Since the heart moves during the cardiac cycle, no single 2-D image location contains the same part of the heart during the entire cycle. Therefore, in order to follow changes in cardiac volume and shape through the entire cycle, the image planes must be interrogated to include all parts of the heart during its entire cycle. When conventional 2-D imaging techniques are used, the relatively poor spatial resolution along the dimension normal to the image planes distorts the apparent boundaries of the cardiac chambers along that dimension. This is particularly problematic in short-axis views, since the very thin cardiac valves cannot be adequately represented without excellent spatial resolution normal to the cardiac valve plane. However, spatial resolution along the normal dimension can be recovered by acquiring a second set of images parallel to that dimension (i.e., normal to the first set of images) and fusing the two sets of 2-D images in a single 3-D representation, as we have done.

The method introduced for fusion of the long-axis and short-axis MR images involves mapping the image slices back into the MR viewing window and estimating image entries that are not obtained by this mapping. The approximation process used in this work is based on a weighted averaging scheme with weights inversely proportional to the distances of voxels with known intensities to the voxel whose intensity is being estimated. This approximation has a smoothness parameter that can be varied to fuse images with different interslice distances.

Computing an entry of the estimated volume image from given image slices requires in the order of N multiplications, where N is the number of voxels whose intensities are known in a small neighborhood of the entry. Neighborhood size $w \times w \times w$ is obtained from the interslice distance d and the smoothness parameter r^2 of the approximation: $w = 2dr^2 - 1$. Assuming the reconstructed image is of size $n \times n \times n$, the algorithm requires in the order of Nn^3 multiplications to construct an isotropic volume image from given long-axis and short-axis image slices. Our implementation of the algorithm on a Sun Sparcstation 10 required about one hour and forty-five minutes to obtain the volume image of Figure 4c ($140 \times 100 \times 178$ voxels) from image slices of Figures 1 and 2 (256×256 pixels).

References

[1] L. Axel, G. T. Herman, J. K. Udupa, P. A. Bottomley, and W. A. Edelstein, "Three-dimensional display of nuclear magnetic (NMR) cardiovascular images," *J. Computer Assisted Tomography,* vol. 7, no. 1, 1983, pp. 172–174.

[2] P. T. Buser, W. Aufermann, W. W. Holt, S. Wagner, B. Kircher, C. Wolfe, C. B. Higgins, "Noninvasive evaluation of global left ventricular function with use of cine nuclear magnetic resonance," *JACC,* vol. 13, no. 6, 1989, pp. 1294–1300.

[3] R. E. Carlson and T. A. Foley, "The parameter r^2 in multiquadric interpolation," *Computers Math. Applic.,* vol. 21, no. 9, 1991, pp. 29–42.

[4] L. D. Cohen, "On active contour models and balloons," *Image Understanding,* vol. 53, no. 2, 1991, pp. 211-218.

[5] G. B. Cranney, C. S. Lotan, L. Dean, W. Baxley, A. Bouchard, and G. M. Pohost, "Left ventricular measurement using cardiac axis nuclear magnetic resonance imaging," *Circulation,* vol. 82, no. 1, 1990, pp. 154–163.

[6] J. S. Duncan, F. A. Lee, W. M. Smeulders, and B. L. Zaret, "A bending energy model for measurement of cardiac shape deformity," *IEEE Trans. Medical Imaging,* vol. 10, no. 3, 1991, pp. 307–320.

[7] R. R. Edelman, R. Thompson, H. Kantor, T. J. Brady, M. Leavitt, and R. Dinsmore, "Cardiac function: Evaluation with fast-echo MR imaging," *Radiology,* vol. 162, no. 3, 1987, pp. 611–615.

[8] T. L. Faber, E. M. Stokely, R. M. Peshock, and J. R. Corbett, "A model-based four-dimensional left ventricular surface detector," *IEEE Trans. Medical Imaging,* vol. 10, no. 3, 1991, pp. 321–329.

[9] S. R. Fleagle, D. R. Thedens, J. C. Ehrhardt, T. D. Sholz, and D. J. Skorton, "Automated identification of left ventricular borders from spin-echo magnetic resonance images," *Investigative Radiology,* vol. 26, no. 4, 1990, pp. 295–303.

[10] G. H. Glover, N. J. Pelc, "A rapid-gated cine MRI technique," in *Magnetic Resonance Annual,* H. Y. Kressel (ed.), Raven Press, New York, pp. 299–333, 1988.

[11] A. Goshtasby and D. A. Turner, "Segmentation of cardiac cine MR images for extraction of right and left ventricular chambers," *IEEE Trans. Medical Imaging,* vol. 14, no. 1, 1995, pp. 56–64.

[12] R. L. Hardy, "Theory and applications of the multiquadrics–biharmonic method," *Computers Math. Applic.,* vol. 19, no. 8/9 1990, pp. 163–208.

[13] C. B. Higgins, W. Holt, P. Pflugfelder, and U. Sechtem, "Functional evaluation of the heart with magnetic resonance imaging," *Magnetic Resonance in Medicine,* vol. 6, 1988, pp. 121–139.

[14] E. J. Kansa, "Multiquadrics– A scattered data approximation scheme with applications to computational fluid dynamics–I," *Computers Math. Applic.,* vol. 19, no. 8/9, 1990, pp. 127–145.

[15] P. Lilly, J. Jenkins, and P. Bourdillon, "Automatic contour definition on left ventriculograms by image evidence and a multiple template-based model," *IEEE Trans. Medical Imaging,* vol. 8, no. 2, 1989, pp. 173–185.

[16] W. E. Lorensen and H. E. Cline, "Marching cubes: A high resolution 3-D surface construction algorithm," *Computer Graphics,* vol. 21, no. 4, 1987, pp. 163–169.

[17] M. Kuwahara and S. Eiho, "3-D heart image reconstructed from MRI data," *Computerized Medical Imaging and Graphics,* vol. 15, no. 4, 1991, pp. 241–246.

[18] P. W. Pflugfelder, U. P. Sechtem, R. D. White, C. B. Higgins, "Quantification of regional myocardial function by rapid cine MR imaging," *AJR,* vol. 150, 1988, pp. 523–529.

[19] M. D. J. Powell, "Radial basis functions for multivariable interpolation: A review," *Algorithms for Approximation,* J. C. Mason and M. G. Cox (eds.), Clarendon Press: Oxford, 1987, pp. 143–167.

[20] U. Sechtem, P. Pflugerfelder, and C. B. Higgins, "Quantitation of cardiac function by conventional and cine magnetic resonance imaging," *Cardiovascular and Interventional Radiology,* vol. 10, 1987, pp. 365–373.

[21] U. Sechtem, P. W. Pflugfelder, R. G. Gould, M. M. Cassidy, C. B. Higgins, "Measurement of right and left ventricular volumes in healthy individuals with cine MR imaging," *Radiology,* vol. 163, no. 3, 1987, pp. 697–702.

[22] W. J. Stratemeier, R. Thompson, T. J. Brady, S. W. Miller, S. Saini, G. L. Wismer, R. D. Okada, R. E. Dinsmore, "Ejection fraction determination by MR imaging: Comparison with left ventricular angiography," *Radiology,* vol. 158, no. 3, 1986, pp. 775–777.

[23] D. Y. Suh, R. L. Eisner, R. M. Mersereau, and R. I. Pettigrew, "Knowledge-based system for boundary detection of four-dimensional cardiac magnetic resonance image sequences," *IEEE Trans. Medical Imaging,* vol. 12, no. 1, 1993, pp. 65–72.

[24] J. Z. Wang, D. A. Turner, and M. D. Chutuape, "Fast, interactive algorithm for segmentation of a series of related images: Application to volumetric analysis of MR images of the heart," *JMRI,* vol. 2, no. 5, 1992, pp. 575–582.

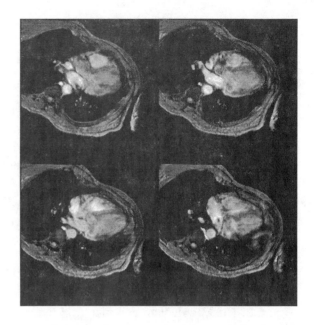

Figure 2. A sequence of long-axis MR images obtained at the end-diastolic phase.

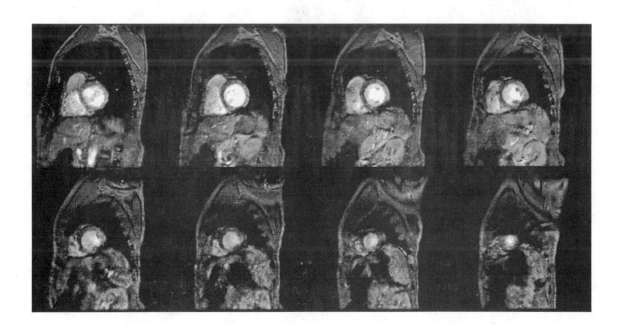

Figure 1. A sequence of short-axis MR images of the heart obtained at the end-diastolic phase.

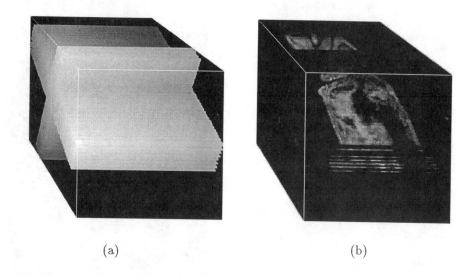

(a)   (b)

Figure 3. The MR viewing window. (a) Planes in the MR window corresponding to the short-axis and long-axis images of Figures 1 and 2. (b) The short-axis and long-axis images after being mapped back to the 3-D MR window.

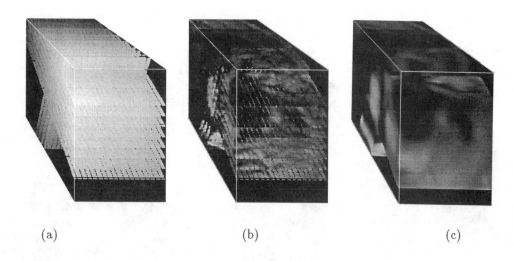

(a)   (b)   (c)

Figure 4. (a), (b) Portions of Figures 3a and 3b, respectively, containing the heart. (c) Volumetric image obtained from image of (b) using the approximation formulas of (4) and (6).

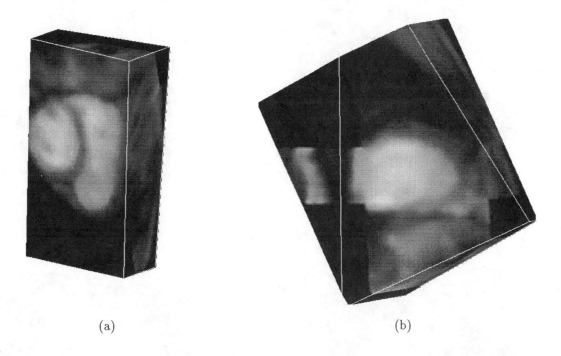

(a)   (b)

Figure 5. (a), (b) Two oblique cross-sections of the image of Figure 4c.

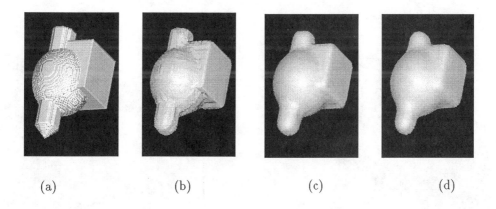

(a)   (b)   (c)   (d)

Figure 6. (a) A synthetic image containing an object composed of a sphere, a cube, a cylinder, and a cone. This image was reduced to a sequence of sixteen image slices parallel to the xy-plane and sixteen slices parallel to the xz-plane. The two image sequences were then fused together by the method described in the paper with $r^2 = 0.5,\ 1.0.$ and 2.0 to obtain images (b), (c), and (d), respectively.

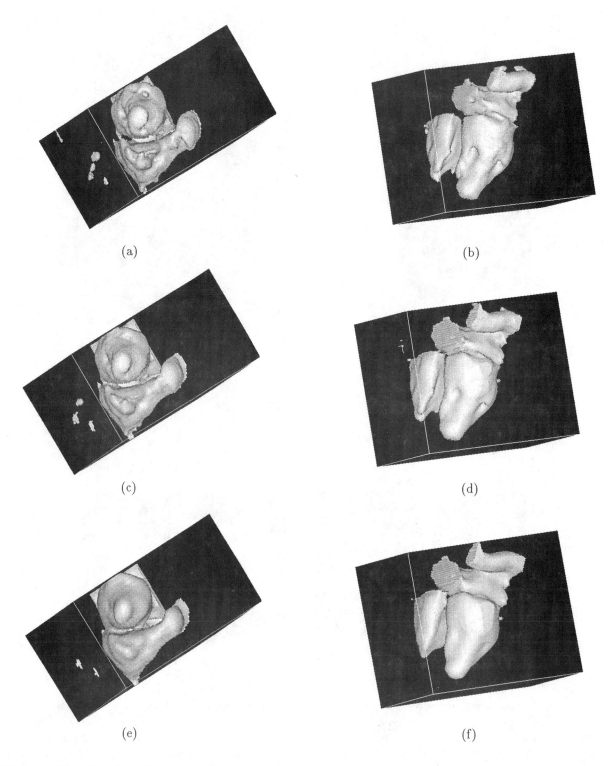

(a)

(b)

(c)

(d)

(e)

(f)

Figure 7. The blood pools when viewed from (a) the cardiac apex, and (b) from the left posterior towards the right anterior of the heart. These images were obtained when parameter r^2 in formula (6) was equal to 0.5. (c)–(d) and (e)–(f) are the same as (a)–(b), except that parameter r^2 was increased to 1.0 and 2.0, respectively.

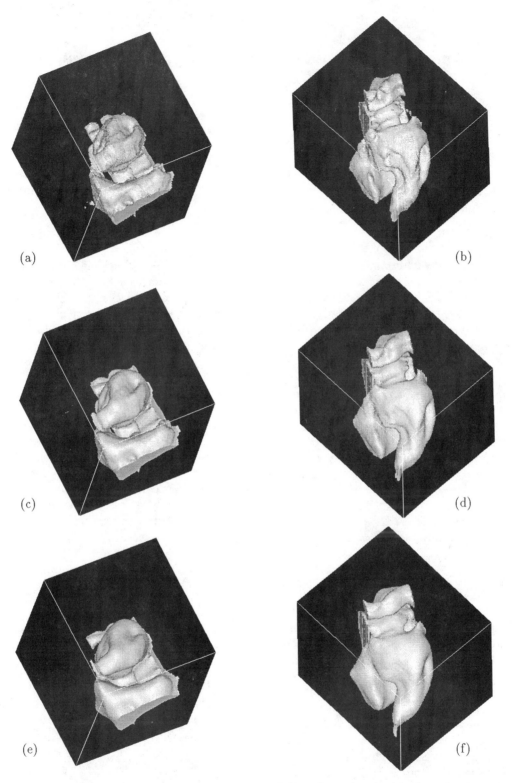

(a)

(b)

(c)

(d)

(e)

(f)

Figure 8. Another example showing the reconstructed blood pools after fusing the long-axis and short-axis MR images from a second patient. Parameters of the image fusion are the same as those used in Figure 7.

Automatic Registration and Alignment on a Template
of Cardiac Stress & Rest SPECT Images

Jérôme Declerck, Jacques Feldmar, Fabienne Betting
Projet EPIDAURE
I.N.R.I.A., B.P. 93
06902 Sophia-Antipolis Cedex, France
Jerome.Declerck@sophia.inria.fr

Michael L. Goris
Division of Nuclear Medicine
Department of Radiology
Stanford University Hospital (Cal. USA)

Abstract

Single photon emission computed tomography (SPECT) imaging is used to assess the location or the extent of myocardial infarction or ischemia.

A method is proposed to decrease the effect of operator variability and morphologically blind sampling in the quantification of scintigraphic myocardial perfusion studies. To effect this, the patient's myocardial images (target cases) are registered automatically over a template image, utilizing non-rigid transformations. The registration method is an adaptation of the Iterative Closest Point algorithm.

Experiments have been conducted on a database including 40 pairs of images selected to obtain a group of image abnormalities and variability. Upon the successful clinical validation of this work, a reliable, operator independent method for the analysis and interpretation of myocardial perfusion scintigraphies will be available.

1. Introduction

Coronary artery disease remains one of the leading causes of death in the developed nations. In a large number of instances, the first symptom is due to a myocardial infarction, and half of the myocardial infarctions cause death. Detecting and preventing it is one of the major goals of modern medicine.

In the normal course of events, infarction follows a more or less progressive narrowing of the coronary artery. At first, the narrowing does not interfere with resting blood flow, but, when during exercise the metabolic demands of the myocardium increases, the narrowed vessel cannot accommodate the required increase in blood flow. The myocardium, normally perfused at rest, becomes ischemic during stress or exercise (increased metabolic demand). This stress ischemia is the phase during which typical symptoms of coronary artery disease occur, and a period when the patient is both at risk for myocardial infarction, and when the disease is amenable to therapy. The classical symptoms are chest pain associated with exercise (typical angina) and changes in the EKG (electro-cardiogram) during exercise. Sometimes the symptoms are less specific (or nearly absent !), and other conditions may mimic the symptoms. The defining diagnostic study is the coronary arteriogram, which reveals narrowing of the coronary arteries, and is needed for the planning and execution of the correcting vascular intervention (coronary artery bypass graft or angioplasty). In view of the aspecificity of the symptoms, and the gravity of the potentially underlying condition, one is faced with the dilemma of performing too many unnecessary coronary arteriograms, and neglecting potentially lethal disease. For those cases in which the combination of risk factors, clinical signs and exercise EKG results are not sufficient to predict a high or low probability of coronary artery disease, an intermediate stratification step is necessary.

Nuclear medicine imaging provides 3D density maps of blood perfusion in a non-invasive way. In the stress-rest study, 2 perfusion maps of the heart muscle are taken: one obtained after the injection of the tracer at rest (rest image) and the other after the injection of the tracer during maximal exercise (stress image). Comparing the two images provides a classification of areas of the myocardium in 3 main classes:

- The intensity distribution is *normal* in both images.

- There are one or more regions with abnormally low count rate densities in both rest and stress images. The abnormality is fixed, and this connotes a myocardial *infarction*, or in some cases a very narrow stenosis, with resting hypoperfusion and a hibernating or stunned myocardium.

- There are one or more regions of low count rate densities in the stress image, but the densities are normal in the rest image. The abnormality is said to be transient, and connotes stress *ischemia*.

212

Proceedings of MMBIA '96

The clinical examination in its current protocol stands in a "de visu" comparison of some central slices of the heart. However, this way of processing, which radiologists are used to, has three main drawbacks:

- the comparison is approximate, because of the lack of accuracy and the subjectivity of the "visual" matching of the two images of the heart,

- only central slices (taken from 3 different directions) are displayed and processed, excluding some intermediate areas,

- it is very hard to accurately compare different sets of images over time in order, for instance, to follow a specific disease or to check if a surgical intervention has been successful.

Various steps in the analysis (segmentation, orientation and centering, registration) have been automated in a variety of ways: [7, 15] define automatic methods to segment the myocardium directly from the transaxial original images, or to define a center and a long axis [2]. Perault et al. [16], inspired by Woods et al. [24], find automatically the rigid registration between the stress and rest images using correlation-based techniques. Venot et al. [22] also use a correlation-based technique with a stochastic sign change criterion to register the images. [18] also use correlation techniques to find a non-uniform scaling transformation to register different hearts. A template is built by normalizing and averaging the resampled images. Some more complicated (free-form) transformations may be found with the intensity-based method described in [20].

The aim of the method proposed in this paper is to provide a reproducible, robust and highly automatic way of comparing the stress and rest perfusion images of the same patient, or images of different patients. We introduce a new 3D registration procedure, allowing a quantitative comparison of stress and rest images. We also introduce a registration with a "template" image of the heart, allowing a quantitative comparison with a model. The article is organized as follows: in section 2, the current clinical examination is described, detailing the various defects of the protocol, our method is explained in section 3 and detailed in sections 4 to 7 and in section 8, some results are presented. We conclude by the perspectives of this work.

2. The Stress-Rest Clinical Examination

In this section, we describe quickly the clinical procedure, a more complete description can be found in [3]. We also discuss the quality of the imaging technique (what is possible to be shown and the inherent defects) and the need of a stable quantification technique in order to obtain a reliable diagnosis.

2.1. SPECT images show 3D perfusion maps

2.1.1 The tracer

A radioactive tracer is injected into a peripheral vein. The tracer has two characteristics: its distribution (*fixation*) in the tissues is proportional to the distribution of tissue blood-flow, and clearance from the blood is rapid enough (a half-life of the order of two minutes) so that most tissue accumulation occurs early.

In some of the tracers the initial distribution changes slowly, until the distribution of the tracer reflects the distribution pools or equilibrium distribution, rather than the flow distribution. This phase is called *redistribution*.

Measuring the amount of tracer in a particular volume indicates the relative level of perfusion of this volume during a relatively short time following the injection. This measure is processed by counting the disintegrations of the radioactive label.

2.1.2 The clinical protocol

For the stress injection the patient is submitted to a physical exercise that increases the myocardial blood flow among other organ flows. The stronger the effort, the more important the need for blood, and hence, if any, the more obvious the perfusion defects. Exercise is continued until the hear rate reaches the maximum predicted heart rate (MPHR = [220 - the age of the patient] beats per minute), or until significant EKG abnormalities appear, blood pressure fails to raise or falls, or the patients feels pain (angor) beyond a certain level. The injection is timed so that exercise will last two minutes after it, to maintain stress kinetics during the larger part of the tissue accummulation.

After the fixation ends and before the redistribution begins is the right time to take the 3D image of the perfusion distribution at stress. The rest image is taken after the redistribution is completed or after a separate injection at rest.

2.2. Acquisition of scintigraphic images

The distribution of the radioactivity within the patient is mapped in a number of projection images. They are taken at equally spaced angles, usually 32 projections over 180 degrees or 64 over 360. The data are stored in a 64x64 matrix, with a pixel size of 6.25 mm x 6.25 mm. A three-dimensional image is reconstructed from the projection data, usually by filtered back-projection. This reconstructed 64x64x64 image is isometric.

The reconstructed image includes the whole thorax of the patient. The heart is extracted as a subset of the original image. A rotation and a translation are performed manually in order to put the heart in a roughly standard position and direction. To avoid including other structures or organs such as the liver, the image is masked through a manually designed shape.

The image is hence smoothed due to this extraction and resizing procedure. Usually, the rest image gives a better definition of the shape of the muscle than the stress image: as a matter of fact, ischemic zones appear as low intensity areas on the stress image, and sometimes do not appear at all. The heart wall is thus more difficult to locate.

2.3. Quantification of myocardial perfusion images

The quantification of scintigraphic myocardial perfusion images is generally based on some form of a polar transformation. In this approach the myocardial densities are sampled from an origin in the center of the cavity, along (evenly spaced) radii.

In one particular application [9] the three-dimensional images are sampled along rays or radii (radial sampling), originating in the center of the left ventricular cavity. Each radius is characterized by its azimuth a and elevation b. The origin of b is the apex, the origin of a is the middle of the lateral wall. A value sampled along the radius $R(a,b)$ is stored in the two-dimensional vector B as in a planispheric projection.

The vector B is therefore a planar image in which central points represent apical locations, peripheral points represent the basal locations. The anterior wall is mapped on top, the inferior wall at the bottom, the septum in the left-hand side of the image. This vector is comparable to the Bull's eye maps described in the literature [6, 12, 13, 21, 23], except for the fact that the distance from the center represents an elevation b in three dimensions, rather than a short axis plane position: the bull's eye map approach interrogates the volume as if it were a set of planes [8].

The effect of a polar transform amounts to a normalization of size and shape [10], since all morphological attributes of the image are reduced to angular coordinates. This normalization allows the comparison between target cases and a population of normal cases and the intercomparison of target cases.

There are four limitations inherent to this approach:

1. Alignment limitation: the effect of the origin location. Structures closer to the origin are relatively oversampled, and perfusion defects appear larger (Fig. 1-a).
2. Alignment limitation: angular shift. If the zero angle is misplaced identical distributions will appear different from each other (Fig. 1-b).
3. Sampling direction. If the lesion is relatively small and not well aligned in relation to the sampling ray direction, the lesion may be underdetected.
4. Non-angular relevant morphology. The proportion of different parts of the myocardium are not necessarily fixed. The base of the heart, with the papillary muscles

may be more or less prominent. Equal angular coordinates do therefore not necessarily map into identical myocardial structures.

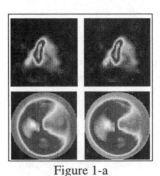 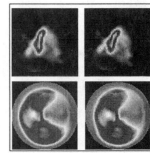

Figure 1-a	Figure 1-b
Effect of origin	**Angular mismatch**
The lateral defect appears smaller if the image is translated laterally (images on the right).	In this case, the same myocardial image has been slightly rotated. The polar maps differ.

Figure 1. Alignment limitations in mapping

Alignment problems are mostly caused by operator variability in identifying the long axis and/or the center point, and attempts have been made to overcome this problem using principal axis orientation [7]. It can be shown however that alignment based on the principal axes of simple geometric forms fitted to the myocardial surfaces does not guarantee stable center points relative to the organ or a stable anatomical alignment [18].

A method is therefore needed which allows registration of target images automatically on a template image whose shape and size may be different, but with general morphological features which are similar. There are two results:

1. If this template is well oriented, the target image will be well oriented, and any small deviation from the ideal orientation will be constant across all target images.
2. Following registration, predefined myocardial segments in the template image can be transferred exactly to the target image. As a result, size and shape normalization are obtained without the need for radial sampling, and regional count rate distributions can be compared from case to case.

3. Description of the method

Since the aim is to compare images between which major density distribution differences may occur, it appears logical to avoid matching algorithms based on density comparisons. Indeed, the goal is not to make densities equal, but to eliminate all size and shape differences while leaving density differences unperturbed. The method we propose is therefore based on shape detectors based on gradients. One expects that gradients would exist even in low density areas. Second, the differences in size and shape between different patient hearts do not allow a straightforward correspondence to be established between an anatomically defined area and the coordinates (x,y,z) of a voxel in each 3D image (stress S, rest R, template T).

The method that we propose splits into two major steps:

- The stress/rest pair of images is matched using a feature-point based method, yielding an affine transformation which defines a correspondence between a point in image S and a point in image R.
- A "template" heart is matched to image S and both S and R images are resampled in its geometry.

After this transformation of the images (the output is a new stress/rest pair S'/R' in a new geometry), the coordinates (x,y,z) of a 3D voxel in any image (stress, rest, template) correspond to the same part of the myocardium and allows quantitative intrapatient and interpatient comparison.

3.1. The matching step

In our method, each matching of two images is a 3 step process:

- automatic extraction of feature points in images R and S, using a Canny-Deriche edge detector [14] in a particular geometry,
- matching of the two sets of points using an adaptation [5] of the iterative closest point method [1, 25]. This yields a 3D deformation function which transforms each point in image S to a point in image R,
- resampling images R and S in the geometry of the image T. Image T and the resampled images are comparable pixel by pixel to measure perfusion differences.

3.2. Two possible approaches

In an ideal situation where the matching with the model is performed perfectly against the stress and rest images respectively, this implicitly also provides the correspondence between the stress and rest images themselves.

In practice, any registration method (and especially one that is 3D non-rigid) is error prone or at least an approximation to the ideal case. We therefore consider the two following possible strategies:

1. - the stress and the rest images are separately matched to the template, producing two resampled images in the geometry of the template,
   - then a match is performed between the 2 resampled images in order to correct the possible mismatches of the template registration.

2. - the stress and the rest images are registered to each other,

- the template is matched to one image (the stress image, for instance), and the pair is resampled in the geometry of the template.

The reasons for choosing Scheme 2 instead of Scheme 1 are twofold:

- Scheme 1 is much more complex and costly than Scheme 2 (3 matching steps versus 2), even if it is theoretically more satisfying and well balanced (between stress and rest).
- As soon as the stress/rest pair shows perfusion maps of the same heart, the geometry of the extracted feature points are similar (even if the intensity distribution is different). Matching the stress/rest pair is hence easier than matching the stress image with the template for which the geometry of the feature points may differ strongly in size and shape. In terms of error accumulation, it is better to do the easiest step first and to end up with the more difficult.

4. Extraction of feature points

4.1. The images

Some characteristics of the scintigraphic images have to be taken into account:

- The densities do not necessarily match the anatomical features since perfusion defects may be present.
- There are high density areas due to the accumulation in other organs (especially the liver). Segmentation solely by thresholding is unlikely to work in general.
- The noise due to the reconstruction from the 32 projections may be important.

4.2. Edge detection in a 3D polar map

The feature points we extract from the image are supposed to feature edges of the heart wall. It would be useless to try to find the precise location of the true limit of the heart wall, because the image shows the heart only in its mean position during acquisition and because spatial resolution is poor. The points we are looking for should be a rough but stable approximation to the myocardial edges.

To detect such feature points, we use an algorithm based on the first derivative of the image by detecting the edges with a Canny-Deriche recursive filter [14] in a particular 3D polar geometry. The 3D polar map is defined as the original image resampled in spherical coordinates (r, θ, ϕ) (Eqn. 1, Fig. 2, top). From a 64x64x64 image, a 128x128x32 image is resampled.

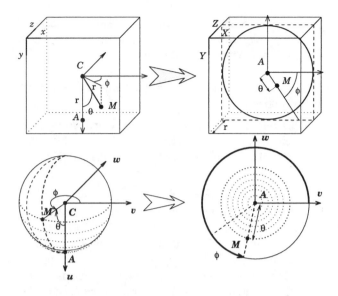

Figure 2. Top, from cartesian (x, y, z) to polar coordinates (X, Y, Z). Bottom, parallels (θ constant) become concentric circles and meridians (ϕ constant) become segments.

$$\begin{cases} X = \theta\,cos(\phi) \\ Y = \theta\,sin(\phi) \\ Z = r \end{cases} \quad (1)$$

The shape of a heart is roughly spherical around the apex and roughly cylindrical around the base. In the 3D polar map, this shape looks like a plate (Fig. 2, bottom).

Extracting edges in this map with a 3D edge detector provides a stable definition of gradient extrema points. Fig. 3 shows intensity profiles along 2 different radii starting from the center of the image.

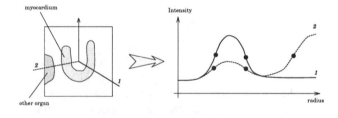

Figure 3. Intensity profiles along 2 different radii. The black dots show on both curves the detected edges.

Because of the mask sometimes used to hide non-cardiac areas, some artificial edges are created, with a very high gradient value (the background noise intensity decreases sharply from roughly 0.1 (normalized value) down to 0 in a one pixel shift). In order to eliminate such artificial extrema, the intensity profile along the radius is modified after the point before the last non-zero intensity point: intensity is set constant after this point (the last non-zero intensity point has a biased value because of the resampling process).

4.3. Filtering the edge points

Some detected edges do not correspond to the heart wall, as shown in the dotted curve in Fig. 3: an edge of another organ has been detected. Therefore, a final step is required: along a radius, on the intensity profile, the first *significant* increasing gradient extremum is likely to belong to the endocardium and the first following *significant* decreasing gradient extremum is likely to belong to the epicardium. Based on this empirical description, we define some constraints to filter incorrect edge points:

1. any edge point in a 15 degree cone around the apicobasal vector is eliminated. This angle value is very low and it is difficult to set correctly for a large database. Such points certainly do not belong to the left ventricle.

2. a large majority of erroneous edge points are eliminated assuming that the filling procedure yields gradient extrema with constant gradient norm along a radius. Such extrema are detected on the deepest plane (32) of the polar map (a high radius value, for which we are sure that no cardiac structure is represented). If there is an edge point for $r = 32$, all the neighboring edge points which have the same gradient norm (tolerating a 0.1 margin due to the smoothing of the edge detection) as this one are eliminated. Experiments with our database have shown that around 80 percent of artificial edge points were removed.

3. the remaining points are sorted with respect to the absolute value of the Z coordinate of the gradient. Thresholding is performed on the contour image in order to eliminate the lowest 20 percent, and only large (> 500 points) connected components are retained.

4. an ordering constraint is applied: we insist on configurations fitting our empirical description and reject edges which we are sure are non-cardiac: we reject every edge point after the first descending gradient extremum which is not too close to the center (a minimum radius of 5 is fixed as a threshold). In Fig. 4, different configurations of intensity profiles are listed with the correspondent algorithmic decision.

Finally, the points are converted back into cartesian coordinates. Fig. 5 and Fig. 6 show the results of feature extraction for different hearts. The proportion of good points is satisfying, the robust matching algorithm is able to cope with remaining outliers.

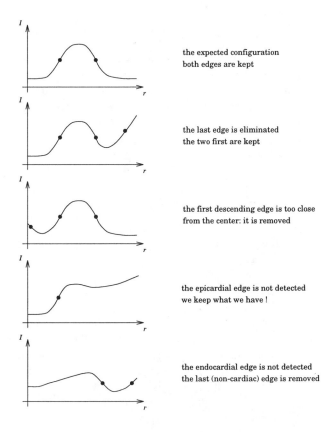

Figure 4. Left, some configurations for the intensity profile along a radius. Right, the consequent decision for the filtering.

5. Robust matching

Edge are detected in both images (stress and rest, or stress and template). We assume that a first derivative extremum in the first image matches with a first derivative extremum in the second image. The matching method is an enhancement of the iterative closest point method, adapted to our problem.

5.1. The matching criterion

We seek a matching function F: given a 3D point M in Image 1, $F(M)$ should be the equivalent 3D point in Image 2. To calculate F, we assume that the image of a feature point in Image1 is a feature point in Image 2. For the other points, an interpolation is made depending of the class of F. We define thus a criterion C:

$$C(F) = \sum_{M_i \in S_1} \|F(M_i) - ClosestPointOnFP_2(F(M_i))\|^2$$

Given a feature point in Image 1, the function F must give a point as close as possible to a feature point in Image 2

(this is what the function $ClosestPointOnFP_2$ calculates). The criterion is the sum of all residual distances extended to S_1, a subset of the feature points in Image 1 for which the matching is considered as being reliable.

5.2. Minimizing the criterion

The minimization process is iterative, given an initial transformation F_0. This initial transformation is chosen in our experiments to be the identity, assuming that the images to be registered are approximately aligned. Each iteration n splits into three steps:

1. For each point M_i, we calculate $F_{n-1}(M_i)$ and we identify its closest feature point in Image 2. We therefore end up with a list of possible matched pairs.

2. We calculate the residual distance for each pair, and we decide whether a pair is reliable or not: we first eliminate pairs for which the residual distance exceeds a fixed threshold. Second, we compute the mean μ and the standard deviation σ attached to the remaining pairs. We then eliminate the points for which the distance is greater than another threshold depending on the distance distribution ($\mu + c.\sigma$, where c can be easily set using a χ^2 table [5]). We get for this iteration a list $S_{1,n}$ of reliable pairs of matched points.

3. We calculate F_n which is the best least squares fit for the pairs of $S_{1,n}$. This new transformation is calculated within a class of acceptable functions (rigid, then affine and finally local spline).

The iterative process stops when a maximum number of iterations is reached, or when $S_{1,n} = S_{1,n-1}$. For further details about this adaptation of the ICP, see [5].

5.3. Definition of the closest point

The matching function $ClosestPointOnFP_2$ takes into account for each point its geometric position and the local direction of the intensity gradient calculated while extracting the edges. Considering 2 points M and N and their intensity gradient vectors $\overrightarrow{n}_M$ and $\overrightarrow{n}_N$ respectively, the distance between them is calculated as follows:

$$d(M, N)^2 = \alpha \|\overrightarrow{MN}\|^2 + \|\overrightarrow{n}_M - \overrightarrow{n}_N\|^2$$

where α is a weighting coefficient.

This double definition of a point (location + direction) refines the matching criterion and makes it more robust in the presence of a crude initialization, for instance.

5.4. The class of transformations

The least squares fit is calculated among a particular class of volume transformations. We choose between:

- rigid (6 parameters define the transformation),
- affine (12 parameters define the transformation),
- local spline, which means that the transformation F is a 3D tensor product of cubic B-splines: if (u, v, w) are the coordinates of F, u is defined as follows:

$$u(x, y, z) = \sum_{i=0}^{n_x-1} \sum_{j=0}^{n_y-1} \sum_{k=0}^{n_z-1} u_{ijk}\, B_{i,K}^x(x)\, B_{j,K}^y(y)\, B_{k,K}^z(z)$$

where we use the following notation:

- n_x : the number of control points in the x direction. This controls the accuracy of the approximation (8 in our experiments).
- (u_{ijk}) : the 3D mesh of control points abscissae. These parameters define the transformation.
- $B_{i,K}^x$: the ith B-spline basis function. Its order is K. The $B_{i,K}^x$ generate the vector space of piecewise K^{th} degree polynomials (see [17]). u is therefore a piecewise K^{th} degree polynomial in each variable x, y and z.

We choose cubic B-splines in our experiments ($K = 3$), because of their regularity properties. For the knots, we used the classic regular mesh.

In the definition of the criterion, a smoothing energy SE is added in order to control the regularity of the solution. This energy is expressed as a second order Tikhonov stabilizer:

$$\int_{\mathbb{R}^3} \left[u_{xx}^2 + u_{yy}^2 + u_{zz}^2 + 2u_{xy}^2 + 2u_{xz}^2 + 2u_{yz}^2 \right]$$

and the same for the other coordinates y and z. This smoothing energy is weighted in the global definition of the least square criterion. [4] gives a more complete description of the local spline transformation. The transformation is defined given a number of $n_x.n_y.n_z$ parameters (= 512 in our experiments).

For our matching problems:

- Matching stress on rest: Because in the stress image, there may be fewer edge points than in the rest image, it is natural to try to find the transformation which deforms the stress edge points to the rest edge points. The shapes of the objects in both images are similar: some differences may appear in size. We define F as an affine transformation. We first apply the algorithm with a rigid transformation in order to have a good initialization and then with an affine transformation. The final result is the affine transformation F which best aligns the stress and rest images. 10 iterations of rigid and 10 of affine are performed.

- Matching template on stress: The size and shapes of the objects are usually different, sometimes, a strong local deformation is necessary. We choose F as a local spline transformation. We first apply the algorithm with a rigid transformation, then with an affine transformation and finally with the local spline. The transformation thus gets more and more degrees of liberty during this progression (rigid, affine, local spline). 10 iterations of rigid, 10 of affine and 6 of local spline are performed.

6. Resampling the rest and stress images

After the matching step, we get a transformation $t_{1\to 2}$ from Image 1 to Image 2. With this transformation, it is possible to build an image Image 2' which is Image 2 resampled in the geometry of Image 1.

Having computed the transformations $t_{T\to S}$ from the template geometry to the stress, and $t_{S\to R}$ from the stress geometry to the rest, it is possible to resample the stress image in the geometry of the template, and by composition ($t_{T\to R} = t_{S\to R} \circ t_{T\to S}$), we resample the rest image in geometry of the template after registration on the stress.

The resampling is a purely geometric transformation, the density counts information is not preserved.

7. Definition of the template

7.1. Our choice

To build the template of the heart, we adapt the previous segmentation process to an image of an average normal healthy heart, and we adapt the values of the parameters to obtain an almost perfect set of points (no gap in the heart wall, no spurious edge points outside the heart wall). This gives an almost ideal set of feature points.

In our experiments, the template is an image of one particular heart which is well defined and in good health.

7.2. A definition of the volume of the LV

Our edge extraction method does not provide a structured set of points. To define the volume of the left ventricle, we used our matching method to deform a structured closed surface on our set of feature points. Because the deformation is smooth, the structure of the surface is conserved. Of course, this definition of the volume has to be clinically validated.

7.3. Possible improvements

Slomka et al. [18] define a template as an average heart among a set of similar hearts after a correlation-based match with a non-uniform scaling transformation. We are currently working on a more sophisticated definition of our template or model image which could support a statistical analysis and classification.

8. Results and discussion

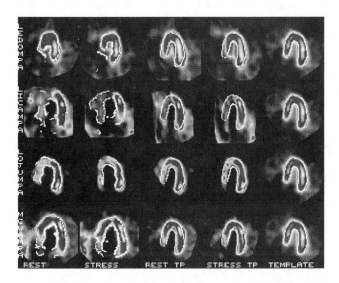

Figure 5. Each row shows a different study. The two left columns show central slices of the rest and stress images before registration. The edge points are overlaid in white. The next two columns show the same images after registration and alignment. The right column shows the central slice of the template. The edge points of the template are overlaid in the images of the right three columns.

8.1. The experimentation on the database

A set of 32 paired stress and rest images has been selected among the studies provided at the Department of Nuclear Medicine of Stanford University Hospital (California, USA). The images were selected to obtain a mixed group of image abnormalities and variations. The method and the parameters have been set with this database.

Another 8 cases (chosen for their disparity in size and shape) were added to the database to make a crude validation of the parameters. A more extensive validation will be processed with a routine database (the studies will not be selected on clinical or pathological characteristics). Our comments in this paper will be limited to morphological and perfusion considerations; quantification and stratification aspects will be discussed in a forthcoming paper.

The images were taken with both Tl 201 and Tc 99m tracers and prealigned manually by an expert (one of the authors). This alignement ensures that the center of the image is inside the cavity of the left ventricle and that the $\overrightarrow{y}$ direction in the image is parallel to the apico-basal vector. The constraints are crucial for our edge extraction step, but they are not hard to satisfy.

8.2. The results

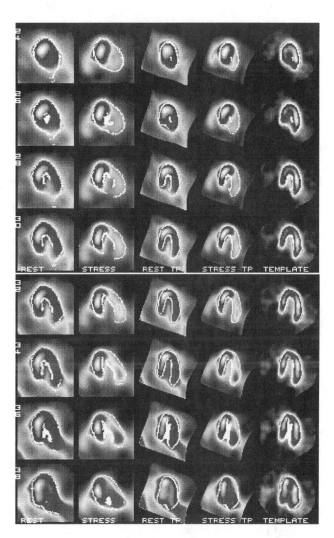

Figure 6. Different transverse slices of patient RYALMPA study. The disposition of the images is identical to fig. 5.

Fig. 5 shows the central frontal slices of the stress and rest images before and after registration and alignment. Each line shows a different patient from our database. The coded name of these patients are written on the left. Some more slices of the 3D images are shown for a particular patient (RYALMPA on fig. 6 respectively).

On the slices (which are only a 2D abstract of a 3D perfusion map), we can appreciate on the left two columns (the original rest and stress images) the differences in sizes and shapes of the patient hearts. In the next two columns, the morphological differences are removed whereas the perfusion information (the intensity level) is conserved.

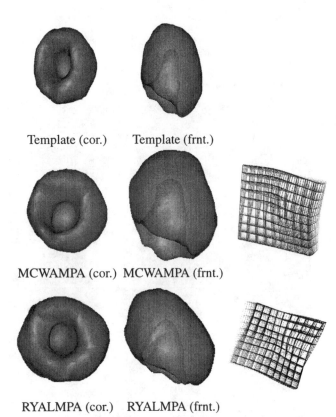

Template (cor.)   Template (frnt.)

MCWAMPA (cor.)   MCWAMPA (frnt.)

RYALMPA (cor.)   RYALMPA (frnt.)

Figure 7. Top, the closed surface of the template. Following lines, this surface deformed to define the boundary of the left ventricle of 2 different hearts, left on a coronal projection and middle on a frontal projection. On the right, a regular grid is deformed by the alignment transformation.

In fig. 6 we can appreciate the robustness of the extraction of the edge points in the stress image of patient RYALMPA. This patient appears to suffer from a large anterolateral ischemia, which is revealed by the difference of intensity in that region between stress and rest images. Despite the fact that the intensity in the ischemic area is low (but not as low as the background noise), it has been possible to detect the cardiac edges.

As far as an expert can appreciate the result of the matching, 80 % of the treated cases give satisfying results: in those cases, the feature points of the template deformed with the matching transformation define a plausible boundary for the left ventricle to an expert eye. For the remaining 20 % (which are difficult cases, according to an expert), some parts of the ventricle are not included in the volume or some non-cardiac areas are included in the volume. It appears that these errors are due, first, to some defects in the segmentation (the basis is not well defined, as for patient LEDOMPA, fig. 5) and second, because the local spline function does not deform sufficiently. Improving the extraction of feature points should lead to a major improvement in the quality of the results; we are currently working on this.

Top line in fig. 7 shows the surface of the template. This surface has been obtained by deforming an isosurface of the template to the feature points with our method. This closed surface could be a definition of the volume of the left ventricle. Fig. 7 shows 2 different hearts at stress (MCWAMPA and RYALMPA) in 2 different projections. These surfaces were obtained by deforming the surface of the template with the deformation computed to match the template on the stress image. The deformation looks regular.

The average time of the whole treatment (edge extractions + matchings + resamplings) is roughly 5 minutes per patient on a DEC Alpha workstation. We are currently working on some optimizations of the source code which could reduce the computational time by at least 50 %.

9. Conclusion

We presented an automated method to register and align images from myocardial perfusion SPECT studies. To reconstruct "better" images, feature points are extracted in stress and rest images, the stress and rest points are matched together using an affine transformation (stress-rest registration) and the stress points are matched to a template using a local spline transformation (alignment). New images are resampled in the geometry of the template.

The method has been tested and implemented on a database of 32 stress-rest studies specifically selected to obtain a sample of image variability and abnormalities. An additional set of 8 cases was used to check the parameters, giving a first appreciation of the validation of the method.

In the future, we will define a clinical validation protocol which will include an experimentation of the method on a large cohort of patients. The method will be validated by demonstrating that after polar sampling, the standard deviation around the mean of the normal case stress polar maps is smaller when this registration method is used, than if the alignment is performed by an experienced operator.

After having validated and eventually improved the method, we will also work on a statistical analysis of the quantification of SPECT myocardial images, inspired by the works of Houston et al. [11] or Strother et al. [19] using Principal Components Analysis.

10. Acknowledgements

We want to thank Focus Medical for their help in making possible the collaboration between the INRIA and the Stanford teams. The Focus team in Grenoble is currently working on the first steps of the industrialization of the method.

We give also special thanks to the teams of the Stanford University Hospital (California, USA) and of the Centre Antoine Lacassagne (Nice, France) for the constructive discussions and comments about the project.

This work was partially supported by regional grant of the Région Provence Alpes Côte d'Azur (doctoral research contract).

References

[1] P. Besl and N. McKay. A Method for Registration of 3D Shapes. *IEEE Transactions on Pattern Analysis and Machine Intelligence*, 14:239–256, Feb. 1992.

[2] J. Cauvin, J. Boire, J. Maublant, J. Bonny, M. Zanca, and A. Veyre. Automated detection of the left ventricular myocardium long axis and center in Thallium-201 single photon emission computed tomography. *European Journal of Nuclear Medicine*, 19:1032–1037, 1992.

[3] J. Declerck, J. Feldmar, M. Goris, and F. Betting. Automatic Registration and Alignment on a Template of Cardiac Stress & Rest SPECT Images. Technical Report 2770, INRIA, Feb. 1996.

[4] J. Declerck, G. Subsol, J.-P. Thirion, and N. Ayache. Automatic Retrieval of Anatomical Structures in 3D Medical Images. In *Computer Vision, Virtual Reality and Robotics in Medicine*, volume 905 of *Lecture Notes in Computer Science*, pages 153–162. Springer-Verlag, Apr. 1995. (Also INRIA Research Report # 2485).

[5] J. Feldmar and N. Ayache. Rigid, Affine and Locally Affine Registration of Free-Form Surfaces. *International Journal of Computer Vision*, In press. (Also INRIA Research Report # 2220).

[6] E. Garcia, J. Maddahi, D. Berman, and A. Waxman. Space/time quantitation of Thallium-201 myocardial scintigraphy. *Journal of Nuclear Medicine*, 22:309–317, 1981.

[7] G. Germano, P. Kavanagh, and H. Su. Automatic Reorientation of three-dimensional transaxial myocardial perfusion SPECT images. *Journal of Nuclear Medicine*, 36:1107–1114, 1995.

[8] M. Goris, S. Boudier, and P. Briandet. Interrogation and display of single photon emission tomography data as inherently volume data. *American Journal of Physiologic Imaging*, 1:168–180, 1986.

[9] M. Goris, S. Boudier, and P. Briandet. Two-dimensional mapping of three-dimensional SPECT data: a preliminary step to the quantitation of Thallium myocardial perfusion single photon emission tomography. *American Journal of Physiologic Imaging*, 2:176–180, 1986.

[10] M. Goris, J. Sue, and M. Johnson. A principled approach to the "circumferential" method for Thallium myocardial perfusion scintigraphy quantitation. In *Noninvasive assessment of the cardiovascular system: diagnostic principle and techniques*. Edward P. Diethrich, John Wright, PSG, Inc., 1982.

[11] A. Houston, P. Kemp, and M. MacLeod. A method for assessing the significance of abnormalities in HMPAO brain SPECT images. *Journal of Nuclear Medicine*, 35:239–244, 1994.

[12] J. Maddahi, K. Van Train, and F. Pringent. Quantitative single photon emission computed Thallium-201 tomography for detection and localization of coronary artery disease: optimization and prospective validation of new technique. *Journal of Am Coll Cardiol*, 14:1689–1699, 1989.

[13] J. Mahmarian, T. Boyce, and R. Goldberg. Quantitative exercise Thallium-201 single photon emission computed tomography for the enhanced diagnosis of ischemic heart disease. *Journal of Am Coll Cardiol*, 15:318–329, 1990.

[14] O. Monga, R. Deriche, and J. Rocchisani. 3D edge detection using recursive filtering: application to scanner images. *Computer Vision Graphics and Image Processing*, Jan. 1991.

[15] R. Mullick and N. Ezquerra. Automatic Determination of LV Orientation from SPECT data. *IEEE Transactions on Medical Imaging*, 14(1):88–99, Mar. 1995.

[16] C. Perault, H. Wampach, and J. Liehn. Three-dimensional SPECT myocardial Rest-Stress substraction images after automated registration and normalization. In K. A. Publisher, editor, *Proceedings of Information Processing and Medical Imaging*, volume 3, pages 391–392, June 1995.

[17] J.-J. Risler. *Méthodes Mathématiques pour la CAO*. Masson, 1991.

[18] P. Slomka, G. Hurwitz, J. Stephenson, and T. Cradduck. Automated alignment and sizing of myocardial Stress and Rest scans to three-dimensional normal templates using an image registration algorithm. *Journal of Nuclear Medicine*, 36:1115–1122, 1995.

[19] S. Strother, J. Anderson, K. Schaper, J. Sidtis, J. Liow, R. Woods, and D. Rottenberg. Principal Component Analysis and the Scaled Subprofile Model Compared to Intersubject Averaging and Statistical Parametric Mapping: I. "Functional Connectivity" of the Human Motor System Studied with O-15 Water PET. *Journal of Cerebral Blood Flow and Metabolism*, 15:738–753, 1995.

[20] J.-P. Thirion. Fast Non-rigid Matching of 3D Medical Images. Technical Report RR 2547, INRIA, May 1995.

[21] K. Van Train, E. Garcia, and J. Maddahi. Improved quantitation of stress/redistribution Tl-201 scintigrams and evaluation of normal limits. In *IEEE transactions on Computers in Cardiology*, 1982.

[22] A. Venot, J. Liehn, J. Lebruchec, and J. Roucayrol. Automated Comparison of Scintigraphic Images. *Journal of Nuclear Medicine*, 27:1337–1342, 1987.

[23] R. Vogel. Quantitative aspects of myocardial perfusion imaging. *Seminars in Nuclear Medicine*, 10:146–155, 1980.

[24] R. Woods, J. Mazziotta, and S. Cherry. MRI-PET registration with automated algorithm. *Journal of Computer Assisted Tomography*, 17:536–546, 1993.

[25] Z. Zhang. Iterative point matching for registration of free-form curves and surfaces. *International Journal of Computer Vision*, 13(2):119–152, Dec. 1994. Also INRIA Research Report #1658.

An Automated Algorithm for Analysis of 2-D Echocardiographic Short-Axis Images: A Brief Overview

David C. Wilson, Edward A. Geiser,
Donald A. Conetta, James M. Murphy, and Dongxing Wang
Department of Medicine
Division of Cardiology
University of Florida
Gainesville, FL 32611
dcw@math.ufl.edu

Abstract

The purpose of this report is to present a brief overview of a computer-based method designed to automatically approximate the epicardial and endocardial borders of the heart for echocardiographic images acquired from the parasternal transthoracic short-axis view. The only user input required is the end diastolic (ED) and end systolic (ES) frame numbers. The method was tested off-line on a developmental database acquired retrospectively from 55 patient studies (2 cycles/patient). The measurements provided by the computer-based method were comparable to those made by 3 expert observers.

1. Introduction

While linear measurements of chamber diameter, and regional wall thickness are frequently made in the clinical setting, time and cost factors discourage the calculation of the chamber area, wall motion, and fractional area change (FAC). The purpose of this report is to briefly describe and evaluate a computer-based algorithm designed to automatically approximate the epicardial and endocardial borders for echocardiographic image sequences acquired from the parasternal transthoracic short-axis view. The only user input required is the the image frame number in the cardiac cycle for the frame at end diastole (ED) and at end systole (ES). Once the borders have been found, the estimation of the two dimensional indicators of cardiac health is immediate. Since the method must produce reliable estimates over a broad range of images, it must be able to not only distinguish endocardium from papillary muscles and mitral valve apparatus, it must be able to also track the myocardium as it contracts, rotates, and translates through a sequence of images despite the fact that part of the signal may have disappeared or changed appearance from one frame to another.

Since the methods of measurement are intended for use in the clinical setting where observers provide the standard, observer estimates are used in the testing and evaluation. Thus, the hypothesis to be tested is: "If measurements made by a computer-based method cannot be distinguished by those made by a number of expert observers, then the new method can be used to replace the observers." While there are numerous ways to quantify this comparison, the results of the algorithm are evaluated on 55 patients (2 cycles/patient) by comparing with measurements made by 3 expert observers using a modification of a method described by Bland and Altman [1] in 64 radial directions emanating from the center of the LV.

2. Overview of the Algorithm

The following steps provide an overview of the algorithm. The details will be discussed in the section 3.

1. Digitize image sequence from video tape for off-line analysis.

2. Determine ED and ES frame numbers.

3. Identify acquisition device.

4. Identify sector scan.

5. Approximate epicardial borders and center point of the LV.

6. Create transformation to polar coordinates.

7. Form 64 radial intensity distributions from the center of the LV.

222

Proceedings of MMBIA '96

8. Form 64 radial Laplace masks from the center of the LV.

9. Use information from radial Laplace masks to identify the endocardial border.

Steps (1) and (2) are performed by a technician or a cardiologist. They are the only processes needed to activate the algorithm. After the ED and ES frame numbers are determined, the algorithm first identifies the device type (3) and the sector scan (4). The search region for the epicardial border is therefore restricted to the interior of the sector scan.

Within the region defined by the sector scan, several large elliptical-arc filters are implemented to estimate the epicardial border. The center of the LV is defined to be the center of the smallest rectangle containing the epicardial contour. Next, a transformation from polar to Cartesian coordinates is established. For a high resolution image (see section 3.1.), the region enclosed by a large circle of radius 150 pixels is divided into 64 equiangular sectors. A normalized intensity histogram is formed for each of the 64 sectors by averaging the pixel intensities across a small circular arc (7). In addition, a binary image is computed by implementing a Laplace-type filter on the computed normalized intensity histogram (8). Using a priori assumptions of the parasternal short-axis view, a variety of different techniques are used to detect key points on the endocardial border in eight equiangular radial directions (9).

3. Methods

The purpose of this section is to describe the computer-based algorithm for estimating the epicardial and endocardial borders during systole. While many details are presented, it is impossible to explain all the reasons behind the decision making. Many of the decisions are made using a priori knowledge and experience that may not be immediately evident.

3.1. Image Acquisition

All parasternal short-axis images in the developmental database were acquired by digitizing from video tape in blocks of 16 frames on the Nova Microsonics ImageVue II DCR using the high resolution ($480 \times 512 \times 1$) option. After acquisition, the image data was transferred to an IBM RS6000 workstation and stored on a disk drive. The image data set includes 55 patient studies with 2 cycles/patient for a total of 110 sequences. This data set, consisting of image sequences selected on the basis of image quality, is the same as that discussed by Wilson, Geiser, et. al. [2, 3].

A excellent quality image in the database is shown in Figure 1. Note that the papillary muscles are close to the endocardial border.

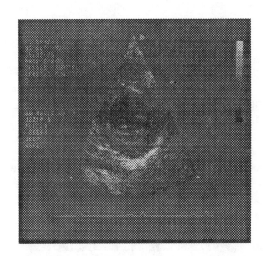

Figure 1. A Typical Short-axis Image

3.2. Assumptions

The following assumptions were made when designing the algorithm.

1. The image is acquired as a transthoracic parasternal short axis image at or near the mid-papillary level.

2. The epicardial and endocardial borders are close to elliptical shapes except possibly across the septum.

3. The center line of the epicardial border is assumed to be within 30° of a vertical line through the center of the LV.

4. The image of the myocardium is of "reasonable size" (cf. section 3.3).

5. The epicardial border along the posterior wall is consistently the most prominent feature in the image.

6. The epicardial border tends to be more prominent than the endocardial border.

When images are acquired using the parasternal short axis view, assumption 2 is usually reasonable. Assumption 3 requires an operator to adjust the transducer appropriately. Assumption 4 can be satisfied by choosing an appropriate depth setting. Assumption 5 is fundamental in identifying the region of interest, which has been discussed previously by Wilson and Geiser [2, 3].

3.3. Sector Scan and Device Types

After the image sequence has been acquired for the systolic portion of the cycle, the user must determine the ED and ES frame numbers. The first step in the algorithm is to determine the device used to acquire the frames. This task is accomplished by checking the location of the colorbar, patient data, and special symbols particular to a certain manufacture's device. The second step is to identify the "background" intensity in the image. The third step is to use a Hough transform together with the background intensity to find the 2 straight lines delineating the sides of the sector. The last step is to identify the elliptical arc comprising the bottom of the sector.

Note that it is always assumed that the LV is enclosed in the sector scan. The fourth assumption given in section 3.2 is that the diameter of the epicardial contour is greater than half the distance between the vertex of the scan and the point of the epicardium furthest from the transducer.

3.4. Epicardial Borders and LV Center Points

The following list indicates the steps used to approximate the epicardial border and the center point of the LV for each frame.

1. Compute posterior circular-arc filter.

2. Compute left and right elliptical-arc filters.

3. Compute anterior elliptical-arc filters.

4. Compute multiple center points.

5. Recompute left and right elliptical-arc filters.

6. Estimate the epicardial border.

Since it has been observed that the interface between the epicardium and the pericardium is invariably the most prominent feature in the image, the first step in border finding is to search for the posterior epicardial estimate [2, 3]. No assumption is made except that the heart is within the sector. The circular arc filters are designed to fit the curved concave up epicardial/pericardial interface along the posterior wall. Another observation of short-axis 2-D echocardiograms has been that the image quality of the frames near ES are better than the image quality of the frames near ED, hence these filters are computed for all frames in the cycle beginning with the ES frame and proceeding backward through time to the ED frame. To reduce computation time and prevent discontinuities in the estimate from one frame to the next, the filters are only computed near the best estimate found in the ES frame. The best posterior estimates are denoted by (x_0, y_p), where x_0 is the same for all frames. The centerline given by the equation $x = x_0$ is the line through the center of the LV and is determined as the column occurring most consistently in these posterior estimates. If the patient's heart exhibits lateral translation during the cycle, then this centerline will also translate.

The second step in border finding is to make a first approximation of the epicardial borders along the lateral walls.

These estimates are above and to the right and left of the best posterior epicardial estimate (x_0, y_p). As with the posterior estimates, these computations are made beginning with the ES frame and proceed backward through time. Since the appearance of the heart in the image may not be a perfect circle, the filters used are elliptical, where the ellipses are symmetric about the centerline and use the posterior estimate (x_0, y_p) to approximate the semi-major axis(ie, the two distances $x_r - x_0$ and $x_0 - x_l$ in Figure 2).

The third step in border finding is to compute the anterior epicardial estimate using elliptical-arc filters together with the right and left estimates. Once again, the computations are made beginning with the ES frame and proceed backward through time.

The fourth step is to determine the center point of the LV. This location is calculated as the point

$$(x_0, y_0) = (x_0, \frac{y_a + y_p}{2}),$$

where y_a is the row occurring most consistently in the anterior estimates and y_p is the associated posterior estimate. In order to track the horizontal translation, the posterior estimates of frame ED and ES are refined. The idea is to define a small window $[x_0 - 5, x_0 + 15] \times [y_p - 1, y_p + 1]$ and call step 1 again in this small region for ED and ES. Suppose the modified center lines are $x = x_{ED}$ for frame ED and $x = x_{ES}$ for frame ES, respectively, then the column of the center line of frame k is defined as

$$x_k = \frac{(k - k_{ES}) * x_{ED} + (k_{ES} - k) * x_{ED}}{k_{ES} - k_{ED}}.$$

The fifth step is to recompute the right and left epicardial elliptical-arc filters, the centers are now the points (x_k, y_0). The filter is actually the integration of two elliptical-arc filters, one from the portion of the image above the center point (ie, the line $y = y_0$.) and one from the portion of image below the center point. The equation of the upper ellipse is based on the point (x_k, y_a), while the equation of the lower ellipse is based on the point (x_k, y_p). Denote the best right and left epicardial estimates by (x_r, y_0) and (x_l, y_0), respectively. Finally, the sixth step is to form the epicardial border for each frame as the union of four elliptical arcs spliced together from the four points (x_k, y_p), (x_r, y_0), (x_k, y_a), and (x_l, y_0).

The notations for four key epicardial points and the center point can be seen in Figure 2. Note that x_0 is written as $X0$, y_0 as $Y0$, etc.

An estimation of the epicardial border and the center point of Figure 1 is shown in Figure 3. Note that the intensity along the posterior wall is extremely high compared to other parts of the image.

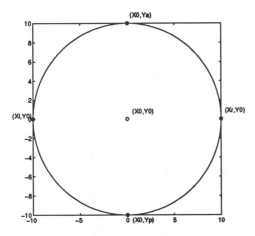

Figure 2. Four Key Points of Epicardial Border

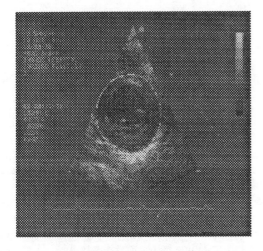

Figure 3. Epicardial Border for LV

3.5. The Endocardial Borders

After the center point and the epicardial border of each frame are computed, a coordinate transformation from polar to Cartesian formats is established. With the lookup table associated with this transformation, the Normalized Radial Intensity Distributions (NRID) and Radial Binary Laplace Masks (RBLM) are created using the estimated center points. A technique effectively using NRID and RBLM is then employed to detect the endocardial border within the region of interest defined by the estimated epicardial borders. The following list indicates the main steps for extracting the endocardial border.

1. Establish coordinate transformation.

2. Form NRID and RBLM using the estimated center points.

3. Use NRID and RBLM to refine the anterior and posterior epicardium.

4. Use NRID and RBLM to compute the anterior endocardium.

5. Use RBLM to compute the posterior endocardium.

6. Use NRID to compute the epicardial and endocardial septum.

7. Use RBLM to adjust the epicardial borders along the lateral walls.

8. Use RBLM to compute the endocardial borders along the lateral walls.

3.6. Transformation to Polar Coordinates

When a 2-dimensional image of the LV is acquired from a parasternal short axis view, the epicardial and endocardial borders can be reasonably approximated by a model spliced together from 4 elliptical arcs. Since the primary motion of the endocardial border is towards the center point of the LV, an analysis carried out along the radial direction is more effective for tracking the endocardial border through time.

The transformation P from polar coordinates to Cartesian is defined by

$$P(r, j) = \{(X_{r,j}, Y_{r,j})\},$$

where $X_{r,j} = \lfloor r * cos(j\theta) \rfloor$, $Y_{r,j} = \lfloor r * sin(j\theta) \rfloor$, and r and j are integers, $0 \leq r \leq R$, $0 \leq j \leq n_s$, $\theta = 360°/n_s$. (The notation $\lfloor x \rfloor$ means the truncation of x to its nearest integer.) The parameters R and n_s are defined as 150 and 512, respectively. Since the diameters of the epicardial contours are infrequently larger than 40mm and since the dimensions of a pixel are roughly $0.5mm \times 0.4mm$, respectively, the mapping P with $R = 150$ and $n = 512$ will guarantee that virtually all of the points within the estimated epicardial border are sampled.

Note that P is a subset of a circle centered at the origin and with radius R. For any point $p_0 = (X_0, Y_0)$, define

$$P + p_0 = \{(X_{i,j} + X_0, Y_{i,j} + Y_0), (X_{i,j}, Y_{i,j}) \in P\}.$$

Assuming p_k is the center point of frame k, further processing will be conducted only in the set $P + p_k$. The reason for adopting an indirect mapping from polar to Cartesian format is that the motion of the center point from ED to ES is considered in the algorithm. A mapping like P therefore works for all frames and can be saved as a lookup table for later reference.

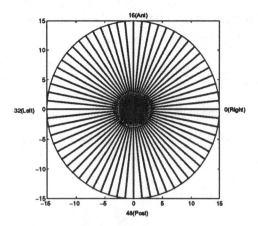

Figure 4. Numbering of Equiangular Sectors

3.7. Histogram Creation

After the LV center point of each frame is computed, a disk of radius 150, centered at the estimated center point, is selected for each frame. The disk is then divided into 64 equiangular sectors, which are graphically displayed in Figure 4.

The tripley indexed array NRID[i][j][r] is filled for each frame i, each sector j, and each radius r by averaging the values on 9 rays emanating from the center of the LV. In other words, sector j is the set

$$S_j = \{(X_{i,l}+X_{0,k}, Y_{i,l}+Y_{0,k}) : 0 \le i \le R, 8j \le l \le 8j+8\},$$

where, $(X_{0,k}, Y_{0,k})$ is the LV center point for frame k.

If there are n_f image frames from end-diastole to end-systole and the upper limit of the radius is 150, then the dimensions of the array NRID is $n_f \times 64 \times 150$.

In order to use both temporal and spatial information to extract borders, a Laplace filter with variant parameters is employed to separate structure from noise. If $N_{i,j,k} = NRID[i][j][k]$ for frame i, ray j, and radius k, then fill the tripley indexed array T by the rule $T_{i,j,k} =$

$$a * N_{i,j,k} + 2 * (N_{i,j-1,k} + N_{i,j+1,k}) -$$
$$(N_{i,j-1,k+r} + N_{i,j,k+r} + N_{i,j+1,k+r}) - 4 * N_{i,j,k-r} -$$
$$(N_{i-1,j-1,k+r} + N_{i-1,j+1,k+r} + 2 * N_{i-1,j,k-1}) -$$
$$(N_{i+1,j-1,k+r} + N_{i+1,j+1,k+r} + 2 * N_{i+1,j,k-1}),$$

where a is 11 for the intermediate frames ($ED+1$ to $ES-1$) and 7 for the frames at ED or ES and the reach r is adjusted depending on the expected wall thickness. In the formula for $T_{i,j,k}$, all terms with subscript $i-1$ are defined as 0 if frame i is at ED and the terms with subscript $i+1$ are 0 if frame i is at ES.

$$\begin{bmatrix} -1 & -1 & -1 \\ \vdots & \vdots & \vdots \\ 2 & <a> & 2 \\ \vdots & \vdots & \vdots \\ 0 & -4 & 0 \end{bmatrix}$$

Figure 5. The Polar Laplace Template for Frame of Interest

$$\begin{bmatrix} -1 & 0 & -1 \\ \vdots & \vdots & \vdots \\ 0 & <0> & 0 \\ \vdots & \vdots & \vdots \\ 0 & -2 & 0 \end{bmatrix}$$

Figure 6. The Polar Laplace Template for adjacent Frames

Note that the array T is filled by applying a shift-invariant operator L_P to the array $N_{i,j,k}$. The operator L_P is constructed as the union of one template of the type indicated in Figure 5 and either one or two of the type indicated in Figure 6. (One is needed if the frame is at ED or ES and two otherwise.) The masks indicated in Figure 6 are to be computed on the preceding and succeeding frames. The value of the variable a is the same as in formula given for $T_{i,j,k}$. The vertical dots represents the value r.

The array T is used to fill the array RBLM[n][64][150] with the rule that RBLM[i][j][k] is 0 if $T_{i,j,k} \le 10$, and 1 otherwise.

All further processing will be restricted to the two arrays: NRID[][][] and RBLM[][][]. (Thus, the array $T_{i,j,k}$ can now be discarded.) The method used to detect the endocardial border is a combination of thresholding, shrinking the searching windows, and a number of direction oriented techniques. Basically, for the regions without confusing intracavity structures, the array NRID is used to identify radial intensity peaks. Usually, the sectors from 45° to 210° (i.e. rays 8 to 36) satisfy this assumption. For the other sectors, the Laplace mask RBLM provides the crucial information.

The Laplace mask is superimposed on an image (see Figure 1) and displayed in Figure 7. Note that the region of dropout across the septum contains a continuous contour in

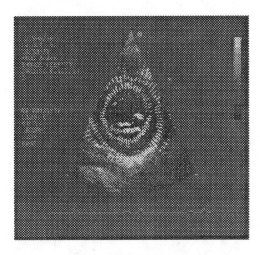

Figure 7. Laplace Mask Imposed on the Original Image

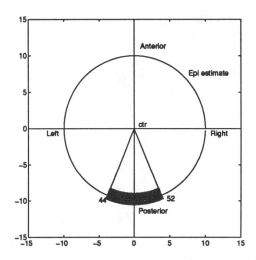

Figure 8. Region for Posterior Epicardial Adjustment

the Laplace Mask. Thus, this operator has the ability to function both as an edge detector and a local threshold operator.

Since even patients with normal function can exhibit small effusions, the array RBLM is used to adjust the epicardial estimate. If the distance between the original posterior epicardium and the center point is d_i for frame i, then the upper band of the searching window is $r_u = (21/20)d_i$. The lower limit of the searching interval is set equal to $r_l = (9/10)d_i$ for the first half of the sequence and $(85/100)d_i$ for the second half of the sequence. A cumulative histogram h_p is computed on RBLM from ray 44 to ray 52 in the defined interval $[r_l, r_u]$. The area marked in Figure 8 is the region for readjusting the initial estimate of the epicardial border along the posterior wall. Since the array RBLM forms a binary image, the histogram h_p has values that range between 0 and 9. The *threshold* is set to be 7 for the first half of the sequence and 6 for the second half. If the histogram at the original estimate of the posterior epicardium, $h_p[d_i]$ is larger than the *threshold*, then adjust d_i to be the first peak of the histogram h_p from r_l to r_u. Here the peak of h_p is defined as the index j such that $h_p[j] \geq max\{threshold, h_p[j-1], h_p[j+1]\}$.

The first step in the computation of the anterior endocardium is to define a search window for each frame. The region for computing the anterior endocardium is marked in the upper part of the Figure 9. Suppose the distance between the anterior epicardium and the center point is d_i for frame i, then the region of the search is set equal to $[d_{ED}/2, (9/10)d_{ED}]$ for ED and $[d_{ES}/3, (9/10)d_{ES}]$ for

ES. For the intermediate frames, the lower and upper limits of the searching interval is a linear average of the corresponding ED and ES limits. The second step for estimating the anterior endocardium is to compute the normalized histogram h_a of a 30° circular arc by averaging ray 13 to ray 19 of the array NRID in the searching window. The threshold is chosen as the sum of the mean and 1/2 of the standard deviation of the histogram. A local peak of the histogram is defined to occur at a distance p from the center if $h_a[p]$ is larger than the threshold and $h_a[p]$ is greater than $h_a[x]$ for $x = p-2, p-1, p, p+1, p+2$. The three largest local peaks in the searching interval are saved and the one with the smallest index (*i.e.* the point is closest to the center) is selected as a candidate for the anterior endocardium. Temporal smoothing and RBLM[][][] are used to refine the anterior estimates. The anterior wall thickness is also estimated by computing the distance between the anterior epicardium and the anterior endocardium.

The first step in the estimation of the posterior endocardial is also the definition of the search window. The region for computing the posterior endocardial position is also shown in Figure 9. For the ED and ES frame, the upper band of the searching interval is the minimum of 9/10 of the epicardial posterior radius, and the radius minus 2/3 of the anterior wall thickness. The lower band of the ES posterior searching region is 1/3 of the posterior epicardial radius, while the lower band of the ED searching region is the maximum of 3/10 of the vertical epicardium diameter and the epicardial posterior radius minus 3/2 of the anterior wall thickness. For the frames between ED and ES, the search regions are the linear average of the regions of ED and ES. For each frame i and each radius r in the search region, a cumulative histogram is computed by summing the values of

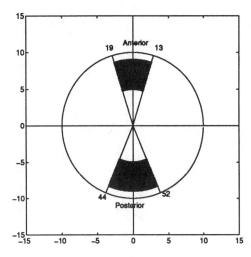

Figure 9. Regions for Computing Anterior and Posterior Endocardium

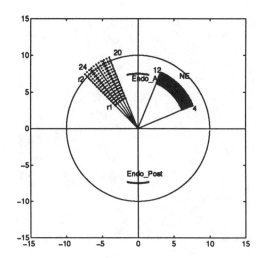

Figure 10. Regions for Computing Septum and Free Wall

RBLM[i][j][r] for $j \in [44, 52]$. The threshold is set equal to 4 for the first half of the sequence and 5 for the second half. Searching towards the center, the algorithm defines the candidate of the endocardial border along the posterior wall to be the first point larger than the threshold. Again, the consistency of the candidates in all frames is checked by the assumption that a border point should not move more than 3mm for two consecutive frames. Posterior wall thickness is computed for all frames after the estimation of the posterior endocardium.

Due to excessive pressure or volume overload from the right ventricle, the epicardial and endocardial borders across the septum represented by rays between 20 and 32 sometimes appear flat. Therefore, summing up an elliptic arc or a circular arc may not accurately estimate the border in this portion of the LV. The approach is to find the midpoint of the septal wall by coupling the search for the epicardial and endocardial structures. Figure 10 shows the search region of the septum. The sectors of interest are rays 20 to 24. As always, a search region needs to be defined in the radial direction. Let the epicardial anterior radius be r_p and the endocardial anterior radius be r_n. In this discussion, the radius means the distance between a specific point and the estimated center point of the LV. The anterior wall thickness is denoted by $t_a = r_p - r_n$. The lower limit for searching for the septal midpoint is $r_l = (9/10)r_n$, while the upper limit is $r_u = (9/10)r_p - t_a/4$. In order to estimate the mid septum radius r_s and the septum wall thickness w_s, the following is computed for each frame i and ray $20 \le j \le 24$,

$$S_{i,j}(k,r) = N_{i,j,k} + 2*(N_{i,j,k+r} + N_{i,j,k-r})$$

$$+ N_{i,j,k+r+1} + N_{i,j,k-r-1}.$$

The estimates r_s and w_s are the values such that

$$S_{i,j}(r_s, w_s/2) =$$

$$max\{S_{i,j}(k,r) : r_l \le k \le r_u, t_a/3 \le r \le (3/5)t_a\}.$$

The midpoint estimates r_s from five rays are then sorted. An estimate is considered consistent with other estimates if it differs no more than 6 units from the previous or the next estimate in the sorted array. Finally, the midpoint estimate which is consistent and closest to ray 24 is chosen as the midpoint estimate of the septum and the associated estimate of the wall thickness w_s is considered to be the septal wall thickness.

For the epicardial border to the left of the center of the LV, a cumulative histogram h_l is computed from radius r_l to r_u using the Laplace mask RBLM by summing up ray 24 to ray 40. The approximate search region is shown on the left side of Figure 11. Each entry in the histogram is an integer between 0 and 17. The threshold is chosen as 12. The lower limit r_l of the search window for the left epicardium is half of the distance between the anterior and posterior endocardium (chamber diameter), while the upper limit r_u is the original epicardial border estimate. If the maximum of $h_l[x]$ for $x = r_l, \ldots, r_u$ is larger than the threshold, then the first estimate of epicardial border is adjusted to the point which attains the maximum.

To evaluate the estimate of the epicardial border to the right of the center point, a region of interest $[r_l, r_u]$ is first defined. This region is indicated in Figure 11. Suppose d_i is the distance of the first estimate of the epicardial border to the right of the center point for frame i, then the lower band

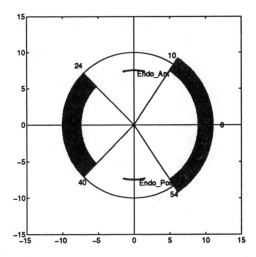

Figure 11. Regions for Epicardial Lateral Wall Readjustment

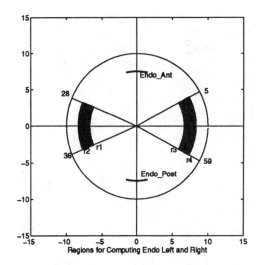

Figure 12. Regions for Computing Lateral Wall Endocardium

r_l is $9d_i/10$ for the first half of the sequence and $85d_i/100$ for the second half. The upper band r_u is defined as $11d_i/10$ for the first half of the sequence and $115d_i/100$ for the second half. Within the interval, a cumulative histogram of the RBLM mask is calculated for the region of ray 0 to ray 10 and ray 54 to ray 64. The value of the histogram is between 0 and 21. The threshold is set to be 15. The readjustment process for this region of the epicardium is the same as the process of adjusting the posterior epicardium.

The last step in the search for the endocardial border is in the region of the lateral walls. Since there are already three wall thickness estimates: anterior, septal and posterior, the median of these three estimates, t_e, is considered as the potential wall thickness of left, right, and in the direction of ray 8. By subtracting t_e from the left and right epicardium, we have the first approximation for the endocardial borders in these regions.

To detect the left endocardium, the radial search region is defined to be $[r-8, r+8]$, where r is the first approximation of the left endocardium. The small band shown in the left side of Figure 12 is the region for computing the left endocardium. The process here is exactly the same as that used in estimating the anterior endocardium except the search region is smaller and the rays of interest are ray 28 to ray 36. If no border is found, the left endocardium remains unaltered from the first estimate.

The first step of extracting the right endocardium is also the definition of the search region. The region of interest is the area containing ray 0 to ray 5 and ray 59 to ray 64. The search limit in radial direction is approximately a 16 pixel

interval centered at the first estimate (cf. Figure 12). The method employed here is the same as the one used to extract the posterior endocardium, except that the threshold for the right endocardium is 5 for the first half of the sequence and 6 for the second half.

After the anterior and right endocardium are computed, the first estimate of the endocardial border in the direction of ray 8 is computed as the midpoint of the elliptical arc connecting the anterior and right endocardial estimates. A 16 pixel search interval is set and centered at the first approximation (cf. Figure 12). The method is the same as the one used for adjusting the right epicardium; that is searching the first peak outward from the center of the LV using rays between 4 and 12. The threshold is 4 for all frames. The method used to identify the endocardium in directions given by ray 40 and ray 54 is similar to the method used to find the posterior endocardium.

Finally, the complete epicardial contours are each formed using a spline fit through the 4 key points, while the endocardial contours are formed using 8 key points. The epicardial and endocardial contours found by the algorithm for the image displayed in Figure 1 are superimposed on the original image and shown in Figure 13.

4. Results and Conclusions

4.1. Results

While it is more typical to present results in terms of uniform or mean border differences, the method used here is

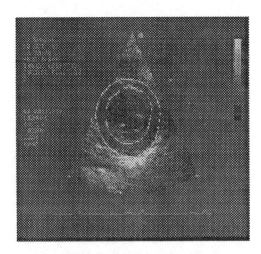

Figure 13. Overlay of ABD Borders

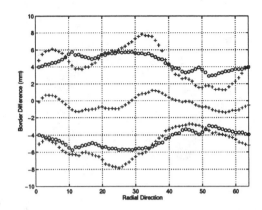

Figure 14. Epicardial Borders at ED: Obs vs ABD

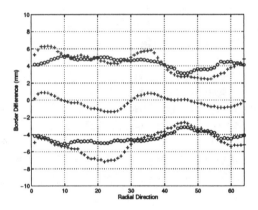

Figure 15. Epicardial Borders at ES: Obs vs ABD

based on confidence intervals in 64 radial directions from the center of the LV. This technique is a variation of a method described by Bland and Altman [1]. It has the benefit of locally integrating the observer and computer estimates. If the confidence intervals for the computer are inside those for the observers, then the new method can replace the observers. In Figures 14-17 the 110 border estimates are compared with those made by 3 expert observers. For all 4 figures the observer borders are plotted using o's and the computer-based borders are plotted using +'s. The middle curve associated with the computer-based borders is the mean of the differences, while the other 2 are the mean ±2SD. The epicardial estimates are compared in Figures 14-15, while the endocardial estimates are compared in Figures 16-17. While it is apparent that the algorithm functions near the level of the observers, it still lacks the consistency of the observers in certain regions. In particular, the comparisons of epicardial estimates show the largest differences in the region of the septum and the RV attachment (directions 10-30) and show the smallest differences along the posterior wall (directions 40-60). The best border comparisons are the endocardial border estimates at ES, where the computer-based methods exhibit less variation than the observers in almost every direction. (Of course, the endocardial contour at ES has the smallest diameter so that in relative terms it remains consistent.) The endocardial border estimates at ED are in good agreement with the observers along the posterior wall (directions 35-64), while some improvement in the region septum and the RV attachment is needed.

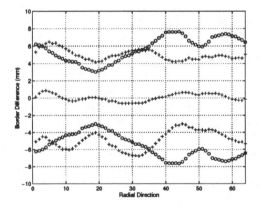

Figure 16. Endocardial Borders at ED: Obs vs ABD

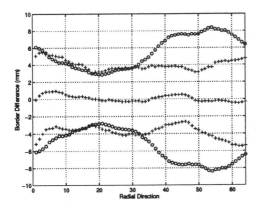

Figure 17. Endocardial Borders at ES: Obs vs ABD

4.2. Conclusions

A computer-based algorithm has been described and evaluated against a serious database of 110 image sequences. While the database consisted of images selected on the basis of image quality, many of the sequences had regions where the epicardium and endocardium was difficult to determine because of noise, other confusing structures, and signal dropout. For these sequences both the observers and automated methods attempted to interpolate across these regions. The observers were able to accomplish this somewhat more consistently than the automated algorithm. In some images the automated method made decisions that were in disagreement with the observers. The next steps are continue to try to improve and test the automated methods and then retest against other more challenging databases containing images of poor quality and that have a greater diversity of image abnormalities represented. However, we already know that the circular arc filter described in section 3.4 has difficulty identifying the epicardial border along the posterior wall for patients with large pericardial effusions. Thus, the method will be of limited utility for patients with this condition. However, even with the imperfections noted, this method consistently and rapidly (in 5-10 seconds on an IBM RISC 6000 workstation) provides measurements that are similar to those of expert observers.

References

[1] J. M. Bland and D. G. Altman, "Statistical methods for assessing agreement between two methods of clinical measurement," *The Lancet*, pp. 307-310, 1986.

[2] D. C. Wilson and E. A. Geiser, *Automatic center point determination in 2-dimensional short-axis echocar-diographic images* Pattern Recognition, vol 25, pp. 893-900, 1992.

[3] D. C. Wilson, E. A. Geiser, and Jun-Hua Li, *Feature extraction in two-dimensional short-axis echocardiographic images* Journal of Mathematical Imaging and Vision, vol 3, pp. 285-298, 1993.

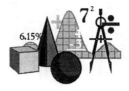

Panel Discussion

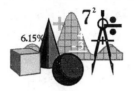

Session 6

Deformable Models II

A Computationally Efficient Shape Analysis via Level Sets

Z. Sibel Göktepe Tari
Mechanical and Industrial Engineering Department
Northeastern University, Boston, MA 02115

Jayant Shah
Mathematics Department, Northeastern University, Boston, MA 02115

Homer Pien
Draper Laboratory, Cambridge, MA 02139

Abstract[1]

In recent years, curve evolution has been applied to smoothing of shapes and shape analysis with considerable success, especially in biomedical image analysis. The multiscale analysis provides information regarding parts of shapes, their axes or centers and shape skeletons. In this paper, we show that the level sets of an edge-strength function provide essentially the same shape analysis as provided by curve evolution. The new method has several advantages over the method of curve evolution. Since the governing equation is linear, the implementation is simpler and faster. The same equation applies to problems of higher dimension. An important advantage is that unlike the method of curve evolution, the new method is applicable to shapes which may have junctions such as triple points. The edge-strength may be calculated from raw images without first extracting the shape outline. Thus the method can be applied to raw images. The method provides a way to approach the segmentation problem and shape analysis within a common integrated framework.

1. Introduction

In recent years, curve evolution has been applied to smoothing of shapes [1,5,13] and shape analysis [6,7,18] with considerable success. The underlying principle is the evolution of a simple closed curve whose points move in the direction of the normal with prescribed velocity. Kimia, Tannenbaum and Zucker [5] proposed evolution of the curve by letting its points move with velocity consisting of two components: a smoothing component proportional to curvature and a constant component corresponding to morphology. Depending on the sign of the

constant component of the velocity, the curve can expand (thus joining two disjoint nearby shapes) or contract (thus separating a dumbbell shape into two separate blobs). The formulation involves one parameter which together with time provides a two-dimensional scale space, called "entropy" scale space of the shape [7]. Keeping track of how singularities develop and disappear as the curve evolves provides information regarding the geometry of the shape in terms of its parts and its skeleton [6,18].

The easiest way to implement curve evolution is by embedding the intial curve as a level curve in a surface and let all the level curves of the surface evolve simultaneously. The advantage is that changes in the topology of the curve are handled automatically, simplifying the data structure. The usual way to embed the curve is by means of the (signed) distance function so that the given curve is defined as the locus of the zero-crossings of the distance function. As the surface evolves, it traces out a three-dimensional volume. Embedded in this volume are the surfaces traced out by the level curves of the initial surface. Numerical scheme of Osher and Sethian [12] may then be used to implement the evolution of the surface. This is how the method is normally used.

In this paper, a simpler and faster method is proposed to obtain essentially the same shape analysis as provided by the method of curve evolution. During the curve evolution, the time t may be thought of as a function over the plane by setting $t(x,y)$ = the time when the evolving curve passes through the point (x,y) if it does and equal to $-\infty$ if it does not, assuming that the evolving curve passes through any point in the plane at most once. Then, the level curves of the surface $t(x,y)$ describe the evolution of the initial curve. (Note however that in a computational framework like the one by Osher and Sethian, the surface $t(x,y)$ is realized as an embedded

[1] This research was partially supported under NIH Grant No. I-R01–NS34189–01.

0-8186-7367-2/96 $5.00 © 1996 IEEE
234
Proceedings of MMBIA '96

surface in a three-dimensional manifold.) In place of the function $t(x, y)$, we propose to use an edge-strength function v whose level curves exhibit properties similar to those of the level curves of t. More specifically, we show that as the constant component of the velocity tends to infinity, the level curves of v obey approximately the same evolution equation as those of t. Function $t(x, y)$ may be thought of as a first order approximation of v. The function v depends on a parameter ρ so that v and ρ parametrize a two-dimensional scale space for the shape analogous to the entropy scale space of Kimia et al. The geometry of the surface defined by v contains information regarding the shape skeleton and the decomposition of the shape into parts.

The alternate framework of the edge-strength function proposed here has a significant computational advantage over curve evolution. First of all, v may be calculated by solving a *linear* diffusion equation which is easy to implement by standard finite difference methods. In contrast, the equation of curve evolution is nonlinear and because the evolving surface develops shocks, standard finite difference methods (for example, central differences) cannot be used. One must use a shock-capturing scheme such as the one proposed by Osher and Sethian in which the direction of the finite difference depends on the direction in which the shock is developing. Secondly, the fact that the surface $t(x, y)$ is realized as the locus of zero-crossings of a three-dimensional manifold adds another layer of computational complexity to the task of locating the singularities of its level curves [18]. Lastly, the new formulation does not require the initial computation of the distance transform.

Another key advantage of the new framework is that it removes the severe restriction imposed by the method of curve evolution on the initial curve, namely, that it must be a simple closed curve. Consequently, the new method may be applied to a collection of curves which need not be disjoint or closed. In particular, the method permits analysis of shapes involving Y-junctions such as the line-drawing of a solid cube and it can be applied to incomplete shape outlines consisting of a collection of disconnected pieces.

Finally, the method proposed here can be applied to raw images and provides an integrated approach to the segmentation problem and shape analysis. A central assumption throughout the discussion above is that the shape outline is already extracted in the form of a closed curve from the raw image. This of course is not an easy task if the image is noisy. A number of recent papers [3,4,8,9,14,15,19] has been devoted to shape recovery from raw images by the method of curve evolution. (See [16] for a discussion and a generalization of these methods.) However, one may calculate the edge-strength function corresponding to shape boundaries directly from the raw image without first segmenting it or resorting to curve evolution for shape recovery. The level curves of this edge-strength function may then be analyzed for shape information. The prime example of such an edge-strength function is the one constructed by Ambrosio and Tortorelli [2] for approximating a segmentation functional.

This paper is organized as follows. In §2, we review curve evolution. The edge–strength function and interpretation of its level curves as a scale space for shapes are described in §3 with illustrative examples. In §4, we define shape skeleton and shape decomposition and show the results for several test cases. In §5, we briefly describe the Ambrosio-Tortorelli approximation of a segmentation functional and apply it to analyze an MRI image.

2. A Review of Curve Evolution

Let Γ be a simple closed curve in the plane. Let $C(p, t) : I \times [0, \infty) \rightarrow \mathbf{R}^2$ be the evolving family of curves where I is the unit interval and t denotes time. (In practice, $\mathbf{R}^2$ is replaced by a bounded domain such as a square.) We require that $C(0, t) = C(1, t)$ for all values of t and the image of $C(p, 0)$ coincides with Γ. Let N denote the inward normal and κ the curvature which is defined such that it is positive when Γ is a circle. Then the evolution of the curve moving inward with velocity $= \alpha + \kappa$ where α is a constant is governed by the equation

$$(1) \qquad \frac{\partial C}{\partial t} = [\alpha + \kappa]N$$

In order to implement the evolution of Γ, assume that Γ is embedded in a surface $f_0 : \mathbf{R}^2 \rightarrow \mathbf{R}$ as the locus of its zero-crossings. For the sake of definiteness, assume that $f_0 < 0$ inside Γ. Let $f(t, x, y)$ denote the evolving surface such that $f(0, x, y) = f_0(x, y)$. Then, in order to let all the level curves of f_0 evolve simultaneously, let f evolve according to the equation (see [6])

$$(2) \qquad \frac{\partial f}{\partial t} = -[\alpha + curv(f)] \|\nabla f\|$$

where

$$(3) \qquad curv(f) = \frac{f_y^2 f_{xx} - 2 f_x f_y f_{xy} + f_x^2 f_{yy}}{\left(f_x^2 + f_y^2\right)^{3/2}}$$

$curv(f)$ is the curvature of the level curves of f. The locus of zeros of $f(x, y, t)$ describes the evolution of Γ.

3. Edge-Strength Function and Scale Space of a Shape

Again, let Γ be a curve in the plane, not necessarily a simple closed curve. We consider the following functional introduced by Ambrosio and Tortorelli [2]:

$$(4) \qquad \Lambda_\rho(v) = \frac{1}{2} \int \int \left\{ \rho \|\nabla v\|^2 + \frac{v^2}{\rho} \right\} dx dy$$

subject to the boundary condition $v = 1$ along Γ. The functional is designed so that as the parameter $\rho \to 0$, $\min \Lambda_\rho(v)$ tends to the length of Γ. The equation of steepest gradient descent for the functional is the linear diffusion equation:

$$(5) \qquad \frac{\partial v}{\partial \tau} = \nabla^2 v - \frac{v}{\rho^2}$$

which is easier to implement than equation (2).

Let v denote the unique minimizer of the functional Λ_ρ. Then, v varies between 0 and 1 and for sufficiently small values of ρ,

$$(6) \qquad v \approx e^{-\frac{d}{\rho}}$$

where d is the (unsigned) distance from Γ. Thus, v may be thought as a blurred version of Γ and ρ as the blurring radius.

In order to relate v to curve evolution, assume that Γ is a simple, closed curve. As shown in Appendix (3) of [11], inside Γ,

$$(7) \qquad v(x,y) = -\rho \left(1 + \frac{\rho \kappa(x,y)}{2} \right) \frac{\partial v}{\partial n}(x,y) + O(\rho^3)$$

where $\kappa(x,y)$ is the curvature of the level curve of v passing through the point (x,y) and n is the direction of the inward normal. Therefore, if we imagine moving from a level curve to a level curve along the normals, then for small values of ρ, a change of Δv in level requires movement

$$(8) \qquad \Delta r \approx -\frac{\rho}{v} \left(1 + \frac{\rho \kappa}{2} \right) (\Delta v)$$

where r denotes the arc length along the gradient lines of v, (the positive direction being the direction of the inward normals). Let $\Delta t = -\frac{\rho^2 \Delta v}{2v}$. (Notice that v is a decreasing function in the direction of the inward normal so that Δv is negative. Functions v and t have the same set of level curves because t is a monotonic function of v.) Passing to the infinitesimals, we get the velocity:

$$(9) \qquad \frac{dr}{dt} \approx \frac{2}{\rho} + \kappa$$

in agreement with equation (1).

A similar argument shows that for moving outward from Γ, the velocity is given by the formula

$$(10) \qquad \frac{dr}{dt} \approx -\frac{2}{\rho} + \kappa$$

That is, the sign of the morphology component of the velocity is reversed. Consequently, the totality of the level curves of v, outside and inside of Γ cover a range of positive and negative values of α in equation (2). However, the proposed method does not extend to the limiting cases, namely, the case of pure morphological evolution obtained by omitting from (1) the curvature term (that is, the limit as $\alpha \to \infty$) and the case of pure smoothing obtained by setting $\alpha = 0$. This is not a serious disadvantage. On one hand, pure morphological evolution is very sensitive to noise which makes inclusion of the curvature term essential; on the other hand, pure smoothing shrinks every shape to a single "round" point and it seems perceptually unnatural to reduce shapes which deviate a great deal from being a circle – shapes such as dumbbells and spirals – to a single point.

Figure 1 shows the scale space obtained by our method for three different shapes. (All the figures in this paper except the figure of a doll in Figure 2 were represented on a 256×256 lattice. The doll figure was on a 128×128 lattice.) The two top rows show the level curves for a duck with ρ equal to 4 and 32. The stronger smoothing effect due to the higher value of ρ is clearly visible. The bottom row of the figure depicts the level curves for the line drawing of a solid cube and a pair of pliers, illustrating the applicablity of the method when the initial shape has junctions and self-intersections.

Figure 2 shows how various shapes evolve and decompose. We used doll and hand image for the purpose of comparison with similar description by the standard curve evolution [7]. Qualitatively, the two descriptions are indistinguishable.

4. Shape Skeleton and Shape Decomposition

In a purely morpholgical evolution, singularities develop as corners and self-intersections form. The locus of these singularities is called the skeleton of the shape. When smoothing is introduced, self-intersections still may develop (due to thinning of narrow necks), but the corners are rounded out. Therefore, when smoothing is present, points of maximum curvature serve as a substitute for corners. In the case of the standard curve evolution, the points of maximum curvature correspond to the points of maximum velocity. Even though this is only approximately true in our formulation, it provides an alternative way of defining shape skeleton, namely, by determining points where $|\nabla v|$ is minimum. (Note that, from Equations (7), (8) and (9), $\frac{dr}{dt} \cdot \left| \frac{\partial v}{\partial n} \right| = \frac{2v}{\rho^2}$ and so maximum velocity corresponds to minimum gradient.) We prefer this alternative because computation of curvature involves second derivatives of v and hence it is more sensitive to noise than $|\nabla v|$.

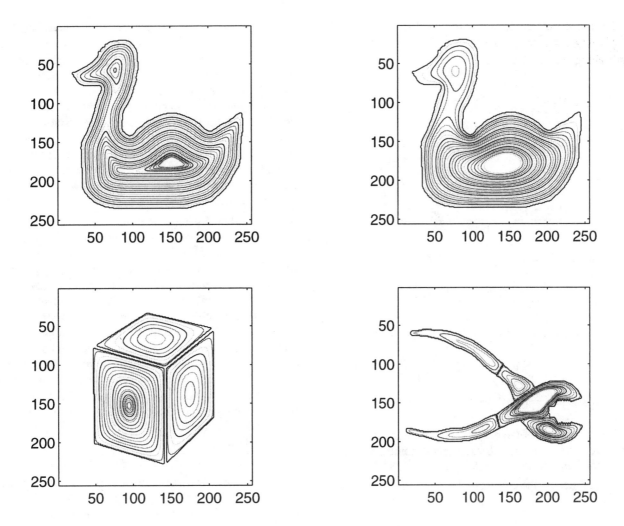

Figure 1: Level Curves
In the top two figures level curves of the duck are shown for the ρ values 4 and 32. The smoothing effect of higher ρ is visible. The two figures on the bottom show the level curves of a line drawing of a solid cube and pliers for ρ = 16. The method is applicable to shapes with triple points and self-intersections.

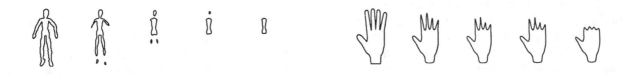

Figure 2: Evolution
The evolution of doll and hand shapes are shown for ρ=4. Qualitatively the behavior is not distinguishable from the behavior of the standard curve evolution. *(We thank B. Kimia and H. Tek from Brown University for the doll image.)*

Let K^+ denote the closure of the set of zero-crossings of $\frac{d|\nabla v|}{ds}$ where $\frac{d^2|\nabla v|}{ds^2}$ is positive. Here, s denotes the arclength along the level curves.

$$(11) \quad \begin{aligned} \frac{d|\nabla v|}{ds} &= v_{\eta\xi} \\ \frac{d^2|\nabla v|}{ds^2} &= v_{\eta\xi\xi} + \frac{v_{\xi\xi}(v_{\xi\xi} - v_{\eta\eta})}{|\nabla v|} \end{aligned}$$

where

$$(12) \quad \begin{aligned} v_{\eta\xi} &= \frac{\left\{ (v_y^2 - v_x^2)v_{xy} - v_x v_y(v_{yy} - v_{xx}) \right\}}{|\nabla v|^2} \\ v_{\xi\xi} &= \frac{\left\{ v_y^2 v_{xx} - 2v_x v_y v_{xy} + v_x^2 v_{yy} \right\}}{|\nabla v|^2} \\ v_{\eta\eta} &= \frac{\left\{ v_x^2 v_{xx} + 2v_x v_y v_{xy} + v_y^2 v_{yy} \right\}}{|\nabla v|^2} \\ v_{\eta\xi\xi} &= \frac{1}{|\nabla v|^3} \{ v_x v_y^2 v_{xxx} + v_y(v_y^2 - 2v_x^2)v_{xxy} \\ &\quad + v_x(v_x^2 - 2v_y^2)v_{xyy} + v_x^2 v_y v_{yyy} \} \end{aligned}$$

(Interestingly, $\frac{1}{|\nabla v|} \frac{d|\nabla v|}{ds}$ is the curvature of the gradient lines.)

Points where the (signed) curvature attains its minimum are also of interest because such points indicate indentations and necks. Therefore,

let K^- denote the closure of the set of zero-crossings of $\frac{d|\nabla v|}{ds}$ where $\frac{d^2|\nabla v|}{ds^2}$ is negative.

Let $K = K^+ \cup K^-$.

Let S denote the set of points where $|\nabla v| = 0$.

The direction of evolution at each point of K is the direction of decreasing v. For a perfect circle, K^+ and K^- are empty and S consists of a single point which is the unique minimum of v. A simple closed curve may be thought of as a deformation of a circle by means of protrusions and indentations. As it evolves towards a more circular shape, K^+ tracks evolution of its protrusions while K^- tracks evolution of its indentations. During the evolution, a protrusion might merge with an indentation, ($d|\nabla v|/ds = d^2|\nabla v|/ds^2 = 0$), joining a branch of K^+ with a branch K^- and terminating both the branches. Of course, more complicated merges between the branches of K^+ and the branches of K^- are also possible and in such a case, a new branch might start from the junction. It is also possible that a branch might bifurcate. This typically happens just before a thinning neck breaks up. As two indentations begin to evolve towards each other, each one gives rise to a branch of K^-. However, as the indentations approach a break-point, they interact and slow down the rate of decay of v. Each branch of K^- splits into three

branches, the middle branch belongs to K^+ and continues towards the break–point while the other two belong to K^-. If a branch is not terminated at a junction, then it will terminate at a point in S. If the point is a minimum point of v, then the evolution has come to rest at that point and it is appropriate to call such a point the center of a part. If the point is not a minimum, then it may signify a change in the topology of the evolving curve, that is, break-up of the shape due to a thinning neck. If the point signifies a change in the topology of the shape, we will call it a saddle point. There are at least two branches of K^+ leaving such a point.

In differential geometric terms, a point in S is either elliptic, hyperbolic and parabolic depending on whether the determinant of the hessian of v, $v_{xx}v_{yy} - v_{xy}^2$, is positive, negative or zero respectively. An elliptic point is always a center and a hyperbolic point is always a saddle point. Parabolic points are more troublesome to classify because of their global nature. We have to analyze the branches of K meeting the parabolic point (or the connected component of S containing the parabolic point in case it is not an isolated parabolic point). If we can find at least two branches of K^+ leaving from the connected component of S containing a given parabolic point, then it is a saddle point. If all the branches of K meeting the connected component containing the parabolic point lead into it, it is a center.

Now we can define the skeleton of a shape.

Definition: The *skeleton* of a shape is the subset of $K^+ \cup S$ which excludes those branches of K^+ which flow into a connected component of S containing a saddle point.

The definition is designed so as exclude the branches of K^+ along which necks of the shape evolve towards a break.

We can also define the segmentation of a shape corresponding to its break-up into parts during evolution due to the presence of narrow necks.

Definition: The segmentation of a shape is the union of branches of K which flow into a saddle point.

Note that since a branch of K^+ may terminate at a junction with a branch of K^-, the skeleton need not be connected. In our description, the skeleton always extends to the boundary while in the purely morphological evolution, a branch starts only after a corner has formed. We could approximate the purely morphological skeleton by deleting from the skeleton defined above all points where the curvature is below a certain threshold. Note also that the definition of segmentation does not deal with protrusions. Significant protrusions such as the fingers of a hand have to be recovered as parts of the shape from the branches of the skeleton.

238

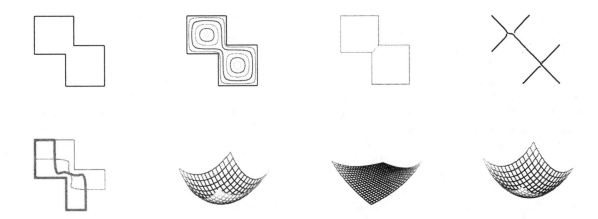

Figure 3:
The top row shows the original shape, its level curves, segmentation and its skeleton. The bottom row shows the singular points. There are three singular points: two eliptic points corresponding to the centers of the squares and one hyperbolic point corresponding to the neck.

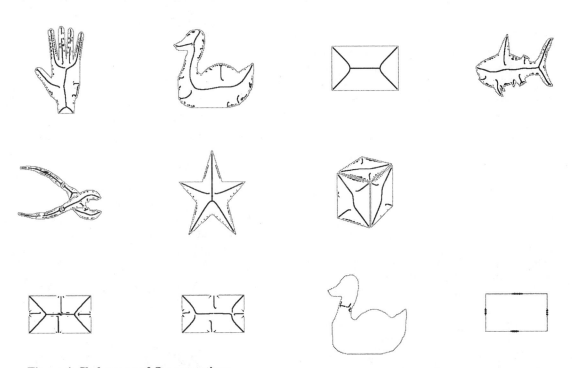

Figure 4: Skeletons and Segmentations
The two rows on the top show the skeletons of various shapes obtained by the method for ρ=16.
The first two figures on the bottom row show the skeleton of an incomplete rectangle for the ρ values 4 and 16. As ρ increases, the branches coming from the gaps terminate earlier. Even for an incomplete contour the skeleton can be obtained. The last two figures on the bottom row show the segmentation. For the incomplete rectangle the segmentation lines actually partition the complement of the shape.

Although the constructions described above were motivated by the example of simple closed curves, they work equally well for more general curves. For example, if the letter C is drawn as an open curve, we can compute its skeleton. If the ends of the letter are sufficiently close, a segmentation line joins the two ends. If the same letter is drawn as a thick shape with a simple closed curve as its boundary, we recover the same information as above and also the medial axis. The point is that v should be computed over the whole plane and the skeleton and the segmentation really describe the complement of Γ. Whether the complement of Γ is connected or not is not relevant to the computation of the skeleton and the segmentation. This property is very useful in particular when the shape boundary is not fully specified. As long as important features of the shape boundary are specified, evolution fills in the gaps and the essential skeleton can be recovered. The missing portions of the boundary are recovered as branches of the segmentation.

This description can be readily translated into the language of the shock grammar of Siddiqi and Kimia [6,18]. The first order shocks are the branches of the skeleton not belonging to S. The second order shocks are the hyperbolic points. The third order shocks correspond to a line of parabolic points. The elliptic points are the fourth order shocks. The rules of the grammar and properties follow easily from the fact that v is monotonically decreasing along the branches of the skeleton and the fact the v is smooth.

In this paper, we have not addressed the issue of assigning a level of significance to each branch of the skeleton and the segmentation. One of the simplest criterion is the "time of extinction", measured in our case by the value of $(1-v)$ when the branch terminates. Another measure of significance could be based on the curvature of the level curves where they intersect the skeleton.

We explain our construction in detail by means of an example of two overlapping squares shown in Figure 3. The shape boundary is given in the top left and next to it are the level curves depicting the evolution of the shape. The shape skeleton (top right) is what one would expect. In the bottom row, we analyze the singularities. The leftmost figure shows the zero–crossings of the x and y derivatives of the edge-strength function v, their intresections corresponding to the singular points where the gradient vanishes. The three figures that follow show the surface corresponding to the edge-strength function in a neighborhood of these singular points. The one in the middle corresponds to the singularity at the neck and the surface at this point is hyperbolic, the other two correspond to the centers of the two squares and the surface there is elliptic.

Figure 4 shows the skeletons and segmentation for various shapes. We get nontrivial segmentation only in the case of the duck figure and the incomplete rectangle. The skeleton for the hand is qualitatively the same as in [18]. The duck is segmented across its neck. Examples of a pair of pliers and the outline of a cube illustrate the effectiveness of the method for complex shapes involving junctions. The incomplete rectangle was obtained by removing a 27 pixel long piece from the middle of each side of the complete rectangle. The skeleton consists of the skeleton of the complete rectangle and four new branches which may be interpreted as the "medial axes" of the gaps in the sides. The larger the value of ρ, the weaker these additional branches. The gaps themselves are filled in by segmentation curves.

In these examples, we didn't do any pruning.

5. Raw Images

Ambrosio and Tortorelli introduced the edge-strength function for obtaining an elliptic approximation of the following segmentation functional introduced in [10]:

(13)
$$E_{MS}(u,B) = \alpha \int \int_{R \setminus B} \|\nabla u\|^2 dx dy$$
$$+ \beta \int \int_R (u-g)^2 dx dy + |B|$$

where R is a connected, bounded, open subset of $\mathbf{R}^2$ (usually a rectangle), g is the feature intensity, B is a curve segmenting R, u is the smoothed image $\subset R \setminus B$, $|B|$ is the length of B and α, β are the weights. Let $\sigma = \sqrt{\alpha/\beta}$. Then, σ may be interpreted as the smoothing radius in $R \setminus B$. With σ fixed, the higher the value of α, the lower the penalty for B and hence, the more detailed the segmentation.

Ambrosio and Tortorelli [2] replace

(14)
$$|B| \text{ by } \frac{1}{2} \int \int_R \left\{ \rho \|\nabla v\|^2 + \frac{v^2}{\rho} \right\} dx dy$$

and

(15)
$$\int \int_{R \setminus B} \|\nabla u\|^2 dx dy \text{ by } \int \int_R (1-v)^2 \|\nabla u\|^2 dx dy$$

The result is the following functional:

(16)
$$E_{AT}(u,v) = \int \int_R \{ \alpha(1-v)^2 \|\nabla u\|^2 $$
$$+ \beta(u-g)^2 + \frac{\rho}{2} \|\nabla v\|^2 + \frac{v^2}{2\rho} \} dx dy$$

As $\rho \to 0$, v converges to 1 at points on B and to zero elsewhere. The corresponding gradient descent equations are:

$$\frac{\partial u}{\partial t} = \nabla \cdot (1-v)^2 \nabla u - \frac{\beta}{\alpha}(u-g)$$

$$(17) \quad \frac{\partial v}{\partial t} = \nabla^2 v - \frac{v}{\rho^2} + \frac{2\alpha}{\rho}(1-v)\|\nabla u\|^2$$

$$\frac{\partial u}{\partial n}|_{\partial R} = 0 \quad \frac{\partial v}{\partial n}|_{\partial R} = 0$$

where ∂R denotes the boundary of R and n denotes the direction normal to ∂R. The solution of these equations gives us the edge-strength function v corresponding to the segmentation locus B without determining B itself.

Notice that equation for each variable is a diffusion equation which minimizes a convex quadratic functional in which the other variable is kept fixed:

Keeping v fixed, the first equation minimizes

$$\int\!\!\int_R \left\{ \alpha(1-v)^2\|\nabla u\|^2 + \beta(u-g)^2 \right\} dx\,dy$$

Keeping u fixed, the second equation minimizes

$$(18) \quad \int\!\!\int_R \{\|\nabla v\|^2$$

$$+ \frac{1 + 2\alpha\rho\|\nabla u\|^2}{\rho^2}\left(v - \frac{2\alpha\rho\|\nabla u\|^2}{1 + 2\alpha\rho\|\nabla u\|^2}\right)^2 \} dx\,dy$$

Thus the edge strength function v is nothing but a nonlinear smoothing of

$$(19) \quad \frac{2\alpha\rho\|\nabla u\|^2}{1 + 2\alpha\rho\|\nabla u\|^2}$$

where u is a simultaneous nonlinear smoothing of g.

Ideally, the edge-strength function v computed from a raw image by equations (17) should be constant along the object boundaries. However this almost never happens due to noise, differing levels of contrast along the object boundaries and the interaction between nearby edges. Therefore, the object boundaries are no longer defined by level curves of v. Typically, we should expect a level curve corresponding to a value of v near its maximum to consist of several connected components, each surrounding a high contrast portion of B. The situation is analogous to the earlier example of the incomplete rectangle

where the shape boundary consists of several disconnected pieces. Note that even in the case of the functional (13), if α is not high enough, then B may not include portions of the object boundary where contrast is too low. The important point is that it is not essential to have the complete shape boundary to compute its essential skeleton. As the evolution progresses, the gaps between the pieces of the boundary are filled in. Thus we still recover an essentially correct skeleton. As the value of α is increased, the skeleton becomes more and more detailed.

In dealing with raw images, the necessity for assigning a level of significance to each branch of the skeleton or the segmentation and for pruning becomes important because of the presence of noise. Since smoothing of the image is minimal near the boundary where v is high, the skeleton tends to be noisier near the boundary. As mentioned before, we have not dealt with this issue in this paper. For the purpose of illustrations in this paper, instead of extracting the skeleton and pruning, we have pruned K^+ near the boundary by simply removing parts of K^+ which have values of v above a manually chosen threshold.

In order to illustrate application of the method to raw images, we present the example shown in Figure 5 and analyze the dark shape in the center of the figure. To compute the edge-strength function by equations (17), we set $\sigma = \rho = 8$ and picked three different values of α, obtaining three different edge-strength functions, v_a, v_b and v_c depicted in the figure. The value of α corresponding to v_a is sufficiently low so that only the corners portions of the central dark area are prominent in the image of v_a. The inner details such as the inner boundaries of the four disjoint corner lobes are smoothed over to a large degree. The value of α was doubled to obtain v_b and doubled again for v_c. At each stage, the edge-strength function becomes more detailed. The figure shows the level curves superimposed on the original image, the set K^+ and its thresholded version as a substitute for the pruned skeleton as explained above. The effect of increasing α is clearly seen in the bottom row of the figure which shows our substitute skeleton. The skeleton in the case of v_a is essentially that of an incomplete rectangle. As α is increased, it becomes more detailed so that the skeleton from v_c depicts the axes of the four lobes more accurately and finds a center for each lobe.

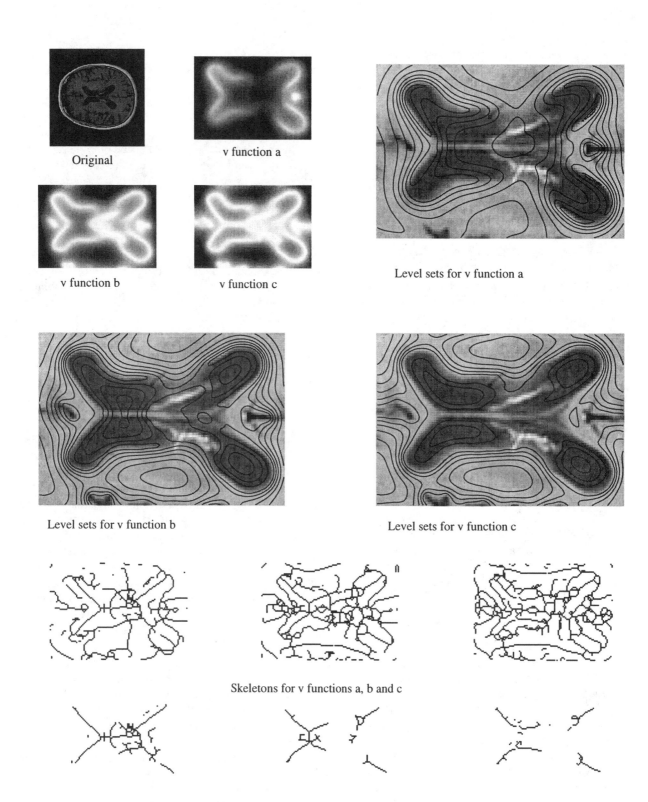

Original

v function a

v function b

v function c

Level sets for v function a

Level sets for v function b

Level sets for v function c

Skeletons for v functions a, b and c

Fig 5: MRI image
(We thank D. Kennedy of the MGH for the mri data)

6. References

[1] L. Alvarez, F. Guichard, P.L. Lions and J.M. Morel: "Axioms and Fundamental Equations of Image Processing", Arch.for Rat.Mech. (1993).

[2] L. Ambrosio and V.M. Tortorelli: "On the Approximation of Functionals depending on Jumps by Quadratic, Elliptic Functionals", Boll. Un. Mat. Ital. (1992)

[3] V. Caselles, F. Catte, T. Coll and F. Dibos: "A Geometric Model for Active Contours", Numerische Mathematik 66, (1993).

[4] V. Caselles, R. Kimmel and G. Sapiro: "Geodesic Active Contours", Fifth International Conference on Computer Vision, (1995).

[5] B.B. Kimia, A. Tannenbaum and S.W. Zucker: "On the Evolution of Curves via a Function of Curvature. I. The Classical Case", J. Math. Anal. and Appl. v.163, no.2, (January, 1992).

[6] B.B. Kimia, A. Tannenbaum and S.W. Zucker: "Shapes, Shocks and Deformations I: The Components of Shape and the Reaction-Diffusion Space", International Journal of Computer Vision, (1992).

[7] B.B. Kimia, A. Tannenbaum and S.W. Zucker: "Entropy Scale-Space", in *Visual Form*, Ed. C. Arcelli et al, Plenum.

[8] S. Kichenassamy, A. Kumar, P. Olver, A. Tannenbaum and A. Yezzi: "Gradient Flows and Geometric Active Contour Models", Fifth International Conference on Computer Vision, (1995).

[9] R. Malladi, J.A. Sethian and B.C. Vemuri: "Shape Modeling with Front Propagation: A Level Set Approach", IEEE-PAMI 17, (1995).

[10] D. Mumford and J. Shah: "Boundary detection by minimizing functionals, I", Proc. IEEE Conf. on Computer Vision and Pattern Recognition, San Francisco (1985)

[11] D. Mumford and J. Shah: "Optimal Approximations by Piecewise Smooth Functions and Associated Variational Problems", Comm. on Pure and Appl.Math., v.XLII, n.5, pp.577-684 (July, 1989).

[12] S. Osher and J. Sethian: "Fronts Propagating with Curvature Dependent Speed: Algorithms based on the Hamilton-Jacobi Formulation", J. Comp. Physics, 79, (1988).

[13] P.J. Olver, G. Sapiro and A. Tannenbaum: "Differential Invariant Signatures and Flows in Computer Vision, A Symmetry Group Approach", Geometry Driven Diffusion in Computer Vision, Kluwer, (1994).

[14] J. Shah: "Uses of Elliptic Approximations in Computer Vision", to appear in *Variational Methods for Discontinuous Structures*, Ed: R. Serapioni and F. Tomarelli, Birkhäuser.

[15] J. Shah: "Shape Recovery from Noisy Images by Curve Evolution" IASTED International Conf. on Signal and Image Processing, (Nov. 1995).

[16] J. Shah: "A Common Framework for Curve Evolution, Segmentation and Anisotropic Diffusion", Proc. IEEE Conf. on Computer Vision and Pattern Recognition, San Francisco (1996).

[17] K. Siddiqi and B.B. Kimia: "Parts of Visual Form: Computational Aspects", IEEE Conf. on Vision and Pattern Recognition, (1993).

[18] K. Siddiqi and B.B. Kimia: "A Shock Grammar for Recognition", Proc. IEEE Conf. on Computer Vision and Pattern Recognition, San Francisco (1996).

[19] H. Tek and B.B. Kimia: "Image Segmentation by Reaction-Diffusion Bubbles", Fifth International Conference on Computer Vision, (1995).

A Geometric Approach to Segmentation and Analysis of 3D Medical Images

R. Malladi,* R. Kimmel,* D. Adalsteinsson,* G. Sapiro,† V. Caselles,‡ J. A. Sethian§

Abstract

A geometric scheme for detecting, representing, and measuring 3D medical data is presented. The technique is based on deforming 3D surfaces, represented via level-sets, towards the medical objects, according to intrinsic geometric measures of the data. The 3D medical object is represented as a (weighted) minimal surface in a Riemannian space whose metric is induced from the image. This minimal surface is computed using the level-set methodology for propagating interfaces, combined with a narrow band technique which allows fast implementation. This computation technique automatically handles topological changes. Measurements like volume and area are performed on the surface, exploiting the representation and the high accuracy intrinsic to the algorithm.

Key words: *Deformable models, minimal surfaces, segmentation, measurements, level sets, narrow-band methods, fast implementation.*

1. Introduction

One of the basic problems in medical imaging is to detect the boundaries of the objects of interest, efficiently represent them, and perform measurements significant for diagnosis, surgery, or other applications. Active contours, initially proposed by Kass *et al.*, and deformable surfaces introduced by Terzopoulos *et al* [44], can be used to solve the first part of this goal, i.e. the segmentation task. These models are based on deforming an initial contour or surface towards the boundary of the object to be detected. The deformation is obtained by minimizing a functional designed such that its (local) minima is obtained at the boundary of the object [4, 44].

Implicit surface-evolution models for medical image segmentation were proposed by Caselles *et al.* [5] and by Malladi *et al.* [28, 29]. In these models, the surface propagates by an implicit velocity containing two terms, one related to the regularity of the deforming shape and the other attracting it to the boundary. The model is given by a geometric flow based on mean curvature motion, and is not the result of minimizing an energy functional. At their core, these models rely on the Osher-Sethian level-set model for evolving surfaces [34, 39]. The level-set approach offers a robust, stable, and efficient numerical algorithm that allows for complex changes in topology, accurate evaluation of curvatures, and straightforward implementation. In addition, fast implementations of this approach were introduced by Adalsteinsson and Sethian [1] and Malladi, Sethian, and Vemuri [30]. In the energy based approach, the flexibility in topology can be obtained only if special tracking procedures are implemented [31, 42]. For details about a wide collection of level-set applications, see [40].

In [6], formal mathematical relation between these two approaches for 2D object detection is shown, proposing the "geodesic active contours." As shown in [6], the geodesic active contours model has the following main properties:

1. It connects energy and curve evolution approaches of active contours.

2. Presents the snake problem as a geodesic computation.

3. Improves existing models as a result of the geodesic formulation.

4. Allows simultaneous detection of interior and exterior boundaries of several objects without special contour tracking procedures.

---

*Mail Stop: 50A-2152, Lawrence Berkeley National Laboratory, University of California, Berkeley, CA 94720

†Hewlett-Packard Labs., 1501 Page Mill Rd., Palo Alto, CA 94304

‡Dept. of Mathematics and Informatics, University of Illes Balears, 07071 Palma de Mallorca, Spain

§Dept. of Mathematics, University of California, Berkeley, CA 94720

244

5. Holds formal existence, uniqueness, and stability results.

6. Stops automatically.

The $2D$ model in [6] was then extended to $3D$ surfaces in [7, 8]. The proposed $3D$ approach has the same important properties as its $2D$ analogous one. The original model in Malladi *et al.* [29] (and in [5]) has also been extended to $3D$ and coupled with fast tube methods for approximating interface position in [24, 27]. In this paper, we combine the model in [7], which is revisited here, with the fast numerical approach first described in [1, 30] and extended to $3D$ in [2, 24, 27] and present a complete approach for $3D$ medical data analysis. Then, following the $2D$ analysis started in [36], we exploit the representation and the high accuracy intrinsic to the algorithm to compute important characteristics such as volume and surface area of the segmented $3D$ medical organs.

We should note that the deformable surfaces model used here is related to a number of previously or simultaneously developed results. It is of course closely related to the works of Terzopoulos and colleagues on energy based deformable surfaces, and the works by Malladi *et al.* and Caselles *et al.* [5, 24, 29]. It is an extension of the $2D$ model derived in [6]; see [7, 8]. The basic equations in this paper, as well as the corresponding $2D$ ones in [6], were simultaneously developed in [20, 21, 41]. In [20, 21], the authors base their approach on gradient flows, while in [41], the development partially follows from the Mumford-Shah segmentation technique [32]. Similar $3D$ models are studied in [45, 46] as well. In [43], the authors work with multiple initializations and multiple parameter-space, partially motivated by the shape theory in [22], using the equations in [5, 28, 29]. In this paper, we develop a complete and fast approach for $3D$ segmentation and area and volumetric measurements on the segmented objects; see Whitaker [46] for fast multi-scale implementation. For more details on the similitude and differences between these approaches, see [6, 7, 8]. The details of tube method for moving $3D$ shapes and a comparison to the traditional full matrix method may be found in [24, 27].

2. Basic approaches of deformable surfaces

The $3D$ deformable surface model was introduced by Terzopoulos *et al.* [44] and further extended by others (e.g. [11, 12, 13]). A parameterized surface $v(r, s) = (x(r, s), y(r, s), z(r, s))$, $(r, s) \in [0, 1] \times [0, 1]$,

is considered, and the energy functional is given by

$$E(v) = \int_\Omega \left[\omega_{10} \left| \frac{\partial v}{\partial r} \right|^2 + \omega_{01} \left| \frac{\partial v}{\partial s} \right|^2 + \omega_{11} \left| \frac{\partial^2 v}{\partial r \partial s} \right|^2 + \right.$$
$$\left. \omega_{20} \left| \frac{\partial^2 v}{\partial r^2} \right|^2 + \omega_{02} \left| \frac{\partial^2 v}{\partial s^2} \right|^2 + P \, dr ds,$$

where $P = - \parallel \nabla v \parallel^2$, or any related decreasing function of the gradient. The first terms are related to the smoothness of the surface, while the last one is responsible for attracting it to the object. The evolution of the surface is expressed via Euler-Largange equations. From an initial surface S_0, generally near the desired $3D$ boundary O, the algorithm tries to deform S_0 towards a local minimum of E.

The geometric models proposed in [5, 29] can easily be extended to $3D$ object detection. Let $Q =: [0, a] \times [0, b] \times [0, c]$ and $I : Q \rightarrow^+$ be a given $3D$ data image. Let $g(I) = 1/(1 + |\nabla \tilde{I}|^p)$, where $\tilde{I}$ a regularized version of I, and $p = 1$ or 2. $g(I)$ acts as an edge detector so that the object boundary we are looking for is ideally given by the equation $g = 0$. Our initial active surface S_0 will be embedded as a level-set [34, 39] of a function $u_0 : Q \rightarrow^+$, say $S_0 = \{x : u_0(x) = 0\}$ with u_0 being positive in the exterior and negative in the interior of S_0. The evolving active surface is defined by $S_t = \{x : u(t, x) = 0\}$ where $u(t, x)$ is the solution of

$$\frac{\partial u}{\partial t} = g(I)|\nabla u|\text{div}\left(\frac{\nabla u}{|\nabla u|}\right) + \nu g(I)|\nabla u|$$
$$= g(I)(\nu + H)|\nabla u|, \qquad (1)$$

with initial condition $u(0, x) = u_0(x)$ and Neumann boundary conditions. Here $H = \text{div}\left(\frac{\nabla u}{|\nabla u|}\right)$ is the sum of the two principal curvatures of the level sets of u, (twice its mean curvature) and ν is a positive real constant. The $2D$ version of this model was heuristically justified in [5, 29]. It contains:

- A smoothing term: Twice the mean curvature in the case of (1). More efficient smoothing velocities as those proposed in [3, 9, 33, 25, 27] can be used instead of H^1.

- A constant balloon-type force similar to [12]; $\nu|\nabla u|$.

- A stopping factor $g(I)$. (Related edge detectors can be used, e.g. [47].) Note that in this model, g must be zero for the surface to stop (see next section).

---

[1]Although curvature flows smooth $2D$ curves [17, 18, 37, 38], a $3D$ geometric flow that smoothes all possible surfaces was not found [33]. Frequently used are mean curvature or the positive part of the Gaussian curvature flows [3, 9].

The sign conventions here are adapted to active contours propagating inwards. For active contours evolving from the inside outwards, we take $\nu < 0$. This is a drawback of this model: the active contours cannot go in both directions (see also [43]). Moreover, we always need to select $\nu \neq 0$ even if the surface is close to the object's boundary.

The goal in [7, 8] was to define a $3D$ geometric model (with level-set formulation) corresponding to the minimization of a meaningful and intrinsic energy functional. It is motivated by the extension of $2D$ geometric model to the geodesic active contours as done in [6] and briefly described in the following section.

3. Weighted minimal surfaces

In [6], a model for $2D$ object detection based on the computation of geodesics in a given Riemannian space was presented. This means that we are computing paths or curves of minimal (weighted) length. That model also shows the exact mathematical relation between energy-based active contours and those based on curvature motion, improving on those approaches. This idea may be extended to $3D$ surfaces [7, 8], computing surfaces of minimal area, where the area is defined in a given Riemannian space. In the case of surfaces, arc-length is replaced by surface area $A = \int \int da$, and weighted arc-length by "weighted" area,

$$A_R = \int \int g(I) da, \qquad (2)$$

where da is the (Euclidean) element of area. Surfaces minimizing A are denoted as *minimal surfaces* [35]. In the same manner, we will denote by minimal surfaces those surfaces that minimize (2). The area element da is given by the classical area element in Euclidean space, while the area element da_r is given by $g(I)da$. Observe that da_r corresponds to the area element induced on a surface of R^3 by the metric of R^3 given by $g_{ij} dx_i dx_j$ with $g_{ij} = g(I)^2 \delta_{ij}$. This is the $3D$ analogue of the metric used in [6] to construct the geodesic active contour model. The energy A_R can be formally derived from the original energy formulation using basic principles of dynamical systems [6, 7, 8], further justifying this model. The basic element of the deformable model will be given by minimizing (2) by means of an evolution equation obtained from its Euler-Lagrange. Let us point out the basic characteristics of this flow.

The Euler-Lagrange of A is given by the mean curvature H, resulting a curvature (steepest descent) flow $\frac{\partial S}{\partial t} = H \vec{N}$, where S is the $3D$ surface and $\vec{N}$ its inner unit normal. With the sign conventions explained above, the corresponding level-set [34] formulation is

$u_t = |\nabla u| \text{div} \left(\frac{\nabla u}{|\nabla u|} \right) = |\nabla u| H$. Therefore, the mean curvature motion provides a flow that computes (local) minimal surfaces [10]. Computing the Euler-Lagrange of A_R, we get

$$\mathcal{S}_t = (gH - \nabla g \cdot \vec{N}) \vec{N}. \qquad (3)$$

This is the basic weighted minimal surface flow. Taking a level-set representation, the steepest descent method to minimize (2), yields

$$\begin{aligned} \frac{\partial u}{\partial t} &= |\nabla u| \text{div} \left(g(I) \frac{\nabla u}{|\nabla u|} \right) \\ &= g(I) |\nabla u| \text{div} \left(\frac{\nabla u}{|\nabla u|} \right) + \nabla g(I) \cdot \nabla u. \quad (4) \end{aligned}$$

We note that comparing with previous geometric surface evolution approaches for $3D$ object detection, the minimal surfaces model includes a new term, $\nabla g \cdot \nabla u$. This term is fundamental for detecting boundaries with fluctuations in their gradient, since it will cause the surfaces to stop even if g is not zero. See [6, 7, 8] for details.

As in the $2D$ case, we can add a constant force to the minimization problem (minimizing volume), obtaining the general *minimal surfaces model* for object detection:

$$\frac{\partial u}{\partial t} = |\nabla u| \text{div} \left(g(I) \frac{\nabla u}{|\nabla u|} \right) + \nu g(I) |\nabla u|. \qquad (5)$$

This is the flow we will use for $3D$ object detection. It has the same properties and geometric characteristics as the geodesic active contours, leading to accurate numerical implementations and topology free object segmentation. The flow also holds important existence and completeness properties. Basically, there is a unique solution to the flow in the viscosity sense, and the flow converges to ideal objects [7, 8] (see also [20, 21]). It is also possible to bound the size of the gaps that can be successfully avoided by the flow [6, 8, 15].

As pointed out in the introduction, see [14, 16, 20, 21, 41, 43, 45, 46] for related approaches and [6, 7, 8, 24, 26, 27] for full comparisons.

4. The Tube method

4.1. Motivation

For a two-dimensional interface evolving in three space dimensions, the level set algorithm is at least an $O(N^3)$ method per time step, where N is the number of points in the spatial direction. One drawback of the technique stems from the expense; by embedding the interface as the zero-level set of a higher dimensional function, a two-dimensional interface problem has been transformed into a three-dimensional problem.

The main idea of the tube method is to modify the level set method so it only affects points close to the region of interest, namely the cells where the front is located. This will save considerable computer time, since it reduces by an order of magnitude the number of points where terms must be evaluated. This is particularly beneficial in cases where there is significant computation to be made at each point, as well as simpler cases involving fronts propagating with a constant normal speed.

Our tube is constructed by choosing points that lie less than some given distance away from the curve. The resulting tube-like domain contains the zero-level set. This method was used before in [29] and described in more detail in [1]. A three dimensional version of the tube method was used in [2].

As an illustration, Figure 1 shows the initial surface for a circle in two dimensions. On the left the surface is defined on a square that contains the circle. On the right the surface is only defined in a neighborhood of the circle.

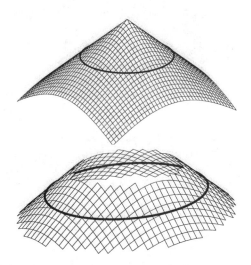

Figure 1. The signed distance function, defined on a square and a tube.

This technique saves memory usage, since all derived quantities, such as curvature and the length of the gradient require less memory than with the full method. The implementation will only store a single copy of the full array. Through careful programming, this too can be eliminated, but at the cost of considerable programming complexity.

4.2. Implementation

The definition of a tube used here is just a set of points inside a rectangular array. There are no restrictions about the shape of the tube, however most of the time it looks like a border around the current front. Initially the surface is defined as the signed distance from the front for all points closer then some predefined maximum value. Outside that tube the surface is constant, chosen to make the surface continuous on all of space.

The front is then moved the same way as in the standard level set method, however only those points belonging to the tube are updated. The tube is rebuilt whenever the front gets too close to an edge. Boundary conditions assume fixed values of u at the tube edge; a more sophisticated implementation is given in [1].

4.3. Speed comparison

To check the speed of the algorithm. we studied the collapse of a sphere with unit speed and according to its curvature. Collapse under mean curvature involves more computation than just the gradient, and better reflects the abilities of the narrow band method. Furthermore, inclusion of such parabolic terms requires smaller time steps than those required by the advection term. The initial sphere is chosen so that it almost fills the computational box. We perform timings with several different time steps and compare the execution time. The full-matrix method and the tube method require approximately the same time when there are 60 cells per side; however, as the number of grid points increases, the narrow band method becomes significantly faster than the full matrix method. Reinitializing the function values in the tube takes up sizable fraction of time but that happens only in the starting stages. The number of reinitializations is independent of the time step, so when the time step is decreased the reinitialization cost becomes a smaller fraction of the total time. We tabulate the execution times of the full matrix and the tube methods until the sphere collapses in Table 1.

5. Experimental results

The experiments described here are based on implementing the level-set flow (4) using the narrow band method [1, 30, 24, 27] and the $3D$ segmentation results are reproduced from Malladi and Sethian [27].

The volume is computed by counting the interior voxels as one volume unit (this is straightforward from the level-sets representation), and proportionally adding the contribution of boundary voxels. Linear

Grid size	$\Delta t=0.8h$	$\Delta t=0.1h$	$\Delta t=0.05h$
The full method			
$60 \times 60 \times 60$	61s	465s	925s
$100 \times 100 \times 100$	480s	3856s	7710s
$150 \times 150 \times 150$	2570s	20500s	41100s
The tube method			
$60 \times 60 \times 60$	49s	115s	182s
$100 \times 100 \times 100$	274s	591s	930s
$150 \times 150 \times 150$	1105s	2240s	3400s

Table 1. Speed comparison between the regular full matrix method and the tube method on a Sun Sparc 10 machine.

interpolation was used in this case, but more precise interpolators can be implemented if better accuracy is needed. The surface area is computed by adding the areas of all the triangles representing the zero level-set, that are extracted from the implicit representation.

The first example presents the segmentation and volume measurement of the soft tissue in a $3D$ CT data of two thighs (see Fig. 2). The computation was done by starting from a collection of spheres inside the thighs and growing outwards thereby reconstructing the thighs and the femur. Fig. 3 presents the final segmentation result in which we can observe the outer surface of the bones and the skin. The $3D$ data is given on a grid of $128 \times 128 \times 61$ which subsequently was mapped onto a unit cube; i.e. $1 \times 1 \times 1$. The measured volume of the soft tissue is 0.268492.

In Fig. 4, the left bone of the first example is extracted by using simple region growing on the segmented thighs. The volume of the bone is measured to be 0.00844465.

In the next example, we present the segmentation results of heart chambers as the heart goes through a diastolic and systolic cycle. The time varying $3D$ MRI heart image data is given on a $256 \times 256 \times 8$ grid. In Fig. 5, we show two cross-sections from the third and sixth data set from our sequence. Again, computation is made to proceed outward from a spherical initilization in the domain. Fig. 6 presents 10 samples of the cycle of a heart beat. The measurements of the area and the volume of each of the segmented heart states are presented in the two graphs in Fig. 7.

6. Concluding remarks

In this paper we presented a complete approach for detecting, representing, and measuring $3D$ medical data, extending work reported in [36, 27]. The med-

ical object is represented as a weighted minimal surface, following [7, 8]. This is computed from geometric measures on the image, via a fast numerical implementation of the level-set approach as in [1, 24, 27]. The high accuracy of the results of the algorithm, enable us to perform measurements like volume and surface area of the detected objects, as was shown in our experiments. Interested readers are invited to visit the web site **http://www.lbl.gov/~malladi** for movies depicting the $3D$ simulations presented in this paper.

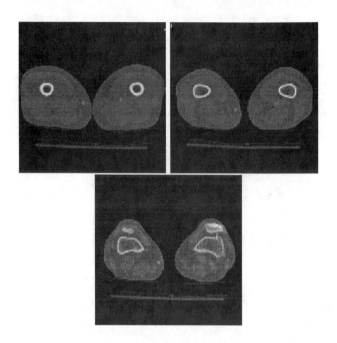

Figure 2. The 5th, 35th, and 59th cross-sections from a CT image of human thighs.

Acknowledgements

The research of RM, RK, DA, and JAS are supported in part by the Applied Mathematical Sciences Subprogram of the Office of Energy Research, U.S. Dept. of Energy under Contract DE-AC03-76SD00098. All calculations shown here were performed at University of California at Berkeley and the Lawrence Berkeley National Laboratory.

References

[1] D. Adalsteinsson and J. A. Sethian, "A fast level set method for propagating interfaces," *J. of Comp. Phys.*, 118:269–277, 1995.

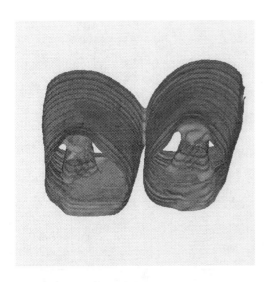

Figure 3. Detection of thighs in $128 \times 128 \times 61$ **CT data images. The volume of the soft tissue was measured to be 0.268492.**

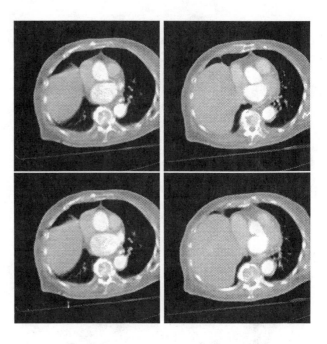

Figure 5. Two cross-sections each from third and sixth heart MRI data set.

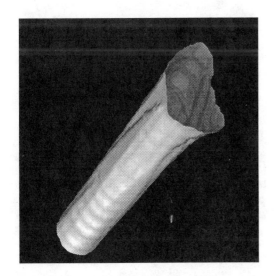

Figure 4. The left thigh bone of Fig. 3, is extracted and its volume is 0.00844465.

[2] D. Adalsteinsson and J. A. Sethian, "A level-set approach to a unified model for etching, deposition, and Lithography II: Three dimensional simulations," *Journal of Comp. Phy.*, Vol. 120, pp. 128-144, 1995.

[3] L. Alvarez, F. Guichard, P. L. Lions, and J. M. Morel, "Axioms and fundamental equations of image processing," *Arch. Rational Mechanics* **123**, 1993.

[4] A. Blake and A. Zisserman, *Visual Reconstruction*, MIT Press, Cambridge, 1987.

[5] V. Caselles, F. Catte, T. Coll, F. Dibos, "A geometric model for active contours," *Numerische Mathematik* **66**, pp. 1-31, 1993.

[6] V. Caselles, R. Kimmel, and G. Sapiro, "Geodesic active contours," to appear *International Journal of Computer Vision*. A short version appears at *ICCV'95*, Cambridge, June 1995.

[7] V. Caselles, R. Kimmel, G. Sapiro and C. Sbert, "Minimal surfaces: A three-dimensional segmentation approach," *Technion Technical Report* **973**, June 1995.

[8] V. Caselles, R. Kimmel, G. Sapiro, and C. Sbert, "Three-dimensional object modeling via minimal

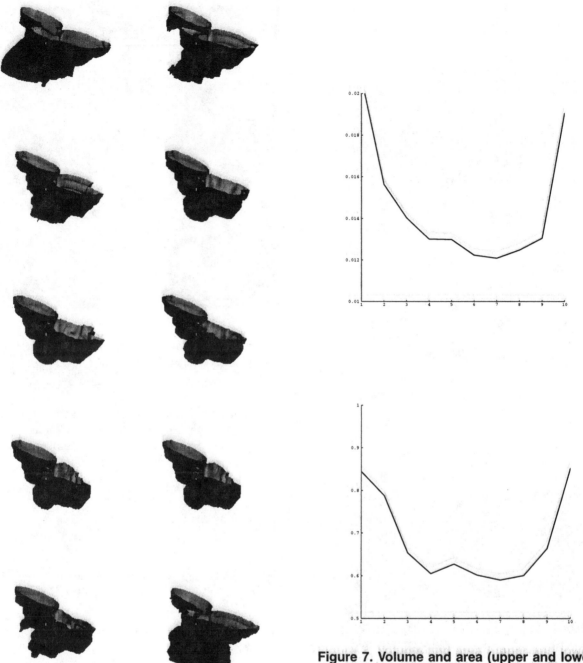

Figure 7. Volume and area (upper and lower graphs) along the heart beat cycle in Fig. 6.

Figure 6. 10 stages along one heart beat, $3D$ segmentation results, presented left`to right top to bottom.

surfaces." *Proc. European Conference on Computer Vision,* Cambridge-UK, April 1996.

[9] V. Caselles and C. Sbert, "What is the best causal scale-space for 3D images?," *SIAM J. on Applied Math,* to appear.

[10] D. Chopp, "Computing minimal surfaces via level set curvature flows," *J. of Comp. Phys.,* 106(1):77–91, 1993.

[11] P. Cinquin, "Un modele pour la representation d'images medicales 3d," *Proc. Euromedicine, Sauramps Medical,* **86,** pp 57-61, 1986.

[12] L. D. Cohen, "On active contour models and balloons," *CVGIP: Image Understanding* **53,** pp. 211-218, 1991.

[13] I. Cohen, L. D. Cohen, and N. Ayache, "Using deformable surfaces to segment 3D images and infer differential structure," *CVGIP: Image Understanding* **56,** pp. 242-263, 1992.

[14] L. D. Cohen and I. Cohen, "Finite element methods for active contour models and balloons for 2D and 3D images," *IEEE Tran. on PAMI* **15**(11), November, 1993.

[15] L. D. Cohen, and R. Kimmel, "Global minimum for active contour models: A minimal path approach," submitted to *IJCV,* 1996; to appear *Proc. CVPR,* June 1996.

[16] P. Fua and Y. G. Leclerc, "Model driven edge detection," *Machine Vision and Applications,* **3,** pp. 45-56, 1990.

[17] M. Gage and R. S. Hamilton, "The heat equation shrinking convex plane curves," *J. Differential Geometry* **23,** pp. 69-96, 1986.

[18] M. Grayson, "The heat equation shrinks embedded plane curves to round points," *J. Differential Geometry* **26,** pp. 285-314, 1987.

[19] M. Kass, A. Witkin, and D. Terzopoulos, "Snakes: Active contour models," *International Journal of Computer Vision* **1,** pp. 321-331, 1988.

[20] S. Kichenassamy, A. Kumar, P.Olver, A. Tannenbaum, and A. Yezzi, "Gradient flows and geometric active contour models," *Proc. ICCV,* Cambridge, June 1995.

[21] S. Kichenassamy, A. Kumar, P.Olver, A. Tannenbaum, and A. Yezzi, "Conformal curvature flows: from phase transitions to active vision," to appear *Archive for Rational Mechanics and Analysis.*

[22] B. B. Kimia, A. Tannenbaum, and S. W. Zucker, "Shapes, shocks, and deformations, I," *International Journal of Computer Vision* **15,** pp. 189-224, 1995.

[23] R. Kimmel, "Curve evolution on surfaces," D. Sc. Thesis, Technion, Israel, June 1995.

[24] R. Malladi, D. Adalsteinsson, and J. A. Sethian, "Fast method for 3D shape modeling using level sets," submitted.

[25] R. Malladi and J. A. Sethian, "Image processing: Flows under min/max curvature and mean curvature," *Graphical Models and Image Processing,* Vol. 58(2), pp. 127–141, March 1996.

[26] R. Malladi and J. A. Sethian, "A unified approach to noise removal, image enhancement, and shape recovery," *IEEE Trans. Image Processing,* to appear, November 1996.

[27] R. Malladi and J. A. Sethian, "Fast level set methods for curvature flow, minimal surfaces, image processing and shape recovery," *Proc. of International Conference on Visualization and Mathematics,* Ed. K. Polthier, Berlin, June 1995, in press, Springer-Verlag.

[28] R. Malladi, J. A. Sethian and B. C. Vemuri, "Evolutionary fronts for topology independent shape modeling and recovery," *Proc. of the 3rd ECCV,* Stockholm, Sweden, pp. 3-13, 1994.

[29] R. Malladi, J. A. Sethian and B. C. Vemuri, "Shape modeling with front propagation: A level set approach," *IEEE Trans. on PAMI,* Vol. 17(2), pp. 158-175, Feb. 1995.

[30] R. Malladi, J. A. Sethian and B. C. Vemuri, "A fast level set based algorithm for topology independent shape modeling," *Journal of Mathematical Imaging and Vision,* Special Issue on Topology and Geometry in Computer Vision, Ed. A. Rosenfeld and Y. Kong, Vol. 6: 2/3, pp. 269–290, April 1996.

[31] T. McInerney and D. Terzopoulos, "Topologically adaptable snakes," *Proc. ICCV,* Cambridge, June 1995.

[32] D. Mumford and J. Shah, "Optimal approximations by piecewise smooth functions and variational problems," *Comm. Pure and App. Math.* **42,** 1989.

[33] P. J. Olver, G. Sapiro, and A. Tannenbaum, "Invariant geometric evolutions of surfaces and volumetric smoothing," *SIAM J. of Appl. Math.*, to appear.

[34] S. J. Osher and J. A. Sethian, "Fronts propagation with curvature dependent speed: Algorithms based on Hamilton-Jacobi formulations," *Journal of Computational Physics* **79**, pp. 12-49, 1988.

[35] R. Osserman, *Survey of Minimal Surfaces*, Dover, 1986.

[36] G. Sapiro, R. Kimmel, and V. Caselles, "Object detection and measurements in medical images via geodesic active contours," *Proc. SPIE-Vision Geometry*, San Diego, July 1995.

[37] G. Sapiro and A. Tannenbaum, "On affine plane curve evolution," *Journal of Functional Analysis* **119:1**, pp. 79-120, 1994.

[38] G. Sapiro and A. Tannenbaum, "Affine invariant scale-space," *International Journal of Computer Vision* **11:1**, pp. 25-44, 1993.

[39] J. A. Sethian, "A review of recent numerical algorithms for hypersurfaces moving with curvature dependent flows," *J. Differential Geometry* **31**, pp. 131-161, 1989.S

[40] J. A. Sethian, "A Review of the Theory, Algorithms, and Applications of Level Set Methods for Propagating Interfaces," in press, Acta Numerica, 1995.

[41] J. Shah, "Recovery of shapes by evolution of zero-crossings," Technical Report, Math. Dept. Northeastern Univ. Boston MA, 1995.

[42] R. Szeliski, D. Tonnesen, and D. Terzopoulos, "Modeling surfaces of arbitrary topology with dynamic particles," *Proc. CVPR*, pp. 82-87, 1993.

[43] H. Tek and B. B. Kimia, "Image segmentation by reaction-diffusion bubbles," *Proc. ICCV*, Cambridge, June 1995.

[44] D. Terzopoulos, A. Witkin, and M. Kass, "Constraints on deformable models: Recovering 3D shape and nonrigid motions," *Artificial Intelligence* **36**, pp. 91-123, 1988.

[45] R. T. Whitaker, "Volumetric deformable models: Active blobs," *Visualization in Biomedical Computing*, pp. 122–134, 1994.

[46] R. T. Whitaker, "Algorithms for implicit deformable models," *Proc. ICCV'95*, pp. 822–827, Cambridge, June 1995.

[47] S. W. Zucker and R. A. Hummel, "A three-dimensional edge operator," *IEEE-PAMI* **3**, pp. 324-331, 1981.

An Integrated Approach for Surface Finding in Medical Images

Amit Chakraborty[1], Lawrence H. Staib and James S. Duncan
Departments of Electrical Engineering and Diagnostic Radiology
Yale University
P.O. Box 208042
333 Cedar Street, New Haven, CT 06520-8042

Abstract

The wide availability of three- dimensional medical images has made their direct analysis a necessity. Accurately segmenting and quantifying structures is a key issue for such images. Conventional gradient- based surface finding however often suffers from a variety of limitations. This paper proposes a surface finding approach that uses in addition to gradient information, region information. This makes the resulting procedure more robust to noise and improper initialization. It uses Gauss's Divergence theorem to find the surface of of a homogeneous region-classified area in the image and integrates this with a gray level gradient-based surface finder. Experimental results show that indeed, as expected, a significant improvement is achieved as a consequence of the use of this extra information. Further, these improvements are achieved with little increase in computational overhead, an advantage derived from the application of Gauss's Divergence theorem.

1. Introduction

Three dimensional image analysis is important especially in the medical imaging domain due to the wide availability and use of three dimensional images from such modalities as magnetic resonance imaging (MRI), computed tomography (CT) and single photon emission computed tomography (SPECT) [12]. In most of these cases, the analysis is comprised of precisely identifying and quantifying structures and abnormalities. Such analysis is important for a variety of tasks such as multimodality image registration, structural measurement of anatomy, deriving priors for image reconstruction in another modality and cardiac motion tracking. Often, it is standard practice is to treat the 3D image as a stack of 2D images (see for example [11]),

thereby reducing it essentially to a 2D image analysis problem. While successful in many cases, the problem with such methods is that they tend to either oversimplify or ignore altogether the true 3D properties of the structures under consideration. Thus, it is important to use 3D image analysis methods for these images.

However, robust identification and measurement of such naturally occurring deformable structures/objects is not always achievable by using a single technique that depends on a single image-derived source of information. Thus, it is our belief that one needs to apply integrated methods that make optimal use of the various sources of information. Most segmentation methods can be divided primarily into region-based and boundary-based approaches. Region-based methods [35, 20, 16, 17, 14, 13, 24, 27], rely on the homogeneity of spatially localized features such as gray level intensity, texture and other pixel statistics. Homogeneity does not necessarily mean identical pixel values within a particular region, rather it means that the variation within a region is of a smaller extent than that between regions. The advantage of such methods is that they rely directly on the gray level image and thus are less susceptible to noise than methods that use derivative information. Also, if the high frequency information in an image is either missing or is unreliable, the segmented images remain relatively unaffected. However, the problem with typical region-based segmentation methods, is that the resulting segmentation depends considerably on the choice of seed points and the region's shape is too dependent on the choice of the actual algorithm used. Also, such methods often result in an over-segmented image. Rule based systems [5] can do better, but are extremely application-specific. Other region-based methods either use probabilistic techniques [14, 22, 19, 4, 13] or use non-linear diffusion methods [24, 27, 1] (see [13] or [24] for the exact mathematical relationship between these methods). The main idea behind these methods is to do what can be termed as *edge-preserved smoothing*. However, isolating objects from the resulting image still requires considerable effort as they also suffer from the problems of poor

---

[1]Currently at Siemens Corporate Research, 755 College Road East, Princeton, NJ 08540 (chakrab@scr.siemens.com).

Proceedings of MMBIA '96

localization and over-segmentation (related to the problem of choosing the appropriate scale).

In contrast to region-based methods, boundary methods primarily use gradient information to locate object boundaries. However, as in the 2D case, boundary finding using only local information in the 3D case is problematic due to the effects of noise, poor contrast, unfavorable viewing conditions, the presence of other objects in the near vicinity, etc. In addition, some of the methods that are applicable in 2D can no longer be used for 3D images. For example, pixel search methods that follow an optimal path through the two dimensional images cannot naturally be extended to three dimensions because the voxels in a surface have no such ordering. Hough transform methods [2] can be used, but for three dimensional images it is very expensive both in terms of storage and computational costs. To overcome these problems, as in the 2D case, the use of whole boundary methods has been advocated. This allows one to augment imperfect image data with shape information provided by a geometric model [30, 33, 29]. The main idea is to form over-constrained estimates that use a few parameters to describe a large number of points.

We adopt the Fourier parameterization of [30, 33, 32] primarily because we consider it suitable for the class of problems that we are looking at and because of its flexibility in using prior information easily, when such information is available. Also, it is a natural extension to our adopted 2D boundary parameterization. Besides the Fourier representation [30, 33, 32] that we describe below after [33] other approaches to three dimensional parametric modeling include generalized cylinders [25], superquadrics [29] hyperquadrics [18], finite element methods [8, 10, 9] etc.

It is key to note however, that while both the region and boundary methods have their advantages and disadvantages their problems are not necessarily identical, i.e. they are not affected in the same way by the various problems. While the presence of noise limits the performance of any image processing algorithm, the region-based methods are less affected than gradient-based boundary finding because the gradient is very noise sensitive. Also, if the high frequency information in the image either is missing or is unreliable, boundary finding is more error-prone compared to region-based segmentation. Shape variations, on the other hand, can be better handled using a deformable boundary finding framework when we consider such variations to be generally around an average shape and such information can easily be incorporated as priors [31]. Further, since conventional boundary finding relies on changes in the gray level, rather than their actual values, it is less sensitive to changes in the gray scale distributions such as shading artifacts over images. Also, gradient-based methods in general do a better job of edge localization. This brings us to the realization that integrated methods are likely to perform better

than either of the methods alone by being able to combine the complementary strengths of these individual methods, as has been pointed out [23, 7].

Unfortunately, however, only a limited amount of previous work has been done, seeking to integrate region and boundary information, and primarily for 2D images. Among the available methods, AI-based techniques have been used where production rules are invoked for conflict removal [23]. Other similar efforts [7, 15] were aimed at integrating region growing with edge-detection rather than finding complex objects. Probability based approaches [14, 22, 4, 13] or the nonlinear diffusion methods [24, 1] achieve integration in the local or dense field sense. Another way of achieving local integration is the reaction-diffusion method [36]. However, the problem of using such local integration methods is that if any one of the processes makes an error (e.g. a false edge), it is propagated to the final solution. Also, a decision regarding the final object boundary in [36] is made by considering the whole space of reaction-diffusion images and somehow choosing one result, something that can get very complicated. Finally, we note that the recent work of [37] has similar motivations as ours even though to our knowledge, extensions to 3D images have not yet been worked out. The algorithm presented here is an extension of our earlier work on integration for boundary finding in 2D images [6].

2. Fourier surface representations

A surface in three dimensions can be represented by three coordinate functions of two surface parameters as $\mathbf{x}(u,v) = (x(u,v), y(u,v), z(u,v))$, where u and v are the free parameters that very over the surface. Since there are two free parameters, a function of two parameters is necessary to describe a surface. The Fourier representation of [30, 33] uses the following basis:

$$
\begin{aligned}
\phi = \{ & 1, \cos mu, \sin mu, \cos lv, \sin lv, \cos mu \cos lv, \\
& \sin mu \cos lv, \cos mu \sin lv, \sin mu \cos lv, ... \\
& (m = 1, 2, ...; l = 1, 2, ...) \}
\end{aligned} \quad (1)
$$

The functions $x(.,.), y(.,.)$ and $z(.,.)$ are composed as a weighted sum of the elements of the above basis and is as follows:

$$
\begin{aligned}
f(u,v) = \sum_{m=0}^{K} \sum_{l=0}^{K} \lambda_{m,l} [& \\
& a_{m,l} \cos mu \cos lv + b_{m,l} \sin mu \cos lv + \\
& c_{m,l} \cos mu \sin lv + d_{m,l} \sin mu \sin lv]
\end{aligned} \quad (2)
$$

where,

$$
\lambda_{m,l} = \begin{cases} 1 & for\ m = 0,\ l = 0 \\ 2 & for\ m > 0,\ l = 0\ or\ m = 0,\ l > 0 \\ 4 & for\ m > 0,\ l > 0 \end{cases}
$$

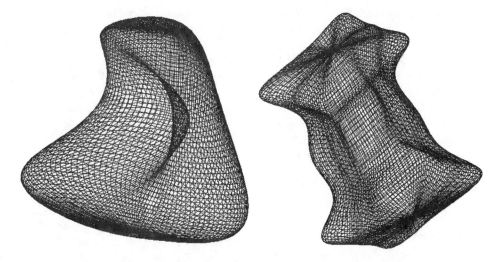

Figure 1. Two closed surface examples using up to four and eight harmonics (taken from [33]).

The series is truncated at K, i.e. only a finite number of harmonics are used. This again is similar to the case in 2D, and is taken to constrain the space of functions. Taken together, the coefficients form the parameter vector,

$$\vec{p} = (a_x, b_x, c_x, d_x, a_y, b_y, c_y, d_y, a_z, b_z, c_z, d_z) \quad (3)$$

The four basic classes of surfaces in three dimensions are tori (closed tubes), open surfaces (with one edge), tubes (open surfaces with two edges) and closed surfaces.

The torus, which is periodic in both the surface variables is formed with the entire basis in equation (1). Closed surfaces, which we are most interested in, is given by the representation:

$$\phi_{closed} = \{1, \sin lv, \cos mu \sin lv, \sin mu \sin lv, ...\} \quad (4)$$

which forces the functions to be constants at $v = 0, \pi, 2\pi$. But this forces the ends to be together as well. The ends need to be separated by adding a weighted term to each coordinate of the form $sin(v - \pi/2)$ resulting in three more additional shape parameters. Two closed surfaces shown in Figure 1 demonstrates the capability of the above mentioned parameterization. We note here that it is also possible to represent open surfaces and tubes by this parameterization, details of which can be found in [33, 32].

3. Region information

The idea here is to classify the image into a number of regions or classes. Thus for each voxel in the image, we need to decide or estimate which class it belongs to. There are a variety of approaches to region based segmentation and while there are differences, the performance does not change from one method to the other considerably. Since the emphasis of this paper lies on an integrated boundary finding approach given the raw image and the region classified image, it does not matter too much which method is being used to get the region classified image as long as the output of that method gives reasonable results.

For our purposes, we use one of the popular methods available in the literature [28, 21], which models the image as a Markov Random Field (MRF) and a Maximum *a posteriori* (MAP) probability approach is used to do the classification. The problem is posed as an objective function optimization, which in this case consists of the *a posteriori* probability of the classified image given the raw data which constitutes the likelihood term, and the prior probability term, which due to the MRF assumption is given by the Gibb's distribution. It can be shown that the MAP objective is equivalent to,

$$x_i = \arg \max_{\{x_i \in l; \, l=1,2,..,L\}} p(y_i|Y_{N/i}, x_i, X_{N/i}) p(x_i|X_{N/i})$$
$$(5)$$

where Y corresponds to the actual image data, X corresponds to the region classified image and l represents the classes in X. The subscript N/i represents the neighborhood of the ith pixel leaving out the ith pixel. A first order neighborhood system having six neighbors (2 neighbors along the three axes) is being used. At every iteration, the probability of a particular pixel being classified to different classes is computed and the pixel is assigned to the class that gives the highest probability. The procedure stops when there is no change between iterations.

4. Integrated surface finding objective function

In this section, we shall define the objective function, optimizing which would result in the estimated surface parameters. The development is similar to our earlier development for 2D images [6].

The input to the problem consists of the actual image I and the region classified image I_s, which is obtained from I after passing it through a region based segmentation step as discussed above. We shall also assume that the interior of the boundary that we are trying to find belongs to a single region in I_s. Let us note here that all that this assumption requires is that the intra region variability should be smaller than the inter region variability. Further relaxations to this can be attained in a similar way as was achieved in the 2D case (see [6] for details). The traditional boundary finding problem does not use the original image directly. Being a gradient based approach, it uses instead the gradient image I_g. As in the Staib and Duncan [33, 30] approach, we use the magnitude of the gradient vector at each voxel location. I_g can be obtained from I either by convolving the input image I with the derivative (taken in the three directions) of a Gaussian kernel and then computing I_g to be the magnitude of the above resulting vector image. Alternatively, one can obtain I_g from I by first convolving with a Gaussian to smooth the effects of noise followed by taking a finite difference approximation to the partial derivatives in the three directions and then calculating the magnitude of the gradient vector at each voxel location. Thus finally, the input to the system is the gradient image I_g and the region classified image I_s.

Parallel to our development for the 2D case, the above surface estimation problem using gradient and region homogeneity information can be posed in the maximum *a posteriori* framework. This is suitable for incorporating *a priori* shape information if available.

Our aim is to maximize $P(\vec{p}|I_g, I_s)$, where as described in the previous section, $\vec{p}$ is the vector of parameters used to parameterize the contour. Now,

$$P(\vec{p}|I_g, I_s) = \frac{P(\vec{p}, I_g, I_s)}{P(I_g, I_s)} \quad (6)$$

$$= \frac{P(I_s|I_g, \vec{p})P(p, I_g)}{P(I_g, I_s)} \quad (7)$$

$$= \frac{P(I_s|I_g, p)P(I_g|\vec{p})P(p)}{P(I_g, I_s)} \quad (8)$$

Thus, ignoring the denominator, which does not change with $\vec{p}$, our aim is to determine (after taking logarithm),

$$\arg\max_{\vec{p}} P(\vec{p}|I_g, I_s) \equiv \arg\max_{\vec{p}} [lnP(\vec{p}) + lnP(I_g|\vec{p})$$
$$+ lnP(I_s|I_g, \vec{p})] \quad (9)$$

In the last equation (9), we have just taken the natural logarithm, which is a monotonically increasing function. Knowledge of I_g may be used to calculate I_s, through the

use of line processes [14, 4]. However, if we do not use that information, we are effectively discarding information rather than assuming extra information. Thus, finally, the above can be written in the following form (assuming that calculation of I_s assumes knowledge of I_g):

$$\arg\max_{\vec{p}} M(\vec{p}, I_g, I_s) = \arg\max_{\vec{p}} [M_{prior}(\vec{p})$$
$$+ M_{gradient}(I_g, \vec{p}) + M_{region}(I_s, \vec{p})] \quad (10)$$

We now explain each of the terms in (10).

The first term in equation (10) corresponds to the prior shape term. When it is non-uniform, it biases the model towards a particular range of shapes. However, since there might be other objects in the image, we would always need an initial estimate of the surface to start the optimization process. The information fusion that we present in this case increases the reliability of the surface finding procedure under increased uncertainty in the initial boundary placement. Experimental results to validate this claim are provided in the results section.

The second term is the gradient likelihood term. It is a measure of the likelihood of the surface being the true object boundary given the gradient image. At each point on the surface, the strength of the boundary is evaluated by the magnitude of the gradient at that particular voxel, given by the gradient image. Thus the likelihood of the whole surface being the true boundary becomes proportional to the sum of the magnitude of the gradients at all the points that lie on the surface boundary. If we assume that the noise can be approximated by a zero mean Gaussian, and further assume that the voxels on the boundary are independent, then we may express the above term in the probability expression as the following area integral (see Staib and Duncan [30, 33] for further details) :

$$M_{gradient}(I_g, \vec{p}) \propto \int\int_{A_{\vec{p}}} I_g(x, y, z)dA \quad (11)$$

where the area element on the surface is given by:

$$dA = |\mathbf{x}_u \times \mathbf{x}_v|dudv \quad (12)$$

The third term in equation (10) is responsible for incorporating the region information into the surface finding framework. The notion is that we expect the bounding surface to surround a homogeneous region. We note that the comments made before regarding the homogeneity assumption are valid here as well. For simplicity's sake, if we assume that we are dealing with an image where the target object is surrounded by a single background, we assign positive values to the interior of the object and negative values outside. If more than two regions are involved, all pixels of the region that needs to be segmented can be assigned a positive value and the remaining ones negative values, the magnitudes of which reflect how much one expects the target region to be dissociated from the remaining regions. Hence, remote regions are expected to have high negative values, representing a larger penalty for including remote points. This way multiple regions can be handled. Once we have associated positive values with the target object and negative values with points that lie outside, a volume integral that sums up all the points inside the surface is taken. Clearly, this integral would be a maximum when the bounding surface is optimally placed over the object. Thus the third term in (10) is given by:

$$M_{region}(I_s, \vec{p}) \propto \int\int\int_{V_{\vec{p}}} I_s(x, y, z) dV \qquad (13)$$

hence finally we have,

$$\arg\max_{\vec{p}} M(\vec{p}, I_g, I_s) = \max_{\vec{p}} [M_{prior}(\vec{p})$$
$$+ M_{gradient}(I_g, \vec{p}) + M_{region}(I_s, \vec{p})]$$
$$\equiv \max_{\vec{p}} \left[M_{prior}(\vec{p}) + K_1 \int\int_{A_{\vec{p}}} I_g(x, y, z) dA \right.$$
$$\left. + K_2 \int\int\int_{V_{\vec{p}}} I_s(x, y, z) dV \right] \qquad (14)$$

where K_1 and K_2 are the weighting constants which signifies the relative importance of the two terms in the above equation.

Of the last two terms in (14), one is an area integral and the other is a volume integral. In general, computing an area integral is much less expensive compared to a volume integral. Thus we would save a lot of computation, especially when we carry out an iterative optimization procedure, if we could convert the volume integral to an area integral which must be computed anyway. The second term which is present in the original surface finding method already involves computation an area integral. Thus the order of the computational complexity is not increased. The above can be done using Gauss' divergence theorem [3] as follows. Let,

$$\mathbf{F}_x(x, y, z) = \frac{1}{3} \int_0^x I_s(\alpha, y, z) d\alpha \qquad (15)$$

$$\mathbf{F}_y(x, y, z) = \frac{1}{3} \int_0^y I_s(x, \beta, z) d\beta \qquad (16)$$

$$\mathbf{F}_z(x, y, z) = \frac{1}{3} \int_0^z I_s(x, y, \gamma) d\gamma \qquad (17)$$

where $\mathbf{F} = (\mathbf{F}_x, \mathbf{F}_y, \mathbf{F}_z)$. We note that the definition of $F()$ is done in such a way that the C^1 continuity requirement in the statement of the above theorem is met. Under the above assumptions, we have,

$$\int\int\int_{V_{\vec{p}}} I_s(x, y, z) dV = \int\int \mathbf{F} \cdot dA \qquad (18)$$

$$= \int\int_{A_{\vec{p}}} \mathbf{F} \cdot (\mathbf{x}_u \times \mathbf{x}_v) du dv$$
$$= 3 \int\int_{A_{\vec{p}}} \mathbf{F}_x(y_u z_v - z_u y_v) du dv$$
$$= 3 \int\int_{A_{\vec{p}}} \mathbf{F}_y(z_u x_v - x_u z_v) du dv$$
$$= 3 \int\int_{A_{\vec{p}}} \mathbf{F}_z(x_u y_v - y_u x_v) du dv$$
$$= \int\int_{A_{\vec{p}}} [\mathbf{F}_x(y_u z_v - z_u y_v) + \mathbf{F}_y(z_u x_v - x_u z_v)$$
$$+ \mathbf{F}_z(x_u y_v - y_u x_v)] du dv \qquad (19)$$

Substituting the above in (14) we finally get,

$$\max_{\vec{p}} M(I_g, I_s, \vec{p}) = \max_{\vec{p}} [M_{prior}(\vec{p})$$
$$+ K_1 \int\int_{A_{\vec{p}}} I_g(x, y, z) dA$$
$$+ K_2 \int\int \mathbf{F} \cdot dA] \qquad (20)$$

Let us note here that the calculation of $\mathbf{F}_x()$, $\mathbf{F}_y()$, and $\mathbf{F}_z()$ are done only once at the start of the optimization process. Also, we note that these calculations merely involve summing up the values of the voxels in the image I_s in the three directions. Further their derivatives, which we need during the optimization process, are the values of the image I_s itself. We mention this to point out that the use of the extra information hardly introduces any extra computational burden.

In the above, we have presented a surface finding procedure that introduces a prior term that incorporates information that we might obtain from region based segmentation. Further, use of Gauss's divergence theorem allows us to reduce the whole problem to computing surface integrals only, rather than both surface and volume integrals.

5. Evaluation and Optimization

The objective function in equation (20), can be evaluated by numerical integration. The gradient of the objective is necessary for optimization. The derivative of the objective is given by,

$$\frac{\partial M}{\partial p_x} = \frac{\partial M_{prior}(\vec{p})}{\partial p_x}$$
$$+ K_1 \int\int_{A_{\vec{p}}} \left[I_g(x, y, z) \frac{\partial}{\partial p_x} |\mathbf{x}_u \times \mathbf{x}_v| \right.$$
$$\left. + \frac{\partial I_g(x, y, z)}{\partial x} \frac{\partial x(\vec{p}, u, v)}{\partial p_x} |\mathbf{x}_u \times \mathbf{x}_v| \right] du dv$$
$$+ 3K_2 \int\int_{A_{\vec{p}}} I_s(x, y, z)(y_u z_v - z_u y_v) \frac{\partial x(\vec{p}, u, v)}{\partial p_x} du dv$$
$$(21)$$

and similarly for y and z. This expression can also be evaluated by numerical integration. Expressions like $\frac{\partial I_g(x,y,z)}{\partial x}$ can be obtained using discrete derivative calculation. Other expressions like $\frac{\partial x(\vec{p},u,v)}{\partial p_x}$ and $\mathbf{x}_u$ and $\mathbf{x}_v$ can be obtained analytically from equations (1) and (2). The derivatives of the prior terms can be obtained in exactly the same way as in the 2D case [31, 33].

Optimization is achieved using the conjugate gradient method which is a local optimization method. For surface finding even local maximization involves a lot of computation. Thus, to avoid even further computational burden, global optimization methods were not considered at the cost, however, of not being able to guarantee global convergence. Since the method is initialized close to the actual location, global optimization methods may not be required.

6. Results

Experiments were carried out both with synthetic and natural images to verify the performance of the above mentioned method. However to evaluate it, we need a method to calculate the error between two surfaces expressed parametrically. We do this using the same definition (given below) as the one used in [33]. The error is defined as the average distance between each point on the estimated surface and the closest point on the true surface. That is, the error between surfaces S and $\hat{S}$ is defined as

$$e(S, \hat{S}) = \frac{\int_{(u,v) \in \hat{S}} \min_{(u',v') \in S} |S(u',v') - \hat{S}(u,v)| dA}{\int_{(u,v) \in \hat{S}} dA}$$

(22)

This can be computed discretely by first taking a distance transform of a binary volume representing the true surface [33]. This is then correlated with the binary volume representing the estimated surface, which gives the minimum distance between the estimated and the true surface. The result is then normalized by the area of the estimated surface.

We first used a synthetic example to evaluate the algorithm developed. This is useful because for this case we had exact knowledge of the true surface boundary. Comparisons of the integrated method were done against the traditional gradient based surface finding approach.

Figure 2 shows a simple synthetic example of a closed surface with added Gaussian noise. The SNR for this image was 1.6. The initial surface was roughly placed on the target object. Clearly, we can observe that the combined method performed better. It can be observed from the wireframe diagrams that the surface finder diverges under these noise conditions when using gradient information alone which is not the case for the integrated method.

Figure 3 shows a comparison of the two methods under increasing noise conditions. Here, the X-axis corresponds to the noise level given by the standard deviation of the noise used. The Y-axis gives a measure of the distance between the estimated surface and the true one using equation (22). Once again, it is obvious that the integrated method is superior under high noise conditions. This upholds our claim that the proposed integrated method is robust to noise which is even more dramatic in 3D.

Now, as for the initialization, Figure 4 shows the performance when the vertical shift was varied from the true position, keeping the initialization for the other parameters fixed. It shows that the integrated method has a larger capture region. In other words, the integrated method converges to the desired target object, which is much further off when compared to the gradient-only case. Thus, the the region within which the initialization must be in order to converge is larger for the integrated algorithm.

In Figure 5, we try out the proposed algorithm on a three dimensional cardiac image of a dog's heart obtained using the Dynamic Spatial Reconstructor (DSR). The DSR is a 3D imaging device based on high speed x-ray computed tomography [26]. One can see that by noting that the integrated method does a better job in capturing the blood pool of the left ventricle (the bright area). The results were confirmed by examination by a cardiologist.

7. Conclusions

We have presented in this paper an integrated method for surface finding using both region and gradient information. As the examples show, the integrated approach is more robust to both increased amounts of noise as well as increasingly displaced initialization of the initial boundary. Thus, there is an improvement over the conventional gradient based boundary finding. It is important to note that this improvement in performance is achieved without significantly increasing the computational burden, due to the appropriate application of Gauss's divergence theorem. Application of this method on real medical images results in noticeable improvement as shown.

However, there remains areas for numerous potential developments. Generating appropriate priors to constrain the search space is very important. Some work in that area has been done in [34]. Extracting more convoluted or multiple objects simultaneously is also interesting in its own right.

References

[1] L. Alvarez, P. Lions, and J. Morel. Image selective smoothing and edge detection by nonlinear diffusion. *SIAM Journal of Numerical Analysis*, 29:845–866, 1992.

[2] D. H. Ballard and C. M. Brown. *Computer Vision*. Prentice Hall, Englewood Cliffs, 1982.

[3] P. Baxandall and H. Liebeck. *Vector Calculus*. Oxford University Press, 1986.

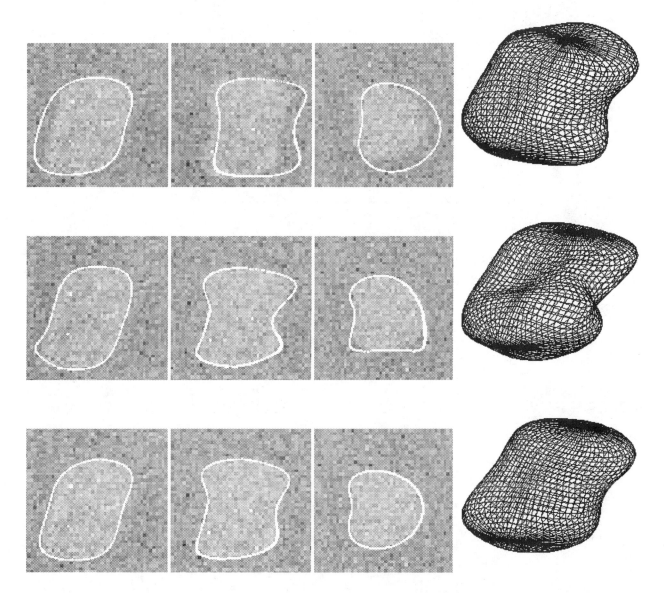

Figure 2. Surface finding for a synthetic image with and without region information. (a)Top: Three perpendicular slices through the 3D image (48 × 48 × 48) are shown with the initial surface along with and the wireframe. (b)Middle: The same slices through the same 3D image are shown with the surface obtained using only the gradient information and the corresponding wireframe. (c)Bottom: The same slices through the same 3D image are shown with the surface obtained using both the gradient and the region information and the corresponding wireframe.

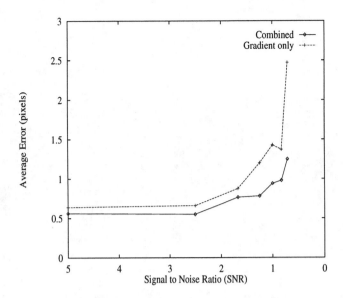

Figure 3. Noise performance of the surface finder with and without region information. Clearly, the combined method is superior.

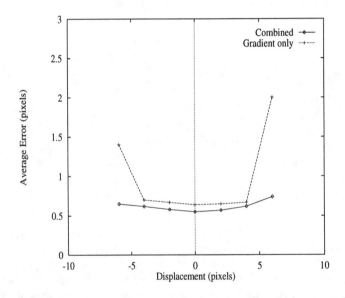

Figure 4. Performance of the surface finder with and without region information under different starting positions. This was varied by shifting the initialization vertically. Clearly, the combined method is superior.

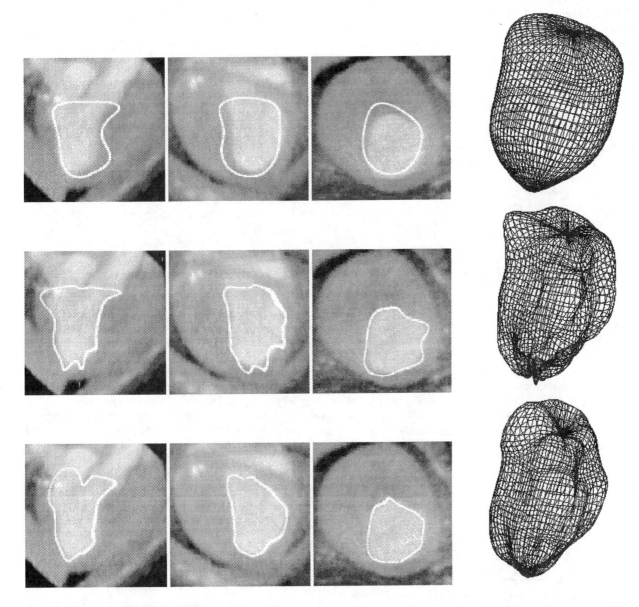

Figure 5. Surface finding for a DSR image of the left ventricle of a canine heart with and without region information. (a)Top: Three perpendicular slices through the 3D image (98 × 100 × 110) are shown with the initial surface and the wireframe. (b)Middle: The same slices through the same 3D image are shown with the surface obtained using only the gradient information and the corresponding wireframe. (c)Bottom: The same slices through the same 3D image are shown with the surface obtained using both the gradient and the region information and the corresponding wireframe.

[4] A. Blake and A. Zisserman. *Visual Reconstruction*. MIT Press, Cambridge, MA, 1987.

[5] P. Burt, T. Hong, and A. Rosenfeld. Segmentation and estimation of region properties through co-operative hierarchical computation. *IEEE Transactions on System, Man and Cybernetics*, 11:802–809, 1981.

[6] A. Chakraborty, L. Staib, and J. Duncan. Deformable boundary finding influenced by region homogeneity. *Proc. Computer Vision and Pattern Recognition*, pages 624–627, 1994.

[7] C. Chu and J. Agarwal. The integration of image segmentation maps using region and edge information. *IEEE Transactions on Pattern Analysis and Machine Intelligence*, 15:1241–1252, 1993.

[8] I. Cohen, L. Cohen, and N. Ayache. Using deformable structures to segment 3D images and infer differential structures. *Computer Vision, Graphics and Image Processing: Image Understanding*, 13:242–263, 1992.

[9] L. Cohen, E. Bardinet, and N. Ayache. Surface reconstruction using active contour models. *Proc. SPIE-93 Conference on Geometric Methods in Computer Vision*, 1993.

[10] L. D. Cohen and I. Cohen. Finite element methods for active contour models and baloons for 2d and 3d images. *IEEE Transactions on Pattern Analysis and Machine Intelligence*, 15, 1993.

[11] T. Cootes, A. Hill, C. Taylor, and J. Haslam. The use of active shape models for locating structures in medical images. In H. H. Barrett and A. F. Gmitro, editors, *Information Processing in Medical Imaging*, pages 33–47. LNCS 687, Springer-Verlag, Berlin, 1993.

[12] P. Ell and B. Holman. *Computed Emission Tomography*. Oxford University Press, Oxford, 1982.

[13] D. Geiger and A. Yuille. A common framework for image segmentation. *International Journal of Computer Vision*, 6:227–243, 1991.

[14] D. Geman and S. Geman. Stochastic relaxation, gibbs distribution and bayesian restoration of images. *IEEE Transactions on Pattern Analysis and Machine Intelligence*, 6:721–741, 1984.

[15] J. Haddon and J. Boyce. Image segmentation by unifying region and boundary information. *IEEE Transactions on Pattern Analysis and Machine Intelligence*, 12:929–948, 1990.

[16] J. Kittler and J. Illingworth. On threshold selection using clustering criteria. *IEEE Transactions on System, Man and Cybernetics*, 15:652–655, 1985.

[17] R. Kohler. A segmentation based on thresholding. *Computer Vision, Graphics and Image Processing*, 15:319–338, 1981.

[18] S. Kumar, S. Han, D. Goldgof, and K. Bowyer. On recovering hyperquadrics from range data. *IEEE Transactions on Pattern Analysis and Machine Intelligence*, 17:1079–1083, 1995.

[19] Y. Leclerc. Constructing simple stable descriptions for image partitioning. *International Journal of Computer Vision*, 3:73–102, 1989.

[20] M. Levine and A. Nazif. Dynamic measurement of computer generated image segmentation. *IEEE Transactions on System, Man and Cybernetics*, 7:155–164, 1985.

[21] B. Manjunath and R. Chellappa. Unsupervised texture segmentation using markov random field models. *IEEE Transactions on Pattern Analysis and Machine Intelligence*, 13:478–482, 1991.

[22] D. Mumford and J. Shah. Boundary detection by minimizing functionals. *Proceedings, IEEE Conf. Computer Vision and Pattern Recognition*, page 22, 1985.

[23] T. Pavlidis and Y. Liow. Integrating region growing and edge detection. *IEEE Transactions on Pattern Analysis and Machine Intelligence*, 12:225–233, 1990.

[24] P. Perona and J. Malik. Scale-space and edge detection using anisotropic diffusion. *IEEE Transactions on Pattern Analysis and Machine Intelligence*, 12:629–639, 1990.

[25] K. Rao and R. Nevatia. Computing volume descriptions from sparse 3d data. *International Journal of Computer Vision*, 2:33–50, 1988.

[26] R. Robb. High speed three-dimensional x-ray computed tomography. *Proc. IEEE*, 71:308–319, 1983.

[27] B. Romeny. *Geometry Driven Diffusion in Computer Vision*. Kluwer, 1994.

[28] B. M. T. Simchony and R. Chellappa. Stochastic and deterministic networks for texture segmentation. *IEEE Transactions on Acoustics, Speech and Signal Processing*, 38:1039–1049, 1990.

[29] F. Solina and R. Bajcsy. Recovery of parametric models from range images: The case for superquadratics with global deformations. *IEEE Transactions on Pattern Analysis and Machine Intelligence*, 12:131–147, 1990.

[30] L. Staib. *Parametrically Deformable Contour Models for Image Analysis*. PhD thesis, Yale University, 1990.

[31] L. Staib and J. Duncan. Boundary finding with parametrically deformable models. *IEEE Transactions on Pattern Analysis and Machine Intelligence*, 14:161–175, 1992.

[32] L. Staib and J. Duncan. Deformable fourier models for surface finding in 3d images. *Proc. Conference on Visualization in Biomedical Imaging (R.A. Robb ed.)*, pages 90–104, 1992.

[33] L. Staib and J. Duncan. Model-based deformable surface finding for medical images. *IEEE Transactions on Medical Imaging*, submitted.

[34] G. Szekely, A. Keleman, C. Brechbuhler, and G. Gerig. Segmentation of 3D objects from MRI volume data using constrained elastic deformations of flexible surface models. In N. Ayache, editor, *Lecture Notes in Computer Science: First International Conference on Computer Vision, Virtual Reality, and Robotics in Medicine*. Springer-Verlag, Nice, France, 1995.

[35] T. Taxt, P. Flynn, and A. Jain. Segmentation of document images. *IEEE Transactions on Pattern Analysis and Machine Intelligence*, 11:1322–1329, 1989.

[36] H. Tek and B. Kimia. Image segmentation by reaction diffusion bubbles. *Proceedings of the International Conference on Computer Vision*, pages 156–162, 1995.

[37] S. Zhu, T. Lee, and A. Yuille. Region competition: Unifying snakes, region growing and bayes/MDL for multi-band image segmentation. *Proceedings of the International Conference on Computer Vision*, pages 416–423, 1995.

Comparison of Multiscale Representations
for a Linking-Based Image Segmentation Model

Wiro J. Niessen   Koen L. Vincken   Max A. Viergever

Imaging Center Utrecht, University Hospital Utrecht,
Heidelberglaan 100, 3584 CX Utrecht, The Netherlands.
E-mail: wiro@cv.ruu.nl

Abstract

Different multiscale generators are qualitatively compared with respect to their performance within a multiscale linking model for image segmentation. The linking model used is the hyperstack that was inspired by linear scale space theory. We discuss which properties of this paradigm are essential to determine which multiscale representations are suited as input to the hyperstack. If selected, one of the main problems we tackle is the estimation of the local scale such that the various stacks of images can effectively be compared. For nonlinear multiscale representations, which can be written as modified diffusion equations, an upper bound can be achieved by synchronizing the evolution parameter. The synchronization is empirically verified by counting the number of elliptic patches at corresponding scales. We compare the resulting stacks of images and the segmentation on a test image and a coronal MR brain image.

1   Introduction

Linear scale space is now a firmly established and well-understood field in computer vision. The last couple of years a number of nonlinear multiscale representations have emerged from different fields, *e.g.*, image dependent diffusion (*i.e.*, an inhomogeneous or anisotropic conduction coefficient), curve/surface evolution and mathematical morphology. Considering the promising results in preserving features at larger scales we consider several of the nonlinear scale spaces as input to the *hyperstack*, a linking model based multiscale segmentation method. The aim of this paper is threefold. First we determine whether the various multiscale representations are suited as input to the hyperstack, considering that it is based upon linear scale space theory. Secondly, we address the question how to synchronize the linear scale parameter with the scale parameter in the nonlinear multiscale representations. Thirdly, the scale spaces and segmentation are compared.

We discuss a number of nonlinear multiscale representations in $2D$ and $3D$, viz: (*i*) Gradient dependent diffusion, (*ii*) Geometric evolutions, (*iii*) Modified geometric evolution, (*iv*) Morphological scale spaces, and (*v*) Wavelet decomposition. We show that the last two are not suitable candidates as input to the hyperstack algorithm. To effectively compare the results of the other approaches we have to relate the levels of a linear scale space to the levels generated by nonlinear scale space constructors. To obtain a rough estimate we regard the approaches as modified diffusion equations with a bounded conduction coefficient. This criterion is qualitatively tested by comparing the number of 'elliptic patches' at corresponding levels with reasonable results.

We present the results on a test image and a medical image in two ways: (*i*) the scale spaces are compared and (*ii*) the segmented images are qualitatively compared. Based on our first series of experiments and validations it is our hypothesis that using nonlinearly blurred levels prior to a linear scale space will yield an improvement in all cases, but with a slightly higher computational burden.

We first review linear scale space theory and its essential properties for the *hyperstack* (section 2). We subsequently review a number of nonlinear multiscale representations (section 3), some of which can effectively be compared after scale synchronization (section 4). Examples in section 5 on a 3D test image and a $2D$ coronal slice of an MR brain qualitatively illustrate the specific properties of the different generators.

2   Linear scale space and the hyperstack

The *hyperstack* is a multiscale image segmentation method originally built upon linear scale space theory. We will first briefly review the hyperstack algorithm and the important linear scale space properties it relies on. This facilitates a comparison with other generators of multiscale representations which will be discussed in the next section.

263

Proceedings of MMBIA '96

2.1 The hyperstack

The hyperstack (for a more detailed description and extensions see [28, 15, 16]) is a linking model based segmentation technique. The entire process requires four steps (see Fig. 2): (*i*) blurring, (*ii*) linking, (*iii*) root labeling, and (*iv*) downward projection.

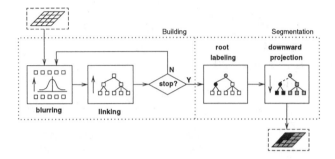

Fig. 2. *Schematic of the hyperstack segmentation process.*

In the blurring phase a stack of images is created. During the linking phase voxels in two adjacent scale levels are connected by so-called child-parent linkages, with an assigned *affection* value based on heuristic and statistical features (see [16] for details). The linking is a bottom-up process such that only parents that have been linked to are considered children in the next linking step. This leads to the typical tree-like structure of linkages through scale space.

If the linking has converged—in the sense that only few parents are left in the top level of the hyperstack—the root labeling takes place. In this phase, the children in the tree with a relatively low affection value are labeled as *roots*, each of which represents a segment in the original image.

Finally, in the down projection phase the actual segments are formed by grouping all the voxels in the ground level that are linked to a single root. This can readily be executed by following the child-parent linkages downwards. Instead of using unique segment values to discriminate between the different segments, it usually gives more attractive segmentations for visual inspection if the mean value within each segment is used.

2.2 Linear scale space theory

Originally, the stack of images in the blurring phase was obtained using a linear scale space representation. It captures the inherent multi-scale nature of image data. By definition, a linear scale space [32, 14] is a one-parameter family of images generated by the linear diffusion equation with the original image as initial condition:

$$\begin{cases} (\frac{\partial}{\partial t} - \triangle)L(\vec{x}, t) &= 0 \\ L(\vec{x}, 0) &= L_0(\vec{x}) \end{cases} \qquad (1)$$

The Green's function of the linear diffusion equation is the Gaussian. Therefore, the analytical solution of (1) is given by:

$$L(\vec{x}, t) = L_0(\vec{x}) \otimes G(\vec{x}, \sigma) \qquad (2)$$

where $\otimes$ denotes convolution and t is related to spatial scale as $t = \frac{1}{2}\sigma^2$. This process can be regarded as having a continuously increasing aperture function (or kernel) G that propagates the initial condition into scale space.

The hyperstack algorithm relies on some essential properties of scale space theory:

- **Causality**: One of the most important features of linear scale space for being a suitable multiscale representation is that it satisfies a maximum principle [13]. When traversing in the positive scale direction no spurious detail is generated [14].

- **Semi-group property**: The Gaussian is closed under convolution. Two consecutive smoothing steps with a kernel are equivalent to one smoothing step of a larger kernel. This property is *essential* for a scale space and it explains why linkages can be made between adjacent levels in scale space.

- **Conservation principle**: The average grey value is conserved under the linear smoothing process. This is important since the linking criterion heavily relies on the grey value of child and parent.

- **Scale invariance**: Modifying the image scale should not affect the results. Therefore, the blurring strategy has to follow an exponential sampling in scale space [9]. Hence, we introduce a natural scale parameter $\tau = n\,\delta\tau$, $n \in \mathbb{N}$, which is related to the absolute scale σ_n at level n by $\sigma_n = \varepsilon \exp(\tau_0 + n\,\delta\tau)$, where τ_0 is the initial scale offset and ε is taken to be the smallest linear grid measure of the imaging device (the *inner scale*).

- **Search Region**: The area in which a parent in level $n + 1$ is selected for a specific child in level n is isotropic [26] and defined by a radius $r_{n,n+1} = k \cdot \sigma_{n,n+1}$, where $\sigma_{n,n+1}$ denotes the relative σ (that corresponds with the transition from level n to level $n + 1$) and k is chosen such that only parents are considered whose intensity has been influenced significantly by the child at hand. Typically, $k = 1.5$.

- **Convergence**: For large scales the image converges to the average grey value. Therefore, a small number of nodes can represent the image establishing convergence of the linkage structure.

3 Nonlinear scale space

A number of nonlinear multiscale representations have appeared in literature. We will briefly comment on five classes: (*i*) variable conductance diffusion (*ii*) geometric evolutions, (*iii*) morphologic scale spaces, (*iv*) a combination of variable conductance diffusion and geometric evolutions and (*v*) wavelet decompositions. We will focus on the question whether these various approaches are suitable candidates for image segmentation using the hyperstack.

3.1 Variable conductance diffusion

The first approach is essentially a modification of the linear diffusion (or heat) equation, first proposed by Perona & Malik [21]. A general form of a diffusion equation with conduction coefficient c is given by:

$$\frac{\partial L}{\partial t} = \nabla \cdot \left(c \, \nabla L \right) \qquad (3)$$

The idea is to choose c such that relevant objects smooth while not affecting one another. An option is to make c a decreasing function of the gradient magnitude [21]:

$$c(\vec{x}, t) = g\left(\|\nabla L(\vec{x}, t)\| \right) = e^{-\left(\frac{\|\nabla L\|}{K} \right)^2} \qquad (4)$$

Here, K is a free parameter that determines the significance of the local gradient. A maximum principle has been proved provided that the solution is C^2. However, there is considerable empirical evidence that the Perona & Malik equation does not exhibit smooth solutions [19, 30]. Therefore, a stack based on the original formulation is not a good candidate as input to the hyperstack algorithm. Instead, we apply a scheme owing to Catté *et al.* [5] in which the gradient in the heat conduction coefficient will be calculated at a certain scale. This implies that insignificant edges (*e.g.*, resulting from high frequency noise) will not be kept. Furthermore, this approach regularizes the equation [5] and satisfies a maximum principle [30]. Note that the formulation is N-dimensional. Since convergence is considerably slower than in the linear scale space approach, convergence is sometimes enforced by a linear blurring process of the higher levels.

3.2 Curve evolution

The second approach to nonlinear scale spaces studies the evolution of curves or surfaces as a function of their geometry, see *e.g.*, [20] and references therein. If we evolve a curve as a function of local geometry and neglect the tangential component, we find:

$$\frac{\partial C}{\partial t} = g(\kappa, \kappa_p, ...)\vec{N} \qquad (5)$$

where κ denotes isophote curvature, κ_p denotes the derivative of curvature with respect to the arc-length parameter p and $\vec{N}$ denotes the normal direction.

In this paper we will consider the case $g = \kappa$, which leads to the well-known Euclidean shortening flow. This particular choice has a very intuitive interpretation if we rewrite it in terms of (v, w)-gauge coordinates (see Fig. 1).

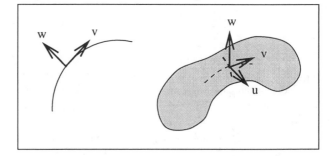

Fig. 1. *Local gauge coordinates in 2D and 3D (w points in the normal direction). In 3D u and v denote the principal curvature directions.*

In this gauge, the v direction denotes the local isophote direction and w denotes the normal direction. The curvature can now be expressed as $\kappa = -L_{vv}/L_w$ (see [8]). This implies the following evolution of the luminance function:

$$\frac{\partial L}{\partial t} = L_{vv} \qquad (6)$$

which can be interpreted as a diffusion equation which only diffuses in the local isophote direction. This equation has been derived independently by Alvarez *et al.* in [2] because of this exact property. The Euclidean shortening flow has important smoothing properties: non-convex curves will evolve into convex curves [11] and from there to a round point [10] in finite time. A main problem of the scheme is that is can not be cast in conservation form: the average grey value is not conserved. However, it does satisfy the semi-group property and we will consider it as input to the hyperstack.

Extensions of curve evolution schemes to $3D$ are not straightforward. Given an isophote surface patch, we can define the orthogonal directions of maximal and minimal curvature (κ_1, κ_2). In literature one has considered evolutions based on the Mean and Gaussian curvature given by the average or product of the principal curvatures. Unfortunately, stability results have only been obtained for convex input surfaces. A dumbbell *e.g.*, develops singularities under Mean curvature flow [25, 12] and Gaussian curvature flow is also unstable for most concave initial surfaces [7].

3.3 Modified geometric evolutions

We consider two approaches which combine contrast dependent diffusion as in the Perona & Malik equation with concepts of geometric evolutions. Weickert [31, 30] considered a heat conduction tensor $\mathbf{D}$ instead of the heat conduction scalar c in (3):

$$\frac{\partial L}{\partial t} = \nabla \cdot \left(\mathbf{D} \, \nabla L \right) \qquad (7)$$

$\mathbf{D}$ is chosen as a function of the local image gradient at a certain scale. It not only defines the *amount* of diffusion but also regulates the *direction* of diffusion, allowing diffusion along edges. This approach has the advantage that it removes noise at edges, which typically remains present in the Perona & Malik equation. The scheme is written in divergence form and therefore the grey value is conserved. Henceforth this scheme is a logical candidate for input to the hyperstack.

Another approach combines geometric evolutions with a contrast dependent speed term [2, 22, 24, 18]:

$$\frac{\partial L}{\partial t} = g(L_w) * L_{vv} \qquad (8)$$

where g is a decreasing function of the image gradient L_w. The approach slows down the diffusion in neighborhoods of large contrast. $g(L_w)$ is typically calculated at a certain scale in order not to preserve noise. Compared to the approach presented by Weickert this approach has the drawback that the average grey value is not conserved.

3.4 Morphological scale spaces

Morphological scale spaces represent stacks of images obtained by dilating/eroding the initial conditions with structuring elements of increasing size. Brockett and Maragos [4], Sapiro *et al.* [23] and Van den Boomgaard and Smeulders [3] considered the differential equations that are solved using these morphological propagators. Morphological dilation of a grey value image $L(\vec{x})$ with a structuring element B is defined as:

$$(L \oplus B)(\vec{x}) = sup\{L(\vec{x} - \vec{y}), \vec{y} \in B\} \qquad (9)$$

If we now consider a continuous (convex!) structuring element $tB, t \in \mathbf{R}$ it can be shown [4, 23, 3] that the scale space representation $L(\vec{x}, t)$ is constructed according to:

$$\frac{\partial L}{\partial t}(\vec{x}, t) = sup\{(\vec{y} \cdot \nabla L)(\vec{x, t}), \vec{y} \in B\} \qquad (10)$$

Hence, dilations and erosions with convex structuring elements satisfy the semi-group property. Although this definitely reflects the scale space behavior of these morphological schemes, it is not easily reconciled with the hyperstack. Consider *e.g.*, a circular structure element B (in this

case we have normal motion in (5); $g(\kappa) = c$ is constant). The structuring elements pushes the initial conditions inward/outward giving rise to a hyperbolic-type evolution equation. This implies that information travels in one direction which is not in accordance with the isotropic search region in adjacent levels of the hyperstack.

Several approaches have tried to construct a multiscale representation based on the morphological operations of openings and closings. Chen and Yan [6] claimed causality since no additional zero-crossings are introduced while moving to coarser scale using the morphological opening operation. However, Nacken [17] constructed a counterexample. Similar as for the dilation/erosion scale space we would like to define a continuous parameter which represents scale in this framework. Alvarez *et al.* tried [1] to write this approach in a differential framework. They consider the opening of $L(\vec{x}$ as $L(\vec{x}, t) = O_t L(\vec{x})$. Now $L(\vec{x}, 2t)$ can be computed as the solution of an erosion of time t followed by a dilation of time t (U denotes the Heavyside function):

$$\frac{\partial \tilde{L}}{\partial s} = U(t - s)(\tilde{L} \ominus B) + U(s - t)(\tilde{L} \oplus B) \qquad (11)$$

The discontinuity at $s = t$ can easily be overcome by slowing down the erosion when s approaches t. However, note that for every $L(\vec{x}, 2t)$ we have to solve (11). The equation does not satisfy the semi-group property. Therefore, we do not know how to relate level n with level $n + 1$ making it questionable whether the approach is a genuine scale space and unsuitable as input to our multiscale linking model.

3.5 Wavelet Decomposition

A wavelet decomposition is by definition not a suitable candidate as input for the hyperstack. Given that wavelets form an orthogonal basis, it follows that data at separate levels are uncorrelated, thus making linkages through the tree useless. Although often coined a shortcoming of linear scale space, the hyperstack fruitfully exploits the redundancy of information in the generated tree.

4 Nonlinear scale spaces and scale

In this section we investigate if we can relate the scales of the levels of a linear scale space to the levels generated by nonlinear scale space constructors. We will consider the regularized Perona & Malik equation and the anisotropic tensor diffusion which were shown to be suitable candidates. Furthermore, we consider the Euclidean shortening flow and modified geometric evolutions, but stress that they suffer from the fact that they do not preserve the average grey value.

Since the Green's function of the abovementioned schemes is unknown, there is no longer an obvious relation between the evolution parameter and the spatial extent of 'some' blurring filter. However, in all cases we constructed evolutions which limited the normal diffusion (note that in the linear case we have a constant diffusion coefficient $c = 1$). The scalar diffusivity c in the Perona & Malik equation (3) and the tensor conductivity $\mathbf{D}$ in (7) are constructed such that $\|c\| \leq 1$ and all eigenvalues of $\mathbf{D}$ have a norm smaller than 1. The Euclidean shortening flow limits the diffusion in the direction defined by the image gradient, which is also true for the modified geometric evolution if $g(L_w) \leq 1$.

We therefore derived an upper bound for the local scale in nonlinear evolution schemes based on the scale corresponding to an equivalent evolution time in the linear diffusion equation. Recall the relation between the evolution parameter and the standard deviation of the Gaussian: $t = \frac{1}{2}\sigma^2$. Instead of using an exponential scale sampling we now use an exponential 'evolution time sampling t' which corresponds to the scale sampling of the linear diffusion equation.

In order to check whether the upper bound is not a too rough estimate for a typical input image we constructed a qualitative verification. We compared the number of 'generic local features' which we measure using the number of 'elliptic patches' [9].

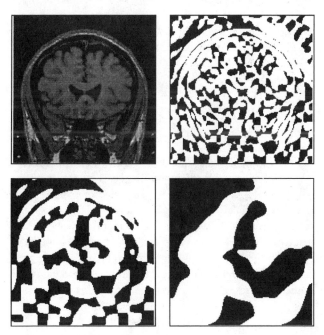

Fig. 3. *Elliptic patches of a* 178×179 *MR image at different scale levels. Shown are (from left to right, top to bottom) the original image and the umbilicity images for* $\sigma = 4, 8, 16$ *pixels, respectively.*

For the two-dimensional case, an elliptic patch is defined as a connected set of pixels in which the umbilicity is positive (see Fig. 3):

$$\frac{\partial^2 L}{\partial x^2} \cdot \frac{\partial^2 L}{\partial y^2} - \frac{\partial^2 L}{\partial x \, \partial y} > 0 \qquad (12)$$

Hence, the decrease in the number of elliptic patches corresponding to any scale space generator should be roughly the same as the decrease for the linear scale space for the synchronization to make sense. In this way, we have defined a qualitative measure to synchronize different scale space generators.

In practice, counting the blob-like structures for a linear scale space is performed by calculating the umbilicity at the corresponding scale. We subsequently scan the resulting image until all the areas satisfying equation (12) have been counted. This is done effectively by a region-growing in each positive valued pixel encountered, after which that region is marked as being 'counted'. The process stops if no more positive valued pixels can be found.

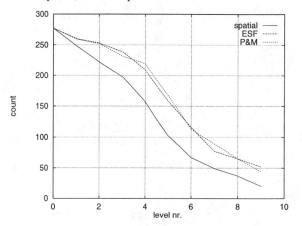

Fig. 4. *Decrease of the number of elliptic patches in the first 9 levels for different scale spaces (left). For the linear scale space we have used* $\delta\tau = \frac{1}{2}\ln 2$. *For the nonlinear scale spaces we have synchronized the corresponding evolution times.*

In Fig. 4, we use the evolution parameter to synchronize the different scale spaces. The linear diffusion does indeed serve as an upper bound for the Euclidean shortening flow and Perona & Malik equation. Note that with respect to this criterion the Perona & Malik equation and Euclidean shortening flow can effectively be compared. In this example the upper bound supplied by the linear diffusion equation remains within reasonable range.

However, the approach presented here is not completely satisfactory. Nonlinear smoothing evolutions can be constructed for certain images in which the upper bound set by linear diffusion is a very rough measure. Weickert [30] proposed a more physical synchronization based on the information content of an image. He constructed a Lyapunov functional which measures *e.g.*, the entropy of an image over scale. This approach can also provide a stopping criterion. The hyperstack itself could also provide a means to synchronize different levels based on the number of segments at each level.

5 Results

We describe the results of applying the different scale space generators to a test image and a coronal MR slice in three ways: (*i*) the generated scale spaces are compared, (*ii*) the stacks are used as input to the hyperstack segmentation algorithm, and the produced segmentations are qualitatively compared and (*iii*) the segmentations are evaluated by an objective measure that we have developed for quantitative analysis and comparison of segmentation results.

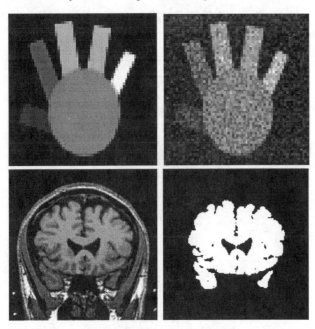

Fig. 5. *Input images to the experiments.*
(a) a slice of the original 3D HAND *image;*
(b) the corresponding slice of the noisy HAND.200 *image;*
(c) the original BRAIN.COR *image;*
(d) the manual segmentation of the ROI;

5.1 Test Image

We created an artificial 3D image (see Fig. 5) containing a hand by using the volumetric object generating package 'THINGS' [27]. The main feature of this package is the simulation of the partial volume artifact by discretizing the specified objects (*i.e.*, ellipsoids, etc.) at sub-voxel level. The original HAND image contains the pixel values 0 (background), 500 (dumb), 800 (forefinger), 1000 (palm of the hand), 1250 (middle finger and ring-finger), and 1500 (little finger). From this artificial image (containing 16 slices of 64×64 pixels) we derived the 'HAND.200'

input image by adding Gaussian noise with standard deviation 200.

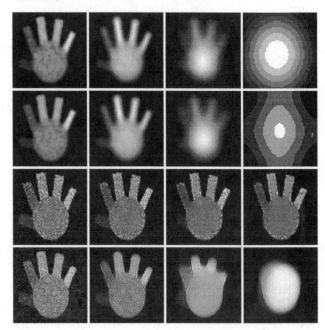

Fig. 6. *A single slice of the* HAND.200 *image shown at different levels of scale for the four different scale space generators. Shown are, from top to bottom:*
(a) Linear scale space, spatial domain (levels 1, 3, 5, 11);
(b) Linear scale space, Fourier domain (levels 1, 3, 5, 11);
(c) Regularized Perona & Malik filter (levels 2, 4, 6, 8);
(d) Euclidean shortening flow filter (levels 2, 4, 6, 8);

5.1.1 The scale spaces

In Fig. 6 the different scale spaces—generated by the methods discussed in this chapter—for the HAND.200 image are shown. More precisely, we extracted one slice of the HAND.200 image at some of the levels of the generated scale spaces to show the scaling function. Note that the detail vanishes at different scales, so for clarity we have chosen different series of scales for every scale space generator. The actual level numbers used have been indicated in the subscript of Fig. 6. We remark the following:

- The boundary effect caused by blurring in the Fourier domain (*i.e.*, data repetition) is much more apparent than in the spatial domain (averaging).

- The regularized Perona & Malik equation preserves the objects' contours best. The thumb disappears first of all fingers, because it has the lowest intensity value. A different (lower) value of K in the equations will better preserve the thumb.

- For the Euclidean shortening flow the absolute image intensities do not affect the local blurring: the curve evolves at the same speed for points with equal curvature.

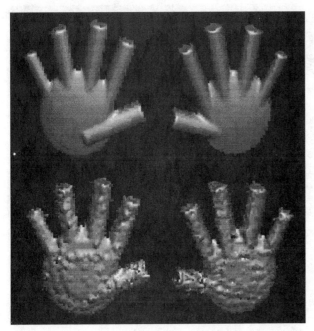

Fig. 7. *Volume renderings of the original* HAND.200 *image and the segmentation of the* HAND.200 *image using the regularized Perona & Malik equation, which performed 'best' according to the objective evaluation measure (see 5.3). The results have been rendered twice to show the front and back sides of the hand.*

5.1.2 The segmentations

A volume rendering of the original HAND image and a segmentation based on the regularized Perona & Malik equation are shown in Fig. 7. In order to enable a visual comparison, the front and back view renderings of the original image are presented simultaneously. The regularized Perona & Malik equation performed best based on a criterion that will be explained in section 5.3, where a quantitative evaluation method for segmentation results is outlined. We do not show the other segmentations since it is hard to detect clear differences (for a detailed comparison see [26]). This is a first indication for the fact that the hyperstack segmentations do not heavily depend on the different scale spaces used.

5.2 Coronal brain image

We compared the different scale space representations for a coronal brain image BRAIN.COR (see Fig. 5). This image contains 178×179 pixels; the corresponding manual segmentation contains two objects. For all experiments

we have used $\delta\tau = \frac{1}{2}\ln 2$. We have also done experiments with a transversal slice of another head (see [29]).

5.2.1 The scale spaces

In Fig. 8 the different scale spaces of the BRAIN.COR image are shown. We see that at larger scales the difference between the spatial and Fourier implementation of linear scale space becomes apparent. It is also obvious that the nonlinear scale space generators preserve features better than in the linear case. However, based on the empirical scale synchronization we conclude that comparing corresponding levels of the regularized Perona & Malik equation and Euclidean shortening flow is justified; the number of elliptic patches is comparable. The different nature of the Euclidean shortening flow and Perona & Malik equation is also apparent. The former is grey value invariant, in contrast to the Perona & Malik equation, where bright image features are better preserved. This can most easily be observed in the ventricle system which—having a considerably lower intensity than its neighboring objects—causes variable conductance diffusion to preserve the ventricles at large scales. In contrast, Euclidean shortening flow considers the ventricles to be objects with high curvature, hence they disappear faster.

5.2.2 The segmentations

In Fig. 9 the four hyperstack segmentations of the white matter are shown. To emphasize the local errors, each (binary) segmentation has been subtracted from the manual segmentation. The pixels in agreement with each other are colored grey, the differences are colored white. Note that 'white' may denote either 'too little' or 'too much' segment. The differences are small and mainly concern the small, disconnected lobe on the right part of the picture. Indeed, small segments and deep inlets are the most difficult parts to segment, owing to the partial volume effect.

5.3 Evaluation

By counting the erroneously segmented pixels in Fig. 9 it is tempting to conclude that the Euclidean shortening flow and regularized Perona & Malik equation perform better than the linear scale spaces (although the differences are small). We have to be careful, however, to interpret these numbers. A manual segmentation will never be 100% correct, and in addition the segmentation task will generally not require a 100% correct result. Therefore, not all the white pixels will have to be corrected to obtain a useful result.

In order to be able to make an objective and quantitative comparison between different segmentations, we have developed a task-driven evaluation method. The task is defined as minimizing the effort of manually editing the segmented image—by using split and merge actions—until a result of satisfactory quality is obtained. See [15] for details.

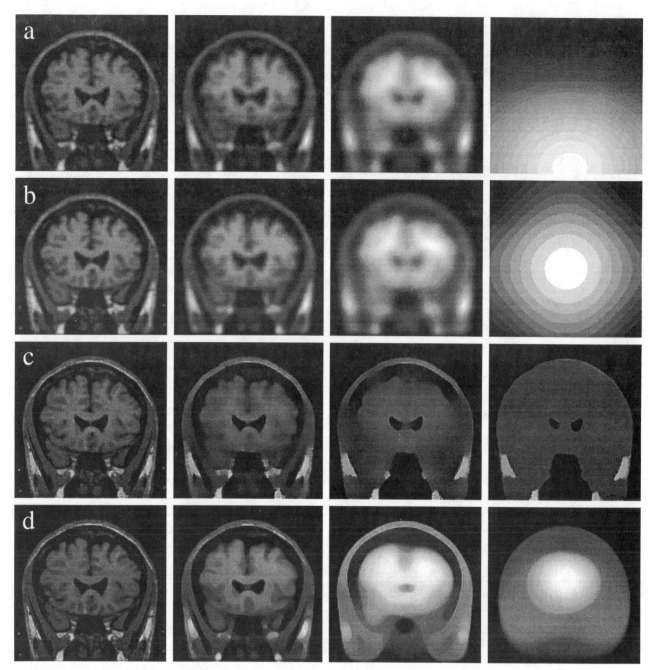

Fig. 8. *The* BRAIN.COR *image shown at different levels of scale for the four different scale space generators.*
(a) Linear scale space implemented in the spatial domain (levels 2, 4, 6, 15);
(b) Linear scale space implemented in the Fourier domain (levels 2, 4, 6, 15);
(c) Regularized Perona & Malik filter (levels 2, 5, 8, 11);
(d) Euclidean shortening flow (levels 2, 5, 8, 11);

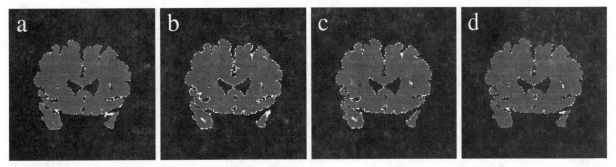

Fig. 9. *Segmentations of the white matter of the* BRAIN.COR *image based on the four different scale space generators. The grey colored areas have been segmented correctly (according to the gold standard), the white colored areas correspond to erroneously segmented pixels. The figures correspond to: (a) Linear scale space implemented in the spatial domain; (b) Ditto, implemented in the Fourier domain; (c) Regularized Perona & Malik equation; (d) Euclidean shortening flow.*

The post-processing editing (PPE) costs do not have an absolute meaning. Rather, they should be compared *relatively* to the costs needed for a complete manual segmentation. The manual costs are calculated by using an entirely homogeneous image as 'segmented image'. Then, the editing costs to change the image to the gold standard correspond precisely to drawing the contours of all segments. The relative PPE costs refer to the ratio of the costs of an automatic segmentation and the costs of a 100% manual segmentation.

For the BRAIN.COR image all relative PPE costs turn out to be significantly smaller than a pure manual segmentation. Moreover, the segmentations based on a linear scale space are slightly more expensive compared to the nonlinear variants [26].

6 Conclusions

In this paper we have investigated a number of multiscale representations as input to the hyperstack, a multiscale linking model. Some approaches were found to be unsuited. A scheme based on multiscale morphological opening/closing operations does not satisfy the essential semi-group property. Multiscale approaches using dilation/erosion have genuine scale space properties but the isotropic search region in the hyperstack segmentation would need to be modified.

Nonlinear diffusion equations which can be written in divergence form can be used as input to the hyperstack. The regularized Perona & Malik equation and the anisotropic tensor diffusion introduced by Weickert [30] seem the most promising candidates. The Euclidean shortening flow satisfies all desirable properties except that it can not be cast in conservation form.

By viewing the processes as limiting the linear diffusion, we derived an upper bound for the scale parameter which we used to synchronize the approaches. Counting the number of elliptic patches at corresponding scales

the synchronization can be empirically verified. For the BRAIN.COR image used in the experiments, this criterion nicely matched the regularized Perona & Malik equation and Euclidean shortening flow.

Finally, we have compared four different scale space generators within the hyperstack framework. Linear scale space implemented both in the spatial and Fourier domain, the regularized Perona & Malik equation, and the Euclidean shortening flow We judged the corresponding segmentations both quantitatively and qualitatively. Based on experiments with artificial and medical images, we conclude that hyperstack segmentation is *in general* not very sensitive to the underlying scale space. Nonetheless, the nonlinear scale space generators based on the regularized Perona & Malik equation and the Euclidean shortening flow perform slightly better on the images.

We are currently evaluating the results for the anisotropic tensor diffusion and the modified geometric evolutions for which we expect further improvement.

7 Acknowledgment

This research is supported by the industrial companies Philips Medical Systems, KEMA, and Shell International Exploration and Production.

References

[1] L. Alvarez, F. Guichard, P. L. Lions, and J. M. Morel. Axioms and fundamental equations of image processing. *Arch. for Rational Mechanics*, 123(3):199–257, September 1993.

[2] L. Alvarez, P.-L. Lions, and J.-M. Morel. Image selective smoothing and edge detection by nonlinear diffusion. II. *SIAM J. Num. Anal.*, 29(3):845–866, 1992.

[3] R. van den Boomgaard and A. Smeulders. The morphological structure of images: The differential equations of morphological scale space. *IEEE Transactions on Pattern Analysis and Machine Intelligence*, 16:1101–1113, 1994.

[4] R. W. Brockett and P. Maragos. Evolutions equations for continuous-scale morphology. In *International Conference on Acoustics, Speech, Signal Processing*. IEEE, 1992.

[5] F. Catté, P.-L. Lions, J.-M. Morel, and T. Coll. Image selective smoothing and edge detection by nonlinear diffusion. *SIAM J. Num. Anal.*, 29(1):182–193, 1992.

[6] M. Chen and P. Yan. A multiscale approach based on morphological filtering. *IEEE Transactions on Pattern Analysis and Machine Intelligence*, 11(7):694–700, 1989.

[7] D. L. Chopp and J. A. Sethian. Flow under curvature; singularity formation minimal surfaces and geodesics. *Jour. Exper. Math*, 2(4):235–255, 1993.

[8] L. M. J. Florack, B. M. ter Haar Romeny, J. J. Koenderink, and M. A. Viergever. General intensity transformations and differential invariants. *Journal of Mathematical Imaging and Vision*, 4(2):171–187, 1994.

[9] L. M. J. Florack, B. M. ter Haar Romeny, J. J. Koenderink, and M. A. Viergever. Linear scale-space. *Journal of Mathematical Imaging and Vision*, 4(4):325–351, 1994.

[10] M. Gage and R. S. Hamilton. The heat equation shrinking convex plane curves. *J. Differential Geometry*, 23:69–96, 1986.

[11] M. Grayson. The heat equation shrinks embedded plane curves to round points. *Journal of Differential geometry*, 26:285–314, 1987.

[12] M. Grayson. A short note on the evolution of a surface by its mean curvature. *Duke Mathematical Journal*, 58(3):555–558, 1989.

[13] R. A. Hummel. Representations based on zero crossings in scale space. In *Proceedings of the IEEE Computer Vision and Pattern Recognition Conference*, pages 204–209, 1986.

[14] J. J. Koenderink. The structure of images. *Biological Cybernetics*, 50:363–370, 1984.

[15] A. S. E. Koster. *Linking Models for Multiscale Image Segmentation*. PhD thesis, Utrecht University, The Netherlands, 1995.

[16] A. S. E. Koster, K. L. Vincken, and M. A. Viergever. Heuristic linking models in multi-scale image segmentation. *Computer Vision, Graphics, and Image Processing*. In press.

[17] P. F. M. Nacken. Openings can introduce zero crossings in boundary curvature. *IEEE Transactions on Pattern Analysis and Machine Intelligence*, 16(6):656–658, 1994.

[18] W. J. Niessen, B. M. ter Haar Romeny, L. M. J. Florack, and M. A. Viergever. A general framework for geometry-driven evolution equations. *International Journal of Computer Vision*. In press.

[19] M. Nitzberg and T. Shiota. Nonlinear image filtering with edge and corner enhancement. *IEEE Transactions on Pattern Analysis and Machine Intelligence*, 14(8):826–833, 1992.

[20] S. Osher and S. Sethian. Fronts propagating with curvature dependent speed: algorithms based on the Hamilton-Jacobi formalism. *J. Computational Physics*, 79:12–49, 1988.

[21] P. Perona and J. Malik. Scale-space and edge detection using anisotropic diffusion. *IEEE Transactions on Pattern Analysis and Machine Intelligence*, 12(7):629–639, 1990.

[22] L. I. Rudin, S. Osher, and E. Fatemi. Nonlinear total variation based noise removal algorithms. *Physica D*, 60:259–268, 1992.

[23] G. Sapiro, R. Kimmel, D. Shaked, B. B. Kimia, and A. M. Bruckstein. Implementing continuous-scale morphology via curve evolution. *Pattern Recognition*, 26(9):1363–1372, 1993.

[24] G. Sapiro, A. Tannenbaum, Y. You, and M. Kaveh. Experiments on geometric enhancement. In *International Conference on Image Processing*, pages 472–475. IEEE, 1994.

[25] J. A. Sethian. Curvature and the evolution of fronts. *Comm. Math. Phys.*, 101:487–499, 1985.

[26] K. L. Vincken. *Probabilistic Multiscale Image Segmentation by the Hyperstack*. PhD thesis, Utrecht University, The Netherlands, 1995.

[27] K. L. Vincken and F. J. R. Appelman. Accurate conversion of geometrical objects to voxel-based images. Report 3DCV 91-20, Utrecht University, 1991.

[28] K. L. Vincken, A. S. E. Koster, and M. A. Viergever. Probabilistic segmentation of partial volume voxels. *Pattern Recognition Letters*, 15(5):477–484, 1994.

[29] K. L. Vincken, W. J. Niessen, A. S. E. Koster, and M. A. Viergever. Blurring strategies for image segmentation using a multiscale linking model. In *IEEE Conference on Computer Vision and Pattern Recognition, CVPR'96*, San Francisco, CA, 1996. IEEE Computer Society Press. Accepted for publication.

[30] J. Weickert. *Anisotropic Diffusion in Image Processing*. PhD thesis, Dept. of Mathematics, University of Kaiserslautern, Germany, January 1996.

[31] J. Weickert. Theoretical foundations of anisotropic diffusion in image processing. In W. Kropatsch, R. Klette, and F. Solina, editors, *Theoretical Foundations of Computer Vision*, volume 11 of *Computing Supplement*, pages 221–236. Springer, Wien, 1996.

[32] A. P. Witkin. Scale space filtering. In *Proc. International Joint Conference on Artificial Intelligence*, pages 1019–1023. Karlsruhe, W. Germany, 1983.

Deblurring the Discrete Gaussian Blur

B. A. Mair and David C. Wilson
Department of Mathematics
University of Florida, Gainesville, FL 32611
bam@math.ufl.edu, dcw@math.ufl.edu

Zoltán Réti
Department of Mathematics
The Pennsylvania State University
University Park, PA 16802
reti@math.psu.edu

Abstract

In 1995 Z. Réti presented a method for deblurring images blurred by the discrete Gaussian. The method is based on theorems borrowed from analytic number theory developed by Gauss, G. Jacobi (1829), and Ramanujan. One advantage of this method over similar ones developed for the continuous domain is that it provides exact formulas for the deblurring convolution. In addition, while deblurring the Gaussian in the continuous domain is an ill-posed inverse problem, deblurring the discrete Gaussian model results in a mathematically well-posed problem. The formulas presented here provide error bounds which relate the quality of the reconstructed image to that of the blurred image. This deblurring method is conveniently expressed in terms of multiplication by Toeplitz matrices whose diagonal entries decrease exponentially, thus rendering the method suitable for numerical approximations. Condition numbers are provided for various choices of σ.

1. Introduction

The purpose of this paper is to provide an error analysis for the discrete deblurring techniques presented by Réti [10]. Since the intent is that these methods would be applied to 2-dimensional images rather than sequences, all results are presented on the space $\ell^2(\mathbb{Z}^2)$. However, the results are valid in any dimension. The reason the reconstruction algorithm is presented in the discrete domain is that if the blurring process is represented by the linear operator T in the space $L^2(\mathbb{R}^2)$, then T fails to have a bounded inverse. This fact can be observed by noticing that if (ω_1, ω_2) represent frequencies in the transform domain, then the multiplier function corresponding to T is $e^{-\sigma^2(\omega_1^2+\omega_2^2)/2}$, which does not have an inverse Fourier transform in the image space. Thus, the problem is ill-posed on the space $L^2(\mathbb{R}^2)$. Consequently, various regularization methods have to be employed to first stabilize the mathematical problem, even before *numerical* stability concerns are addressed [2, 6, 7, 12, 9]. These regularization methods rely on determining an appropriate degree of regularization, either from apriori information, or, more usually from the data. The quality of the reconstructed image is extremely sensitive to this degree of regularization, and the data-based methods [13] always result in a significant computational burden. The work in [3] demonstrates that the operator T does have a bounded inverse when the domain is enlarged to the space of regular tempered distributions. In [11], this approach is used to obtain an exact method of inverting T in this larger space, by successive convolutions with derivatives of the Gaussian.

In this paper, we consider the discrete mathematical model of Gaussian blur [8, 10]. In this model, images are represented as square summable, doubly indexed sequences, so $\ell^2(\mathbb{Z}^2)$, represents the space of all images, and the blurring operator A_σ is represented by the discrete convolution of an image with the tensor product sequence $w_\sigma \otimes w_\sigma$, where w_σ is the discretely sampled Gaussian filter. By considering the corresponding Fourier series of an image, we show (Section 2) that this convolution operator can be lifted to a multiplication operator on the space $L^2(\mathbb{T}^2, \frac{ds\,dt}{4\pi^2})$, of square integrable functions on the two dimensional torus, with Lebesgue measure normalized so that the surface area of the torus is one. (Recall that the torus can be represented as the Cartesian product of the unit circle with itself.) Unlike the continuous case, the reciprocal of this multiplier function does represent a bounded operator on $L^2(\mathbb{T}^2, \frac{ds\,dt}{4\pi^2})$. Thus, this discrete model produces a mathematically well-posed problem, which does not need any regularization methods or extension of domain techniques.

This paper presents an exact method of deblurring the discrete Gaussian based on results in the theory of q-series [1, 4, 10]. In particular, by using the Jacobi Triple Product Identity, we obtain (Section 3) the condition number of the blurring operator, which relates the quality of the reconstructions to that of the blurred image.

By using a special case of the q-binomial theorem [4] we obtain the reciprocal of the multiplier function as a product of two Fourier series, one of which is the discrete Fourier transform of a causal linear filter, and the other corresponding to an anticausal linear filter (with the same coefficients as the causal). Thus, the proposed inversion technique consists of multiplying the rows (transposed), and then the resulting columns by a matrix product $L_\sigma^T L_\sigma$, and then by a normalizing factor Q_σ. Kimia and Zucker [8] also obtain an exact deblurring procedure in terms of multiplication. With their procedure, deblurring is achieved by multiplying by $K^T D K$ where K is a lower triangular matrix, and D is a diagonal matrix. However, K is *not* Toeplitz, whereas our L_σ is Toeplitz, and D is *not* a constant multiple of the identity. Thus it is not as easily implemented as ours. In our method, the unavoidable *numerical* ill-conditioning of the deblurring process is isolated in a single normalizing term that only needs to be calculated in the final step of the deblurring process. Furthermore, the diagonal entries of L_σ decrease exponentially as one moves away from the main diagonal, which consists entirely of ones. Thus, truncation of these infinite matrices yields a well-conditioned numerical deblurring procedure for a wide range of values of the variance. This range of values for the variance are also obtained.

2. Mathematical Model

As usual, we denote an image by a sequence of values $\{f(m,n)\}_{m,n=-\infty}^\infty$ which is square summable. So the image space is

$$\ell^2(\mathbb{Z}^2) = \left\{ f : \sum_{m,n=-\infty}^\infty |f(m,n)|^2 < \infty \right\}$$

For any $\sigma > 0$, the one dimensional discrete Gaussian blur with mean zero and variance σ^2 is obtained by convolution with the sequence

$$w_\sigma(n) = \frac{1}{\sqrt{2\pi}\,\sigma} \exp\left(-\frac{n^2}{2\sigma^2}\right) \qquad (1)$$

Hence, the blurred images that we consider in this paper are of the form

$$g = A_\sigma f \qquad (2)$$

where the operator $A_\sigma : \ell^2(\mathbb{Z}^2) \to \ell^2(\mathbb{Z}^2)$ is defined by

$$A_\sigma f(m,n) = \sum_{j,k=-\infty}^\infty f(m-j,n-k)w_\sigma(j)w_\sigma(k) \qquad (3)$$

The key to this method is that this discrete convolution operator on sequence space, is equivalent (via the Fourier transform $\mathcal{F}$) to a multiplication operator on the space of square integrable 2π−periodic functions, with normalized surface

measure, which is denoted by $L^2(\mathbb{T}^2, \frac{ds\,dt}{4\pi^2})$. Thus, by defining the operator $M_\sigma : L^2(\mathbb{T}^2, \frac{ds\,dt}{4\pi^2}) \to L^2(\mathbb{T}^2, \frac{ds\,dt}{4\pi^2})$ as

$$(M_\sigma H)(s,t) = W_\sigma(s)W_\sigma(t)H(s,t) \qquad (4)$$

we obtain that the blurring in sequence space $g = A_\sigma f$ is equivalent to the multiplication in the dual space $G = M_\sigma F$. Precisely,

$$\mathcal{F}(M_\sigma F) = A_\sigma(\mathcal{F}F) \qquad (5)$$

Hence, if the multiplier function $W_\sigma \otimes W_\sigma$ is never zero, we can hope to invert the operator M_σ by simple division, and then project this inverse onto the image space by the Fourier transform. This technique is made possible by explicit representations for W_σ and its reciprocal, that are well known in the theory of q-series [4]. These explicit representations also enable us to obtain sharp error bounds which predict the quality of the resulting reconstruction from the quality of the approximation of the blurred image and the variance of the blur.

3. Invertibility of Blurring Operators

By using the Jacobi Triple Product Identity [4] we demonstrate that both blurring operators A_σ and M_σ, have bounded inverses. In addition we use this number theoretic representation of W_σ to calculate their norms and condition numbers, which give vital information on the accuracy of the reconstruction procedure which will be obtained in the next section.

For notational convenience, we define

$$q = e^{-1/(2\sigma^2)}$$

so that

$$W_\sigma(t) = \frac{1}{\sqrt{2\pi}\,\sigma} \sum_{n=-\infty}^\infty q^{n^2} e^{int}$$

Then by [4], we obtain

$$W_\sigma(t) = \frac{1}{\sqrt{2\pi}\,\sigma} \prod_{k=1}^\infty (1-q^{2k})(1+q^{2k-1}e^{it})(1+q^{2k-1}e^{-it}) \qquad (6)$$

A simple calculation produces

$$W_\sigma(t) = \frac{1}{\sqrt{2\pi}\,\sigma} \prod_{k=1}^\infty (1-q^{2k})(1+2q^{2k-1}\cos(t)+q^{4k-2}) \qquad (7)$$

Thus, we obtain the following result.

Lemma 3.1. For all t, $0 < W_\sigma(\pi) \le W_\sigma(t) \le W_\sigma(0) < \infty$.

Theorem 3.1 $\|A_\sigma\| = \|M_\sigma\| = W_\sigma(0)^2$.

Proof: By using (5) and the fact that the Fourier transform $\mathcal{F}$ is an isomorphism we know that for any $f \in \ell^2(\mathbb{Z}^2)$ there is an $F \in L^2(\mathbb{T}^2, \frac{ds\,dt}{4\pi^2})$ such that

$$\|A_\sigma f\| = \|A_\sigma \mathcal{F}F\| = \|\mathcal{F}(M_\sigma F)\| = \|M_\sigma F\| \quad (8)$$

The first equality in (3) follows immediately. Now, for any $F \in L^2(\mathbb{T}^2, \frac{ds\,dt}{4\pi^2})$, by Lemma 3.1, we obtain

$$
\begin{aligned}
\|M_\sigma F\|^2 &= \int_0^{2\pi} \int_0^{2\pi} W_\sigma(s)^2 W_\sigma(t)^2 F(s,t)^2 \frac{ds\,dt}{4\pi^2} \\
&\leq W_\sigma(0)^4 \|F\|^2.
\end{aligned}
$$

Thus, $\|M_\sigma\| \leq W_\sigma(0)^2$. Now, let $\{F_n\}$ be a sequence in $L^2(\mathbb{T}^2, \frac{ds\,dt}{4\pi^2})$ of unit norm, which converges weakly to the point mass at the origin, which implies that $\|M_\sigma F_n\|$ converges to $W_\sigma(0)^2$. This argument completes the proof.

Theorem 3.2 A_σ and M_σ have bounded inverses on $\ell^2(\mathbb{Z}^2)$ and $L^2(\mathbb{T}^2, \frac{ds\,dt}{4\pi^2})$ respectively, which satisfy

$$\|A_\sigma^{-1}\| = \|M_\sigma^{-1}\| = W_\sigma(\pi)^{-2}. \quad (9)$$

Furthermore, for all $F \in L^2(\mathbb{T}^2, \frac{ds\,dt}{4\pi^2})$

$$M_\sigma^{-1}(F)(s,t) = W_\sigma^{-1}(s) W_\sigma^{-1}(t) F(s,t). \quad (10)$$

Proof: By Lemma 3.1, it is clear that multiplication by $W_\sigma^{-1} \otimes W_\sigma^{-1}$ is a well-defined linear operator on $L^2(\mathbb{T}^2, \frac{ds\,dt}{4\pi^2})$, so (10) follows. From Lemma 3.1 and an argument similar to that in the proof of Theorem 3.1, it is easy to see that $\|M_\sigma\| = W_\sigma(\pi)^{-2}$. Now, define the map $B_\sigma : \ell^2(\mathbb{Z}^2) \to \ell^2(\mathbb{Z}^2)$ by $B_\sigma f = \mathcal{F}(M_\sigma^{-1} \mathcal{F}^{-1} f)$. Then, by using (5), it follows that $B_\sigma = A_\sigma^{-1}$ so that $\|A_\sigma^{-1}\| = \|M_\sigma^{-1}\|$ is again a result of the properties of the Fourier transform.

Thus, to deblur, we can simply apply the *continuous* operator A_σ^{-1} to the blurred image, and we are assured that the reconstruction will be a good approximation to the original image, even if the blurred image contains other random errors. This setting contrasts with that of the continuous convolution model [7, 11], where the inverse operator is severely discontinuous. In that case, one has to employ various regularization techniques which lead to reduced numerical efficiency of any numerical reconstruction algorithms, and introduce many other serious theoretical and practical complications, such as determining the appropriate degree of regularization.

Now, to estimate the resulting errors in our deblurring procedure, just as for matrix equations, we compute the condition number [5] of the operator A_σ, defined to be $\|A_\sigma\|\|A_\sigma^{-1}\|$. By using the representation (6) in (3) and (9), we obtain this condition number as

$$C_\sigma = \prod_{k=1}^\infty \left(\frac{1 + q^{2k-1}}{1 - q^{2k-1}} \right)^4. \quad (11)$$

While the following result is immediate, it is necessary to explain the introduction of the term corrupted. The reason for this introduction is that while an image in $\ell^2(\mathbb{Z}^2)$ may have compact support(i.e. all but a finite number of terms equal to zero), its blurred image will not. In particular, if an image is defined on a finite rectangular array with m rows and n columns, then its blurred image will necessarily have infinitely many non-zero entries. Of course, in practice the choice is always made to clip the blurred image to also have m rows and n columns. This clipped image is the image referred to with the term corrupted. Of course, the term corrupted could easily be extended to include any noise that has been introduced into the blurred image. Because information has been lost when noise is introduced, the deblurring of the corrupted image will not be able to recover the original image exactly. The purpose of the error estimates is to determine just how close the reconstruction process has come to recovering the original image.

Theorem 3.3 Suppose $\tilde{g}$ is a corrupted blurring of an image f, so that $\tilde{g} \approx g$ where g is the blurred image of f, then

$$\frac{\|A_\sigma^{-1}\tilde{g} - f\|}{\|f\|} \leq C_\sigma \frac{\|\tilde{g} - g\|}{\|g\|} \quad (12)$$

4. Exact Deblurring Procedure

In this section we demonstrate our method of deblurring by obtaining an exact representation of the operator A_σ^{-1} on image space. As in the previous section, the principal tool used here is a result from the theory of q-series [4]. In the notation of [4] a special case of the q-binomial theorem is

$$
\begin{aligned}
\frac{1}{(z;q)_\infty} &= \sum_{n=0}^\infty \frac{1}{(q;q)_n} z^n, \quad \text{where} \\
(z;q)_n &= \prod_{k=1}^n (1 - q^{k-1}z) \quad \text{if } n \geq 1, \text{ and } (z;q)_0 = 1
\end{aligned}
$$

By replacing q by q^2 and z by $-qe^{it}$, we obtain

$$\prod_{k=1}^\infty (1 + q^{2k-1}e^{it})^{-1} = \sum_{n=0}^\infty (-1)^n \frac{q^n}{(q^2;q^2)_n} e^{int} \quad (13)$$

Applying (13) to (6), and recalling that $q = e^{-1/(2\sigma^2)}$, we obtain the Fourier series for $W_\sigma(t)^{-1}$ as follows. If Q_σ is defined by the rule

$$Q_\sigma = \sqrt{2\pi}\,\sigma \prod_{k=1}^\infty (1 - q^{2k})^{-1}, \quad (14)$$

and

$$
\begin{aligned}
h_\sigma(n) &= (-1)^n q^n \prod_{k=1}^n \left(1 - q^{2k}\right)^{-1} \quad \text{if } n \geq 1 \quad (15) \\
h_\sigma(0) &= 1, \quad (16)
\end{aligned}
$$

then

$$W_\sigma(t)^{-1} = Q_\sigma \sum_{n=0}^{\infty} h_\sigma(n) e^{-int} \cdot \sum_{n=0}^{\infty} h_\sigma(n) e^{int}. \quad (17)$$

Thus, to deblur a one dimensional Gaussian blurred signal, simply convolve it with the filter u_σ defined by

$$u_\sigma(n) = h_\sigma(n), \text{ if } n \geq 0, \text{ and } u_\sigma(n) = 0, \text{ if } n < 0 \quad (18)$$

and then convolve with the filter

$$\tilde{u}_\sigma(n) = h_\sigma(-n), \text{ if } n \leq 0, \text{ and } \tilde{u}_\sigma(n) = 0, \text{ if } n > 0 \quad (19)$$

and then multiply by Q_σ. Of course, theoretically, that is equivalent to convolving the blurred signal with the convolution filter

$$v_\sigma = Q_\sigma \tilde{u}_\sigma \star u_\sigma \quad (20)$$

Thus, for one dimensional signals, our deblurring procedure can be written as

$$Q_\sigma L_\sigma^T L_\sigma g \quad (21)$$

where L_σ is the lower triangular Toeplitz matrix having (m, n)-th entry, $h_\sigma(m-n)$.

To deblur a two dimensional image $\tilde{g}$ which is "close" to some blurred image $A_\sigma f$, we apply the above deblurring procedure on the rows and then the columns of $\tilde{g}$. In terms of our deblurring operator A_σ on the image space $\ell^2(\mathbb{Z}^2)$, this can be written as

$$A_\sigma^{-1} \tilde{g}(m,n) = \sum_{j,k=-\infty}^{\infty} \tilde{g}(m-j, n-k) v_\sigma(j) v_\sigma(k) \quad (22)$$

5. Numerical Properties

To apply our deblurring procedure, we will of course need to compute the entries in a truncation of the matrix L_σ. Thus, it is important to investigate the numerical properties of the matrix L_σ.

In this section, our deblurring process is viewed as the iterative application of matrix multiplication with the Toeplitz matrices L_σ and L_σ^T, first on the columns (of course, transposed) of the blurred image, then on the resulting column of entries, and finally a multiplication by the scalar quantity Q_σ^2.

First, we observe that the main diagonal entries of L_σ are all 1, and the entries on the n-th subdiagonal are all $h_\sigma(n)$. Hence, by using (15), the successive sub-diagonals are easily computed by the following recurrence formula

$$h_\sigma(n) = -\frac{q}{1 - q^{2n}} h_\sigma(n-1), \text{ for } n = 1, 2, \ldots \quad (23)$$

The numerical properties of the entries in L_σ, will be described by properties of the terms

$$a_\sigma(n) = |h_\sigma(n)| \quad (24)$$

which satisfy

$$a_\sigma(n) = r_\sigma(n) a_\sigma(n-1), \text{ for } n \geq 1, \text{ where } r_\sigma(n) = \frac{q}{1 - q^{2n}} \quad (25)$$

Since $0 < q < 1$, then

$$r_\sigma(n+1) < r_\sigma(n) \text{ for all } n \geq 1. \quad (26)$$

So, there exists an integer $N_\sigma \geq 1$, such that

$$r_\sigma(n) > 1 \text{ if } n < N_\sigma \text{ and } r_\sigma(n) \leq 1 \text{ if } n \geq N_\sigma \quad (27)$$

Thus we find that

$$a_\sigma(0) < a_\sigma(1) < \cdots < a_\sigma(N_\sigma - 1) \quad (28)$$

and

$$a_\sigma(N_\sigma - 1) \geq a_\sigma(N_\sigma) > a_\sigma(N_\sigma + 1) > \cdots \quad (29)$$

By using (25), (26), (27), and setting $t_\sigma = r_\sigma(N_\sigma)$ we obtain the following

Theorem 5.1 There exists $0 < t_\sigma < 1$, such that for all σ,

$$|h_\sigma(n)| \leq t_\sigma^{n-N_\sigma} |h_\sigma(N_\sigma)|, \text{ for } n = 1, 2, \ldots. \quad (30)$$

Thus, the diagonal entries of the lower triangular matrix L_σ decrease exponentially after the index N_σ.

Since the results in this paper depend heavily on number theoretic properties, it may not be surprising that the golden mean

$$\gamma = \frac{\sqrt{5} + 1}{2} \quad (31)$$

plays a role in the numerical properties of the deblurring process.

Theorem 5.2 The sequence $\{|h_\sigma(n)|\}$ is decreasing if and only if $0 \leq \sigma \leq (2 \log \gamma)^{-1/2}$.

Proof: From (27), $\{|h_\sigma(n)|\}$ is decreasing if and only if $N_\sigma = 1$. Now, $q/(1-q^2) \leq 1$ if and only if $q^2 + q - 1 \leq 0$ if and only if $q \leq \gamma^{-1}$. The result follows by using $q = e^{-1/(2\sigma^2)}$.

We now summarize the important numerical properties of the matrix L_σ.

Theorem 5.3

1. L_σ is a lower triangular Toeplitz matrix with main diagonal all ones, and the entries on the n-th subdiagonal can be computed recursively by multiplying the value of the entries on the $(n-1)$-st subdiagonal by $-q(1-q^{2n})^{-1}$.

2. The subdiagonal entries of L_σ eventually decrease exponentially.

3. If $\sigma \leq (2 \log \gamma)^{-1/2} \approx 1.0193$, then the subdiagonal entries of L_σ decrease exponentially in value as one moves away from the main diagonal, and their values are all less than 1.

Now, from (11) we see that as $\sigma \to \infty$ (i.e. $q \to 1$), the condition number $C_\sigma \to \infty$, so this deblurring problem is ill-conditioned. In the work of Kimia and Zucker [8], this ill-conditioning appears the diagonal matrix D, but in our process, it appears in the computation of the *single* term Q_σ which is the final computation necessary to complete the proposed deblurring.

Table 1 contains numerical values of the standard deviation σ, and the corresponding values of the condition number C_σ, and the final factor, Q_σ^2, for the deblurring process applied to a two dimensional image.

TABLE 1

σ	C_σ	Q_σ^2
0.1	1.0000e+00	6.2832e-02
0.2	1.0000e+00	2.5133e-01
0.3	1.0314e+00	5.6550e-01
0.4	1.4225e+00	1.0092e+00
0.5	3.0330e+00	1.6311e+00
0.6	8.7586e+00	2.5931e+00
0.7	3.1502e+01	4.2290e+00
0.8	1.3842e+02	7.2088e+00
0.9	7.4106e+02	1.2961e+01
1.0	4.8334e+03	2.4693e+01
1.1	3.8404e+04	4.9992e+01
1.2	3.7173e+05	1.0772e+02
1.3	4.3834e+06	2.4729e+02
1.4	6.2968e+07	6.0524e+02
1.5	1.1019e+09	1.5800e+03
1.6	2.3491e+10	4.4007e+03
1.7	6.1008e+11	1.3081e+04
1.8	1.9302e+13	4.1500e+04
1.9	7.4394e+14	1.4055e+05
2.0	3.4930e+16	5.0820e+05

It is clear from this table that if $\sigma \geq 1.2$, the condition number C_σ of the blurring operation is so large that deblurring without strong apriori knowledge of the desired image, is a risky procedure. For $\sigma \leq 2$, we only need the first 200 terms to compute the values in the infinite product defining Q_σ to double precision.

Note that when q is close to 1, it will be impossible to accurately compute the entries in very large truncations of L_σ. However, for $\sigma \leq 2$, this is not a problem, even for 512×512 images, since the values of q^{1024} are very small.

References

[1] G. E. Andrews, *The Theory of Partitions*, Addison-Wesley Pub. Co., Reading Mass., 1976.

[2] J. Baumeister, *Stable Solution of Inverse Problems*, Friedr. Vieweg & Sohn, Wiesbaden, Germany, 1987.

[3] L. M. J. Florack, B. M. ter Haar Romeny, J. J. Koenderink, and M. A. Viergever, "Images: Regular tempered distributions," *Proc. NATO Advanced Research Workshop Shape in Picture - Mathematical description of shape in greylevel images; NATO ASI Series F*, vol. 126, pp. 651-660, Springer, Berlin, 1994.

[4] G. Gasper and M. Rahman, *Basic Hypergeometric Series*, Cambridge University Press, 1990.

[5] G. Golub and C. Van, *Matrix Computations, Second Edition*, Johns Hopkins Press, Baltimore, 1989.

[6] C. W. Groetsch, *The Theory of Tikhonov Regularization for Fredholm Equations of the First Kind*, Pitman Inc., Boston, 1984.

[7] R. A. Hummel, B. B. Kimia, and S. W. Zucker, "Deblurring Gaussian blur," *Computer Vision, Graphics, and Image Processing*, vol. 38, pp. 66-80, 1987.

[8] B. B. Kimia and S.W. Zucker, "Analytic inverse of discrete Gaussian blur," *Optical Engineering*, vol. 32, pp. 166-176, 1993.

[9] B. A. Mair, "Tikhonov regularization for finitely and infinitely smoothing operators," *SIAM J. Math. Anal.*, vol. 25, pp. 135-147, 1994.

[10] Z. Réti, "Deblurring an image blurred by the discrete Gaussian," *Applied Math. Letters*, vol. 8, pp. 29-35, 1995.

[11] B. M. ter Haar Romeny, L. M. J. Florack, M. de Swart, J. Wilting, and M. A. Viergever, "Deblurring Gaussian blur," *SPIE* vol. 2299, pp. 139-148, 1994.

[12] A. N. Tikhonov and V. Y. Arsenin, *Solutions of Ill-Posed Problems*, John Wiley, New York, 1977.

[13] G. Wahba, *Spline Models for Observational Data*, SIAM, Philadelphia, PA, 1990.

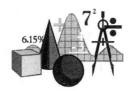

Session 7

Shape

Landmark Methods for Forms Without Landmarks:
Localizing Group Differences in Outline Shape

Fred L. Bookstein
University of Michigan, Ann Arbor, Michigan
fred@brainmap.med.umich.edu

Abstract

Procrustes superposition and the thin-plate spline, each principally developed within the context of discrete landmark data, can be combined in a novel adaptive filter for detecting localized group differences of outline shape.

1. Summary

When one extended curve is relaxed along another by minimizing bending energy of the associated thin-plate spline [1], small-scale variation along the curve is strongly attenuated with respect to variation at larger scales. There results a sort of low-pass filter for shape differences along the average curve. A seemingly complementary (high-pass) filter for group shape difference has always been implicit in the Procrustes method itself. Should two samples of shapes differ in the mean position of just one point, one good signal detector is the Procrustes residual of the point in question after superposition using the whole of the data set. The more central the point, the better this detector. Large-scale shape variation within groups serves as colored noise reducing the power of this filter; in the presence of such variation, detection is more effective if the Procrustes fit is restricted to smaller neighborhoods of the target point than would be used if the variation were uncolored (as in the fundamental Kendall model).

To the extent that the spectra of these two filters are complementary, we gain considerable data-analytic power by applying them as a pair in series. The spline relaxation of every specimen curve against an average has the effect, more or less, of filtering out tangential differences of group mean shape within "small" neighborhoods. We can thereupon specialize the Procrustes filters, too, to smaller neighborhoods than those that would most effectively detect shifts of ordinary landmarks not free to slide along curves. After joint spline relaxation of all the curves against a common average, a radius for an adaptive δ-filter (center-to-periphery contrast) is set separately at each homologous curve element. The radius chosen is simply the neighborhood size for which the component of Procrustes residual difference normal to the curve is the highest multiple of its own standard error.

Estimated in this way, an underlying model of localized group difference of curves suits data to the extent that the signal-to-noise ratio being maximized looks corrugated: sharply peaked along the curve but only gently graded as a function of radius. In one small data set lying conveniently to hand (the shape of the corpus callosum in a psychiatric sample of parasagittal MR images), the dependence of signal on radius and locus fits this characterization well.

The combination of spline-driven and Procrustes-based filters describes differences among sets of these abstracted images in a manner encouragingly similar to what underlies the familiar anisotropic diffusions and contrast-of-Gaussians filters of conventional (i.e., non-biometrical) medical image analysis. At the same time, the biometrics driven by these adaptive matched filters is both more realistic and more powerful than landmark-based treatment of the same structures. The increase in power owes partly to the concentration of degrees of freedom in one single direction normal to the mean curve and partly to the restriction of linear combinations to clusters of neighboring "landmarks."

2. Introduction

Over the last decade, previously scattered or fragmentary tactics and techniques from medical image analysis, multivariate statistics, and computational geometry have been interwoven very effectively in a newly standardized praxis for landmark data. This *morphometric synthesis* binds together the Riemannian structure of David Kendall's shape space, multivariate statistical maneuvers in the tangent space at the Procrustes average form, and graphical approaches for vi-

279

sualizing a wide variety of signals in the resulting data sets. The synthesis brings to the analysis of medical images a biometrical spirit—a concern for optimal description of causes and effects—that was hitherto limited to the more esoteric reaches of evolutionary biology. Its power and its promise have been reviewed recently [2–6] and will not be revisited here.

The power of the synthesis for scientific description, however, has thus far typically been bound to the very demanding abstraction of *landmark point data*. This is inconvenient for a number of reasons. Such data cannot at present be supplied automatically with any reliability, but instead require the scientist either to locate these loci herself or continually to correct the erroneous selections produced by automatic algorithms. Landmark data seem unavailable for large extents of scientifically important images, and for others, such as renderings of the human cerebral cortex, landmarks cannot be declared with assurance to correspond across reasonable ranges of normal adult variation (to say nothing of disease states). Most seriously, the discrete structure of landmark data does not particularly suit the actual formal content of biomathematical and biotheoretical explanations, which tend to concern extended organs and structures better quantified by integrals like surface area or volume or image contents over such extended regions.

The two techniques at the core of the synthesis are the Procrustes-projection construction of shape coordinates and the visualization of localized shape phenomena by thin-plate spline. One of the synthesis's main foundations is the elementary observation that "the partial warps are Procrustes-orthonormal"—that the two techniques, however different their origins, agree in one crucial geometric aspect that permits a formally fruitful interplay. There have been several previous attempts to extend these techniques from the somewhat constricted domain of landmarks to curving form more generally. The thin-plate spline, for instance, has been extended to incorporate arbitrary information about affine derivatives [7] and curvature [8–9], to treat whole extended curves spanning landmarks [10], and, just recently, to handle curves in a manner formally wholly independent of landmarks [1]. Procrustes analysis is likewise being extended to whole curves (see, for instance, [11]). But in these extensions there has not hitherto been any formal coherence analogous to the theorem binding together the two approaches for landmarks.

This essay introduces such a combination of these tools for a problem that has not previously been formalized: the task of localizing group differences in data from curving forms that, while not featureless, nev-

ertheless need not have any punctate landmarks anywhere along the arcs. We will proceed by construing each component of the synthesis, the spline and the Procrustes fit, as a gently nonlinear filter. We will find the filters to be related by a directional complementarity of band-pass characteristics, so that the power of the Procrustes-based filter is greatly heightened after a spline-based preprocessing.

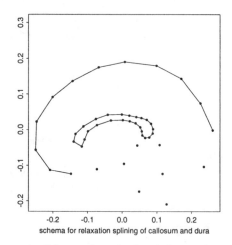

schema for relaxation splining of callosum and dura

Figure 1. Scheme for relaxing information about curving form of a parasagittal brain section: eight landmark points, a callosal arc of 26 points, and a calvarial/dural arc of 12 points. Only the callosal arc is used in this paper, but assignments of homology are based on a spline relaxation that involves the other structures as well. The geometry here corresponds to the Procrustes mean shape. The head is facing *left*.

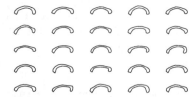

Figure 2. Our data set: 25 26-point polygons around the callosal border as traced by W. D. K. Green. Medical staff, first twelve forms; schizophrenics, last thirteen. Sample and planes selected by John DeQuardo, Adult Psychiatry Unit, University of Michigan. The bulbosity at the rightmost (posterior) end is named "splenium"; the one at the left (anterior), "genu."

The data set to be used to exemplify the localization technique of this paper has been exploited previously to demonstrate landmark-based techniques [6, 12]. The original images are single parasagittal slices selected from clinical MR brain scans of 12 doctors and

13 patients from the Adult Psychiatry Unit, University of Michigan Hospitals. Previous analyses began with a data set of 13 landmarks located by John De-Quardo, MD; the discrimination was sharpened after I included four additional intersects placed around the inner boundary of the corpus callosum. But of the original 13 landmarks, three were already positioned rather arbitrarily along that arc, and two others lay with equal arbitrariness along the falx cerebri. Green [1] deleted those five landmarks in favor of augmenting the data set by tracings of the two arcs in full. For the complete feature set, the average of all 25 forms, against which each case has been relaxed, is shown in Figure 1. From this scheme we will use only the callosal outline itself, a polygon of 26 quasilandmarks in each of the forms. The 25 polygons are shown in Figure 2. (Owing to limitations in the original images, Green chose to intentionally blunt the rostrum of corpus callosum, which otherwise would appear as a right-facing cusp at their lower left.) The first twelve pertain to the doctors; the last thirteen, their patients.

3. Spline relaxation and quasilandmarks

At the core of the technique of spline relaxation along curves [13–14, 1] is a rearrangement of the familiar spline equations. Classically, let U be the function $U(\vec{r}) = r^2 \log r$, and consider a reference shape (in practice, a sample Procrustes average) with landmarks $P_i = (x_i, y_i)$, $i = 1, \ldots, k$. Writing $U_{ij} = U(P_i - P_j)$, build up matrices

$$K = \begin{pmatrix} 0 & U_{12} & \ldots & U_{1k} \\ U_{21} & 0 & \ldots & U_{2k} \\ \vdots & \vdots & \ddots & \vdots \\ U_{k1} & U_{k2} & \ldots & 0 \end{pmatrix}, \quad Q = \begin{pmatrix} 1 & x_1 & y_1 \\ 1 & x_2 & y_2 \\ \vdots & \vdots & \vdots \\ 1 & x_k & y_k \end{pmatrix},$$

and

$$L = \begin{pmatrix} K & Q \\ Q^t & O \end{pmatrix}, \quad (k+3) \times (k+3),$$

where O is a 3×3 matrix of zeros. The thin-plate spline $f(P)$ having heights (values) h_i at points $P_i = (x_i, y_i)$, $i = 1, \ldots, k$, is the function

$$f(P) = \sum_{i=1}^{k} w_i U(P - P_i) + a_0 + a_x x + a_y y$$

where $W = (w_1, \ldots, w_k, a_0, a_x, a_y)^t = L^{-1} H$ with $H = (h_1, h_2, \ldots, h_k, 0, 0, 0)^t$. Then we have $f(P_i) = h_i$, all i: f interpolates the heights h_i at the landmarks P_i. Moreover, the function f has minimum **bending energy** of all functions that interpolate the heights h_i in

that way: the minimum of

$$\iint_{\mathbf{R}^2} \left(\left(\frac{\partial^2 f}{\partial x^2} \right)^2 + 2 \left(\frac{\partial^2 f}{\partial x \partial y} \right)^2 + \left(\frac{\partial^2 f}{\partial y^2} \right)^2 \right)$$

where the integral is taken over the entire picture plane. The value of this bending energy is

$$\frac{1}{8\pi} W^t H = \frac{1}{8\pi} H_k^t L_k^{-1} H_k,$$

where L_k^{-1}, the *bending energy matrix*, is the $k \times k$ upper left submatrix of L^{-1}, and H_k is the corresponding k-vector of "heights" $(h_1, h_2, \ldots, h_k)$.

A plane-to-plane interpolation is couched as a Cartesian pair (f_x, f_y) of these functions based in the same matrix L and for which f_x uses a vector H_x of x-coordinates of a target form and f_y uses a vector H_y of y-coordinates. The bending energy being minimized is now the quadratic form $H_x^t L_k^{-1} H_x + H_y^t L_k^{-1} H_y$.

This last formulation is the key to extending the method so that some of the target landmarks are freed to slide along lines. Let there be a "nominal set" of right hand landmarks $Y_1^0, \ldots, Y_k^0$ collected coordinate-wise as the vector $Y^0 = (Y_{1x}, \ldots, Y_{kx}, Y_{1y}, \ldots, Y_{ky})$, the concatenation of the two vectors H of the preceding treatment. We now seek the spline of one set of landmarks $X_1 \ldots X_k$ onto another set of landmarks $Y_1 \ldots Y_k$ of which a sublist $Y_{i_1} \ldots Y_{i_m}$ are free to slide away from their nominal positions $Y_{i_j}^0$ along directions $u_j = (u_{jx}, u_{jy})$.

To minimize the bending energy $Y_x^t L_k^{-1} Y_x + Y_y^t L_k^{-1} Y_y$ as the landmarks Y_{i_j} of the sublist range over lines $Y_{i_j}^0 + t_j u_j$, collect the parameters $t_1, \ldots, t_m$ in a vector T and the directional constraints $u_1, \ldots, u_m$ in a matrix of $2k$ rows and m columns in which the (i_j, j)-th entry is u_{jx} and the $(k+i_j, j)$-th entry is u_{jy}, otherwise zeroes. The task is now to minimize the form

$$Y^t \begin{pmatrix} L_k^{-1} & 0 \\ 0 & L_k^{-1} \end{pmatrix} Y \equiv Y^t \mathbf{L}_k^{-1} Y$$

over the hyperplane $Y = Y^0 + UT$. The solution to this familiar *generalized* or *weighted least squares* problem is achieved for parameter vector

$$T = -\left(U^t \mathbf{L}_k^{-1} U \right)^{-1} U^t \mathbf{L}_k^{-1} Y^0.$$

Figure 3 demonstrates this computation for a little scheme of 11 "landmarks." The starting form is at upper left, the original target form at upper right, together with the classical (unrelaxed) spline. All 11 points here are free to slide, and I have chosen to let each slide on its "escribed chord," the line parallel to the join of its two immediate neighbors. The fully relaxed spline is shown at lower left. (The original positions of the landmarks are shown as asterisks through which the directions of relaxation cut as indicated.) The superposition at lower right shows that we have saved almost 75% of the bending energy of the spline without deviating much from the original form except at the sharp bottom corners. In practice, forms will have far smaller exterior angles and shifts will be quite a bit less than those shown here.

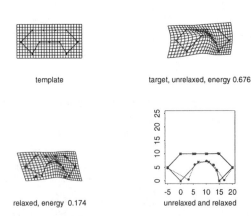

template   target, unrelaxed, energy 0.676

relaxed, energy 0.174   unrelaxed and relaxed

Figure 3. The geometry of relaxation by thin-plate spline. Upper left, a "template" or starting form of 11 points. Upper right, arbitrary set of pre-assigned homologues, with the ordinary thin-plate spline interpolating these point-pairs. Lower left: landmarks after a relaxation along escribed chords (short segments shown through starting positions). Lower right: the principal effect of the relaxation is the counter-rotation of the opposing curve segments at center, as viewed in the regularization of the grid at its center between upper right and lower left panels.

The bending energy matrix L_k^{-1} has a spectrum of $k-3$ nontrivial principal warps [14] usefully characterized by a hierarchy of spatial scales. In any minimization such as this, the high-energy terms will be relaxed preferentially in relation to the low-energy terms to the extent that they are spanned by the subspace over which the minimization is occurring. In the example here, the region of highest energy in the initial warp lies in the arch of the form, and the relaxation has concentrated its visible effect there, relaxing landmarks of the upper arc to the right, the lower arc, to the left.

In the context of curving outlines, the vectors u_j assembled in the constraint matrix U are themselves differences (here, $Y_{i+1} - Y_{i-1}$; in [1], $Y_i - Y_{i\pm 1}$) of the nominal landmark set. Because **L** is evaluated at the nominal positions P_i of the quasilandmarks, the optimization must be an iterative one. After a relaxation along a chord direction as just demonstrated, the target point is projected back down onto the curve, perhaps a new chord direction is computed, and all computations repeated until convergence. But because U is already entailed in the matrix $U^t \mathbf{L}_k^{-1} U$ that is inverted in the course of computing T, the resulting filter would have been (gently) nonlinear in the nominal data even if the algorithm were not already iterative in this way.

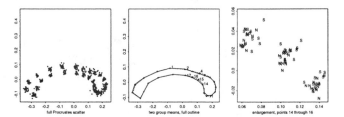

full Procrustes scatter   two group means, full outline   enlargement, points 14 through 16

Figure 4. Procrustes analysis of the whole callosal form. Left: conventional scatter of Procrustes-fit coordinates (least-squares superposition to an average). Center: group mean contours in this registration, with some landmark numbers indicated. Solid line, normals; dashed line, schizophrenics. Right: enlargement of scatters at points 14, 15, and 16. N, normals; S, schizophrenics. The difference at point 15 is significant at about the 2% level by ordinary T^2 test.

The data of Figure 2 have already been preprocessed by this algorithm using the landmark-and-arc scheme of Figure 1 and relaxing with respect to the affine-controlled superposition average of Green [1]. The outlines in Figure 2 collect the resulting loci for the 26 points around the corpus callosum. These points do not have local definitions—they are not landmarks in any of the senses of Bookstein [14]—but each set of 26 minimizes the bending energy of the spline representing its deviation from their common average. Because each of these 26 points represents a spline of the same point of the average, we will refer to them here as *quasilandmarks* analogous to the "computed homologues" introduced in [15]. The reader should keep in mind, nevertheless, that they were computed globally, outline by outline, as a joint representation of the whole corporeal outlines on which they lie. Presently we shall see whether they bear any information about local features of those outlines.

Even though the assumptions of the Kendall null model are unlikely to obtain, the usual Procrustes scatter, Figure 4, of our 25 callosal shapes is an image of mostly well-behaved only modestly noncircular scatters at the 26 separate quasilandmarks. The outlying points at lower right center derive from one callosum of extremely recurved splenium, the form at the right in the third row of Figure 2.

[The Procrustes scatter is the most useful general tool of landmark-based morphometrics [16, 2]. Procrustes was a Greek bandit who standardized the size of his victims by stretching or shrinking them to fit his guest bed. Somewhat more vicariously, standardize each of a pair of forms to centroid at the origin and Centroid Size (sum of squares about the centroid) equal to 1. Then the squared Procrustes distance between the two forms, a distance that is a function solely of their two shapes, can be taken as the minimum sum-of-squares of distances between corresponding landmarks over the rotation group. For a sample of more than two forms, there is a Procrustes average form with respect to which the sum of squared Procrustes distances is a global minimum. And when each of the forms of the sample, recentered at the centroid of the average, is superimposed over this average by the rotation and rescaling that jointly minimize its own distance from that average, the resulting positions of the landmarks, called *Procrustes fit coordinates* or *Procrustes residuals*, become a very useful set of variables for the multivariate description of shape variation in the vicinity of the average. In this paper all "average shapes" will be produced by averaging these residuals within groups. For more on Procrustes fit coordinates, see [5, 6].]

The group means, at center, indicate a series of alternating deviations between the patient and the normal group mean outlines, of which the largest displacement normal to the common tangent is at point 15. The right panel in the figure shows scatters by group at points 14, 15, and 16. In this registration, the difference at point 15 (N's vs. S's) is significant separately (by Hotelling's T^2) at $p \sim .02$.

The weak signal we just detected at point 15 seems to lie approximately normal to the outline shape in that vicinity, just where the spline relaxation should have left it. (Indeed, the group difference seems nearly perpendicular to the average curve except around point 11, which lies close to true landmarks (Figure 1) not drawn here but exerting a tug on the relaxed position of these quasilandmarks.) But in fact the original relaxation along this gently curving segment of arc could well have been overridden by aspects of the Procrustes fit that incorporate information at a relatively great distance. Variations in genu, the structure at the far left, will displace the entire form in ways that have nothing to do with the shape difference in the vicinity of point 15 but which nevertheless contribute to the residual we just inspected. Since there are such group differences at the other end, best to exclude them from

our judgment of what's happening at point 15.

We experiment, then, with a different starting Procrustes fit: just half the form, the "back half," as in Figure 5. The individual shifts and rotations to the average, and the individual scaling with respect to a Centroid Size, have been recomputed *de novo*. The net effect is mainly to alter the superposition of the mean contours, not to change the mean shapes of these half-outlines; but, of course, the variances of individual landmark positions and their covariances with group are altered as well. The scatter of residuals, at left, is qualitatively unchanged from the earlier version, but the residual at point 15 (coded scatter in center) now has a T^2 that is nearly twice as large, with $p \sim .0015$, which has become promising. A plot showing the original polygonal outlines, far right, confirms this tendency of separation for the locus at which the outlines transect their approximate shared "normal" near point 15. "On the average," the perturbing effect of including distant points in the Procrustes fit seems to have been ameliorated quite a bit by the simple decision to ignore the entire region of genu. Notice, also, that point 15 now lies quite near the centroid of the Procrustes landscape within which we are fitting; that was not the case in Figure 4.

One can experiment in this wise for quite a while. Different subarcs of the outline give rise to different estimates of "the shift at point 15" that mostly align with the normal to the mean curve there and that rise and fall with the delimitation of arcs to either side in an obscure fashion. It seems clear, nevertheless, that (a) there *is* a group mean difference of the shape of these outlines "at point 15," if only we were clever enough to persuasively operationalize such a claim, and (b) the Procrustes superposition is somehow related to a useful tool for extracting that description.

4. An adaptive local filter for differences athwart curves

The way out of this perplexity consists in reconceptualizing the Procrustes-based T^2 as a signal detection filter complementing that already supplied by the relaxation spline. In this construal, the signal being sought is the shift of one quasilandmark on a background of a subset of the others presumed unchanging in mean position—a very special case of the "resistant residual" familiar to the morphometric community [16]. Any mean shift signal will be passed through the "Procrustes projection" [17] like any other quasilinear shape signal. This projection attenuates more or less as the landmark suspected of shift lies near to or far from the centroid of the mean Procrustes form. Thus we should be searching in neighborhoods centered over the target landmark.

The preliminary spline-relaxation step has augmented the power of this filter in a very suggestive way. Because of the severe anisotropy of its spectrum, one can assume any local changes along the curve to be negligible by comparison with those across the curve; hence the Procrustes filter needs to be read only in one single direction, the direction normal to the mean curve.

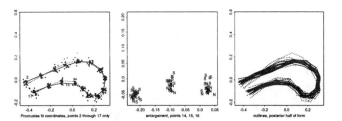

Figure 5. The same for "the posterior half" of the form, rotated to its own Procrustes horizontal. Left: Means and Procrustes-fit coordinates. Center: enlargement for points 14, 15, and 16. As a multiple of its own standard error, the difference at point 15 is 40% larger than it was in Figure 4. Right: superposition of original outline polygons indicates the extent of separation at point 15 normal to the shared tangent direction.

There remains the concern of neighborhood *size*, which I handled so cavalierly in Figure 5 by cutting the form in half. This matter will turn out to be a wholly empirical question: there is good reason to expect intermediate maxima for the power of filters like these, but no simple parametric models for estimating what the most useful radius might be.

A plausible analogy for the problem of setting this neighborhood radius could cut through the peculiar nonlinearities of the present setting—the splines, the rescalings entailed by Procrustes fits—for a model from a much more familiar domain: random processes over the integers of the real axis. Figure 6 shows the setup: two samples of functions over a wide interval of integers centered at $x = 0$. The function has expected value 0 at every value except $x = 0$; there, one group has expected value 0, the other, some nonzero value α (here, .6). The observations vary around this expected value by the sum of two processes of quite different spatial scales. One is a completely uncorrelated process of Gaussian noise i.i.d. $N(0, \sigma^2)$, at each point of the domain. The other is a process of very long-range order indeed—for each case an independent nor-

mal deviate ϵ_i, distributed as $N(0, \tau^2)$, multiplying an exact parabola $y = x^2$ applying throughout the domain. (Here $\sigma^2 = .01, \tau^2 = .001$.) The figure displays one realization of this composite process for two groups of 25. The small-scale process is intended as the analogue of ordinary edge-location noise, while the long-range order corresponds to large-scale shape differences or signals from other parts of the tissue under study.

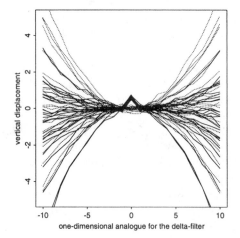

Figure 6. Analogue for the proposition that Procrustes δ-filters will have greatest power at some intermediate aperture width. The functions here are a superposition of uncorrelated noise of variance .01 and multiples of x^2 by Gaussians of variance .001 over a mean shift of .6 at the single argument 0 (obvious sharp peak at center). The two groups are shown in two different line textures. The text derives the optimal neighborhood width for detecting the peak at 0. This optimal interval is $(-4, 4)$, smaller than one might expect, owing to the pernicious effect of the long-range order in the quadratic term.

By analogy with our Procrustes-based search for a normal deviation, in this setup we apply a filter that contrasts the value of the function at 0 to its average value across some neighborhood of zero. This is the "δ-filter" having coefficients

$$(2m)^{-1}(\overbrace{-1, \dots, -1}^{m}, \ 2m, \ \overbrace{-1, \dots, -1}^{m})$$

centered at 0. As m varies, the filter will supply an estimate $\hat{\alpha}$ of the mean shift α at 0 whose error variance is a function of m having a proper minimum somewhere. In fact, the variance of the filter output for the single case is $\sigma^2 + (2m)^{-2}(2m\sigma^2 + m(m + 1)(2m + 1)\tau^2/3)$, which is minimized for $m = \sqrt{\frac{3}{2}\frac{\sigma^2}{\tau^2} + \frac{1}{2}}$. For the values of σ^2 and τ^2 here, this yields $m \sim 4$: an interval of only about one-sixth of the width of the plot around the target point 0. From there on out, as m increases by 1 the contribution of the long-range term ϵx^2 adds new variance of order $\tau^2/3$—note this does *not* drop with increasing m—that is no longer compensated by the increase in precision (which goes as $\sigma^2/2m^2$) of the baseline engendered by the longer sampling interval over which the contrast with $f(0)$ is accrued.

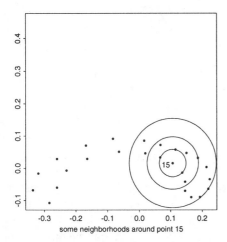

Figure 7. Three neighborhoods around quasi-landmark 15, the point of greatest interest. Smallest: consecutive triangle on the outline; the radius is indistinguishable from that of the three-neighbor neighborhood, which extends to the closest point on the other side of the isthmus. Intermediate: the optimal neighborhood according to the algorithm described in the text (optimum of signal-to-noise ratio of the δ-filter). Outer circle: the "back half" of the form, Figure 5, is also the neighborhood of point 15's 15 closest neighbors.

Back in the domain of morphometrics, this model of quadratic growth (the function x^2) for long-range or large-scale effects is qualitatively quite plausible—growth-gradients, the largest partial warps, and other realistic candidates have always been modeled by such supralinear scaling [14, Secs. 7.3–7.4]. If the analogy of a filter balancing competing sources of variance is valid, and if true group differences in the form of the curve are this local, then they might be found by neighborhood-centered center-vs.-periphery searches of adaptive Procrustes radius neither too large (the whole form) nor too small (single consecutive triangles of edge-points).

Such reflections eventually lead us to a heuristic search over the set of $k(k-2)$ potential neighborhoods consisting, simply enough, of all the lists of j nearest neighbors of each landmark in turn, $j = 2, 3, \ldots, k-1$. (The hierarchy of neighborhoods is computed from the Procrustes average shape.) The case $j = k-1$ is the full least-squares Procrustes residual with which we be-

gan (Figure 4). Figure 7 indicates a set of three other such neighborhoods around point 15, the point we are finding so interesting. The smallest and the second-smallest are indistinguishable in this case, as the callosal form is so narrow at its isthmus; the outer circle happens to span the half-form we already considered in Figure 5. The circle of intermediate radius, corresponding to a neighborhood of seven neighbors, will turn out to give the optimal signal-to-noise ratio for the δ-filter. It continues to be the case that fits to different neighborhoods use different Procrustes superpositions, varying not only shift and rotation but also the rescaling to unit Centroid Size.

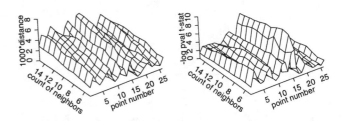

Figure 8. Response surfaces corresponding to performance of the δ-filter at all points for a range of neighborhood sizes. Left: distance between group mean Procrustes fit coordinates, scaled to Figure 4. Right: the surface of log tail-probability of the t-ratio (signal-to-noise ratio) of the δ-filter corresponding. This is the surface texture referred to in the text as "corrugated." The obvious ridge is aligned with point 15.

The model that is being estimated by this heuristic search is a close analogue for Figure 6 in the context of Procrustes-registered shape. We presume a common grand mean shape around which specimens vary by large-scale processes, by small-scale noise, and by one single displacement of a small stretch of outline. The large-scale noise is treated as nuisance variation; one imagines it to include affine variation along with the sort of bending spanned by the first few *partial warps* [14, 2]. A preliminary relaxation to the Procrustes average by thin-plate spline has concentrated tangential variation at these larger scales. Both the small-scale noise model and the displacement of the single point are presumed normal to the averaged outline. Estimation is by maximizing S/N as captured by t-test of the component of the target point's Procrustes residual normal to the mean outline there.

For the set of all 26 quasilandmarks, tail-probability of the associated t-ratio for displacement normal to the curve is shown as a surface in two panels of Figure 8. (The vertical axis here is minus log probability merely to stretch out the interesting region a bit: this transform is just a little better than quadratic in the t-ratio itself.) This surface shows one clearly dominant locus of group mean difference, exactly at point 15, the point that has intrigued us all along. Also, the global texture of this surface manifests a sort of corrugation that supports our overall model. The center-versus-periphery Procrustes filter output is very robust to variation of neighborhood size but highly sensitive to position along the curve.

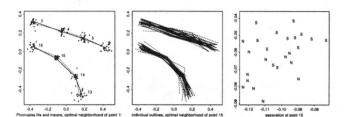

Figure 9. Analysis for the optimal neighborhood around point 15. Left: group mean outlines and Procrustes scatter. Center: individual outlines. Right: output of the δ-filter at point 15. All panels are in the coordinate system of the entire form, Figure 4.

The signal-to-noise ratio of the filter atop point 15 is gently maximized at neighborhood size 8. This neighborhood, already indicated in Figure 7, corresponds to the Procrustes fits and the scatter in Figure 9. The filter output here now separates the groups quite effectively. In fact, the group separation is 174% of the mean within-group variation in this normal direction. The T^2 is nominally significant at $p \sim .0004$; but the appropriate test has now become a simple Student's t of 4.9 in the normal direction, which is significant here at .000066. Thus there is no longer any doubt either about the significance of the finding or about its localization.

The dominant ridge of Figure 8 can be graphed more informatively as a sequence of points corresponding to those same discrete steps of radius back in the original Procrustes space of the full shape, Figure 10. The mean shift (left panel) of point 15 continually rises with neighborhood count right up to a maximum corresponding to the full Procrustes fit in Figure 4. In the context of the analogy for functions on the real line, Figure 6, this increase might have been expressing the effect of some nuisance group mean difference in the variate ϵ times a coefficient (net "large-scale effect") that asymptotes for $m \to 26$ instead of continuing to increase monotonously. But back in the world of morphometrics, Figure 10, the direction of this difference is remarkably stably aligned with the normal to the mean curve over the full range of neighborhood sizes, confirming that we are dealing with a well-defined signal at small scale normal to the variation that the spline already relaxed to large scale.

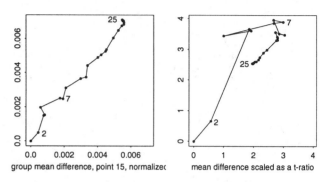

Figure 10. Contrast between Procrustes and statistical geometry of the δ-filter, for the complete sequence of neighborhood sizes at point 15 only. Left: trajectory of group mean difference in the plane of Figure 4. The group separation increases with neighborhood size. Right: rescaling of the left side to a t-ratio (division by within-group variability). Beyond the scale of the smallest neighborhoods, noise rises faster than signal strength with increasing neighborhood size, as it does also in the one-dimensional analogue in Figure 6. Numbers on the figure are counts of neighbors; the plots begin with difference zero for the single pair (all shapes the same).

Yet the noise in that shift, *estimated by these δ-like filters*, rises over neighborhood aggrandizement at a faster rate than the ability of Procrustes averaging to produce better estimates of that signal. A maximum of the signal-to-noise ratio emerges at the neighborhood of size 8 (right panel). The largest jump is from the two-neighbor neighborhood (a simple triangle of three consecutive points) to the three-neighbor version, which (Figure 7) incorporates an anchor from the other "side" of the structure under study. Some additional improvements in signal detection become possible as the relevant arcs grow a bit longer separately, but we have maxxed out by the neighborhood of size 8; thereafter, the signal (growth of mean shift) no longer keeps pace with the large-scale noise.

5. Discussion

5.1. Why does this work?

The model underlying the filter here contrasts strongly with the basic distributional model for Procrustes-type analyses of discrete landmarks. Our standard landmark methods [2–6, 14] cast a 26-"landmark" data set like this one into a 48-dimensional space of shape phenomena within which a strenuous symmetry is enforced a priori. Variation tangential to and normal to outlines must be weighted equally, and group differences are modeled as equally plausible regardless of the direction along which they lie in this space. For instance, every set of three landmarks, neighboring or not, is considered an equally likely locus of some potentially crucial aspect of shape discrimination. In this context, the best single overall multivariate test statistic is Goodall's omnibus F-ratio [18]. For the data here its value is 1.32 on 48 and 1104 d.f., significant at $p \sim 0.07$ only. That was, in essence, a single test of the displacement between mean curves in Figure 4 with respect to the net degree of variation around those means aggregated over all the "landmarks" separately. Because the F could not take into account the concentration of the finding (Figure 8), it was blocked from finding anything particularly implausible about the configuration of group differences as a whole.

Inasmuch as the data were produced by a preliminary spline relaxation, we know that at every quasilandmark one dimension of the Procrustes residual has been strongly smoothed with respect to the model of isotropic Gaussian noise that might otherwise be applied [19–20]. According to Figure 8, any substantial group difference in the direction of "residual variation," variation perpendicular to the mean curve, seems concentrated along one short stretch of the outline. The finding seems to extend over at most two consecutive quasilandmarks and to be quite stable over variations of neighborhood size. We certainly gain power if we select over a cycle of $k = 26$ possible foci of shift in this way rather than an entire $2k - 4 = 48$-dimensional sphere of potential features, and we gain yet more power from the restriction to a single direction of shape change. The count of 26 quasilandmarks here is arbitrary, but changes won't much alter the Goodall F; the issue is one of localization, not dimensionality.

The nuisance variables associated with the $k(k-2)$ recenterings and rescalings of the Procrustes fits underlying the δ-filter are handled quite neatly by the strategy of attending only to the comparisons at the centers. While large-scale shape transformations strongly affect Procrustes residuals of points away from the center, they do not much alter fitted positions of quasiland-

marks near the centers of small neighborhoods. The preliminary spline fit will attenuate some dimensions of these nuisance effects even more strongly.

At the same time, there is more structure here in the callosum example than would be seen in the equivalent finding for normal displacement somewhere along a simple circular template. The callosum is elongated, and except at splenium and genu, its relatively bulbous ends, most of the neighborhoods considered by these δ-filters span both sides of the boundary (cf. Figure 7). The specific finding at point 15, Figure 9, is a reshaping of the entire neighborhood of eight points there. It is partially an erosion or thinning at point 15, partially a sharpened bending of the boundary in the immediate vicinity. That the filter produces a finding only at point 15, not at the comparable point 4 across the local axis of the form, suggests that even though the neighborhood straddles the two sides of this form, our particular finding is rather distant from anything that might be produced by direct characterization of medial structure in the original image, such as by the UNC method of "cores." Nevertheless, there is a hint, perhaps clearest in Figure 5, that at a larger scale this strip may be considered to have been shifted "on both sides."

5.2. Similar approaches

The adaptive filter optimization here is partly analogous to two otherwise disparate techniques that have been the subject of previous discussions in the literature of medical image analysis. Techniques of *anisotropic diffusion* [21] modify images toward the equilibration of picture content within regions without allowing information to diffuse across sharp boundaries. They thus achieve part of the purpose of the processing here—an enhancement of the signal normal to the boundary, by flattening gradients elsewhere—without the corresponding relaxation along the boundary that seems the key to the success of our filter. That lacuna is understandable, of course, in that these diffusion techniques deal with analysis of pictures one at a time, whereas what is relaxed by the spline is not a property of any single image, but of a pair or a whole data set of instances in relation to a template or an average.

The δ-filter method here can be considered as a limiting case of a *contrast-of-annuli* filter. (In fact, because the Procrustes fit tends to leave less residual at points farther from the center, its weight profile is qualitatively not altogether dissimilar from that of the classical contrast-of-Gaussians. In light of the strongly anisotropic nature of the preliminary spline processing, these annuli or Gaussians are better taken not as circular but as severely elongated in the direction of the edge under study. The combined method here can be thought of as an even larger-scale adaptation of such contrasts to the accidents of curvature at some distance—it is as if the edge were straightened before these parametrically simple filters were applied.

But the estimator here is *not* the limit of analogous techniques for localization of shape change applying to the context of actual landmark data. The partial warps, eigenfunctions of the bending-energy matrix L_k^{-1} introduced in Section 2, supply an orthogonal basis for shape variation around any Procrustes mean. After an initial affine term, there are 23 pairs of these warps expressing variation in a full circle of directions at *some* location and *some* scale. For most quasilandmarks of the outline, there will be no single term anywhere in the partial warp basis corresponding to its shift against its immediate neighbors. A modification of the typical thin-plate visualization (warping of squared graph paper) could highlight bending in the normal direction—perhaps a "grid" of parallel curves to either side of the averaged outline—but any associated statistical method would have to resemble the δ-filter here.

5.3. Implications

The δ-filter method postulates a radical divergence of correlation scale between within-group and between-group shape variation. Within-group variation is "very long-range," especially in the metric of bending energy; between-group variation is modeled here as wholly uncorrelated, a process of displacement (the actual scientific signal of interest) at one single point over a background of white noise (digitizing jitter) of even smaller amplitude. Though this often corresponds to our understanding of certain anatomical anomalies as focal processes, it would be simple to modify the analogue in Figure 6 to incorporate a spectrum of some finite width for that signal instead: an inner correlation dimension of two or three points, perhaps. In the morphometric context, this corresponds to a larger family of filters in which the δ-function is replaced by a central contrasting core of somewhat larger support. There is a bit of evidence for such an alternative in the present data set, in which point 14 seems to "follow" point 15 up the wall of the filter signal surface (Figure 8) for neighborhoods beyond a certain size. Slightly alter the analogue, Figure 6, so that the central peak rises from zero with a width $2k$, $k > 0$. The variance of the δ-filter is not changed thereby, but the signal becomes $[2m - (k - 1)]\alpha/2m$ instead of α. For small k there is still an internal maximum for the signal-to-noise ratio

as a function of m. I expect a similar robustness to apply in the morphometric context.

To be able to treat curving form by landmark methods without requiring their acquisition in landmark-anchored form would be a significant step forward in the morphometrics of biomedical images. For many three-dimensional data sets, for instance, representation is by the method of *ridge curves* or *crest lines* [22–23], which extract reliable three-dimensional loci at which the surface is locally most like a sharp edge. Statistical methods for analysis of such data have hitherto either been limited to very simple parametric models—rigid motion, polynomial warping—or have required the extraction of specific landmark points specimen by specimen (typically, curvature maxima along these curves). Such landmarks are typically much noisier than the arcs on which they lie. The combination of the spline relaxation and local orthogonal filtering makes it possible to analyze such curves *as a whole*, by assigning quasilandmarks that describe the relation to a template without requiring any geometric semantics of characterization upon the individual form. In this aspect these new methods are converging with other approaches to form-comparison from McGill, Washington University, and elsewhere, in which parametrization of the individual form is subordinated to parametrization of the relation to a template. For landmark data sensu stricto, these parametrizations are identical a priori: the points of shape space serve equally well as vector specifications of the corresponding splines [5].

The δ-filter method here will sustain valid findings to the extent that the simplistic model driving it is an adequate preliminary representation of the information discriminating the image groups under study: discrete group differences of small scale masked by long-range order. A model this specific for "comparative image content" is consistent with one tendency of medical image reports often found in the applied literature even though it corresponds to no previous method of image analysis. Our filter may, for instance, be helpful in studies of myocardial wall motion, the effect of disease on which has often been modeled as local defect of "motion" with respect to a globally twisting shape change at quite large scale (e.g., [24]). It may also be helpful in more detailed consideration of the shapes of fluid-filled cavities such as the cerebral ventricles (D. Dean, pers. comm.), or other complex shapes having subtle but crucial functional implications, shapes that have hitherto proved refractory to analyses that followed conventional image-by-image processing.

Acknowledgement. Preparation of this contribution was supported by NIH grants DA–09009 and

GM–37251 to Fred L. Bookstein. The former grant is jointly supported by the National Institute on Drug Abuse, the National Institute of Mental Health, and the National Institute on Aging as part of the Human Brain Project. All the statistical graphics were produced in the Splus package available from Math-Soft, Inc., Seattle. The callosal outline data were acquired by Bill Green using an experimental version of his program package `edgewarp` that will eventually be available by FTP from the directory `pub/edgewarp` on `brainmap.med.umich.edu`.

References

[1] W. D. K. Green. Spline-based deformable models. Pp. 290–301 in R. Melter, A. Wu, F. Bookstein, and W. D. K. Green, eds., *Vision Geometry IV*. S. P. I. E. *Proceedings*, vol. 2573, 1995.

[2] F. L. Bookstein. Metrics and symmetries of the morphometric synthesis. Pp. 139–153 in K. V. Mardia and C. A. Gill, eds., *Proc. Current Issues in Statistical Shape Analysis*. Leeds University Press, 1995.

[3] F. L. Bookstein. The Morphometric Synthesis for landmarks and edge-elements in images. *Terra Nova* 7:393–407, 1995.

[4] F. L. Bookstein. The morphometric synthesis. To appear in J. Rosenberger, ed., *Proc. 27th Conference on the Interface between Computer Science and Statistics*. American Statistical Association, 1995.

[5] F. L. Bookstein. Biometrics, biomathematics, and the morphometric synthesis. *Bulletin of Mathematical Biology* 58:313–365, 1995.

[6] F. L. Bookstein. Biometrics and brain maps: the promise of the Morphometric Synthesis. To appear in S. Koslow and M. Huerta, eds., *Neuroinformatics: An Overview of the Human Brain Project. Progress in Neuroinformatics*, vol. 1. Hillsdale, NJ: Lawrence Erlbaum, 1996.

[7] F. L. Bookstein and W. D. K. Green. A feature space for edgels in images with landmarks. *Journal of Mathematical Imaging and Vision* 3:231–261, 1993.

[8] J. A. Little and K. Mardia. Edgels and tangent planes in image warping. Pp. 263–270 in L. Marcus et al., eds., *Proc. NATO Advanced Study Institute on Morphometrics*. New York: Plenum.

[9] K. V. Mardia, J. Kent, C. Goodall, and J. Little. Kriging and splines with derivative information. *Biometrika*, to appear.

[10] C. B. Cutting, D. Dean, F. Bookstein, B. Haddad, D. Khorramabadi, F. Zonnefeld, and J. McCarthy. A three-dimensional smooth surface analysis of untreated Crouzon's disease in the adult. *Journal of Craniofacial Surgery* 6:444–453, 1995.

[11] P. D. Sampson, F. Bookstein, F. Sheehan, and E. Bolson. Eigenshape analysis of left ventricular outlines from contrast ventriculograms. Pp. 211–233 in L. Marcus et al., eds., *Proc. NATO Advanced Study Institute on Morphometrics*. New York: Plenum, 1996.

[12] F. L. Bookstein. How to produce a landmark point: the statistical geometry of incompletely registered images. Pp. 266–277 in R. Melter, A. Wu, F. Bookstein and W. D. K. Green, eds., *Vision Geometry IV*. S. P. I. E. *Proceedings*, vol. 2573, 1995.

[13] F. L. Bookstein. Principal warps: Thin-plate splines and the decomposition of deformations. *I.E.E.E. Trans. Pattern Analysis and Machine Intelligence* 11:567–585, 1989.

[14] F. L. Bookstein. *Morphometric Tools for Landmark Data*. Cambridge University Press, 1991.

[15] F. L. Bookstein, B. Chernoff, R. Elder, J. Humphries, G. Smith, and R. Strauss. *Morphometrics in Evolutionary Biology*. Acad. Natural Sciences of Philadelphia, 1985.

[16] F. J. Rohlf and D. Slice. Extensions of the Procrustes method for the optimal superposition of landmarks. *Systematic Zoology* 39:40–59, 1990.

[17] J. T. Kent. Current issues for statistical inference in shape analysis. Pp. 167–175 in K. V. Mardia and C. A. Gill, eds., *Proc. Current Issues in Statistical Shape Analysis*. Leeds University Press, 1995.

[18] C. R. Goodall. Procrustes methods in the statistical analysis of shape. *J. Royal Statistical Society* B53:285–339, 1991.

[19] D. G. Kendall. Shape-manifolds, procrustean metrics, and complex projective spaces. *Bull. London Mathematical Society* 16:81–121, 1984.

[20] K. V. Mardia. Shape advances and future perspectives. Pp. 57–75 in K. V. Mardia and C. A. Gill, eds., *Proc. Current Issues in Statistical Shape Analysis*, Leeds University Press, 1995.

[21] P. Perona, T. Shiota, and J. Malik. Anisotropic diffusion. Pp. 73–92 in B. M. ter Haar Romeny, ed., *Geometry-Driven Diffusion in Computer Vision*. Dordrecht: Kluwer, 1994.

[22] D. Dean, L. Marcus, and F. Bookstein. Chi-square test of biological space curve affinities. Pp. 235–261 in L. Marcus et al., eds., *Proc. NATO Advanced Study Institute on Morphometrics*. New York: Plenum, 1996.

[23] J.-P. Thirion. The extremal mesh and the understanding of 3D surfaces. Pp. 3–12 in *Proc. IEEE Workshop on Biomedical Image Analysis*. Los Alamitos, CA: Computer Society Press, 1994.

[24] J. C. McEachen, II, A. Nehorai, and J. Duncan. A recursive filter for temporal analysis of cardiac motion. Pp. 124–133 in *Proc. IEEE Workshop on Biomedical Image Analysis*. Los Alamitos, CA: Computer Society Press, 1994.

Shape Reconstruction from an Endoscope Image by Shape-from-Shading Technique for a Point Light Source at the Projection Center

Koichiro DEGUCHI   Takayuki OKATANI

Faculty of Engineering, University of Tokyo,
7-3-1, Hongo, Bunkyo-ku, Tokyo 113 Japan

E-mail: deguchi@meip7.t.u-tokyo.ac.jp

Abstract

This paper describes an approach to reconstructing a shape from it's shaded image in the case where a point light source is at the projection center. This condition well approximates the imaging system of an endoscope. In this case, the image gray level depends on not only the gradient of the object surface but also the distance from the light source to each point on the surface. To deal with this difficulty, we introduce the evolution equation for equal-range contours on the surface. Propagating this contour by solving the equation, we can reconstruct a shape. Experimental results for real medical endoscope images of a human stomach inner wall show feasibility of this method, and present a promising technique for morphological analysis of tumors on human inner organs.

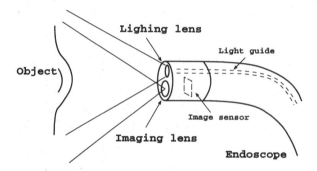

Figure 1. An endoscope and its imaging system. Image sensor and lighting mechanism are included in its head.

1. Introduction

To reconstruct 3D object shape from its image has been a main subject of computer vision researches. The problem described in this paper is a medical application of such a shape reconstruction by a new algorithm of *shape from shading*. Here, our objective is to reconstruct 3D shape of an inner wall of human stomach, for example, from its endoscope images. **Fig.1** shows a sketch of an endoscope system taking an image. If accurate 3D shapes of the object can be obtained from medical endoscope images, it enables easily, for example, quantitative evaluations and morphological studies on shape of tumors.

The problem of shape reconstruction from endoscope images has been conventionally studied with a stand point of *shape from motion* (or *shape from image sequence*) using a sequence of images obtained by moving the endoscope [1],[2]. In such an approach, first, some feature points are extracted from images, then their correspondences are established within the image sequence, and finally the object shape and the relative motion to the endoscope are obtained using shape from motion techniques.

Our previous approach [1] employing so-called the factorization method for shape from image sequence technique produced good rough global 3D sketch of human stomach inner wall.

These approaches assume that the object is rigid. For the medical application described above, however, the motion of the inner wall of stomach, for example, is not strictly rigid, so that this assumption does not hold for most cases. Moreover, generally for images of inner stomachs, it is difficult to extract many fine feature points and track them to make correspondences stably in a long image sequence. As the result, fine morphological structures cannot be reconstructed by these method.

Here, we employ shape from shading approach and intend to reconstruct the object fine shape from shadings. This approach has a possibility to obtain 3D shape of a nonrigidly moving object more stably.

Research of the shape from shading has long history, and many shape reconstruction algorithms have been proposed in the literatures. However, almost of them are not available for our problem. This is because almost of the conventional approach treats shadings generated by a light source locating at an infinitely far distance resulting parallel illumination light. Furthermore, it employs simple orthogonal projection models for the imaging system. These assumptions do not hold for real endoscope images, because the light source is near to the object and considered to be a point. For such a case, the shading on the object depends not only on the gradient of its surface but also on the distances to the surface points from the light source (Generally, the lighting intensity is proportional to the squared reciprocal of the distance. This assumption of infinite far light source is for a uniform illumination intensity for all the object surfaces).

Fig.2 shows a photograph of an endoscope head. The imaging lens and the light source lens are located very near. So that, an endoscope is well approximated by an imaging system having a point light source at the projection center. This approximation has an advantage to solve the problem of shape from shading by a point light source, because the directions from an object surface point to the light source and the projection center are considered to be same. At the same time, the distances to them are also same.

In this paper, using this advantage, we propose a new algorithm to reconstruct object shape from endoscope images. We construct an imaging model of the endoscope and introduce the evolution equation for equal-range contours on the object surface based on the shading model. Propagating this contour by solving the equation, we can reconstruct the shape. To select an initial contour for the propagation and also to avoid the intrinsic ambiguities of shape from shading, we utilize the rough global 3Dsketch obtained by our previous shape from image sequence method in [1].

The introduction of the evolution equation to solve shape from shading problem was initiated by Kimmel *et al.* [3, 6]. But they only applied to the conventional cases of far light source and orthogonal projection. Here, we extend the algorithm to a case of near point light source and perspective projection.

The experimental results applying the algorithm to real endoscope images show its promising availability

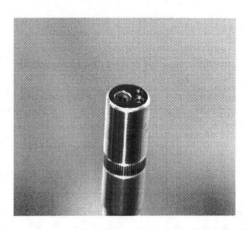

Figure 2. The head of an endoscope. The diameter of this endoscope is 12mm. Larger circular hole at the left side is the object lens of the image sensor, and two smaller holes at the right are the lenses to radiate light.

for the shape reconstruction.

2. Formulation of the Shape from Shading

In this section, first, we briefly review the conventional techniques of shape from shading to point out problems of their applicability. Then, we formalize our problems in contrast with them.

2.1. Factors determining shape from shading

Let us denote the object surface by a (continuous) function $z(x, y)$, which express the depth to the surface at (x, y) with respect to image coordinate system. An image, which is expressed as a brightness distribution $E(x, y)$, is determined by three conditions, that is, physical refrectance of the object surface, the gradient of the surface at (x, y) and the lighting condition. In many cases, the brightness of the surface is determined only by the three relative angles spanned between the three vectors shown in **Fig.3** and the distance to the light source. The shape from shading is the technique to recover the depth $z(x, y)$ from the image intensity $E(x, y)$ by using these conditions.

To simplify the problem, most of the conventional approach to the shape from shading assumed; 1) the orthogonal projection for the imaging model, and 2)

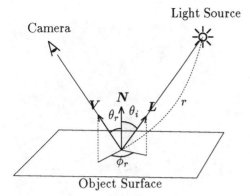

Figure 3. Vectors determining the reflectance of the object surface

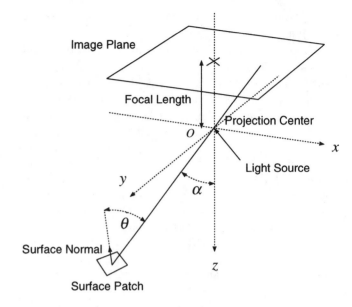

Figure 4. Optical system with a point light source at the projection center

the light source at infinitely far distance. The second assumption is importnat for these techniques. It makes needless to consider the distances from the light source to the surface point. This means all surface points have same distance to the light source, which results in a uniform illumination intensity for all the object surface points. This makes the problem fairly simple.

2.2. The light source at the projection center

For our problem of shape reconstruction from endoscope image shading, such an artificial simplification no longer holds. The light source and the object surface are near, and the shading depends on the distance from the light source to the surface point by point.

We employ an optical system shown in **Fig.4** for the imaging model of the endoscope, where an ideal point light source is at the projection (lens) center (which is the coordinate origin), and the projection is of the full perspective (not orthogonal).

Real endoscope image has distortions produced by its lens. We need lens calibration and preprocessing for an image to correct the distortions to apply this model. We also developed a method for this correction, but here we omit the description on the preprocessing.

Now, let us express the object surface using polar coordinates as $r(\alpha, \beta)$ where α is the elevation angle and β is the azimuth angle of the line of sight as shown in Fig.4. That is, a surface point is expressed by $(\alpha, \beta, r(\alpha, \beta))$. α and β span within $[0 : \pi/2)$ and $[0 : 2\pi)$, respectively.

Let us also assume that the object surface has homogeneous reflectance and has not multiple reflections. The focal length of the lens is denoted by f.

For a surface point, let the angle between surface normal (denoted by $\boldsymbol{n}$) and the direction of line of sight (denoted by $\boldsymbol{v}$) be denoted by θ (See Fig.4). Because the range r to this point from the origin is just the distance from the light source, the gray level of the image of this point is expressed after some normalization as

$$
\begin{aligned}
E(x,y) &= \frac{F(\cos\theta)}{r^2} \\
&= \frac{F(\boldsymbol{n} \cdot \boldsymbol{v})}{r^2}
\end{aligned}
\tag{1}
$$

where $F(\cos\theta)$ expresses the reflectance of the surface with respect to θ. If this function is known and monotonic, the surface gradient θ with respect to the line of sight can be obtained from r and $E(x,y)$ by using its inverse of F^{-1}

Here, we use this relation between the distance to a surface point from the origin and the gradient of the surface at the point. In our proposed method, we derive an evolution equation ([3], [4], [5], [6]) considering the shape reconstruction as an initial value problem of a partial differential equation. The details are described in the next section.

3. A Solution Based on an Evolutional Equation of Equal-Range Contours

In our proposed method, we introduce an evolution equation with respect to the equal-range contours of the surface, which describes the relation between the gray level of the image of a surface point, the range to the point and the gradient of the surface at the point. Then, we solve this equation to reconstruct the total object shape.

3.1. Equal-range contours

First, we assume the function $r(\alpha, \beta)$, which represents the shape of the object surface, is of one-valued and smoothly continuous. Then, let us consider a spatial contour curve that consists of object surface points of $r = $ const. We call this curve a *equal-range contour* of the object surface. When we denote this constant with t, the contour is given as

$$C(t) = \{(\alpha, \beta, r(\alpha, \beta)) \ \text{s.t.} \ r(\alpha, \beta) = t\} \qquad (2)$$

As shown in **Fig.5**, the curve $C(t)$ can be considered as a crossing of the object surface with a sphere whose center is at the origin and radius is t. The figure shows schematically equal-range contours of $C(t_1), C(t_2), \ldots, C(t_n)$ for the radii t as $t_1, t_2, \ldots, t_n$, respectively.

3.2. Derivation of the evolutional equation

Now, given an equal-range contour $C(t)$ with a range t, we derive contour $C(t+\Delta t)$ with $t+\Delta t$ using the image $E(x, y)$. We introduce another expression of qual-range contour $C(t)$ using a parameter s as

$$C(s, t) = \{(\alpha(s, t), \beta(s, t), t)\} \qquad (3)$$

where s is the contour length from some fixed contour point (or its monotonic function) and $s \in [0, S)$.

We are interested in $\alpha(s, t+\Delta t)$ and $\beta(s, t+\Delta t)$ with $t + \Delta t$. The parameter s is set to be common between $C(s, t)$ and $C(s, t + \Delta t)$ at the respective points along the normal direction of the contours.

For a surface point $(\alpha(s, t), \beta(s, t))$ on a equal-range contour $C(s, t)$, as shown in **Fig. 6**, let us denote the normal vector of the surface at this point with $\boldsymbol{n}$, the tangential vector of the contour with $\boldsymbol{t}$ and the angle between the normal vector $\boldsymbol{n}$ and the line of sight to this point with θ. The most important fact is that the vector $\boldsymbol{t}$ is also tangential of the spherical surface whose center is the origin. This means that $\boldsymbol{t}$ is vertical to the line of sight. Utilizing this fact, we can evolve

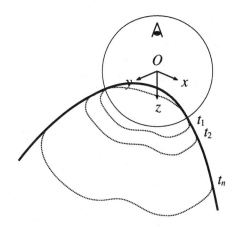

Figure 5. Equal-range conoturs

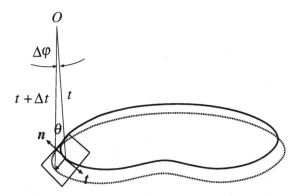

Figure 6. Evolution of the equal-range conoturs

the contour along with the object surface to the normal direction of the contour.

Evolving the point $(\alpha(s, t), \beta(s, t))$ in the direction normal to both $\boldsymbol{n}$ and $\boldsymbol{t}$, the angle $\Delta\varphi$ that spans the evolution viewed from the origin becomes

$$\Delta\varphi = \frac{\Delta t}{t \tan\theta} \qquad (4)$$

Defining $\boldsymbol{n}_p \equiv \boldsymbol{t} \times \boldsymbol{n}$, and using orthogonal curved coordinate bases $\boldsymbol{e}_\alpha$, $\boldsymbol{e}_\beta$ and $\boldsymbol{e}_r$ for the polar coordinates, the increments $\Delta\alpha$ and $\Delta\beta$ in the evolution for α and β, respectively, are expressed by

$$(\Delta\alpha, \Delta\beta) = \Delta\varphi \left(\boldsymbol{n}_p \cdot \boldsymbol{e}_\alpha, \frac{\boldsymbol{n}_p \cdot \boldsymbol{e}_\beta}{\sin\alpha} \right) \qquad (5)$$

Rewriting this in forms of differentials,

$$\begin{bmatrix} \alpha_t(s, t) \\ \beta_t(s, t) \end{bmatrix} = \frac{1}{t \tan\theta} \begin{bmatrix} \boldsymbol{n}_p \cdot \boldsymbol{e}_\alpha \\ \boldsymbol{n}_p \cdot \boldsymbol{e}_\beta / \sin\alpha \end{bmatrix} \qquad (6)$$

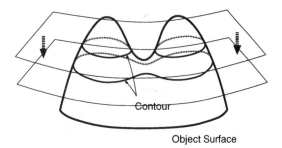

Figure 7. An example where two contours join into one equal-range contour

where $\tan\theta$ is given by the image gray level $E(x,y)$ as

$$\tan\theta = \sqrt{\frac{1}{(F^{-1}(t^2 E(x,y)))^2} - 1} \qquad (7)$$

from the equation (1). This is the evolution equation that just we are interested in.

3.3. Level set method

From a given initial contour, evolving the equal-range contours according to the equation of (6), the equal-range contour at t will be obtained. That is, solving the evolution equation, we obtain the object surface reconstructed from the image. However, this method has some difficulties.

The first difficulty arises for cases, as shown in **Fig.7**, where a non-smooth point of the contour (singular point) for an even smooth surface may exist when, for example, two or more contours join into one contour, or conversely one contour divides into two or more contours. At the point of such singularity, the normal direction of the contour cannot be defined and the right hand side of the evolution equation of (6) becomes meaningless. For this case, generally, global smooth solutions of the object surface are difficult to obtain.

Other than this case, we ocasionally have intrinsic ambiguous solutions. The shape from shading from one image allows alternate solutions such as shown in **Fig.8**, for example. From the shown shading image we cannot distinguish between two surface shapes shown in the figure. This makes reconstruction be difficult for some geometrically complex surface shapes. To avoid this type of intrinsic ambiguity, we use the result of our shape from image sequence technique devoloped in [1]. We aiready have a rough global 3D sketch of the object surface by this method. For this latter ambiguity can

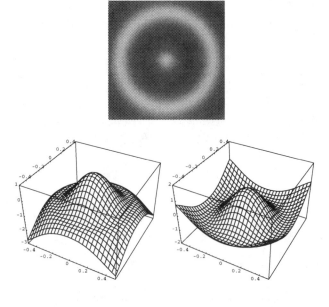

Figure 8. An example where two shapes cannot be discriminated from their image shadings

be overcome by referring the result to select a correct solution.

The second difficulty arises from that, practically, the image gray levels are given only at lattice sample points. The equal-range contour is generally a free curve, so that, in the solution of (6), image points that are not at just the lattice points must be considered. For example, to evaluate $\tan\theta$ in (7), we must refer the image gray level $E(x,y)$. But the coordinates (x,y) are not necessarily just of a lattice sample point, because the values x and y are given according to the object shape. For such a case, we must employ an interpolation of some gray level samples at the lattice points.

To overcome both difficulties for numerical solutions, a combination of level set method and a viscosity solution approach is proposed ([7],[8]) in the field of material science.

In the level set method, next *Hamilton-Jacobi* equation (called the *level set equation*) is employed for equal-range contours,

$$\phi_t + H(x,y,t,\phi_x,\phi_y) = 0 \qquad (8)$$

by introducing a level function $\phi(x,y,t)$. The solution contour of the evolution equation of (6) at t is given as the zero-crossing of this ϕ as

$$\phi(x,y,t) = 0 \qquad (9)$$

where $\phi(x, y, t)$ is the solution of the level set equation (8).

By this method, also a contour having singular points can be expressed using a smooth function of ϕ. Moreover, as is described later, numerical solution can be carried out only based on the image sampling points (x, y). To adding this, by employing the next idea of viscosity solution, the solution is always given uniquely, except for the previous mentioned intrinsic cases for which we employ the results of shape from image sequence method.

3.4. Viscosity solutions

The idea of the viscosity solution of a partial differential equation was introduced as a so-called *weak solution* based on the maximal principle [7, 9, 10]. (The name "viscosity" does not make sense for our problem.) Its definition is given as;

> A continuous function $v(x, y, t)$ is called a *viscosity subsolution*, if, for an arbitrary function ψ, $v - \psi$ has the maximum value at $(\bar{x}, \bar{y}, \bar{t})$, then
> $$\psi_t + H(x, y, v, \psi_x, \psi_y) \geq 0 \qquad (10)$$
> at this point.

> A *viscosity supersolution* is defined by replacing "maximum" by "minimum" and $\geq$ by $\leq$, respectively, in the above definition. The solution which is a viscosity subsolution and, at the same time, a supersolution is called a *viscosity solution*.

We can obtain the viscosity solution of (8) by numerical methods ([9],[7]), and the existence theory [10] guarantees its global uniqueness. Therefore, our solution of (6) is summarised that, derive the corresponding level set equation first, then obtain its viscosity solution by a numerical method.

3.5. Derivation of the level set equation

Following Osher[8], we derive the level set equation for (6). We rewrite our basic equation (1) including the normalization coefficient σ as

$$E(x, y) = \sigma \frac{F(\cos \theta)}{r^2}$$
$$= \sigma \frac{F(\boldsymbol{n} \cdot \boldsymbol{v})}{r^2} \qquad (11)$$

and assume the reflectance function F is a unit function, for the simplicity, which means that the object surface is Lambertian.

The object shape is represented with a range function r from the origin, but we employ the image coordinates x and y as parameter variables such as $r(x, y)$.

A point on the object surface corresponding to an image coordinates (x, y), denoted by a vector $\boldsymbol{r}(x, y)$, is given as

$$\boldsymbol{r}(x, y) = \frac{r(x, y)}{\sqrt{x^2 + y^2 + f^2}}(-x, -y, f) \qquad (12)$$

The normal vector of the surface $\boldsymbol{n}$ at this point is given as

$$\boldsymbol{n} = \frac{\boldsymbol{r}_x \times \boldsymbol{r}_y}{\|\boldsymbol{r}_x \times \boldsymbol{r}_y\|} \qquad (13)$$

and the unit vector of the direction of its line of sight $\boldsymbol{v}$ is

$$\boldsymbol{v} = -\frac{\boldsymbol{r}}{r} \qquad (14)$$

Substituting these into (11), we obtain a form of a partial differential equation as a form of

$$G(x, y, r, r_x, r_y) = 0 \qquad (15)$$

Then, an equation that the level set function $\phi(x, y, t)$ must satisfy has the form when $\phi = 0$ as [8]

$$G(x, y, t, \frac{-\phi_x}{\phi_t}, \frac{-\phi_y}{\phi_t}) = 0 \qquad (16)$$

Arranging this equation we finally obtain the next level set equation

$$\phi_t = -\frac{tE(x, y)\sqrt{A(B\phi_x^2 + C\phi_y^2 + 2xy\phi_x\phi_y)}}{f\sqrt{\sigma^2 - t^4(E(x, y))^2}} \qquad (17)$$

where $A \equiv f^2 + x^2 + y^2$, $B \equiv f^2 + x^2$, and $C \equiv f^2 + y^2$.

3.6. Numerical method for solution

To summarize the algorithm to obtain equal-range contours from a shading image (cf. **Fig.9**):

1. Give an initial equal-range contour on the object surface.

2. Select a function $\phi(x, y, t_0)$ which has next properties:

   (a) $\phi(x, y, t_0) = 0$ gives the initial contour.

   (b) $\phi(x, y, t_0) < 0$ within the area bounded by the initial contour.

   (c) $\phi(x, y, t_0) > 0$ out of the area bounded by the initial contour.

   (d) $\phi(x, y, t_0)$ is Lipsitz continuous.

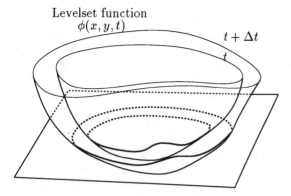

Levelset function
$\phi(x, y, t)$

Figure 9. Evolution of equal-range contour using levelsets.

3. For all lattice points on the image, evolve the ϕ according to (17) and iterating the method to obtain its viscosity solution.

4. For every nth iteration, obtain a level set of $\phi(x, y, t_0 + n\Delta t) = 0$.

The details of the numerical methods for the viscosity solution are discussed in [9], [7]. In those methods, the partial differentials in (17) with respective t are approximated by simple first order differences, and the spatially partial differentials with respect to x and y are approximated by, for example,

$$\phi_x^2 = (\min(D_x^-, 0))^2 + (\max(D_x^+, 0))^2 \qquad (18)$$

Where D_x^- represents the backward difference of ϕ with respect to x, D_x^+ the forward difference and so on.

3.7. Obtaining the initial equal-range contour

To employ proposed method, we must have at least one equal-range contour initially, then evolving this contour we obtain total object shape. We obtain this initial contour using the gray level distribution of the image as in [3]. If there is an isolated maximum gray level point which is a specular point and the range to this point can be estimated, we can construct a proper initial contour around this point. This is because at the maximum gray level point or the specular point the direction of the surface normal is just that of the line of sight to this point. So that we can introduce a ring contour within the neighbor of the maximum gray level point as an initial equal-range contour. For

proper selection of the initial contour, our already obtained rough global 3D sketch helps much.

In the experiments, we selected one such point on the object surface, and estimated or assumed the range to this point, then, introduced a closed contour within the neighbor of this point as an initial equal-range contour.

4. Experimental results

Fig.10 shows experimental simulation for a computer generated image. (a) is the original image consisting of 64×64 pixels. (b) shows obtained equal-range contours obtained at every iteration. In this figure, the contours are mapped on the image coordinates (x, y). (c) is the result of the object shape reconstruction, and (d) shows the reconstruction errors.

We have applied the proposed method for some real medical endoscope images. **Fig.11** shows a result of object shape reconstruction. (a) shows the original image of an inner wall of human stomach taken by a medical endoscope also having 64×64 pixels. (b) shows its obtained equal-range contours, and (c) is the result of the shape reconstruction. (d) shows the mapping of the original texture of (a) on the reconstructed 3D shape.

Fig.12 shows anothor result of an experiment for real endoscope image.

5. Conclusions

An algorithm is proposed to reconstruct the object shape from shadings of endoscope images, where the optical imaging system is considered to have a point light source at the projection (lens) center. For this optical system, the conventional shape from shading methods that assume the light source is at infinitely far make no sense. We introduce an equal-range contour on the object surface to which the distance from the point light source is constant. Then evolving this contour according to the gray level of image shading and obtain total object shape. The experimental results show promising availability for real endoscope image applications.

However, we need an initial equal-range contour which corresponds to an initial condition of the given differential equation. For this problem to obtain proper initial contours and accurate object shapes, we combined shape from image sequence algorithm using time series of images to our proposed algorithm of shape from shading.

References

[1] K.Deguchi *et al.* 3-D Shape Recognition from Endoscope Image Sequences by The Factorization Method. *MVA '94: IAPR Workshop on Machine Vision Applications*, Kawasaki, pp. 455–459, 1994.

[2] N. Oda, J. Hasegawa, T. Nonami, M. Yamaguchi and N. Ohyama. Estimation of the surface topography from monocular endoscopic images. *Optics Communications*, Vol. 109, pp. 215–221, 1994.

[3] R. Kimmel and A. M. Bruckstein. Tracking level sets by level sets: A method for solving the shape from shading problem. *Computer Vision and Image Understanding*, Vol. 62, No. 2, pp. 47–58, 1995.

[4] A. M. Bruckstein. On shape from shading. *Comput. Vision, Graphics, Image Process.*, Vol. 44, pp. 139–154, 1988.

[5] E. Rouy and A. Tourin. A viscosity solutions approach to shape-from-shading. *SIAM J. Numer. Anal.*, Vol. 29, No. 3, pp. 867–884, 1992.

[6] R. Kimmel, et al. Shape from shading: Level set propagation and viscosity solutions. *Int. J. of Comput. Vision*, Vol. 16, pp. 107–133, 1995.

[7] S. Osher and C. W. Shu. High-order essentially nonoscillatory schemes for Hamilton-Jacobi equations. *SIAM J. Numer. Anal.*, Vol. 28, No. 4, pp. 907–922, 1991.

[8] S. Osher. A level set formulation for the solution of the Dirichlet problem for Hamilton-Jacobi equations. *SIAM J. Math. Anal.*, Vol. 24, No. 5, pp. 1145–1152, 1993.

[9] S. Osher and J. A. Sethian. Fronts propagating with curvature-dependent speed: Algorithms based on Hamilton-Jacobi formulations. *J. Comput. Phys.*, Vol. 79, pp. 12–49, 1988.

[10] M. G. Crandall, H. Ishii and P. -L. Lions. User's guide to viscosity solutions of second order partial differential equations. *Bull. Amer. Math. Soc.*, Vol. 27, pp. 1–67, 1992.

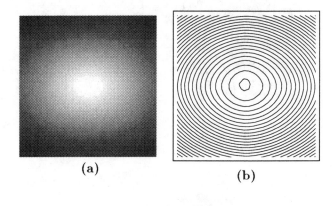

(a)   (b)

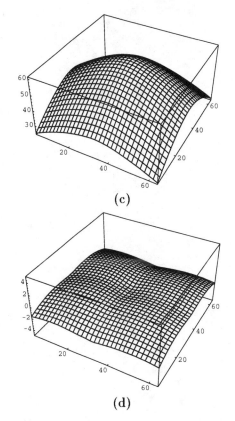

(c)

(d)

Figure 10. Result of experimental simuration for a computer generated image. (a) Original image, (b) Reconstructed equal-range contours, (c) Reconstructed 3D object shape, and (d) Shape reconstruction errors.

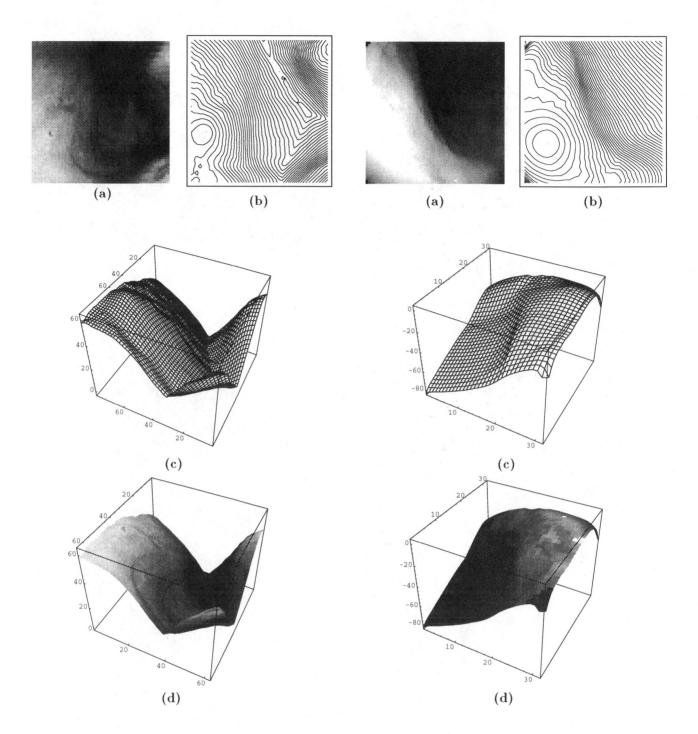

Figure 11. An example of 3D shape reconstruction from a medical endoscope image. (a) Original endoscope image of inner wall of human stomach, (b) Reconstructed equal-range contours, (c) Reconstructed shape of inner wall of human stomach, and (d) texture mapped display of (c) with the original image of (a).

Figure 12. Another example of 3D shape reconstruction from a medical endoscope image. (a) Original endoscope image of inner wall of human stomach, (b) Reconstructed equal-range contours, (c) Reconstructed shape of inner wall of human stomach, and (d) texture mapped display of (c) with the original image of (a).

On Computing Aspect Graphs of Smooth Shapes from Volumetric Data

Alison Noble and Dale Wilson
Department of Engineering Science
University of Oxford
Oxford OX1 3PJ, England
{noble,dale}@robots.ox.ac.uk

Jean Ponce
Beckman Institute
University of Illinois
Urbana IL 61801, USA
ponce@cs.uiuc.edu

Abstract

In this paper we address the problem of computing the aspect graph of an object from volumetric image data, with applications in medical image analysis and interpretation. Anatomical surfaces are assumed to be smooth and are identified as the zero set of a three-dimensional density function (e.g., a CT, MR, or ultrasound image). The orthographic-projection aspect graph is constructed by partitioning the view sphere at infinity into maximal regions bounded by visual event curves. These events are the intersections of the view sphere with surfaces ruled by singular tangent lines that graze the object's surface along a set of critical curves. For each visual event the proposed algorithm constructs a new density function from the original one and its derivatives, and computes the corresponding critical curve as the intersection of the object's surface with the zero set of the new density function. Once the critical curves have been traced, the regions of the sphere delineated by the corresponding visual events are constructed through cell decomposition, and a representative aspect is constructed for each region by computing the occluding contour for a sample viewing direction. A preliminary implementation of the proposed approach has been constructed and experiments with synthetic data and real medical data are presented. Extensions to the sectional imaging case are also discussed.

1. Introduction

Despite the increasingly widespread use of volumetric images in the medical domain, many every-day clinical applications still primarily involve 2D image acquisition modalities, corresponding to either projections (e.g., X-ray radiographs) or cross-sections (e.g., X-ray CT slices) of 3D anatomical objects. This is particularly true in real-time applications, such as routine echocardiographic examinations, or endovascular surgery, for example. Thus, the automated analysis of 2D images remains an important step toward computer-aided clinical interpretation. At the same time,

being snap-shots of 3D anatomical structures, the 2D images record some of the geometric characteristics of these objects. It is therefore important to develop general tools for robustly and efficiently selecting the 2D views which capture the most important features of a 3D object. Efficiency is particularly relevant in visualization and image database applications [44], and robustness is critical for automated segmentation and geometry measurements.

Consider, for example, the every-day problem faced by a radiographer who has to view many images of a patient taken at slightly different viewing angles. It would be advantageous to reduce the number of images presented to a minimal set conveying distinct informations about the object, but there is currently no reliable way of quantifying the similarities between adjacent views. Further, tasks such as picking a good X-ray view for looking at the structure of an aneurysm, or adjusting the angle of an ultrasonic probe to get a good echogram (i.e., a minimally obstructive slice) of the heart of a foetus require considerable clinical expertise. It would clearly be interesting to simplify this process to the level where, for example, a clinical assistant can readily be trained to acquire high-quality echograms of a foetus heart, or going one step further, to design an active imaging sensor adaptively controlling the probing direction of a sensor to get the best view of an internal organ with minimal human assistance. One of the aims of our work is to investigate new ways to perform view selection to ultimately achieve the latter goal.

A key point here is that a 3D object can look very different depending on the choice of image acquisition angle or slice location. Put another way, shape characterization from 2D projections or slices is not stable, which can lead to mis-diagnosis. Further, the automated selection of stable views is particularly important for tasks such as segmenting "identical" slices of a patient acquired at different times or performing volumetric measurements from 2D views. Finally, methods for 3D reconstruction from a sparse set of views [43] would also benefit from an improved understanding of how to select critical images.

Proceedings of MMBIA '96

Within the field of computer vision, Koenderink and Van Doorn introduced twenty years ago a mathematical object representation, called the *aspect graph* [21, 22], which identifies the set of all qualitatively distinct (projection) views of an object. In the medical domain, Kergosien [16, 17] has suggested that aspect graphs may be a natural tool for representing and visualizing anatomical surfaces. However, his work has mostly focussed on the theory of aspect graphs rather than their implementation. The main contribution of this paper is to propose an algorithm for computing the aspect graph of a smooth object from real volumetric medical data. Unlike previous approaches, this algorithm does not depend on an intermediate parameterization of the surface –a particularly attractive feature for medical images which frequently have a complex form.

More precisely, the surface of the object is assumed to be smooth, and it is identified as the zero set of a three-dimensional density function. Its aspect graph is constructed by partitioning the view sphere at infinity into maximal regions bounded by visual event curves. These events are the intersections of the view sphere with surfaces ruled by singular tangent lines that graze the object's surface along a set of critical curves. For each visual event the proposed algorithm constructs a new density function from the original one and its derivatives, and computes the corresponding critical curve as the intersection of the object's surface with the zero set of the new density function. Once the critical curves have been traced, the regions of the sphere delineated by the corresponding visual events are constructed through cell decomposition, and a representative aspect is constructed for each region by computing the object's occluding contour for a sample viewing direction.

In the rest of this paper we firstly recall the theoretical underpinnings of aspect graphs, and then outline the algorithms underlying our approach. Finally we present preliminary results and their implementation for synthetic and real data. We are currently completing the full implementation.

2. Background

2.1. Aspect Graphs

The aspect graph [22] is a qualitative, viewer-centred representation which enumerates all possible appearances of an object. The range of possible viewpoints is partitioned into maximal regions, in which each point yields an identical aspect. The change in appearance at the boundary between regions is called a visual event. The maximal regions and the associated aspects form the nodes of an aspect graph, whose arcs correspond to the visual event boundaries between adjacent regions.

Since the invention of aspect graphs by Koenderink and Van Doorn [21, 22] in the mid-seventies, much research has

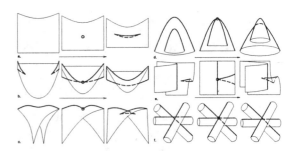

Figure 1. Local events: a. lip, b. beak-to-beak, c. swallowtail. Multi-local events: d. tangent crossing, e. cusp crossing, f. triple point. The transitions take place from left to right, the singularities being indicated by small circles.

been devoted to the problem of constructing these objects from various other geometric representations. Indeed, one may find implemented algorithms for computing the aspect graphs of polyhedra [41, 48, 42, 32, 47, 12, 39] as well as solids bounded by curved surfaces, including quadrics [5], surfaces of revolution [23, 9, 10], and algebraic surfaces [35, 36, 31].

A recurrent criticism of aspect graphs is that their size is unwieldy: indeed, a polyhedron with n faces has an aspect graph of size $O(n^6)$ under orthographic projection and $O(n^9)$ under perspective projection [32, 12], and a solid bounded by n algebraic patches of degree d has $O(n^{12}d^{12})$ distinct aspects under orthographic projection and $O(n^{18}d^{18})$ aspects under perspective projection (these numbers reduce respectively $O(n^6d^{12})$ and $O(n^9d^{18})$ for surfaces homomorphic to polyhedra) [37, 30]. Taking the finite resolution of digital images into account does not always reduce the aspect graph size, and in fact may increase it [11, 40].

Despite these concerns, aspect graphs remain an intriguing and potentially promising object representation for computer vision, and it is important to understand whether it is possible to construct the aspect graph of complex natural objects which are neither polyhedra nor algebraic surfaces. This is one of our motivations for proposing in this paper an algorithm for computing the aspect graph of an object from volumetric data (e.g., CT or MR images). As stated earlier, our other primary motivation is, of course, to investigate the adequacy of the aspect graph to medical image analysis.

2.2. Visual events

In this section, we recall the pertinent results from catastrophe theory that form the theoretical basis for the construction of aspect graphs [46, 22, 15, 1, 4, 34].

The image contours of smooth objects are the projection of surface curves (occluding contours) where the visual ray grazes the surface. From most viewpoints, the contour is a piecewise-smooth curve whose only singularities are cusps and t-junctions, and its structure is stable with respect to viewpoint, i.e., it does not change when the camera position is submitted to a small perturbation. From some viewpoints, however, almost any perturbation of the viewpoint will alter the contour topology. A catalogue of these "visual events" has been established by Kergosien [15] for smooth surfaces observed under orthographic projection (Figure 1).

Under this camera model, the range of possible viewpoints (viewing directions) is two-dimensional and can be modelled as a view sphere at infinity. The visual events in Kergosien's catalogue lie along curves on the view sphere. They occur when the viewing direction has high-order contact with the observed surface along certain characteristic curves [1, 19, 20]. When contact occurs at a single point on the surface, the event is said to be local; when it occurs at multiple points, it is said to be multi-local. A catalogue of visual events is also available for piecewise-smooth surfaces [46, 34], but we will restrict our discussion to smooth surfaces in this paper.

2.3. Local Events

A smooth surface may exhibit three types of local events: swallowtail, beak-to-beak, and lip (Figure 1a-c). During a swallowtail transition, a smooth image contour forms a singularity and then breaks off into two cusps and a t-junction. In a beak-to-beak transition, two distinct portions of the contour meet at a point in the image. After meeting, the contour splits and forms two cusps. Finally, in a lip transition, a closed contour appears out of nowhere, with the formation of two cusps.

A swallowtail occurs when the viewing direction is an asymptotic direction at some point on a flecnodal curve of the surface; both beak-to-beak and lip events occur when the viewing direction is an asymptotic direction on a parabolic curve [1, 19, 20]. Flecnodal points are inflections of the projection of the asymptotic curves into the tangent plane, and parabolic points are zeros of the Gaussian curvature [49].

2.4. Multi-local Events

These events occur when two or more surface points project onto the same contour point. There are three types of multi-local events: triple point, tangent crossing, and cusp crossing (Figure 1d-f). A triple point is formed by the intersection of three contour segments. A tangent crossing occurs when two contours meet at a point and share a common tangent. Finally, a cusp crossing occurs when the projection of a contour cusp meets another contour.

A multi-local event is characterized by a curve defined in a high-dimension space, or equivalently by a family of surface curves. For example, a triple point occurs when three occluding contour points are aligned with the viewing direction. Sweeping the supporting line while maintaining three points of contact generates a developable surface which intersects the original surface along a family of three curves. In the process, the direction of the line traces a visual event curve on the view sphere. The case of tangent and cusp crossings is similar, but only two surface curves are involved.

3. Approach

As shown in [31], constructing the aspect graph of a smooth object can be decomposed into four steps: (1) tracing the parabolic, flecnodal, limiting bitangent, asymptotic bitangent, and tritangent curves (critical curves) on the object surface, (2) mapping these curves onto the view sphere curves (visual events) representing the corresponding singular (asymptotic and bitangent) directions, (3) constructing a cell decomposition of the view sphere into maximal regions bounded by visual events, and (4) constructing a sample view for each region.

The most difficult and costly step is the initial construction of the five surface curves: steps (2) and (3) only involve classical algorithms such as line sweeps, and step (4) is essentially an exercise in computer graphics.

In this section we present a simple approach for constructing critical curves from volumetric data. It is based on the idea of representing surfaces as the zero set of some density function. Constructing an explicit representation of the critical curves thus reduces to tracing the intersection of two level sets: the surface of the object itself, and the zero set of the "equation" of the critical curve. This can be done using the marching lines algorithm for example [45].

3.1. Surfaces, Density Functions and Blurred Derivatives

Let us suppose without loss of generality that the data is given as a density function $D : I^3 \to \mathbb{R}$, where $I \subset \mathbb{R}$ is some interval of the real line, the surface of the object of interest being given by the level set $D(\boldsymbol{x}) = 0$, where $\boldsymbol{x} = (x, y, z)^T \in I^3$.

Note: throughout, x, y, z subscripts denote partial derivatives with respect to the corresponding variables.

Since it is defined as a level set, the surface can be extracted with sub-voxel precision and a correct topology using the marching cubes algorithm [24].

To estimate the differential geometry of a surface, the classical computer vision approach is to parameterize this surface then use either analytical or numerical methods to compute partial derivatives of the parameterization [33, 2]. Here we propose instead to follow Koenderink's suggestion and compute the (*blurred*) derivatives of the density function itself [20, Chapter 9.4] by convolving this function with the derivatives of a Gaussian. This has the advantage of replacing a potentially ill-conditioned numerical differentiation process by a well-conditioned integration one.

Specifically, following Koenderink's notation, if

$$G_{000}(\boldsymbol{x}, \sigma) = \frac{1}{(\sigma\sqrt{2\pi})^3}e^{-|\boldsymbol{x}|^2/4\sigma^2}$$

denotes the three-dimensional Gaussian kernel, and if

$$G_{klm} = \frac{\partial^{k+l+m}}{\partial x^k y^l z^m}G_{000}$$

denotes a partial derivative of this kernel, then the corresponding blurred derivative of D is

$$\frac{\partial^{k+l+m}}{\partial x^k y^l z^m}(G_{000} * D) = G_{klm} * D.$$

It should be noted that a similar approach has been proposed independently by Monga, Benayoun and Faugeras [27], Thirion and Gourdon [45], and Monga, Lengagne and Deriche [28] with medical applications in mind. In particular, Monga, Lengagne and Deriche [28] propose to improve the efficiency of the computation of the blurred derivatives by using the recursive approximation of a Gaussian filter introduced by Deriche [6].

3.2. Algorithmic Tools

In this paper, we will be interested in extracting from volumetric data the locus of points where one, two, or three density functions are zero. We will assume throughout that all intersections are transversal ones, thus the zero sets of one, two, and three density functions are respectively surfaces, curves, and isolated points.

A polyhedral approximation of the zero set of a single density function can be found with sub-voxel precision and a consistent topology by using a case analysis of possible intersections of surfaces with the faces of a cube and linear interpolation between adjacent vertices of the image grid. This is the basis for the marching cubes algorithm of Lorensen and Cline [24].

The marching cubes technique has been extended to finding the intersection of two density zero sets by Thirion and Gourdon [45]. Their approach relies once again on a case analysis and linear interpolation between edge points.

Finally, if the polyhedral approximation of the surface passing through a voxel and the polygonal approximation of a curve passing through the same voxel have been constructed, it is a simple matter to determine whether and where the three level sets associated to the surface and the curve intersect within the voxel, once again using linear interpolation.

Our algorithm relies on these three capabilities. In particular, we will trace the critical curves corresponding to visual

events by intersecting the level sets $D = 0$ and $F = 0$, where F is a function of D and its partial derivatives. We derive the various "equations" (i.e., the density functions F) corresponding to the various critical curves in the next two sections.

3.3. Constructing the Local Event Curves

Here we recall the equations for asymptotic directions, parabolic curves, and flecnodal curves. See [31, 29] for details. Given these equations, the corresponding curves can be traced using the marching lines algorithm, as explained in the previous section.

Asymptotic Directions An asymptotic direction $\boldsymbol{v} = (\alpha, \beta, \gamma)^T$ at a point $\boldsymbol{x} = (x, y, z)^T$ lies in the tangent plane and has second-order contact with the surface. It is thus characterized by:

$$\begin{cases} \alpha D_x + \beta D_y + \gamma D_z = 0, \\ \alpha^2 D_{xx} + \beta^2 D_{yy} + \gamma^2 D_{zz}, \\ +2\alpha\beta D_{xy} + 2\beta\gamma D_{yz} + 2\alpha\gamma D_{xz} = 0. \end{cases} \quad (1)$$

Parabolic Curves As shown in [49], the parabolic curves are given by the intersection of the surfaces $D(\boldsymbol{x}) = 0$ and $P(\boldsymbol{x}) = 0$, where

$$\begin{aligned} &D_x^2(D_{yy}D_{zz} - D_{yz}^2) + D_y^2(D_{xx}D_{zz} - D_{xz}^2) \\ &+D_z^2(D_{xx}D_{yy} - D_{xy}^2) \\ &+2D_xD_y(D_{xz}D_{yz} - D_{zz}D_{xy}) \\ &+2D_yD_z(D_{xy}D_{xz} - D_{xx}D_{yz}) \\ &+2D_xD_z(D_{xy}D_{yz} - D_{yy}D_{xz}) = 0. \end{aligned} \quad (2)$$

For each point $\boldsymbol{x}$ along a parabolic curve, there is only one asymptotic direction, which is given by (1).

Flecnodal Curves A surface point $\boldsymbol{x}$ on a flecnodal curve has third order contact with a line along an asymptotic direction $\boldsymbol{v} = (\alpha, \beta, \gamma)^T$ [1]. Thus $\boldsymbol{x}$ and $\boldsymbol{v}$ are characterized by (1) and

$$\begin{aligned} &\alpha^3 D_{xxx} + \beta^3 D_{yyy} + \gamma^3 D_{zzz} + 3\alpha^2\beta D_{xxy} \\ &+3\alpha\beta^2 D_{xyy} + 3\beta^2\gamma D_{yyz} + 3\beta\gamma^2 D_{yzz} \\ &+3\alpha^2\gamma D_{xxz} + 3\alpha\gamma^2 D_{xzz} + 6\alpha\beta\gamma D_{xyz} = 0. \end{aligned} \quad (3)$$

The constraints (1) and (3) define three homogeneous polynomial equations in the coordinates of $\boldsymbol{v}$, hence resultants [38, 7, 25] can be used to eliminate these coordinates and construct a single equation $F(\boldsymbol{x}) = 0$ in $\boldsymbol{x}$ only: briefly, resultants generalize determinants to the non-linear algebraic case. A square homogeneous system of linear equations admits a non-trivial solution if and only if its determinant (which is a function of the equations' coefficients only) is zero. Likewise, a square homogeneous system of polynomial equations admits a non-trivial solution if and only if its resultant (which is also a function of the equations' coefficients only) is zero. See [14] for a modern treatment of resultants and other tools from elimination theory.

It should be noted that, although it is possible to compute F *symbolically* by constructing the Dixon resultant of the three equations [7], this resultant contains 1851 terms, each of them is a function of the first, second, and third derivatives of D. An alternative is to keep the resultant in determinant form, and, as proposed by Manocha [26] and explained below, to evaluate it *numerically* when necessary.

Manocha has constructed an implementation of the Macaulay resultant [25], which is expressed as the ratio of the determinants of two matrices. Instead of computing the Macaulay resultant symbolically, Manocha's program constructs the Macaulay matrices, whose entries are polynomial expressions in the first, second, and third derivatives of D in our case. The Macaulay resultant output by the program is $F = \mathrm{Det}(M_1)/\mathrm{Det}(M_2)$, where M_1 is the matrix shown in Figure 2 and $\mathrm{Det}(M_2) = D_x^4$. Instead of evaluating F symbolically, we compute the derivatives for each data point, then substitute the corresponding values in M_1 and M_2, then evaluate the two determinants numerically, using a linear algebra package such as LINPACK [8] for example.

Constructing the Local Events   Once discrete approximations of the parabolic and flecnodal curves have been traced using the marching lines algorithm, it is a simple matter to compute the asymptotic directions along these curves using Eq. (1), which in turn yields discrete approximations of the visual event curves on the unit sphere.

3.4. Constructing the Multi-Local Event Curves

For the multi-local events, things are a bit different, since the corresponding curves are defined by pairs or triples of points. We take advantage of the fact that there is only a finite (possibly zero) number of bitangents going through any surface point to reduce the problem of computing the multi-local events to computing the intersection of two zero sets.

Computing Bitangents   Consider a given point x_0 in the volume of interest, and let $D_0 = D(x_0)$. The point x_0 is on the surface S_0 defined by $D(x) = D_0$. A bitangent to S_0 in x_0 grazes this surface at a second point x_1 verifying the three equations

$$
\begin{cases}
D(x_1) = D_0, \\
(x_1 - x_0) \cdot \nabla D(x_0) = 0, \\
(x_1 - x_0) \cdot \nabla D(x_1) = 0.
\end{cases}
\tag{4}
$$

For a fixed point x_0, these three equations admit in general a finite number of solutions, which can be found with sub-voxel accuracy as follows: voxel-precision solutions

are first found by looking for common zero-crossings of the three equations. Sub-voxel localization is then achieved by approximating each of the three equations by a trilinear function within the voxel and computing the common zeros of the three trilinear functions using Newton-Raphson iterations (since it can be assumed that the candidate voxel is already a good guess). An alternative would be to directly intersect the zero sets of the three equations, as suggested in Section 3.2.

It should be noted that the bitangent directions define on the surface a vector field, similar to the vector fields defined by the principal directions and asymptotic directions. As in the asymptotic direction case, there is in general an even number of bitangent directions at each point, except at singular points where there is an odd number of bitangents (limiting bitangents and tritangents).

Limiting Bitangents   Once all of the solutions have been found, we compute for each of them the value of

$$
l(x_0, x_1) = \frac{(\nabla D(x_0) \times \nabla D(x_1)) \cdot (x_1 - x_0)}{|\nabla D(x_0)||\nabla D(x_1)||x_1 - x_0|},
$$

which is simply equal to the sine of the angle between the two surface normals (when the two points form a bitangent exactly). We then choose the solution x_1^* minimizing $|l(x_0, x_1)|$, and finally set $L(x_0) = l(x_0, x_1^*)$. The limiting bitangent curve is found by intersecting the surfaces $D(x) = 0$ and $L(x) = 0$.

Asymptotic Bitangents   The case of asymptotic bitangents is similar. Consider a hyperbolic point x and the associated asymptotic direction a (assumed to have been normalized to unit length). For each of the potential bitangent points x_1 found earlier, we compute the value of

$$
a(x_0, x_1) = \frac{(a \times (x_1 - x_0)) \cdot \nabla D(x_0)}{|x_1 - x_0||\nabla D(x_0)|},
$$

which is simply the sine of the angle between the vectors a and $x_0 - x_1$ (when the two point exactly form a bitangent). We then choose the solution x_1^* minimizing $|a(x_0, x_1)|$, and finally set $A(x_0) = a(x_0, x_1^*)$. The asymptotic bitangent curve is then found by intersecting the surfaces $D(x) = 0$ and $A(x) = 0$.

Tritangents   Here we must consider pairs of solutions, say x_1 and x_2. We compute for each of these pairs the value of

$$
t(x_0, x_1, x_2) = \frac{((x_1 - x_0) \times (x_2 - x_0)) \cdot \nabla D(x_0)}{|x_1 - x_0||x_2 - x_0||\nabla D(x_0)|},
$$

which is simply the sine of the angle between the vectors $x_1 - x_0$ and $x_2 - x_0$ (when the points x_0 and x_i actually

$$M_1 = \begin{pmatrix}
D_x & D_y & D_z & 0 & 0 & 0 & 0 & 0 & 0 & 0 & 0 & 0 & 0 & 0 & 0 \\
0 & D_x & 0 & D_y & D_z & 0 & 0 & 0 & 0 & 0 & 0 & 0 & 0 & 0 & 0 \\
0 & 0 & D_x & 0 & D_y & D_z & 0 & 0 & 0 & 0 & 0 & 0 & 0 & 0 & 0 \\
0 & 0 & 0 & D_x & 0 & 0 & D_y & D_z & 0 & 0 & 0 & 0 & 0 & 0 & 0 \\
0 & 0 & 0 & 0 & D_x & 0 & 0 & D_y & D_z & 0 & 0 & 0 & 0 & 0 & 0 \\
0 & 0 & 0 & 0 & 0 & D_x & 0 & 0 & D_y & D_z & 0 & 0 & 0 & 0 & 0 \\
0 & 0 & 0 & 0 & 0 & 0 & D_x & 0 & 0 & 0 & D_y & D_z & 0 & 0 & 0 \\
0 & 0 & 0 & 0 & 0 & 0 & 0 & D_x & 0 & 0 & 0 & D_y & D_z & 0 & 0 \\
0 & 0 & 0 & 0 & 0 & 0 & 0 & 0 & D_x & 0 & 0 & 0 & D_y & D_z & 0 \\
0 & 0 & 0 & 0 & 0 & 0 & 0 & 0 & 0 & D_x & 0 & 0 & 0 & D_y & D_z \\
0 & 0 & 0 & D_{xx} & 0 & 0 & 2D_{xy} & 2D_{xz} & 0 & 0 & D_{yy} & 2D_{yz} & D_{zz} & 0 & 0 \\
0 & 0 & 0 & 0 & D_{xx} & 0 & 0 & 2D_{xy} & 2D_{xz} & 0 & 0 & D_{yy} & 2D_{yz} & D_{zz} & 0 \\
0 & 0 & 0 & 0 & 0 & D_{xx} & 0 & 0 & 2D_{xy} & 2D_{xz} & 0 & 0 & D_{yy} & 2D_{yz} & D_{zz} \\
0 & D_{xxx} & 0 & 3D_{xxy} & 3D_{xxz} & 0 & 3D_{xyy} & 6D_{xyz} & 3D_{xzz} & 0 & D_{yyy} & 3D_{yyz} & 3D_{yzz} & D_{zzz} & 0 \\
0 & 0 & D_{xxx} & 0 & 3D_{xxy} & 3D_{xxz} & 0 & 3D_{xyy} & 6D_{xyz} & 3D_{xzz} & 0 & D_{yyy} & 3D_{yyz} & 3D_{yzz} & D_{zzz}
\end{pmatrix}$$

Figure 2. The matrix used in the construction of the Macaulay resultant.

form bitangents for $i = 1, 2$). We then choose the solutions x_1^* and x_2^* minimizing $|t(x_0, x_1, x_2)|$, and finally set $T(x_0) = t(x_0, x_1^*, x_2^*)$. The tritangent curve is then found by intersecting the surfaces $D(x) = 0$ and $T(x) = 0$.

Efficiency Concerns Computing the limiting bitangent curve requires computing L, with a potential cost of n^2, where n is the number of data points. This cost can be lowered by considering only the points where $|D(x)| \leq \epsilon$, where ϵ is a threshold set by the user, and by mapping the surface normals onto a tessellated Gaussian sphere (see [20] for a discussion of related issues). For limiting bitangents, the idea is as follows: store in each sphere bucket the identity of all points whose normal falls into it; for each surface point, form a candidate pair by retrieving all points falling in the same bucket; verify that the candidate pairs actually form a limiting bitangent. Using the same device, all pairs of points forming asymptotic bitangents can be retrieved in $O(n\sqrt{m})$ time, where n is now the number of surface points, and m is the number of cells of the tessellated sphere (usually, m is smaller than n), while all triples of points forming tritangents can be retrieved in $O(n^2)$ time.

Constructing the Multi-Local Events Once the critical curves have been constructed, polygonal approximations of the corresponding visual event curves on the view sphere are easily constructed, either by directly using the bitangents computed during the construction of the new density functions, or by refining these by recomputing the bitangents at the curve points estimated at the end of the process.

4. Remaining Steps of the Algorithm

Once the critical curves have been computed, two steps of the algorithm remain to be performed: the decomposition of the sphere into maximal regions bounded by the visual event curves, and the construction of a representative aspect per region. Both are relatively simple.

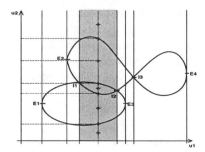

Figure 3. An illustration of the cell decomposition algorithm in the (u_1, u_2) plane. The points E_i are the curve extrema, and the points I_i are curve intersections. The intervals of the u_2 axis are associated with the shaded interval of the u_1 axis. The corresponding samples are shown as small crosses.

4.1. Cell Decomposition

We parameterize the view sphere by the latitude and longitude angles (say u_1 and u_2) and perform cell decomposition in the u_1, u_2 domain. The algorithm is classical, and it is divided into the following steps (Figure 3):

1. Compute all curve extrema in the u_1 direction.

2. Compute all intersections among pairs of curves.

3. Compute all intersections of the curves with the vertical lines orthogonal to the u_1 axis at the extremal and double points.

4. For each interval of the u_1 axis delimited by these lines, do the following:

    4.1. Intersect a vertical line which passes through the midpoint of the u_1-interval with the curves, to obtain a sample point on each branch of each curve.

    4.2. Sort the sample points in increasing u_2 order.

    4.3. March along each curve from its sample point to its intersection points with the vertical lines found in step 3.

    4.4. Two consecutive branches of the curve projections within an interval of u_1 and the segments parallel to

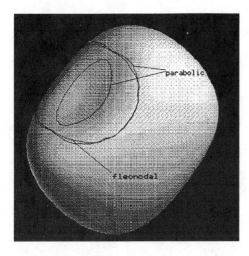

Figure 4. An isosurface for the smoothed dimple volume with computed flecnodal and parabolic curves are indicated. (image size 64x64x64 voxels, $\sigma^2 = 2.0$).

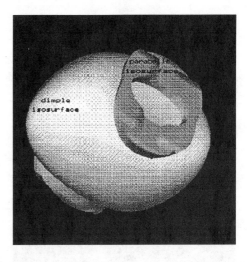

Figure 5. The dimple isosurface and its corresponding "parabolic" isosurface. The intersection shown here defines the parabolic curves on the surface of the dimple.

the u_2 axis joining their endpoints bound a region of the (u_1, u_2) plane.

A sample point can be found for each region as the midpoint of the samples of the bounding curve branches. Maximal regions are found by merging all regions adjacent along line segments parallel to the u_2 axis.

4.2. Aspect Computation

We finally compute the aspect of the surface corresponding to the sample viewing direction associated with each region. This is essentially a computer graphics task: given the viewing direction v, we can compute the occluding contour as the intersection of the surface $D = 0$ with the surface $\nabla D \cdot v = 0$. This can be done again through marching lines. An alternative would be to start with one view and use the known transitions corresponding to each visual event to update the view as you cross the visual event. This is more elegant but a bit more difficult.

5. Implementation and Results

We are in the early stages of the implementation of our algorithm, and so far have only computed results for the local events: parabolic and flecnodal surface curves, and the visual events on the unit sphere for the parabolic curves, accompanied by the corresponding aspects. We are in the process of implementing the rest of the algorithm. Here we present preliminary results on synthetic data (for which the geometry of the surface curves and visual events is known and can be used to validate our experiments) as well as real SPECT data for a heart.

5.1. Synthetic Example Using an Algebraic Surface

In this first example the volumetric density function is defined by

$$D(x) = (4x^2 + 3y^2)^2 - 4x^2 - 5y^2 + 4z^2 - 1.$$

The zero set of this function is the "dimple" surface, previously used by Petitjean [29] in the calculation of the aspect graph for algebraic surfaces. The isosurface of the dimple is shown in Figure 4, with the computed parabolic and flecnodal curves labelled. Figure 5 shows the intersection of the two volumes which defines the parabolic curves on the dimple surface.

The asymptotic directions at the parabolic curve points plotted on the unit sphere, are shown in Figure 6. For this example, the computation of asymptotic directions at the flecnodal points turns out to be quite difficult because the flecnodal points lie close to the parabolic points. Since the data is discrete, it is possible to end up calculating asymptotic directions in an elliptic region of the surface! However, this is a problem in our current implementation and not in the fundamentals of the algorithm. Clearly, one solution would be to move to analysing a higher resolution data set.

The (transparent) aspects of the dimple surface are shown in Figures 7(a)-(d). The corresponding viewing direction are labelled in Figure 6. The aspects are consistent with those calculated algebraically by Petitjean [29].

5.2. Real Data

Finally we present results for a real SPECT data set of a human heart. The smoothed surface is shown in Figure 8, with the flecnodal and parabolic curves overlayed on the

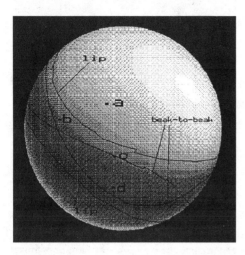

Figure 6. The visual events (asymptotic directions) for the parabolic points are overlayed on the unit sphere. Labels (a)-(d) refer to the viewing directions corresponding to the aspects in Figure 7.

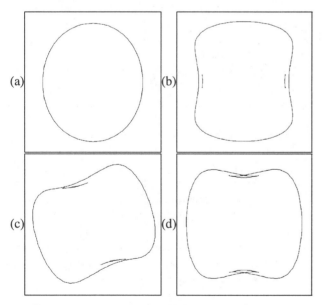

Figure 7. Transparent aspects for the dimple surface.

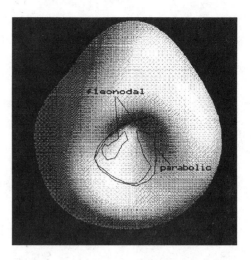

Figure 8. An isosurface for the smoothed SPECT volume of a human heart with flecnodal and parabolic curves overlayed. (image size 64x64x64 voxels, $\sigma^2 = 4.0$).

surface. The asymptotic directions at the parabolic curve points are displayed on the unit sphere in Figure 9. As for the dimple surface the asymptotic directions at the flecnodal points have, as yet, proven difficult to compute accurately.

The (transparent) aspects of the heart surface are displayed in Figures 10(a)-(e). The corresponding viewing directions are labelled in Figure 9. The aspects show a beak-to-beak event as the viewing direction swings around from position (e) to (c), or from (a) to (c). Intuitively, from the shape of the SPECT heart surface there should be views for which no "lip" is visible, and only a single outline of the heart can be seen. We attribute a lack of the case in our results to the omission of a parabolic curve on the heart surface. This may be because such a curve is shorter than the minimum length threshold required as an input parameter by the marching lines algorithm. We have yet to verify that this is the case.

6. Discussion

We have presented an algorithm for computing the aspect graph of a smooth surface defined as the zero set of a volumetric density distribution.

It should be noted that the same tools can be used to compute a related object representation proposed by Kergosien [17] for visualization purposes in the medical domain. Kergosien has shown that the structure of parallel planar sections of a surface is in general stable with respect to small variations in the parameters of the family of sectioning planes, and only changes for sectioning planes parallel to the tangent plane at a parabolic point or to a limiting bitangent plane. Thus the techniques developed in this paper can directly be

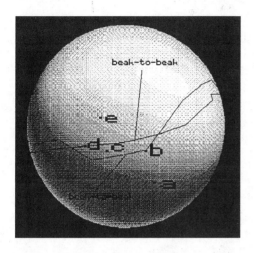

Figure 9. The visual events for the parabolic curves on the surface of the heart overlayed on the unit sphere. Labels (a)-(e) refer to the viewing directions corresponding to the aspects in Figure 10.

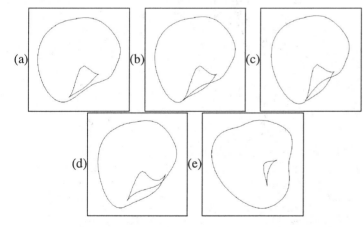

Figure 10. Transparent aspects for the SPECT heart surface.

applied to computing a "sectional aspect graph" that captures the structure of parallel sections of the surface as well as its catastrophic changes.

Interestingly, when the volumetric data has been obtained from a series of X-ray images (sinograms) through CT reconstruction, and the parabolic and limiting bitangent curves are the only critical curves of interest (as in the sectional aspect graph case), it is possible to compute these curves directly from the (segmented) sinograms without having to actually perform CT reconstruction: the idea is to exploit the fact that limiting bitangents and parabolic lines manifest themselves in image contours as bitangents and inflections [18]. Thus detecting and tracking these features over time provides us with information about three-dimensional shape. The method is described in detail in [13] in the context of video image sequences.

Finally, we have not touched on the issue of how to compute aspect graphs of curved objects at different resolutions. Some interesting new theoretical result by Bruce, Giblin and Tari have shed some new light on this topic [3] and we plan to look at the computability of their classification in future work.

Acknowledgements: Jean-Philippe Thirion is thanked for providing the authors with his implementation of the marching lines algorithm.b Jean Ponce was supported in part by the National Science Foundation under Grant IRI-9224815.

References

[1] V. Arnol'd. Singularities of systems of rays. *Russian Math. Surveys*, 38(2):87–176, 1983.

[2] P. Besl and R. Jain. Segmentation through variable-order surface fitting. *IEEE Trans. Patt. Anal. Mach. Intell.*, 10(2):167–192, March 1988.

[3] J. Bruce, P. Giblin, and F. Tari. Parabolic curves of evolving surfaces. *Int. J. of Comp. Vision*, 17(3):291–306, 1996.

[4] J. Callahan and R. Weiss. A model for describing surface shape. In *Proc. IEEE Conf. Comp. Vision Patt. Recog.*, pages 240–245, San Francisco, CA, June 1985.

[5] S. Chen and H. Freeman. On the characteristic views of quadric-surfaced solids. In *IEEE Workshop on Directions in Automated CAD-Based Vision*, pages 34–43, June 1991.

[6] R. Deriche. Recursively implementing the Gaussian and its derivatives. Technical Report 1893, INRIA, 1992.

[7] A. Dixon. The eliminant of three quantics in two independent variables. *Proc. London Mathematical Society, Series 2*, 7:49–69, 1908.

[8] J. Dongarra, J. Bunch, C. Moler, and G. Stewart. *LINPACK User's Guide*. Philadelphia, 1979.

[9] D. Eggert. *Aspect Graphs of Solids of Revolution*. PhD thesis, University of South Florida, Dec. 1991.

[10] D. Eggert and K. Bowyer. Perspective projection aspect graphs of solids of revolution: An implementation. In *IEEE Workshop on Directions in Automated CAD-Based Vision*, pages 44–53, June 1991.

[11] D. Eggert, K. Bowyer, C. Dyer, H. Christensen, and D. Goldgof. The scale space aspect graph. *IEEE Trans. Patt. Anal. Mach. Intell.*, 15(11):1114–1130, 1993.

[12] Z. Gigus, J. Canny, and R. Seidel. Efficiently computing and representing aspect graphs of polyhedral objects. *IEEE Trans. Patt. Anal. Mach. Intell.*, 13(6), June 1991.

[13] T. Joshi, J. Ponce, B. Vijayakumar, and D. Kriegman. Hot curves for modelling and recognition of smooth curved 3d shapes. In *Proc. IEEE Conf. Comp. Vision Patt. Recog.*, pages 876–880, Seattle, WA, June 1994.

[14] D. Kapur and Y. Lakshman. Elimination methods: An introduction. In D. K. B. Donald and J. Mundy, editors, *Symbolic and Numerical Computation for Artificial Intelligence*, pages 45–88. Academic Press, 1992.

[15] Y. Kergosien. La famille des projections orthogonales d'une surface et ses singularités. *C.R. Acad. Sc. Paris*, 292:929–932, 1981.

[16] Y. Kergosien. Generic sign systems in medical imaging. *IEEE Computer Graphics and Applications*, 11(5):46–65, 1991.

[17] Y. Kergosien. Topology and visualization:from generic singularities to combinatorial shape modelling. In T. Kunii and Y. Shinagawa, editors, *Modern Geometric Computing for Visualization*, pages 31–54. Springer-Verlag, 1992.

[18] J. Koenderink. What does the occluding contour tell us about solid shape? *Perception*, 13:321–330, 1984.

[19] J. Koenderink. An internal representation for solid shape based on the topological properties of the apparent contour. In W. Richards and S. Ullman, editors, *Image Understanding: 1985-86*, chapter 9, pages 257–285. Ablex Publishing Corp., Norwood, NJ, 1986.

[20] J. Koenderink. *Solid Shape*. MIT Press, Cambridge, MA, 1990.

[21] J. Koenderink and A. V. Doorn. The singularities of the visual mapping. *Biological Cybernetics*, 24:51–59, 1976.

[22] J. Koenderink and A. V. Doorn. The internal representation of solid shape with respect to vision. *Biological Cybernetics*, 32:211–216, 1979.

[23] D. Kriegman and J. Ponce. Computing exact aspect graphs of curved objects: solids of revolution. *Int. J. of Comp. Vision*, 5(2):119–135, 1990.

[24] W. Lorensen and H. Cline. Marching cubes: a high resolution 3D surface construction algorithm. *Computer Graphics*, 21:163–169, 1987.

[25] F. Macaulay. *The Algebraic Theory of Modular Systems*. Cambridge University Press, 1916.

[26] D. Manocha. *Algebraic and Numeric Techniques for Modeling and Robotics*. PhD thesis, Computer Science Division, Univ. of California at Berkeley, 1992.

[27] O. Monga, S. Benayoun, and O. Faugeras. From partial derivatives of 3D density images to ridge lines. In *Proc. IEEE Conf. Comp. Vision Patt. Recog.*, pages 354–359, Champaign, IL, 1992.

[28] O. Monga, R. Lengagne, and R. Deriche. Extraction of zero-crossings of the curvature derivatives in volumic 3D medical images: a multi-scale approach. In *Proc. IEEE Conf. Comp. Vision Patt. Recog.*, pages 852–855, Seattle, WA, 1994.

[29] S. Petitjean. Computing exact aspect graphs of curved objects bounded by smooth algebraic surfaces. Master's thesis, University of Illinois at Urbana-Champaign, 1992.

[30] S. Petitjean. *Géométrie énumérative et contacts de variétés linéaires: application aux graphes d'aspects d'objets courbes*. PhD thesis, Institut National Polytechnique de Lorraine, 1995.

[31] S. Petitjean, J. Ponce, and D. Kriegman. Computing exact aspect graphs of curved objects: Algebraic surfaces. *Int. J. of Comp. Vision*, 9(3), 1992.

[32] H. Plantinga and C. Dyer. Visibility, occlusion, and the aspect graph. *Int. J. of Comp. Vision*, 5(2):137–160, 1990.

[33] J. Ponce and J. Brady. Toward a surface primal sketch. In T. Kanade, editor, *Three-dimensional machine vision*, pages 195–240. Kluwer Publishers, 1987.

[34] J. Rieger. On the classification of views of piecewise-smooth objects. *Image and Vision Computing*, 5:91–97, 1987.

[35] J. Rieger. The geometry of view space of opaque objects bounded by smooth surfaces. *Artificial Intelligence*, 44:1–40, 1990.

[36] J. Rieger. Global bifurcations sets and stable projections of non-singular algebraic surfaces. *Int. J. of Comp. Vision*, 7(3):171–194, 1992.

[37] J. Rieger. On the complexity and computation of view graphs of piecewise-smooth algebraic surfaces. Technical Report FBI-HH-M-228/93, Universität Hamburg, 1993.

[38] G. Salmon. *Modern Higher Algebra*. Hodges, Smith, and Co., Dublin, 1866.

[39] W. Seales and C. Dyer. Constrained viewpoint from occluding contour. In *IEEE Workshop on Directions in Automated "CAD-Based" Vision*, pages 54–63, Maui, Hawaii, June 1991.

[40] I. Shimshoni and J. Ponce. Finite resolution aspect graphs of polyhedral objects. In *10th Israeli Symposium on Artificial Intelligence*, pages 505–514, Ramat Gan, Israel, 1994.

[41] J. Stewman and K. Bowyer. Aspect graphs for planar-face convex objects. In *Proc. IEEE Workshop on Computer Vision*, pages 123–130, Miami, FL, 1987.

[42] J. Stewman and K. Bowyer. Creating the perspective projection aspect graph of polyhedral objects. In *Proc. Int. Conf. Comp. Vision*, pages 495–500, Tampa, FL, 1988.

[43] S. Sullivan, A. Noble, and J. Ponce. On reconstructing curved object boundaries from sparse sets of x-ray images. In N. Ayache, editor, *First Int. Conference on Computer Vision, Virtual Reality, and Robotics in Medicine*, Lecture Notes in Computer Science, pages 385–396, Nice, France, April 1995. Springer-Verlag.

[44] H. Tagare, F. Vos, C. Jaffe, and J. Duncan. Arrangement: A spatial relation between parts for evaluating similarity of tomographic section. *IEEE Trans. Patt. Anal. Mach. Intell.*, 17(9):880–893, September 1995.

[45] J. Thirion and G. Gourdon. The 3D marching lines algorithm and its application to crest lines extraction. Technical Report 1672, INRIA, 1992.

[46] C. Wall. Geometric properties of generic differentiable manifolds. In A. Dold and B. Eckmann, editors, *Geometry and Topology*, pages 707–774, Rio de Janeiro, 1976. Springer-Verlag.

[47] R. Wang and H. Freeman. Object recognition based on characteristic views. In *International Conference on Pattern Recognition*, pages 8–12, Atlantic City, NJ, June 1990.

[48] N. Watts. Calculating the principal views of a polyhedron. CS Tech. Report 234, Rochester University, 1987.

[49] C. Weatherburn. *Differential geometry*. Cambridge University Press, 1927.

Synthesis of an Individualized Cranial Atlas with Dysmorphic Shape

Gary E. Christensen[12], Alex A. Kane[1], Jeffrey L. Marsh[12], and Michael W. Vannier[21]

Department of Surgery[1] and Mallinckrodt Institute of Radiology[2]

Washington University School of Medicine, St. Louis, Missouri 63110

Abstract

A new method for non-rigid registration of a normal infant CT head atlas with CT data of infants with abnormal skull shape is presented. An individualized atlas is synthesized by computing a volume transformation from the normal atlas to the target data set shape. This process begins rigidly by eliminating translation and rotation differences and proceeds non-rigidly to eliminate anatomical shape differences. Operator specified anatomical landmarks are used to find the initial rigid transformation. Non-rigid registration is achieved by constraining the transformation by the low frequency modes of vibration of a 3D linear-elastic solid while minimizing the squared intensity difference between atlas and target CT image volumes. Results are presented in which the CT atlas was transformed into the shape of several infants with various types of craniofacial deformities.

1. Introduction

Electronic atlases of normal individuals have been generated for several adults, especially in the head by Höhne [11], and for the entire human body as part of the National Library of Medicine Visible Human Project [18]. Electronic atlases of the head in infants and children, especially those with cranial deformities, have not been reported.

Tools that adapt a normal electronic atlas to match a specific individual wherein the atlas is transformed volumetrically to the target individual's shape have emerged and found application in neuromorphometry [2, 10], multimodality fusion [15], and locating regions of interest [3, 6, 7, 8, 17].

Atlas matching tools which produce an individualized labeled volume avoid the necessity for tedious and error prone segmentation and labeling. In general, these tools have been applied only in data sets from mature normal adults.

This paper reports on development of new methodology to synthesize individualized atlases corresponding to well known types of major craniofacial deformities, including sagittal synostosis, bilateral coronal synostosis, and unilateral coronal synostosis. Since these deformities are usually treated with surgery in infancy or early childhood, a new electronic CT atlas of the head was created using scans from a three month old female whose skull shape was normal.

The goal of this study was to test extensions of previously developed tools [3, 15] based on Grenander's global shape models [9] in craniofacial dysmorphology. Specifically, we sought to test the feasibility of generating electronic atlases in cases with major skull deformities and evaluate the quality of the results.

If successful, individualized atlases of dysmorphic individuals could simultaneously provide automatic segmentation and labeling of craniofacial anatomy as well as a quantitative description of the dysmorphic features thereby facilitating treatment and evaluation.

2. Problem Statement

An anatomical atlas is an annotated collection of images, charts, or tables that systematically illustrates biological structure for all or part of an organism. In our case, the atlas is a spatial array of CT scan data (voxel-based attenuation measurements with associated tissue type (bone or not bone) and labels derived from a volumetric CT scan of a normal 3 month old female head. The atlas annotations (knowledge base) provide a basis for understanding the relevant anatomy. However, due to the labor intensive nature of creating an atlas knowledge base, only one atlas from a population is usually produced. This paper addresses the problem of synthesizing individualized atlases given a target CT data set and a topologically equivalent electronic atlas. The atlas is individualized by finding the transformation that changes its shape to match the target CT volume and then using that transformation to map the atlas knowledge base onto the target CT volume as shown

309

in Fig. 1. In addition, the atlas transformation can be used to quantitatively assess the absolute shape characteristics of the target CT as well as its shape differences compared to the atlas. It is therefore possible to use the atlas transformation to locate and measure areas of abnormality in the target CT data set. Ideally, synthesizing an individualized atlases in this manner can provide the following information regarding a patient's anatomy based their on CT data set.

Individualized Atlas

- Bone and soft-tissue segmentation
- Anatomical landmarks and suture locations
- Geometric information such as distances, angles, volumes, and curvatures
- Connectivity
- Text description of dysmorphology
- Treatment options and procedures
- Links to relevant medical literature

Atlas Transformation

- Location of abnormality
- Magnitude of abnormality
- Shape of abnormality
- Measure of asymmetry
- Change in shape

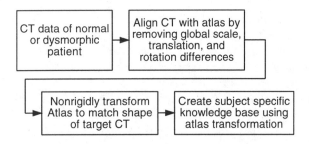

Figure 1. Synthesis of an Individualized Atlas.

The atlas is described mathematically on the domain Ω as a vector valued function $A(x) = (A_1(x), \ldots, A_N(x))$ for $x \in \Omega \subset R^3$. The modality A_1 corresponds to a 3D CT data set of the atlas anatomy where the other $N-1$ modalities correspond to the knowledge base of the atlas, i.e., A_2 could correspond

to a bone segmentation, A_3 could correspond to a collection of anatomical landmarks, etc. The notation T will be used to represent the CT modality of the atlas and is referred to as the template.

Problem Statement: Given a target CT data set $S(x)$, find the optimal transformation $h(x)$ in some sense that transforms the shape of the atlas template $T(x)$ into that of $S(x)$ while maintaining the topology of $T(x)$ for $x \in \Omega$. The individualized atlas is generated by applying the transformation h to the atlas A, i.e., the individualized atlas is given by $A(h(x))$.

3. Construction of the Atlas

The construction of the atlas consisted of defining the atlas coordinate system, selecting a data set for the atlas, and defining the information in the atlas knowledge base.

3.1. The Atlas Coordinate System

The first step in constructing an atlas requires definition of the coordinate system, a reference frame that assigns each anatomic structure a specific location. The reference system facilitates measurement of distances and angles between standardized anatomic (cephalometric) landmarks, curvatures, volumes, and other shape measures.

The atlas coordinate system is defined by an origin and three orthonormal basis vectors. The coordinate system was defined to correspond to the normals of the Frankfort Horizontal plane (FH), the Median Sagittal or MidSagittal Plane (MSP), and the Coronal Plane, see Figs. 2 and 3. The FH is a horizontal plane represented in profile by a line between the *orbitale*, the lowest point on the margin of the orbit, and the *porion*, the highest point on the margin of the auditory meatus. Its definition as the standard orientation for depicting human skulls was initially adopted at the 13th General Congress of German Anthropologists (the "Frankfort Agreement"), Frankfurt-am-Main, 1882, and subsequently by the International Agreement for the Unification of Craniometric and Cephalometric Measurements, Monaco, 1906 [12]. The MSP is perpendicular to the FH and is defined as the plane of symmetry that passes through the head from front to back dividing it into right and left halves. The Coronal Plane is defined perpendicular to the FH and MSP dividing the head into anterior and posterior parts.

The origin of the coordinate system was selected as the *basion*, the midpoint of the anterior border of the foramen magnum in the midsagittal plane (see Fig. 2). This point was chosen because it is almost always

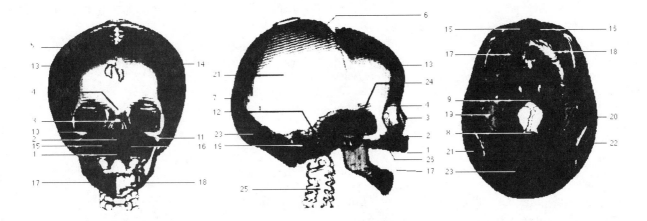

Figure 2. Front, side, and bottom views of the 3 month old infant, CT atlas skull. Landmarks: 1. prosthion, 2. subnasale, 3. rhinion, 4. nasale, 5. top of metopic suture, 6. bregma, 7. lambda, 8. opisthocranion, 9. basion, 10. right orbitale, 11. left orbitale, 12. right porion. Bones: 13. & 14. R./L. frontal bone, 15. & 16. R./L. maxilla, 17. & 18. R./L. mandible, 19. & 20. R./L. temporal bone, 21. & 22. R./L. parietal bone, 23. occipital bone, 24. sphenoid bone, 25. vertebral column. 26. R. zygomatic bone.

3.2. The Atlas CT Data

A CT data set of a normal 3 month old female was chosen as the atlas template and was selected from the craniofacial image archive at the Cleft Palate and Craniofacial Deformities Institute (CPCDI) of St. Louis Children's Hospital at Washington University Medical Center. This data was collected using a Siemens Splus S Spiral CT scanner at $0.49 \times 0.49 \times 2.0 \text{ mm}^3$ resolution forming a $512 \times 512 \times 82$ voxel volume.

The CT data volume was aligned with the atlas coordinate system using the rigid registration procedure described in Section 4.1. In this procedure, the CT data was resampled such that the voxel lattice of the new CT volume corresponded to the Frankfort horizontal, midsagittal, and coronal planes of the data.

The CT data is stored in the atlas at three different resolutions—low, medium, and high—corresponding to voxel dimensions of $1.96 \times 1.96 \times 2.0$, $0.98 \times 0.98 \times 1.0$, and $0.49 \times 0.49 \times 0.49 \text{ mm}^3$, respectively, in a $251 \times 251 \times 200 \text{ mm}^3$ domain Ω. The low resolution $128 \times 128 \times 100$ voxel volume was used as the template for individualizing the atlas; the medium resolution $256 \times 256 \times 200$ voxel volume was used to visualize the atlas CT before and after transformation; and the high resolution volume (stored as a $285 \times 345 \times 335$ voxel subvolume) was used to create precise manual segmentations of the atlas anatomy and for generating high resolution segmentations of the target CT data sets.

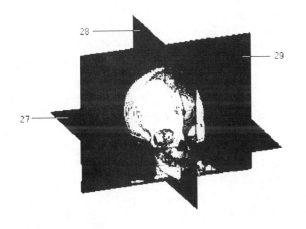

Figure 3. Coordinate system of 3 month old infant, CT atlas skull. Planes: 27. Frankfort horizontal plane, 28. medial sagittal plane, 29. coronal plane.

present in normal and abnormal anatomies. Another possible choice for the origin is the center of the sella turcica which is used in a majority of the cephalometric literature. This point was not used due to the difficulty in trying to locate the center of this cup-like structure in 3D [16].

3.3. The Atlas Knowledge Base

The atlas knowledge base for this project consisted of 13 landmark coordinates and the segmentations of 17 major bones of the skull (see Figure 2). The bone segmentations were generated by careful manual segmentation performed by an anatomic expert (A.A.K.) using Analyze^{TM} software. The CT data was converted from 16-bit to 8-bit data by linearly mapping the intensity range of 600-2200 to 0-255; intensities below 600 where mapped to zero, and intensities above 2200 were mapped to 255. Bone was segmented from soft-tissue using a threshold of 85-255 and manually partitioned into individual skull bones. In the future, additional structures will be added to the knowledge base as needed.

4. Individualizing the Atlas

The atlas is individualized for a particular target CT data set using a two-step process as shown in Fig 1. First, a rigid transformation s applied that removes rotation and translation differences between the target and the atlas. Next, a non-rigid transformation based on a linear-elastic solid model is used to accommodate anatomical shape differences between the target data set and the atlas.

4.1. Rigid Registration

Rigid registration of a CT data set to the atlas coordinate system consists of finding a translation vector and a rotation matrix. The translation vector is determined by computing the difference between the coordinates of the origin in the atlas and the corresponding landmark in the target data set.

The rotation matrix is determined by estimating the equations of the Frankfort horizontal, midsagittal, and coronal planes in the CT data set and calculating the three angles required to rotate these orthogonal planes onto the voxel lattice. Landmarks are used to define points on one of the three planes and least-squares estimation is used to estimate the equation of a plane that best fits the landmarks. The second plane is found in a similar manner but is constrained to be perpendicular to the first. The orientation of the third plane is constrained to be perpendicular to the first two planes and is therefore completely determined by the first two planes There are six different possible orderings for determining the equations of the planes, each of which gives a slightly different procedure for finding the rotation matrix. Rather than enumerating all six procedures, only the case corresponding to finding the MSP

first and the FH second is presented. The procedures for the other five cases can be derived in a similar manner.

The transformation that rigidly registers a CT data set to the atlas coordinate system finding the MSP followed by the FH can be written as

$$q = R_x R_y R_z (p - p_0) + p_1 \qquad (1)$$

where

$$R_x = \begin{bmatrix} 1 & 0 & 0 \\ 0 & \cos\phi & \sin\phi \\ 0 & -\sin\phi & \cos\phi \end{bmatrix}, \quad R_y = \begin{bmatrix} \cos\theta & 0 & \sin\theta \\ 0 & 1 & 0 \\ -\sin\theta & 0 & \cos\theta \end{bmatrix},$$

$$R_z = \begin{bmatrix} \cos\gamma & \sin\gamma & 0 \\ -\sin\gamma & \cos\gamma & 0 \\ 0 & 0 & 1 \end{bmatrix},$$

are rotation matrices about the x, y, and z-axis, respectively. Points $p = [x, y, z]$ are mapped to points $q = [x', y', z']$ and $p_1 = [x_1, y_1, z_1]$ is the origin of the atlas and $p_0 = [x_0, y_0, z_0]$ is the origin in the target data set. The angles ϕ, θ, and γ rotate the data set so its data voxel lattice corresponds to its Frankfort horizontal plane (FH), midsagittal plane (MSP), and coronal plane. Notice that the translation vector aligns the origin of the data set with that of the atlas anatomy.

In a normal anatomy the landmarks that define the FH are the porions and the orbitales; the landmarks used to define the MSP were the prosthion, subnasale, rhinion, nasale, the top of the metopic suture, bregma, lambda, opisthocranion, and basion (see Fig. 2). Finding landmarks to define the FH and MSP is more complicated for dysmorphic (abnormal) skulls, due to asymmetries and missing landmarks. For the SS and BCS results presented in Section 5, all of the landmarks above were used to define the FH and MSP due to the symmetry of these deformities. However due to the asymmetry of the UCS data set, only the prosthion, subnasale, and basion were used to define the MSP and the left porion and left orbitale were used to define the FH.

The equation of the MSP is determined as follows. Let the set $\{(x_1, y_1, z_1), \ldots (x_n, y_n, z_n)\}$ denote the coordinates of the n landmarks used to define the MSP. The equation of the MSP can be written as $ax + by + cz = d$ where $a + b + c = 1$. Combining these equations, we get n equations (one for each landmark) of the form $z_i - a(z_i - x_i) - b(z_i - y_i) - d = 0$ for determining the unknown constants a, b, and d. Provided that $n \geq 3$, we can formulate the following

312

least-squares problem

$$\min_v (u - Wv)^2 =$$

$$\min_{a,b,d} \left(\begin{bmatrix} z_1 \\ \vdots \\ z_n \end{bmatrix} - \begin{bmatrix} (z_1 - x_1) & (z_1 - y_1) & 1 \\ \vdots & \vdots & \vdots \\ (z_n - x_n) & (z_n - y_n) & 1 \end{bmatrix} \begin{bmatrix} a \\ b \\ d \end{bmatrix} \right)^2. \quad (2)$$

The solution of this minimization problem is

$$\hat{v} = (W^T W)^{-1} W^T u \quad (3)$$

(see pg. 83 of Luenberger [14]). Using this estimate of a, b, and c, we can find the angles θ and γ that rotate the MSP plane such that its normal vector (a, b, c) is aligned parallel to the x-axis, i.e.,

$$\begin{bmatrix} \cos\theta & 0 & \sin\theta \\ 0 & 1 & 0 \\ -\sin\theta & 0 & \cos\theta \end{bmatrix} \begin{bmatrix} \cos\gamma & \sin\gamma & 0 \\ -\sin\gamma & \cos\gamma & 0 \\ 0 & 0 & 1 \end{bmatrix} \begin{bmatrix} a \\ b \\ c \end{bmatrix}$$

$$= \begin{bmatrix} \cos\theta & 0 & \sin\theta \\ 0 & 1 & 0 \\ -\sin\theta & 0 & \cos\theta \end{bmatrix} \begin{bmatrix} a' \\ 0 \\ c \end{bmatrix} = \begin{bmatrix} a'' \\ 0 \\ 0 \end{bmatrix}. \quad (4)$$

The solution of this equation is

$$\gamma = \tan^{-1}\left(\frac{b}{a}\right) \quad \text{and} \quad \theta = \tan^{-1}\left(\frac{c}{a'}\right) \quad (5)$$

where $a' = a\cos\gamma + b\sin\gamma$.

The equation of the FH plane can now be determined as follows. Let $\{(x_1, y_1, z_1), \ldots (x_m, y_m, z_m)\}$ denote the coordinates of the m landmarks used to define the FH. These landmarks are rotated by θ and γ to get the new coordinates in which the MSP is perpendicular to the x-axis, i.e.,

$$\begin{bmatrix} \tilde{x}_i \\ \tilde{y}_i \\ \tilde{z}_i \end{bmatrix} = \begin{bmatrix} \cos\theta & 0 & \sin\theta \\ 0 & 1 & 0 \\ -\sin\theta & 0 & \cos\theta \end{bmatrix} \begin{bmatrix} \cos\gamma & \sin\gamma & 0 \\ -\sin\gamma & \cos\gamma & 0 \\ 0 & 0 & 1 \end{bmatrix} \begin{bmatrix} x_i \\ y_i \\ z_i \end{bmatrix}$$

The equation of the FH plane can be written as $ax + by + cz = d$ where $a + b + c = 1$ and $a = 0$. The condition $a = 0$ ensures that the FH plane will be perpendicular to the MSP. Combining these equations, we get m equations of the form $\tilde{z}_i - b(\tilde{z}_i - \tilde{y}_i) - d = 0$. Provided that $m \geq 2$, the least-squares estimate of FH is given by

$$\min_v (u - Wv)^2 = \min_{b,d} \left(\begin{bmatrix} z_1 \\ \vdots \\ z_m \end{bmatrix} - \begin{bmatrix} (z_1 - y_1) & 1 \\ \vdots & \vdots \\ (z_m - y_m) & 1 \end{bmatrix} \begin{bmatrix} b \\ d \end{bmatrix} \right)^2$$

which has solution given by Eq. 3. The angle ϕ that rotates the FH such that its normal $(0, b, c)$ is parallel

to the z-axis satisfies

$$\begin{bmatrix} 1 & 0 & 0 \\ 0 & \cos\phi & \sin\phi \\ 0 & -\sin\phi & \cos\phi \end{bmatrix} \begin{bmatrix} 0 \\ b \\ c \end{bmatrix} = \begin{bmatrix} 0 \\ 0 \\ c' \end{bmatrix}$$

implying

$$\phi = \tan^{-1}\left(-\frac{b}{c}\right). \quad (6)$$

4.2. Non-Rigid Registration Using a Linear-Elastic Model

Non-rigid registration of the atlas is accomplished by finding the displacement field $u(x) = x - h(x)$ that minimizes the energy functional

$$E_1(u) = \frac{1}{2\sigma^2} \int_\Omega (T(x - u(x)) - S(x))^2 dx$$

$$+ \frac{1}{2} \int_\Omega |Lu(x)|^2 dx \quad (7)$$

where σ is a constant and L is a linear operator. The first term on the right-hand-side corresponds to a cost of the intensity mismatch between the template and target CT volume. The second term is a regularization term that maintains the topology of the template by penalizing rough displacement fields. We simplify Eq. 7 by representing u by its eigenfunction decomposition $u(x) = \sum_{i=1}^d \mu_i \phi_i(x)$ where $L\phi_i(x) = \lambda_i \phi_i(x)$. The functions ϕ_i are the eigenfunctions of L and have eigenvalue λ_i. Substituting the eigenfunction expansion of u into Eq. 7 gives a new energy function

$$E_2(\mu) = \frac{1}{2\sigma^2} \int_\Omega (T(x - u(x)) - S(x))^2 dx + \frac{1}{2} \sum_{i=1}^d \lambda_i^2 \mu_i^2$$

in terms of the coefficients $\mu = [\mu_1, \ldots, \mu_d]^T$. The problem now becomes that of finding μ that minimizes $E_2(\mu)$. The solution of this problem is found by gradient decent

$$\mu_i^{k+1} = \mu_i^k - \Delta[S(x) - T(x - u(x))] \left.\frac{\partial T}{\partial \mu_i}\right|_{x-u(x)} - \Delta\lambda_i^2 \mu_i \quad (8)$$

The linear operator L used in this work was the linear elastic operator $Lu(x) = \alpha\nabla^2 u(x) + \beta\nabla(\nabla \cdot u(x))$ with boundary conditions $\left.\frac{\partial u_i}{\partial x_i}\right|_{(x|x_i=k)} = u_i(x|x_j = k) = 0$ for $i, j = 1, 2, 3$; $i \neq j$; $k = 0, 1$; and $x \in \Omega = [0, 1]^3$. The notation $(x|x_i = k)$ is defined as $x \in \Omega$ such that $x_i = k$, $\nabla = [\frac{\partial}{\partial x_1}, \frac{\partial}{\partial x_1}, \frac{\partial}{\partial x_1}]$, and

$\nabla^2 = \nabla \cdot \nabla$. Thus as first reported in [3], the displacement field has the form

$$u(x) = \sum_{n=1}^{3} \sum_{\nu \in S(d)} \mu_{n,\nu} \phi_{n,\nu}(x). \qquad (9)$$

where

$$S(d) = \{(i,j,k) \mid i+j+k > 0 \quad \text{and} \quad 0 \le i,j,k, \le d\}$$

$$\phi_{1,\nu}(x) = \eta_1 [ig_{1,\nu}(x), jg_{2,\nu}(x), kg_{3,\nu}(x)]^T$$
$$\phi_{2,\nu}(x) = \eta_2 [-jg_{1,\nu}(x), ig_{2,\nu}(x), 0]^T$$
$$\phi_{3,\nu}(x) = \eta_3 [ikg_{1,\nu}(x), jkg_{2,\nu}(x), -(i^2+j^2)g_{3,\nu}(x)]^T$$

$$g_{1,\nu}(x) = \cos i\pi x_1 \sin j\pi x_2 \sin k\pi x_3$$
$$g_{2,\nu}(x) = \sin i\pi x_1 \cos j\pi x_2 \sin k\pi x_3$$
$$g_{3,\nu}(x) = \sin i\pi x_1 \sin j\pi x_2 \cos k\pi x_3 \qquad (10)$$

$\eta_1 = \sqrt{8/(i^2+j^2+k^2)}$, $\eta_2 = \sqrt{8/(i^2+j^2)}$, and $\eta_3 = \eta_1\eta_2\sqrt{1/8}$. The eigenvalues for $\phi_{n,\nu}$ are $\lambda_{1,\nu} = -\pi^2(2\alpha+\beta)(i^2+j^2+k^2)$ and $\lambda_{2,\nu} = \lambda_{3,\nu} = -\pi^2\alpha(i^2+j^2+k^2)$. A limitation of this model and others such as the membrane model $Lu(x) = \nabla^2 u(x)$ or the biharmonic model $Lu(x) = \nabla^4 u(x)$ is that they are only valid for small deformations [1]. These limitations can be overcome using a fluid model [4] for atlas transformations requiring large nonlinear deformations.

This minimization problem can be interpreted probabilistically as the maximum a posteriori estimate of μ for the density $p(\mu) = \frac{1}{Z}e^{-E_2(\mu)}$. It is also possible to find the conditional mean estimate of μ as in [3, 15].

The parameters used to generate the experimental results were $\sigma = 0.01$, $\alpha = 0.1$, and $\beta = 0$. The template and study intensities were normalized from 0-255 to 0-1. The gradient decent Eq. 8 was run for 300 iterations; $d = 1$ initially and $d = d + 1$ every 40 iterations which gave a final transformation with 2187 degrees of freedom. Increasing the number of basis functions allows a multiresolution solution that matches larger structures before smaller structures and requires less computation time then if all 300 iterations were performed for $d = 8$. The step size of the gradient decent was normalized as the number of basis functions was increased by setting $\Delta = 2.0 \times 10^{-11} \times (\sum_{n=1}^{3} \sum_{\nu \in S(d)} \lambda_{n,\nu}^2)^{-1}$. The computation of the linear-elastic transformation for the $128 \times 128 \times 100$ voxel template and study required approximately 2.75 hours using a 128×128 MasPar MP-2 massively parallel computer. All final transformations had a globally positive Jacobian over Ω and therefore preserved the topology of the template [5].

5. Results

Three individualized atlases of infants with abnormal skull shapes were generated to test the atlas registration algorithm. Figures 4, 5, and 6 show the skull of the target CT data volumes (top row) and the skull of the transformed atlas (bottom row) for the craniofacial deformities of sagittal, bilateral coronal, and unilateral coronal synostosis. Abnormal skull shape due to sagittal synostosis (SS) is characterized by an anterior-posterior elongation and left-right narrowing of the skull. Abnormal skull shape due to bilateral coronal synostosis (BCS) is characterized by an anterior-posterior shortening and left-right widening of the skull. In contrast to SS and BCS skull shapes which are relatively symmetric about the midsagittal plane, unilateral coronal synostosis (UCS) skull shape is asymmetric about the midsagittal plane.

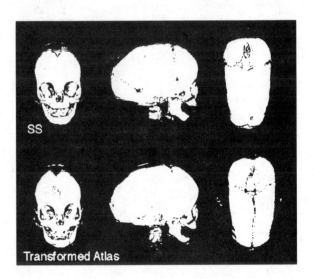

Figure 4. Front, right, and top views of the skull of an infant with sagittal synostosis (top row) and the skull of the transformed atlas (bottom row). Note: This transformation was constrained only to match bone and soft tissue in the CT volumes and not the sutures (the gaps between bones). Therefore, the shape of the transformed atlas skull matches very well with the shape of the patient skull, but the sutures do not necessarily match.

Visual inspection of the individualized atlases in these figures shows a good correspondence between the ensemble skull shape of the target data set and the individualized atlas. This demonstrates that the linear-elastic model had enough degrees of freedom to match

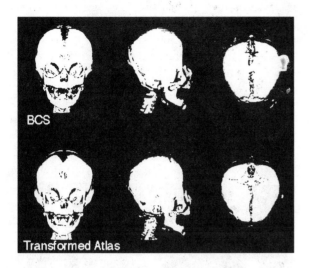

Figure 5. Front, right, and top views of the skull of an infant with bilateral coronal synostosis (top row) and the skull of the transformed atlas (bottom row). See note in Fig. 4.

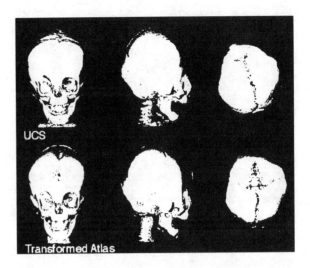

Figure 6. Front, right, and top views of the skull of an infant with unilateral coronal synostosis (top row) and the skull of the transformed atlas (bottom row). See note in Fig. 4.

the ensemble shape of the three abnormally shaped skulls. Notice that even the shape of the orbits of the individualized UCS atlas matches the shape of the orbits in the UCS target data set. These results also demonstrate that it is possible to transform an atlas of a normal infant head into the shape of an abnormal infant head in these three cases.

The intensity absolute error performance of the matching algorithm was determined quantitatively and visually. Table 1 tabulates the intensity absolute difference between the target CT volume and the atlas template CT volume before and after transformation. Notice that the intensity absolute difference was reduced to approximately 25 % of its original value after transformation. Figure 7 shows the absolute difference images between the target CT data set and the atlas before (top row) and after transformation (bottom row) for the BCS individualized atlas. This figure demonstrates that the reduction of the absolute difference to 25 % of its original value is enough to give good alignment of the the target and individualized template data sets. If a better alignment of the atlas and target is required, a higher dimensional transformation such as described in [4] could be used to refine these linear-elastic transformations.

Figures 4, 5, and 6 also demonstrate that the atlas registration method described in this paper does not accommodate the shape of each individual skull bone. This can be seen by comparing the skull sutures (the

Table 1. Performance of Registration

Experiment	Normalized Intensity Absolute Error		
	Before	After	% difference
Atlas to SS	1.54×10^5	4.38×10^4	28.4
Atlas to BCS	2.28×10^5	3.55×10^4	15.6
Atlas to UCS	2.07×10^5	5.40×10^4	26.1

gaps between the bones of the skull) of the individualized atlas and the target CT data set. Notice that none of the sutures necessarily agree between the target and the atlas. This limitation is expected because the similarity energy or cost (see Eq. 7) used to match the atlas and target is only a function of CT volume intensity. Therefore only subvolume differences between the atlas template and target contribute to the matching energy. Substructures such as points, lines, and surfaces have zero measure (zero energy) in this volume integral and thus have no effect on the the matching procedure. In the future, we intend to overcome this limitation by adding constraints to the transformation that match landmarks and sutures [13].

Another observation that can be made from these figures is that the individualized atlas contains all of the skull sutures while the target data sets do not.

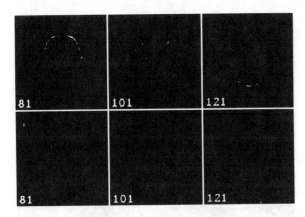

Figure 7. Top row shows absolute difference subtraction images between the untransformed atlas and BCS patient (see Fig. 5) for 3 axial slices. Bottom row shows the absolute difference subtraction images between the transformed atlas and BCS patient for the same 3 slices as the top row.

Each of the three abnormalities shown are caused by fusion (obliteration) of one or more sutures which therefore is (are) missing in the target. The sagittal suture is missing in SS, both coronal sutures are missing in BCS, and one of the coronal sutures is missing in UCS. The reason that the all of the sutures are present in the individualized atlases is that all of the sutures are present in the atlas and therefore must be present in the transformed atlas because of the topology preserving nature of the transformation.

Selected slices of the 3D displacement fields that generated the SS, BCS, and UCS individualized atlases are shown in Figures 8, 9, and 10, respectively. The top, middle, and bottom rows of these figures show the x, y, and z-components of the atlas transformation, respectively, superimposed on the corresponding axial CT slices of the target data set. White corresponds to a large positive displacement, medium-gray to zero displacement, and black to a large negative displacement. These transformation images can be interpreted in the following manner. In Figure 8, the x-component of slice 81 (top row) shows that the atlas was compressed left-to-right, the y-displacement of slice 81 (middle row) shows the atlas was stretched front-to-back, and the z-component (bottom row) shows no displacement top-to-bottom for the atlas to match the patient data.

Comparison of the y-displacement fields of Figures 8 and 9 shows that these displacements are inverted accounting for the elongation front-to-back in the SS individualized atlas and the compression front-to-back

in the BCS individualized atlas. The asymmetry of the displacement fields in Figure 10 were necessary to generate the asymmetry of the UCS individualized atlas.

These volume transformation give a quantitative measure of the distance from each point in the target to a corresponding point in the atlas; they therefore measure the shape change between the target and the atlas. Future work is planned that will use these volume transformations to measure and quantify abnormal anatomical shapes.

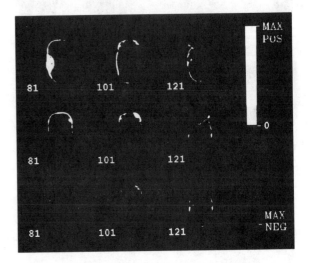

Figure 8. The atlas was compressed left-to-right, stretched front-to-back, and had very little displacement top-to-bottom for the atlas to match the patient data shown in Fig. 4. Key: Top, middle, and bottom rows show the x, y, and z-components of the atlas transformation, respectively, superimposed on three axial CT slices of the patient. The CT slices go from top to bottom of the head as the slice number increases. White corresponds to a large positive displacement and black to a large negative displacement.

Finally, Figure 11 shows the automatic segmentation generated for the SS individualized atlas. This segmentation was generated by applying the atlas transformation to the knowledge base of the atlas. This figure is intended to demonstrate the feasibility of mapping the atlas knowledge base and not as an accurate segmentation of the bones in the target data set. In the future when the individual bones of the atlas are constrained to match the corresponding bone in the target (see above), the automatic segmentation should give a precise segmentation of the bones in the target data set.

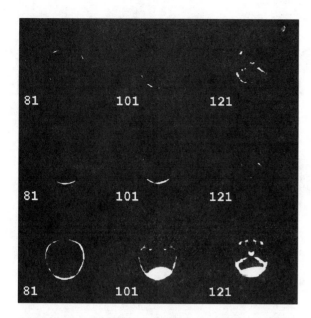

Figure 9. The atlas was compressed front-to-back, slightly compressed left-to-right, and the bottom-rear of the skull was displaced up for the atlas to match the patient data shown in Fig. 5. See key in Fig. 8.

6. Summary and Conclusions

After applying the new method for nonrigid registration of the normal female infant's CT head atlas to the CT data sets of infants with abnormal skull shape, the results were displayed visually and the moduli for displacement fields computed and viewed in multiplanar displays. Operator specification of anatomic landmarks demonstrated a high degree of consistency along the target and transformed atlases showing that the procedure is robust to even high degrees of skull asymmetry.

7. Acknowledgments

This research was supported in part by a grant from The Whitaker Foundation and by the Craniofacial Imaging Laboratory, St. Louis Children's Hospital, Washington University Medical Center.

References

[1] R. Bisplinghoff, J. Marr, and T. Pian. *Statics of Deformable Solids*. Dover Publications, Inc., 1965.

[2] F. Bookstein. *Morphometric Tools for Landmark Data*. Cambridge University Press, New York, 1991.

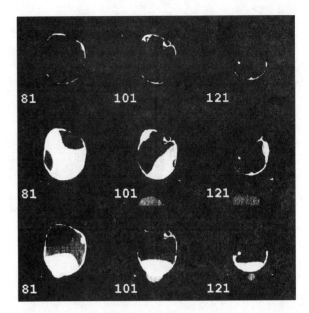

Figure 10. The transformation of the atlas to match the patient data shown in Fig. 6. Notice that the only x-displacement (top row) occured at the top-right portion of the skull, the asymmetry of the y-displacement (middle row) results from the asymmetry of the patient's skull, and the z-displacement (bottom row) shows that the back of the skull was lifted up while the front of the skull was pushed down. See key in Fig. 8.

[3] G. Christensen, R. Rabbitt, and M. Miller. 3D brain mapping using a deformable neuroanatomy. *Physics in Medicine and Biology*, 39:609–618, 1994.

[4] G. Christensen, R. Rabbitt, and M. Miller. Deformable templates using large deformation kinematics. *IEEE Transactions on Image Processing*, To appear in September, 1996.

[5] G. Christensen, R. Rabbitt, M. Miller, S. Joshi, U. Grenander, T. Coogan, and D. V. Essen. Topological properties of smooth anatomic maps. In Y. Bizais, C. Braillot, and R. D. Paola, editors, *Information Processing in Medical Imaging*, volume 3, pages 101–112. Kluwer Academic Publishers, Boston, June 1995.

[6] R. Dann, J. Hoford, S. Kovacic, M. Reivich, and R. Bajcsy. Evaluation of Elastic Matching Systems for Anatomic (CT, MR) and Functional (PET) Cerebral Images. *Journal of Computer Assisted Tomography*, 13(4):603–611, July/August 1989.

[7] A. Evans, W. Dai, D. Collins, P. Neelin, and S. Marret. Warping of a computerized 3-d atlas to match brain image volumes for quantitative neuroanatomical and functional analysis. *Image Processing*, SPIE 1445:236–246, 1991.

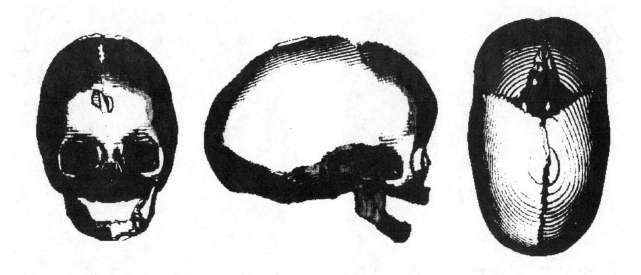

Figure 11. Individualized atlas for sagittal synostosis provides automatic segmentation and labeling (original in color to denote labels of each cranial bone).

[8] T. Greitz, C. Bohm, S. Holte, and L. Eriksson. A computerized brain atlas: Construction, anatomical content, and some applications. *Journal of Computer Assisted Tomography*, 15(1):26–38, Janurary/February 1991.

[9] U. Grenander. *General Pattern Theory*. Oxford University Press, 1993.

[10] J. Haller, G. Christensen, S. Joshi, J. Newcomer, M. Miller, J. Csernansky, and M. Vannier. Hippocampal MR morphometry by pattern matching. *Radiology, in press*.

[11] K. Höhne, M. Bomans, M. Reimer, and R. Schubert. A 3D anatomical atlas based on a volume model. *IEEE Comput. Graphics Appl.*, 12(4):72–78, 1992.

[12] S. Jablonski. *Illustrated Dictionary of Dentistry*. W.B. Saunders Company, Philadelphia, 1982.

[13] S. C. Joshi, M. I. Miller, G. E. Christensen, A. Banerjee, T. A. Coogan, and U. Grenander. Hierarchical brain mapping via a generalized dirichlet solution for mapping brain manifolds. *Vision Geometry IV*, SPIE 2573:278–289, 1995.

[14] D. Luenberger. *Optimization by Vector Space Methods*. John Wiley and Sons, New York, 1969.

[15] M. Miller, G. Christensen, Y. Amit, and U. Grenander. Mathematical textbook of deformable neuroanatomies. *Proceedings of the National Academy of Sciences*, 90(24):11944–48, Dec. 1993.

[16] Y. Sagawara, K. Harii, and S. Hirabayashi. Analysis of craniofacial asymmetry using accurate three-dimenional coordinates on the skull. In K. H. et al., editor, *Transactions of the 11th Congress of the International Confederation of Plastic, Reconstructive and Aesthetic Surgery*, page 33. Kugler Publications, New York, 1995.

[17] S. Sandor and R. Leahy. Towards automated labelling of the cerebral cortex using a deformable atlas. In Y. Bizais, C. Braillot, and R. D. Paola, editors, *Information Processing in Medical Imaging*, volume 3, pages 127–138. Kluwer Academic Publishers, Boston, June 1995.

[18] V. Spitzer, M. Ackerman, A. Scherzinger, and D. Whitlock. The visible human male: A technical report. *Journal of the American Medical Informatics Association*, 3(2), Mar/Apr 1996.

Shape Bottlenecks and Conservative Flow Systems

Jean-François Mangin
Service Hospitalier
Frédéric Joliot, CEA
4, place du général Leclerc
91401 Orsay Cedex, France
mangin@uriens.shfj.cea.fr

Jean Régis
Service de Neurochirurgie
Fonctionnelle et Stéréotaxique
C.H.U. La Timone
254 rue Saint Pierre
13005 Marseille, France

Vincent Frouin
Service Hospitalier
Frédéric Joliot, CEA
4, place du général Leclerc
91401 Orsay Cedex, France
frouin@uriens.shfj.cea.fr

Abstract

This paper proposes an alternative to mathematical morphology to analyze complex shapes. This approach aims mainly at the detection of shape bottlenecks which are often of interest in medical imaging because of their anatomical meaning. The detection idea consists in simulating the steady state of an information transmission process between two parts of a complex object in order to highlight bottlenecks as areas of high information flow. This information transmission process is supposed to have a conservative flow which leads to the well-known Dirichlet-Neumann problem. This problem is solved using finite differences, over-relaxation and a raw to fine implementation. The method is applied to the detection of main bottlenecks of brain white matter network, namely corpus callosum, anterior commissure and brain stem.

1. Introduction

1.1. Bottlenecks and mathematical morphology

Shape bottlenecks have been widely used in mathematical morphology to decompose complex objects in simpler parts. The usual approach is the following. First, the whole object is eroded in order to get disconnection of its different parts at the bottleneck level (see Fig. 1 and 2). Then parts of interest are reconstructed in order to recover their original shapes. In fact, the reconstruction process itself can be performed according to two slightly different points of view. When only specific object parts are of interest, the connected components corresponding to these parts are selected as seeds using problem dedicated procedures. Then a dilation of limited size (usually the size of the previous erosion) is applied conditionally to the initial object. This kind of approach is used today by a number of teams in order to segment the brain in 3D T1-weighted MR images [14]. For other applications, the reconstruction process is applied until convergence, which means that the final result is simply a generalized Voronoï diagram constructed for the set of selected seeds. Such an approach can be applied for instance to segment brain white matter in four main parts corresponding to brain and cerebellum hemispheres (see Fig. 1 and 3).

With a modern point of view, this kind of morphological deconnection schemes could be related to the decomposition obtained using the reaction/diffusion space [12]. Indeed morphological erosion can be related to an evolutionary partial differential equation corresponding to pure reaction [3].

During these morphological segmentation processes, few attention is given to shape bottlenecks for themselves. However, in medical imaging, shape bottlenecks have often an important anatomical meaning which justifies their detection. For instance, the corpus callosum, which is morphologically the bottleneck which links both brain hemispheres, has been intensively studied for morphometric purpose (male/female differences...) and is a subject of increasing interest in image processing [7, 19]. Therefore usual morphological deconnection schemes are sometimes not sufficient to analyze complex anatomical shapes. A decomposition in parts and bottlenecks is then required. Extending the morphological approach with this purpose is possible. For instance junction points of the Voronoï diagram are a first kind of representation of bottlenecks but it appears difficult to master their localization. Indeed, the diagram is highly dependent on the choice of the discrete distance used to construct it, on the kind of structuring element used for erosion and on the shape of the bottleneck. Moreover, junction point sets do not really represent bottlenecks because they do not share the initial object dimension (3D objects give usually 2D junctions). This problem could be addressed through the study of a new object constituted by the difference between the initial object and a morphological opening of the initial object (the result of a limited re-

Proceedings of MMBIA '96

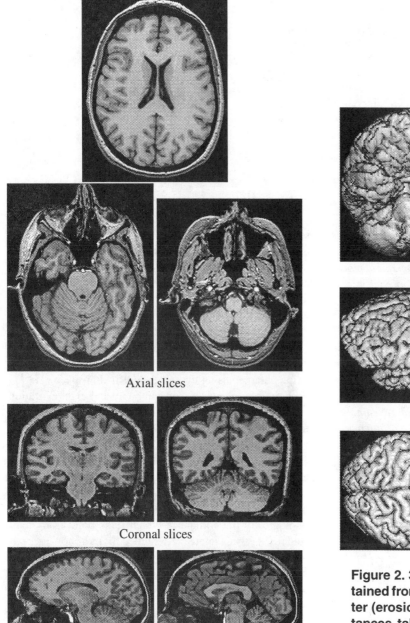

Axial slices

Coronal slices

Sagittal slices

Figure 1. A few slices of a T1 weighted MR image acquired with a Signa GE 1.5 T. (124 slices, 1mm slice thickness, 0.9mm pixel size)

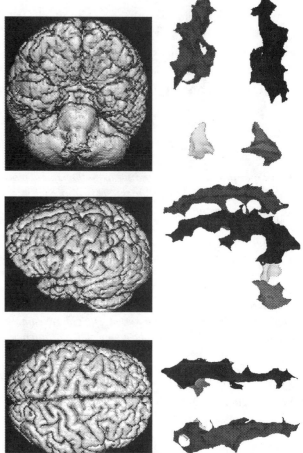

Figure 2. 3D renderings of the four seeds obtained from a 7mm erosion of brain white matter (erosion computed using 3D chamfer distances taking into account voxel anisotropy [13])

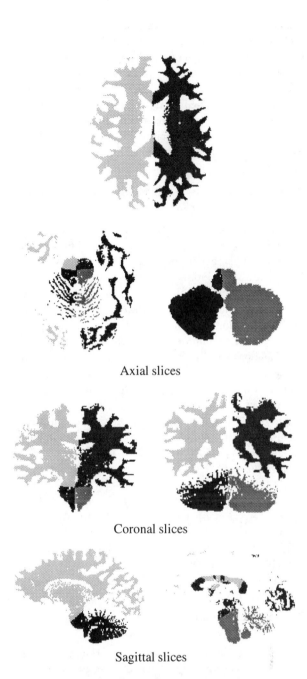

Axial slices

Coronal slices

Sagittal slices

Figure 3. A few slices of a generalized Voronoï diagram of brain white matter computed for 4 seeds obtained from a 7mm erosion. Erosion and Voronoï diagrams have been computed using anisotropic chamfer distances taking into account voxel anisotropy. Brain white matter has been simply segmented by thresholding a presegmented brain obtained by standard mathematical morphology [14].

construction of seeds as described in first paragraph). Indeed this new object should include bottlenecks which could be detected using the Voronoï diagram junctions mentioned above as seeds. Unfortunately difficulties could occur with convoluted objects because bottlenecks could be connected to other fine parts of the initial object removed during the opening.

1.2. White matter network of the brain

In this paper we propose a different approach to address shape bottleneck detection. This approach is inspired by the anatomical nature of brain white matter bottlenecks. White matter of brain hemispheres is mostly made up by association and commissural fibers which interconnect different cortical areas [15]. Commissural fibers interconnecting cortical regions of both hemispheres cross mainly in the corpus callosum and the anterior commissure (see Fig. 4). Other commissures generally interconnect internal nuclei. They are usually difficult to identify because of MR image resolution.

Several reasons call for an important development of studies of brain white matter network in the future. There is a relative lack of knowledge of this network. In the human brain, long association systems are mainly known from gross dissection. Almost nothing is known on their inter-individual variability. Nevertheless, experimental literature gives a fairly complete account of these connections in primate. Information on the fiber tracts should become of crucial importance for the interpretation of functional images originating from positron emission tomography (PET), magnetic resonance imaging (fMRI) and especially magneto-encephalography (MEG) and electro-encephalography (EEG), because of their accurate temporal resolution (ms). Moreover, the organization of callosal connections gives an insight into myelo- and cytoarchitecture, which results in a direct delimitation of functional areas [6, 18]. Detection of long association fibers could also be of fair importance for neurosurgical planning and morphometric studies. Lastly, new imaging methods allow the detection of fiber tract orientation. Indeed magnetic resonance diffusion tensor imaging shows the anisotropic diffusion of water in anisotropic tissues which is related to fiber tract direction [4].

1.3. Conservative flow systems

Usual T1 or T2-weighted MR images do not allow the fiber tract tracking but we will propose a way of highlighting some white matter network bottlenecks. Let us consider for instance information transmission between left hemisphere cortex and right hemisphere cortex. All information has to cross using commissural fibers. Hence, information flow

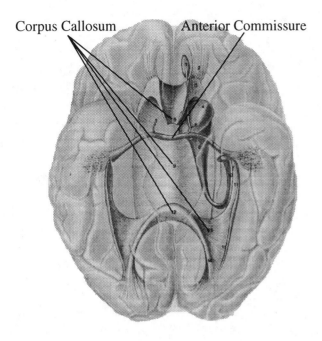

Corpus Callosum   Anterior Commissure

Figure 4. Commissural connections of the teleencephalon as seen from the basal side of the brain [15].

should be higher in commissures than anywhere else. In order to apply this idea we have to simulate a steady state of information transmission in order to get an image of information flow in white matter. This phenomenon can be modelized using partial differential equations, such a model being clearly a huge simplification of reality. Since information sources are only located outside white matter, the information transmission process has a conservative flow inside white matter. Let $i(x, y, z)$ denote the information potential[1] located at point x, y, z. Whatever the domain Ω included in white matter, the following result is true:

$$\int_{\Sigma} \vec{\text{grad}}\, i \cdot \vec{n}\, d\Sigma = 0 \, , \qquad (1)$$

where $\Sigma = \partial\Omega$ and $\vec{n}$ denotes the normal oriented towards Ω exterior. The usual transformation of Eq.1 obtained from Green formula gives:

$$\int_{\Omega} \text{div}(\vec{\text{grad}}\, i)\, dxdydz = 0 \, . \qquad (2)$$

Since Eq.2 is true for any Ω we get the well-known Laplace equation (assuming regularity of i):

$$\triangle i = 0 \, . \qquad (3)$$

---

[1] We use here the term "information potential" with a very arbitrary meaning...

Hence the detection of white matter bottlenecks between both cerebral hemispheres could be inferred from the solution of the Laplace equation with appropriate boundary conditions. In the following we address the discretization of this equation for a domain of arbitrary shape and the boundary condition choice. Then we describe the resolution by a raw to fine process and over-relaxation. Lastly we present some experiments with real data aiming at the detection of corpus callosum, anterior commissure and brain stem.

2. Discrete formulation of the Laplace equation

The Laplace equation is one of the fundamental equations of physics, mechanics and applied mathematics. Indeed, it is the prototype of elliptic linear homogeneous equations. Therefore its resolution has been intensively dealt with in literature [8]. Three kinds of problem rely on Laplace equation according to boundary conditions. If i value is imposed on the whole domain boundary, we get a Dirichlet problem. If $\partial i/\partial n$ value is imposed on the whole boundary, we get a Neumann problem. Lastly, let Σ denote the domain boundary with $\Sigma = \Sigma_1 \cup \Sigma_2$ (subsets with non null areas). If i value is imposed on Σ_1 and $\partial i/\partial n$ value is imposed on Σ_2, we get a Dirichlet-Neumann problem. The idea presented in introduction will lead to Dirichlet-Neumann problems. Indeed this idea consists in the simulation of information transmission from a boundary subset $H \subset \Sigma$ towards another subset $L \subset \Sigma$. With this purpose, we set $i = h$ on H, $i = l$ on L, and $\partial i/\partial n = 0$ on $\Sigma - (H \cup L)$, where h and l are constant values with $h > l$. Hence $\Sigma_1 = H \cup L$ and $\Sigma_2 = \Sigma - (H \cup L)$. Existence and unicity of the solution of continuous Dirichlet-Neumann problems is a well-known result (with a sufficient regularity of boundary conditions). We will now address the discrete formulation of a Dirichlet-Neumann problem with a domain of arbitrary shape.

2.1. Finite differences

Assuming the regularity of the solution, partial derivatives are classically approximated using finite differences. Indeed such an approach is sufficient for our purpose and much simpler than finite elements with a domain of arbitrary shape. From the discretization of Laplacian operator, we get for Ω interior the usual consistent second order discrete Laplace equation:

$$\frac{1}{h_x^2}(i(x - 1, y, z) - 2i(x, y, z) + i(x + 1, y, z)) \qquad (4)$$

$$+\frac{1}{h_y^2}(i(x, y - 1, z) - 2i(x, y, z) + i(x, y + 1, z))$$

$$+\frac{1}{h_z^2}(i(x, y, z - 1) - 2i(x, y, z) + i(x, y, z + 1)) = 0 \, ,$$

where h_x, h_y, h_z correspond to voxel sizes. It should be noted that this numerical scheme has to be viewed as a network of 6-connected points of which values are related by Eq. 5. Indeed, since we deal with domains of arbitrary shape, a real discretization should involve a discretization step largely smaller than voxel sizes. In the following, for the sake of simplicity, we assume $h_x = h_y = h_z$. Then Eq. 5 amounts to the simple relation:

$$i(x, y, z) = \frac{1}{6} \sum_{M \in N_6(x,y,z)} i(M) , \qquad (5)$$

where $N_6(x, y, z)$ denotes 6-neighborhood of point (x, y, z).

2.2. Dirichlet-Neumann boundary conditions

The discrete version of Dirichlet boundary condition is straightforward:

$$\forall M \in H \; i(M) = h \; ; \; \forall M \in L \; i(M) = l \qquad (6)$$

The discrete version of Neumann boundary condition is far more problematic, especially for a domain defined by a binary image, because a lot of points do not have a clear normal partial derivative. The usual approach consists in substituting normal second order partial derivatives by tangential second order partial derivatives using the Laplace equation [8]. Let M be a boundary point, namely a point of which 6-neigborhood is not included in Ω. Let d be the "local dimension" of Ω at that point, namely the number of grid directions for which at least one 6-neighbor of M belongs to Ω. Lastly let $\mathcal{N}$ (respectively $\mathcal{T}$) be the set of directions with only one 6-neighbor N in Ω (respectively two 6-neighbors T_1, T_2). A solution to deal with difficult situations where cardinal($\mathcal{N}$)> 1 consists in imposing a null first partial derivative in each direction of $\mathcal{N}$ (simple cases where cardinal($\mathcal{N}$)$= 1$ are naturally processed). Then for any point N we can write

$$i(N) = i(M) + \frac{h^2}{2} \frac{\partial^2 i}{\partial x_N^2}(M) + O(h^3) ,$$

where x_N is the direction of N. Summing over $\mathcal{N}$ we get

$$
\begin{aligned}
\sum_{\mathcal{N}} i(N) &= \text{card}(\mathcal{N})i(M) + \frac{h^2}{2} \sum_{\mathcal{N}} \frac{\partial^2 i}{\partial x_N^2}(M) + O(h^3) \\
(\text{Laplace}) &= \text{card}(\mathcal{N})i(M) - \frac{h^2}{2} \sum_{\mathcal{T}} \frac{\partial^2 i}{\partial x_T^2}(M) + O(h^3) \\
&= \text{card}(\mathcal{N})i(M) \\
&\quad - \frac{h^2}{2} \sum_{\mathcal{T}} \frac{1}{h^2}(i(T_1) - 2i(M) + i(T_2)) + O(h^2),
\end{aligned}
$$

because $f(x+h) + f(x-h) - 2f(x) = h^2 f''(x) + O(h^4)$ (x_T is a direction of $\mathcal{T}$, card($\mathcal{N}$) denotes $\mathcal{N}$ cardinal). Finally we get the following second order discrete version of Neumann condition:

$$\forall M \in (\Omega - (H \cup L))$$

$$i(M) = \frac{1}{d} \sum_{\mathcal{N}} i(N) + \frac{1}{2d} \sum_{\mathcal{T}} (i(T_1) + i(T_2)) . \qquad (7)$$

2.3. Successive over relaxation

The Dirichlet-Neumann problem reduces now to a huge linear system through Eq. 5, 6 and 7. We solve this system using the usual iterative scheme corresponding to successive over relaxation. The process is initialized by

$$\forall M \in (\Omega - (H \cup L)) \quad i^0(M) = \frac{h+l}{2} . \qquad (8)$$

Then the iterative process can be written

$$\forall M \in (\Omega - (H \cup L)), \quad \forall k \geq 0 \qquad (9)$$

$$i^{(k+1)}(M) = (1-w) \, i^k(M) + w \sum_{N \in N_6(M)} \alpha_N(M) \, i^k(N),$$

where $\alpha_N(M)$ is a coefficient given by Eq. 5 or 7 or zero if $N \notin \Omega$, and $1 < w < 2$. Convergence of this kind of process for domains with simple shapes is well-known [8]. Convergence in the case of domains defined by complex binary images is questionable even if in practice we did not run into problems. Indeed, as mentioned above, our discretization step seems too large to hope a good approximation of the continuous case. Moreover, convergence speed is very difficult to assess because with convoluted domains large wavelength oscillations could require a large number of iterations to disappear. Nevertheless this last problem can be forgotten because we do not need an exact solution for our purpose.

A 2D illustration of the result of successive over relaxation is proposed in Fig. 5. High and low potential Dirichlet conditions have been imposed on parts of left and right hemisphere white matter surface ($h = 5000$, $l = 1000$). These parts have been simply defined by a geodesic distance to the left most and right most points. Successive over-relaxation has been applied with $\omega = 1.5$ and 1000 iterations. The corpus callosum is clearly highlighted in the information flow image. The information potential image shows that the iterative process has not fully converged in some very fine brain convolutions, which has no consequence on bottleneck detection. This image shows also that isopotential lines are orthogonal to white matter surface which tends to show that our Neumann boundary conditions have been respected.

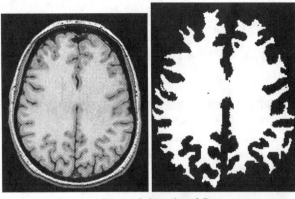

raw data and domain of flow

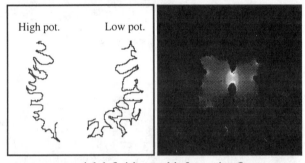

High pot.   Low pot.

potentiel definition and information flow

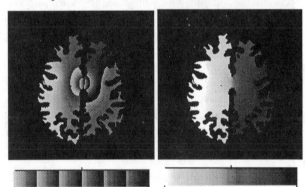

information potential

Figure 5. 2D illustration of the bottleneck detection method. High and low potential Dirichlet conditions have been fixed on parts of left and right hemisphere white matter surface. The corpus callosum is clearly highlighted in the information flow image.

2.4. Diffusive process

In order to interpret our iterative process independently of the continuous problem, another point of view related to diffusion on a regular network seems preferable. In fact iterative process (9) turns out to almost correspond to the well-known integration scheme of the diffusion equation [17, 11, 3]. Indeed Eq. 9 can be written

$$i^{(k+1)}(M) = i^k(M)$$
$$+ w \sum_{N \in N_6(M)} \alpha_N(M) \left(i^k(N) - i^k(M)\right) \quad (10)$$

(in all cases $\sum_{N \in N_6(M)} \alpha_N(M) = 1$). Hence similarity with diffusive processes is straightforward:

$$i^{t+\Delta t}(N) = i^t(N)$$
$$+ \Delta t \sum_{N \in N_6(M)} c(N, M)(i^t(N) - i^t(M)) , \quad (11)$$

where $c(N, M)$ would be a conduction coefficient. In fact some differences remain for "corner points", namely points with cardinal($\mathcal{N}$)> 1, where some $\alpha_M(N) \neq \alpha_N(M)$. This observation led us to question our discretization of Neumann boundary condition. Therefore we tried a slightly different scheme which could be interpreted as "geodesic isotropic diffusion":

$$\forall M \in (\Omega - (H \cup L)) \quad i^{(k+1)}(M) = i^k(M)$$
$$+ w \sum_{N \in N_6(M) \cap \Omega} \frac{1}{6} \left(i^k(N) - i^k(M)\right) \quad k \geq 0 , \quad (12)$$

Up to now, we have observed no significative differences between the results of schemes 9 and 12, but further work has to be done on this subject. It should be noted that an important difference remains with standard diffusion. Indeed thanks to boundary conditions and since we are only interested in the steady state, we can use a larger integration constant Δt than usual bounds for stability [11]. Stationary boundary conditions drive then the evolutionary diffusive process toward a steady state.

3. Applications

We will now propose a few applications of ideas developed above for the detection of main white matter network bottlenecks. In all cases, the domain corresponding to white matter has been defined by thresholding a presegmentation of the brain in a T1-weighted MR image using standard mathematical morphology [14].

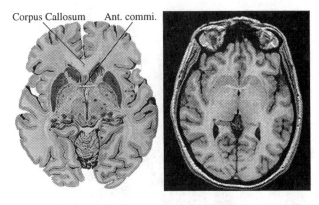

Corpus Callosum   Ant. commi.

Figure 6. Anterior commissure in atlas of Nieuwenhuys [15] and in real MR slice

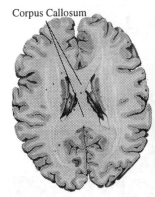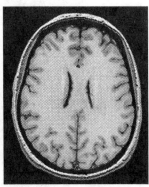

Corpus Callosum

Figure 7. Corpus callosum in atlas of Nieuwenhuys [15] and in real MR slice

3.1. Raw to fine resolution

In order to get reasonable computation times, the iterative process defined above has been implemented using a raw to fine approach. Indeed, the over relaxation scheme requires about 1000 iterations before reasonable convergence with highly convoluted objects, which costs more than one hour of computation on a conventional workstation for a 3D binary object including several million points. Hence, most iterations are performed at highest levels of a resolution pyramid which allows us to obtain convergence in less than 10mn on conventional Sun Sparc stations. It should be noted that the iterative process could be implemented easily on massively parallel architectures, like usual diffusive schemes. The resolution pyramid is computed classically. Resolution of the 3D binary image is reduced level by level (by a factor 2) using median filtering which preserves as far as possible initial shape. All experiments presented further have been obtained using a 4 level resolution pyramid. The number of iterations performed at each level, from the lowest resolution to the finest, are 1000, 800, 200, 100 (these choices have been fixed empirically, a serious study of these parameter influence is far beyond the scope of the paper). The highest level is initialized according to Eq. 6. Other levels are initialized by the result of respective previous level.

3.2. Corpus callosum and anterior commissures

The first experiment aimed at the detection of the corpus callosum and the anterior commissure, which is an important landmark in the field of functional imaging, because it allows transformation towards the widely used Talairach referential [9, 10, 20]. Fig. 4, 6 and 7 give a good idea of the anatomical nature of the two structures of interest. These structures interconnect both cortical hemispheres. An automatic approach has been recently proposed in order to

detect intersection between anterior commissure and inter-hemispheric plane using 2D scene analysis [2].

Two different boundary conditions have been tried for this experiment. The first one consists in the definition of two sub-parts of hemispheric white matter surfaces using a threshold (60 grid bonds) on a geodesic distance to left most and right most points (see Fig. 5). The second one consists in using seeds of both hemispheres obtained by erosion (cf. introduction and Fig. 2). This second approach is less satisfying because it does not correspond any more to the simulation of information transmission between both cortical hemispheres. Nevertheless, it is interesting because of its generic aspect. Indeed, such an approach can be combined with the usual morphological approaches in any case where bottleneck detection is of interest. For both boundary condition choices, high and low potential values have been fixed to 5000 and -5000.

Fig. 8 and 9 propose a glimpse of the result for the first choice. The anterior commissure and the corpus callosum are clearly highlighted in information flow images. A third domain of high flow is located in the brain stem. This domain includes posterior commissure and other fibers which actually inter-connect the tele-encephale (brain hemispheres) and the cerebellum. These three main areas can be sorted according to mean value, highest value and volume after segmentation by hysteresis thresholding. Another way of using this result could stemmed from the intersection with inter-hemispheric plane which can be detected independently [2, 5] (this could turn out to be a better approach for morphometric studies [7] because the 3D volume of commissures is dependent on the chosen threshold). Lastly small areas of high flow can be observed near Dirichlet boundary conditions. These areas could be removed by postprocessing according to their highest values and distance to boundary. Fig. 10 proposes the result for the second choice, which presents less parasitic high flow areas

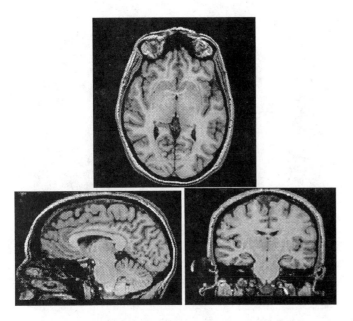

Figure 8. Three orthogonal slices of raw data

near boundaries. This could stem from the fact that seed boundaries are less convoluted than white matter surface. Lastly, Fig. 11 proposes a 3D rendering of the corpus callosum detected as the largest connected component over a high threshold in the first choice information flow image.

3.3. Brain stem

Another experiment has been done in order to detect brain stem as bottleneck between teleencephalon and cerebellum. Low and high potential Dirichlet boundary conditions have been simply applied respectively to the 20 top most and the 20 bottom most slices. Fig. 12 shows that the situation is more complex than for corpus callosum because of the presence of a "bulb" called pons in the middle of brain stem.

4. Conclusion

In this paper we have presented an alternative to mathematical morphology to analyze complex shapes. This approach aims mainly at the detection of shape bottlenecks which are often of interest in medical imaging because of their anatomical meaning. The detection idea consists in simulating the steady state of an information transmission process between two parts of a complex object in order to highlight bottlenecks as areas of high information flow. This information transmission process is supposed to have a conservative flow which leads to the well-known Dirichlet-Neumann problem. Hence, a new application of partial differential equations (PDE) to image processing has been

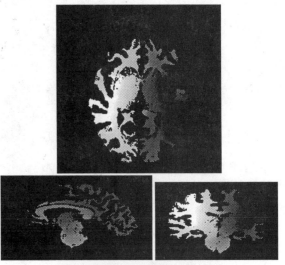

information potential

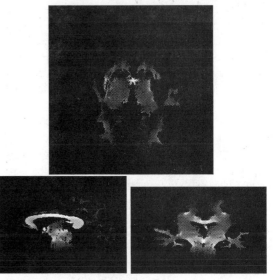

information flow

Figure 9. Detection of corpus callosum and anterior commissure: High and low potential Dirichlet boundary conditions have been fixed on parts of the left and right hemisphere white matter surfaces. Three orthogonal slices of information potential and information flow during the steady state are displayed. The anterior commissure and the corpus callosum are clearly highlighted in information flow images.

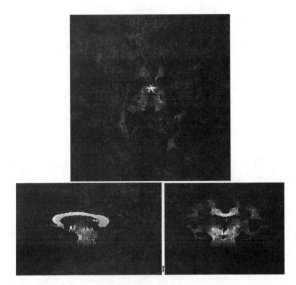

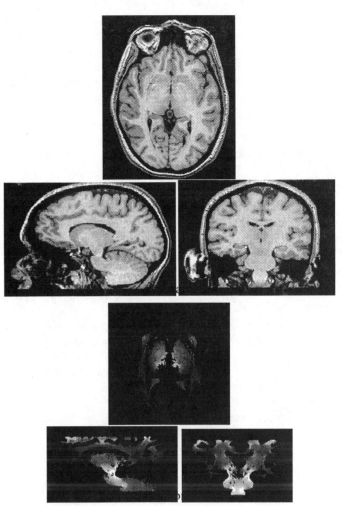

Figure 10. Same results as in Fig.9 with different boundary conditions. High and low potential Dirichlet boundary condition have been fixed on both seeds of brain hemispheres given by an initial erosion of 7mm (cf. Fig. 3). This result presents less parasitic high flow areas.

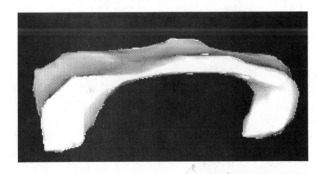

Figure 11. 3D rendering of corpus callosum detected as the largest connected component over a high threshold in the information flow image. The rendering relies on an initial triangulation according to the method described in [1]

Figure 12. Detection of brain stem as bottleneck between teleencephalon and cerebellum (3 orthogonal slices). Low and high potential Dirichlet boundary conditions have been simply applied respectively to the 20 top most and the 20 bottom most slices. The result shows that the situation is more complex than for corpus callosum because of the presence of a "bulb" (namely the pons) in the middle of brain stem.

found. Like some other applications of PDE to this field, the idea consists in defining a problem which steady state is of interest for the segmentation purpose. A similar idea has been proposed for instance in the case of anisotropic diffusion through the addition of a term expressing the deviation between original and filtered image to the diffusion scheme [16]. Applications have been proposed dedicated to the detection of brain white matter network bottlenecks. The result are promising but further work has to be done in order to study robustness of the method.

References

[1] M.-E. Algorri and F. Schmitt. Deformable models for reconstructing unstructured 3D data. In N. Ayache, editor, *CVRMed'95 Nice, France*, volume 905 of *LNCS*, pages 420–426. Springer-Verlag, 1995.

[2] P. Allain, J. M. Travère, J. C. Baron, and D. Bloyet. Accurate PET positioning with reference to MRI and neuroanatomical data bases. In K. U. et al., editor, *Quantification of Brain Function. Tracer Kinetics and Image Analysis in Brain PET*, pages 401–408. Elsevier Science, 1993.

[3] L. Alvarez, P.-L. Lions, and J.-M. Morel. Image selective smoothing and edge detection by nonlinear diffusion: II. *SIAM Journal of Numerical Analysis*, 29(3):845–866, 1992.

[4] P. J. Basser, J. Mattiello, and D. LeBihan. MR diffusion tensor spectroscopy and imaging. *Biophysical Journal*, 66:259–267, 1994.

[5] M. E. Brummer. Hough transform detection of the longitudinal fissure in tomographic head images. *IEEE Transactions on Medical Imaging*, 10(1), Mar. 1991.

[6] S. Clarke and J. Miklossy. Occipital cortex in man: organization of callosal connections, related myelo- and cytoarchitecture, and putative boundaries of functional visual areas. *J. Comp. Neurol.*, 298:188–214, 1990.

[7] C. Davatzikos, M. Vaillant, S. M. Resnick, J. L. Prince, S. Letovsky, and R. N. Bryan. A computerized approach for morphological analysis of the corpus callosum. *Journal of Computer Assisted Tomography*, 20(1):88–97, 1996.

[8] D. Euvrard. *Résolution numérique des équations aux dérivées partielles*. Masson, 1988.

[9] P. T. Fox, S. Mikiten, G. Davis, and J. L. Lancaster. *Brainmap: a database of human functional mapping*, chapter 9, pages 95–105. Functional Neuroimaging: Technical Foundations, Academic Press, 1994.

[10] K. J. Friston. *Statistical Parametric Mapping*, chapter 8, pages 79–91. Functional Neuroimaging: Technical Foundations, 1994.

[11] G. Gerig, O. Kübler, R. Kikinis, and F. A. Jolesz. Nonlinear anisotropic filtering of MRI data. *IEEE Trans. on Medical Imaging*, 11(2):221–232, 1992.

[12] B. B. Kimia, A. R. Tannenbaum, and S. W. Zucker. Shapes, shocks, and deformations I: the components of two-dimensional shape and the reaction-diffusion space. *International Journal of Computer Vision*, 15:189–224, 1995.

[13] J.-F. Mangin, I. Bloch, J. Lopez-Krahe, and V. Frouin. Chamfer distances in anisotropic 3D images. In *VII European Signal Processing Conference, Edimburgh, Scotland*, pages 975–978, Sept. 1994.

[14] J.-F. Mangin, V. Frouin, I. Bloch, J. Regis, and J. López-Krahe. From 3D magnetic resonance images to structural representations of the cortex topography using topology preserving deformations. *Journal of Mathematical Imaging and Vision*, 5(4):297–318, 1995.

[15] R. Nieuwenhuys, J. Voogd, and C. vanHuijzen. *The Human Central Nervous System, a Synopsis and Atlas*. Springer-Verlag, 1988.

[16] N. Nordström. Biased anisotropic diffusion – a unified regularization and diffusion approach to edge detection. *Image Vision Comput.*, 8(4):318–327, 1990.

[17] P. Perona and J. Malik. Scale-space and edge detection using anisotropic diffusion. *IEEE Trans. on Pattern Analysis and Machine Intelligence*, 12(7):629–639, 1990.

[18] J. Régis. Anatomie sulcale profonde et cartographie fonctionnelle du cortex cérébral. Thèse de doctorat en médecine, Université d'Aix-Marseille II, 1994.

[19] G. Székely, A. Kelemen, C. Brechbühler, and G. Gerig. Segmentation of 3D objects from MRI volume data using constraint elastic deformations of flexible Fourier surface models. In N. Ayache, editor, *CVRMed'95, Nice, France*, volume 905 of *LNCS*, pages 495–505. Springer-Verlag, 1995.

[20] J. Talairach and P. Tournoux. *Co–Planar Stereotaxic Atlas of the Human Brain. 3–Dimensional Proportional System: An Approach to Cerebral Imaging*. Thieme Medical Publisher, Inc., Georg Thieme Verlag, Stuttgart, New York, 1988.

Contour Model Guided Image Warping for Medical Image Interpolation

Wen-Shiang Vincent Shih[†], Wei-Chung Lin[†], and Chin-Tu Chen[*]

[†]Department of Electrical Engineering and Computer Science, Northwestern University
Evanston, IL 60208
[*]Department of Radiology, The University of Chicago
Chicago, IL 60637

Abstract

An interpolation method using contours of organs as the control parameters is proposed to recover the intensity information in the physical gaps of serial cross-sectional images. In our method, contour models are used for generating the control lines required for the image warping algorithm. Contour information derived from this contour-model-based segmentation process is processed and used as the control parameters to warp the corresponding regions in both input images into compatible shapes. In this way, the reliability of establishing the correspondence among different segments of the same organs is improved and the intensity information for the interpolated intermediate slices can be derived more faithfully. In comparison with the existing intensity interpolation algorithms that only search for corresponding points in a small physical neighborhood, this method provides more meaningful correspondence relationships by warping regions in images into similar shapes before resampling to account for significant shape differences. Experimental results show that this method generates more close to realistic and less blurred interpolated images especially when the shape difference of corresponding contours is significant.

1. Introduction

The resolution of data obtained from medical imaging modalities has the characteristics that the slice thickness is usually much larger than the pixel size within a single slice, and the gap between slices is usually much larger than the in-plane resolution. The non-isotropic resolution in these images will adversely affect subsequent visualization and analysis processes. To enhance the qualitative and quantitative accuracy of visualization and analysis, a suitable interpolation process, in which the original data are interpolated to meet the isotropic resolution requirement, is called for.

In this paper, we propose an interpolation method, Morphological Field Morphing, that utilizes the shape descriptions of the organs in the source image slices to guide the recovery of the intensity information in the physical gaps of serial cross-sectional medical images. In our method, the contour information derived from a contour-model-guided image segmentation process is used as the control parameters to perform image warping, which deforms the corresponding regions on two source data slices into the same shape. With corresponding organ regions in both data slices being deformed into compatible shapes, the reliability to locate different segments of the same organs is improved and the intensity information for the interpolated intermediate slices can be filled in more faithfully. The remainder of this paper is organized as follows. In the next section, a survey of image interpolation is provided. Then, the proposed interpolation method is described. This is followed by the presentation of the experimental results and the comparison with the existing whole-image intensity interpolation methods. Section 5 gives our conclusions.

2. Background

Classical image interpolation procedures fall into three main categories: contour-based, intensity-based and shape-based interpolations. Contour-based interpolation [1-11] takes a set of binary images containing cross-sectional boundaries of objects segmented from the intensity-value data and generates a new set of interpolated binary sequence representing the surface of the objects. Intensity-based interpolation [12, 22] takes the original voxel intensity values and generates a new set of interpolated voxel intensities. Shape-based interpolation [13-19] takes a set of binary images representing cross-sections of objects segmented from the intensity-value data and performs morphological interpolation between the shapes of the contours.

In contour-based interpolation (or surface reconstruction), the cross-sections are usually represented as a set of oriented contours derived from a segmentation process and the goal is to determine the intermediate contours by reconstructing smooth surfaces covering the exteriors of the set of given contours. To obtain a unique solution, assumptions have to be made at three different levels corresponding to the three major tasks of surface reconstruction. First, contour association must be explicitly available to specify which contours on one slice are to be connected to which contours on the adjacent slice. Second, contour matching that relates the points on one contour to the points on the other associated contour must be established using some predetermined rules, e.g., shortest Euclidean distance, and evaluated using a heuristic matching function such as maximal volume, minimal surface, or minimal span length. Third, given the correspondence between vertices, an interpolating surface, e.g., a set of triangular patches, has to be constructed [19]. Besides the feature selection problem, association problem, correspondence problem, branching and merging problem, and surface fitting problem to be addressed in this approach, one major drawback for applying this approach to medical image processing is the loss of detailed anatomical information. Since only the information from contours of selected features is used in the interpolation process, critical information in the form of image intensity variation would be lost.

In comparison with the contour-based approach, relatively fewer researches were conducted to improve the intensity-based interpolation techniques. The goal of intensity-based interpolation is to reconstruct a three-dimensional continuous signal from the original samples from the data slices. The most widely used intensity interpolation technique is linear interpolation. Other intensity interpolation methods use higher order interpolation kernels such as bi-cubic, tri-linear, tri-cubic, and polynomial splines. In general, higher order interpolations can produce smoother images because more sample values are used in the estimation [22]. However, there are several drawbacks to these deterministic methods. First, they can assume only a single type of variability in intensity, such as linearity. Data variation assumptions can lead to inaccurate estimation if the actual variation is not the same as the assumed variation. Second, there is no control parameters in these deterministic methods. Even when estimation errors are detected, there is no way to incorporate high-level knowledge into the estimation process to make corrections. Third, since the calculation of the estimated value only takes a limited number of data

points within a small physical neighborhood. When there is any noticeable shape variation between two images, these methods will choose semantically incorrect corresponding data points and produce wrong estimation. The work by Goshtasby et al. [12] tries to improve the correspondence with a local matching process similar to pair-wise stereo imaging matching. However, this improvement only works for simple images where geometrical variation is small.

Instead of using the binary cross-sectional information to reconstruct a smooth interpolating surface, a shape-based interpolation scheme uses the geometric properties of the cross-sections and generates a set of interpolating cross-sections directly. Raya and Udupa's method [13] and Herman's method [14] calculate the interpolating cross-sections by interpolating the distance to the cross-sectional boundary. These methods establish contour association by assuming that the corresponding regions do overlap, and the result is a distance map according to the segmentation threshold value selected. In the work by Lin et al. [15], a variant of the elastic matching method of Burr's [17-18] is proposed to iteratively interpolate new intermediate cross-sectional contours for filling the gaps between one start and one or more goal contours by deriving a "force field" acting on the start contour to distort it to be similar to the goal contours, and an "onion peeling-off" intensity filling operation is proposed to calculate the content of the interpolated region. Due to the complex nature of the dynamics of the force field, this method is only suitable for simple cross-sectional shapes, and the interpolated images are blurred by the signal averaging operation. Vandermeulen et al. [19] propose an interpolation method that is limited neither by the shape of the cross sections nor by the topology of the object by reconstructing a binary volume under the assumption that the inter-plane surface must be entirely situated in the difference volume. Shape-based algorithms are deterministic and produce satisfactory results when their assumptions are fulfilled, which may not be always true in medical images.

Image metamorphosis is the combination of generalized image warping with cross-dissolution between image elements and is typically used as an animation tool for deforming from one image to another. As the metamorphosis proceeds, the first image is gradually distorted and is faded out, while the second image starts out totally distorted toward the first and is faded in. For image warping, the mesh warping technique [20] uses spline mapping in two dimensions and a rubber-sheet mental model can be used for predicting the distortion behavior. However, since every point exerts the same amount of influence as each of the other points in this method, it is sometimes difficult for the animators to decide which control points to choose and where to place them to avoid undesirable results. To improve the expressiveness of the warping control specification, a "field morphing" technique is proposed by Beier et al. [21]. In this approach, everything that is specified with control lines is moved exactly as the animator wants it to move, and everything else is blended smoothly based on those positions. Adding new control line segments increase control in that area without affecting things too much everywhere else. While the warping algorithms are straightforward, the major problem is that 2D morphing is still a very manual and time-consuming process. It relies heavily on the animators to specify each control point and line to generate desired results and avoid the "ghost effect" mentioned in Beier et al.'s [21] work.

Our proposed method not only provides a way to automatically specify control lines required for the field morphing process, which at this time is still accomplished mostly by hand, but also reduces the high time-complexity for calculating the image warp in the field morphing process by a hierarchical decomposition process.

3. The proposed interpolation method

To estimate the locations and intensities of pixels that would appear in the nonexistent intermediate slices, this method can be divided into the following steps. First, we use a contour model initialized with a pre-segmented atlas slice to extract the contours of the features of interest and establish correspondence relationships between contours using contour models. Second, perform contour interpolation using one of the shape-based morphological interpolation method to generate intermediate contours. Then, the contours are converted into directed and matched polygon pairs to be used as control parameters in the field morphing process, and the area of influence for each contour polygon is determined using a hierarchical decomposition process. Finally, these contour-based control polygons are used to perform field morphing interpolation to fill in the intensity information. These steps will be addressed in detail next.

3.1 Segmentation using contour models

The use of energy-minimizing curves known as "snakes" to extract the boundaries of regions of interest in images has been introduced in [23] and improved by various researchers [24-29]. These contour models have been proven effective for locating the contours of feature regions in complex images. These active contour models deform under the action of internal and external forces attracting the curve toward detected edges by means of an

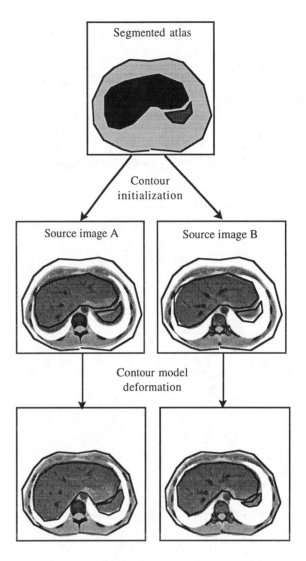

Figure 1. Segmentation using contour models.

attraction potential, which are influenced by image-derived forces and by forces intrinsic to the shape of the contour. In our method, we use a variation of the active contour model, progressive contour model, proposed in the work by Lin et al. [30]. This method uses the internal component of the contour energy to impose the smoothness constraints on the displacements of deformation instead of on the shape of the contour, and the external component of the contour energy to locate the correspondence for the contour through a predetermined correspondence mapping.

For the corresponding regions of interest in two consecutive source cross-sectional images, one initial contour is specified from a pre-segmented atlas image, such as the example shown in Fig. 1. When a segmented reference atlas image set is available, a linear transformation process is applied to the atlas image to make sure that the scales and locations of the initial contours are appropriate. When interpolating a stack of images slices without a reference atlas image set, one slice is chosen and segmented with manually initialized contour model. This segmented image is then used to initialize the selected slice and its adjacent slices. After its adjacent slices are segmented, they in turn can be used to initialize

their adjacent slices. Having chosen an appropriate initial contour set, two copies of the initial contour set are deformed independently to fit on the boundary of the corresponding regions in the two input image slices as shown in Fig. 1. At the end of this step, the contours of the regions of interest are extracted, and the operator or human expert may inspect the segmentation result and make some adjustment if necessary. One such special case that may need human intervention is when the tissue only exists in one of the input images and there is no corresponding region in the other image. The contour model will then not be able to find appropriate region to extract. One of the solutions to accommodate this situation is to make sure that a very small corresponding region is manually assigned in the image where the tissue is missing, and the interpolated result of the tissue area will then appear as if it is contracting from the tissue area to this region in the interpolated image.

3.2 Hierarchical decomposition process

One major drawback in the original field morphing process [21] is that it does require a lot of time-consuming computations because the weighting functions governing the effect of each control line segment are not local and all control line segments need to be referenced for every pixel. As more control lines are specified, more computation is required. To improve the performance, a hierarchical decomposition process is proposed to localize the weighting function evaluation process.

A segmented image can be considered as a set of regions $\Re = \{R_i | i = 0, 1, 2, \ldots, n\}$, where R_i is the i-th region in the segmented image and is surrounded and defined by the contour C_i. Due to the segmentation process, for any two different regions, either they do not overlap or one contains the other, i.e.,

$$\begin{cases} R_i \cap R_j = \phi, or \\ R_i \subset R_j, or \qquad R_i \in \Re, R_j \in \Re, i \neq j \qquad (1) \\ R_i \supset R_j \end{cases}$$

With this property, we can then represent the segmented image with a tree structure where the nodes represent the regions and the branches the contours. An example is given in Fig. 2. When calculating the warp, each region needs only reference its exterior and directly connected interior contours. For example, in Fig. 2, the pixels that are in region R_2 but not in R_3 or R_4 only need to reference contour C_2, C_3, and C_4.

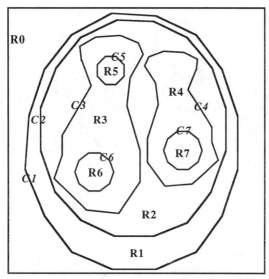

(a) A segmented image

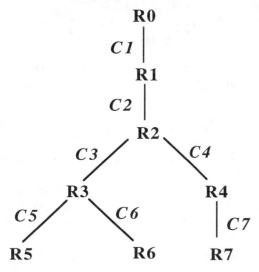

(b) The corresponding tree-representation

Figure 2. An example of hierarchical decomposition.

3.3 Control-polygon interpolation

With the information gathered in the previous steps, we can now perform field morphing to blend the two source images. Each intermediate image I is defined by a set of contour polygons derived by interpolating the contours of the two segmented images. Since we use the same initial contours for segmenting the two source images, the vertex correspondence can be easily maintained and the interpolated polygonal contours are generated by using one of the following three methods, vertex interpolation, edge center and orientation interpolation or the star-skeleton representation [31].

For vertex interpolation, vertices on intermediate contour are calculated by linearly interpolating the corresponding vertices on the two contours to be interpolated. Edge center and orientation interpolation are accomplished by linearly interpolating the center and the orientation of each pair of corresponding edges. In star-skeleton representation, a star polygon is defined as a polygon for which there exist a point, the star point, from which all the other points in the polygon are visible. Let P denotes all the points in a polygon. A point $v \in P$ is visible from a point $w \in P$ if the line segment $[v, w]$ is contained in P. The star-skeleton representation scheme decomposes the polygons to be interpolated into star-polygon pieces and represents each piece with its vertices and the star point, and then joins the star points with a planar skeleton graph. The interpolation process is accomplished by first interpolating between the skeletons to determine the interpolated star points, and then calculating positions of the vertices of the star polygon pieces from the start point by interpolating the distances and angles with respect to the star points accordingly. Detailed discussion about the star-skeleton representation can be found in [31]. In our application, star-skeleton representation is employed when significant rotational transformation is necessary and the star polygon decomposition for non-star shapes is specified manually.

3.4 Intensity filling using field morphing

To fill in the intensity information for image I, both source images are distorted toward the position of the contour-based control lines in image I. Then, the two deformed images are blended with a weighted-averaging function to generate the image I. The pixel correspondence relationship between the distorted image and the source image is defined in the following fashion. Each corresponding pair of lines PQ and $P'Q'$ on the polygonal contours in the two images define a local coordinate mapping from one image to the other. For the destination pixel coordinate X, its corresponding source image pixel X' is defined as follows [21]:

$$u = \frac{(X - P) \cdot (Q - P)}{\|Q - P\|^2} \quad (2)$$

$$v = (X - P) \cdot Unit\_Perp(Q - P) \quad (3)$$

$$X' = P' + u \cdot (Q' - P') + v \cdot Unit\_Perp(Q' - P') \quad (4)$$

where the value u is the position along the line normalized by the distance between two end points, the value v is the distance from the line, and $Unit\_Perp()$ returns a unit-length vector that is perpendicular to the input vector.

In essence, each line segment PQ defines a local coordinate system with two vectors, the vector $(Q - P)$ and a unit-length vector along the direction that is perpendicular to the vector $(Q - P)$. The region of influence of this local coordinate system is the set of regions directly above and below the contour that line PQ is on in the hierarchical decomposition tree. With the local coordinate systems defined, we can reformulate the warping problem as follows. Given a global coordinate system G and a set of local coordinate systems C_1, C_2,..., C_n in G, a point X has different coordinates with respect to different coordinate systems.

$$X = (x, y)_G = (u_{c_1}, v_{c_1})_{C_1} = (u_{c_2}, v_{c_2})_{C_2} = ... = (u_{c_n}, v_{c_n})_{C_n} \quad (5)$$

The coordinate transformation among these coordinate systems is given by

$$\begin{aligned}(x, y)_G &= (u_{c_1}, v_{c_1})_{C_1} * M_{C_1} + T_{C_1} \\ &= (u_{c_2}, v_{c_2})_{C_2} * M_{C_2} + T_{C_2} \\ &= \cdots \\ &= (u_{c_n}, v_{c_n})_{C_n} * M_{C_n} + T_{C_n}\end{aligned} \quad (6)$$

$$M_{C_i} = \begin{bmatrix} (Q_{C_i} - P_{C_i})_G \\ Unit\_Perp(Q_{C_i} - P_{C_i})_G \end{bmatrix} \quad (7)$$

$$T_{C_i} = (P_{C_i})_G \quad (8)$$

where M_{C_i} is the matrix of the two vectors that define the coordinate systems C_i, i.e., the vector $(Q - P)$ and a unit-length vector along the direction perpendicular to the vector, and T_{C_i} is the origin of the coordinate systems C_i, i.e., P.

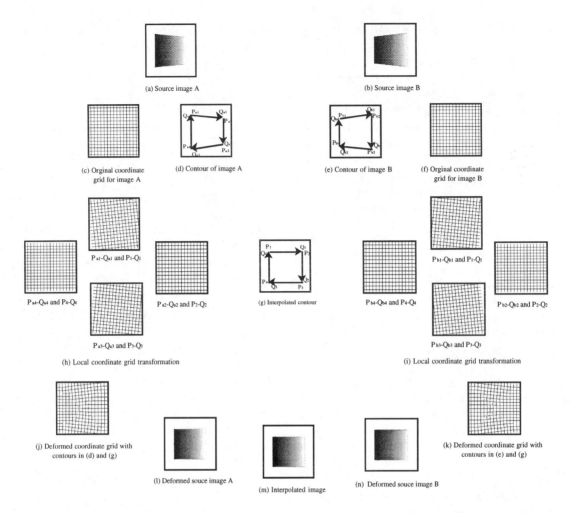

Figure 3. Intensity filling process based on weighted local coordinate systems.

When these local coordinate systems C_1, C_2,..., C_n change to C_1', C_2',..., C_n', we calculate the corresponding point X' for X as follows.

$$X' = \frac{\sum_{i=1}^{n} w_i \cdot \left[(u_{C_i}, v_{C_i}) * M_{C_{i'}} + T_{C_{i'}} \right]}{\sum_{i=1}^{n} w_i} \quad (9)$$

$$w_i = (a + distance)^{-b} \quad (10)$$

where the *distance* is the shortest distance from the point X to the line segment *PQ*, the parameter *a* is a very small number to specify the maximum weight when the distance is zero, and the parameter *b* is used to control the rate of influence degradation.

The detailed algorithm is given in the Appendix and an example to illustrate the local coordinate systems is given in Fig. 3. Figs. 3(a) and 3(b) are the source images to be interpolated. Figs. 3(d) and 3(e) are the contours of the source images in Figs. 3(a) and 3(b), respectively, and Figs. 3(c) and 3(f) are the grid images used to demonstrate the coordinate transformation. Fig. 3(g) is the interpolated contour of the contours in Figs. 3(d) and 3(e). Figs. 3(h) and 3(i) are the transformation demanded by each pair of contour edge. For example, the upper right grid in Fig. 3(h) is determined by the edge pair P_{a1}-Q_{a1} and P_1-Q_1. Since P_{a1}-Q_{a1} needs to be rotated and shrunk to fit on P_1-Q_1, the transformed grid appears to be rotated counterclockwise. Figs. 3(j) and 3(k) are the deformed coordinates calculated with Equation (9). Figs. 3(l) and 3(m) are the results of the source images being deformed into the same shape. Finally, Fig. 3(m) is the result of the interpolation.

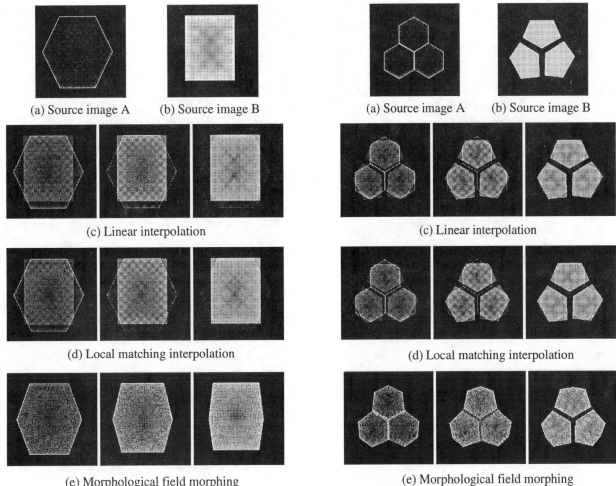

(a) Source image A   (b) Source image B

(c) Linear interpolation

(d) Local matching interpolation

(e) Morphological field morphing

Figure 4. Interpolation example - simple topology.

(a) Source image A   (b) Source image B

(c) Linear interpolation

(d) Local matching interpolation

(e) Morphological field morphing

Figure 5. Interpolation example - complex topology.

The underlying rationale behind using contours as control lines to perform field morphing is as follows. First, the most important and intriguing property of field morphing algorithm [21] is that pixels near the control lines are moved along with the lines and pixels far away from the control lines are influenced by the lines according to the distance form the pixel to the lines. Second, in image processing, it is widely recognized that the most noticeable features to human eyes in images usually occur at the points with high gradient magnitudes, which are also where the contour or boundary points usually locate. Therefore, using contours as the control lines will guarantee that the boundary of the interpolated object will conform to the interpolated boundary generated by the shape-based morphological interpolation algorithms, and intensity information will be filled in under the control of these contours. Since the line segments on the contour

polygons do not intersect each other, one of the most important benefits from using contours as the control lines is that the "ghost effect" mentioned in the work by Beier et al. [21] can be vastly avoided.

4. Experimental results

In this section, we present the results obtained with morphological field morphing interpolation and compare them with the results obtained with linear interpolation and Goshtasby's [12] interpolation method.

Several sets of synthetic images are used in the experiments. The images in Fig. 4 are the interpolation of a scene of simple topology. Fig. 4(a) and Fig. 4(b) are a pair of source images to be interpolated. Fig 4(c) is the result of linear interpolation. The images in Fig 4(d) are generated with Goshtasby's [12] method. Even though

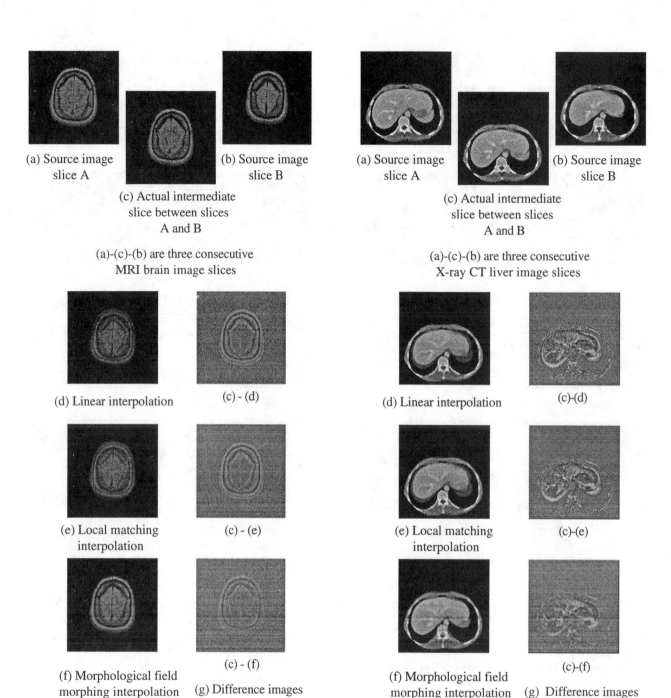

(a) Source image slice A

(b) Source image slice B

(c) Actual intermediate slice between slices A and B

(a)-(c)-(b) are three consecutive MRI brain image slices

(d) Linear interpolation

(c) - (d)

(e) Local matching interpolation

(c) - (e)

(f) Morphological field morphing interpolation

(c) - (f)

(g) Difference images

Figure 6. Comparison among different interpolated slices of MRI images.

(a) Source image slice A

(b) Source image slice B

(c) Actual intermediate slice between slices A and B

(a)-(c)-(b) are three consecutive X-ray CT liver image slices

(d) Linear interpolation

(c)-(d)

(e) Local matching interpolation

(c)-(e)

(f) Morphological field morphing interpolation

(c)-(f)

(g) Difference images

Figure 7. Comparison among different interpolated slices of CT images.

several different parameter settings were tried, we found that the matching process failed to perform satisfactorily when the intensity pattern is complex and the pixels cannot locate their matches in the neighborhood. The result shows that it only looks as good as linear interpolation in such cases. In Fig. 4(e), we can see that by using morphological field morphing, the shape and the

intensity can be smoothly interpolated. The images in Fig. 5 are the results of interpolation of a scene of more complex topology that involves branching.

A set of real cross-sectional consecutive MRI brain images is shown in Figs. 6(a), 6(c) and 6(b). The images in Figs. 6(a) and 6(b) are used as the source images while Fig. 6(c) is the actual image data slice between Fig. 6(a) and Fig. 6(b) that can be used as a reference to evaluate the interpolated result. Fig. 6(d) is the result of linear interpolation, Fig. 6(e) is the result of local matching interpolation, and Fig. 6(f) is the interpolated image from morphological field morphing. Fig. 6(g) is the difference images of 6(c) and 6(d), 6(c) and 6(e), 6(c) and 6(f). These difference images are calculated by the addition of medium intensity value, i.e., half of maximum intensity value minus minimum intensity value, to half of the difference value. Another set of cross-sectional consecutive X-ray CT liver images is shown in Fig. 7. In Figs. 6 and 7, we can easily notice that the morphological field morphing algorithm does produce better interpolated results. In Fig. 6(g), Fig. 7(g), and Table 1, we can see that the standard deviation of the intensity difference of the results from the morphological field morphing algorithm and the actual intermediate slice is much smaller than those from the other two methods.

Image	Mean	Std. Dev.
(6(c) - 6(d)) / 2 + 128	126.73	9.17
(6(c) - 6(e)) / 2 + 128	127.14	8.83
(6(c) - 6(f)) / 2 + 128	127.54	4.36
(7(c) - 7(d)) / 2 + 128	127.38	19.27
(7(c) - 7(e)) / 2 + 128	127.54	18.55
(7(c) - 7(f)) / 2 + 128	128.42	12.03

Table 1. Statistic information of the difference images in Figure 6(g) and Figure 7(g).

5. Conclusions

In this paper, we proposed an intensity interpolation method that is superior to the straightforward methods, such as linear or tri-linear interpolation, since it incorporates high-level knowledge, i.e., contour information, in the interpolation process. In comparison with the existing intensity interpolation algorithms that consider only points in a very small physical neighborhood, this method warps the data images into similar shapes and tries to provide more meaningful correspondence relationships. The intensity filling process does generate more realistic results, especially when the local intensity variation is significant, due to the use of warping to distort source images and the avoidance of the smoothing operation proposed in Liang's [12] method. Also, this method can interpolate the whole image instead of only the regions of interest. This method also provides a way to utilize high-level knowledge to help automatically generate reasonable control lines for field morphing.

References

[1] E. Kepell, "Approximating Complex Surfaces by Triangulation of Contour Lines," *IBM Journal of Research and Development,* 19, pp. 2-11, 1975.

[2] H. Fuchs, Z. Kedem, and S. Uselton, "Optimal Surface Reconstruction from Planar Contours," *Comm. ACM,* Vol. 20, No. 10, pp. 693-702, 1977.

[3] H. Christiansen and T. Sederberg, "Conversion of Complex Contour Line Definitions into Polygonal Element Mosaics," *Computer Graphics,* Vol. 13, No. 3, pp. 187-192, 1978.

[4] Y. Wang and J. Aggarwal, "Surface Reconstruction and Representation of 3-D scenes," *Pattern Recognition,* Vol. 19, No. 3, pp. 197-207, 1986.

[5] J. D. Boissonnat, "Shape Reconstruction from Planar Cross Sections," *Computer Vision Graphics and Image Processing,* 44, pp. 1-29,1988.

[6] N. Kehtarnavaz, L. Simar, and R. De Figuerido, "A Systatic/Semantic Technique for Surface Reconstruction from Cross-Sectional Contours," *Computer Vision Graphics and Image Processing,* 42, pp. 399-409, 1988.

[7] S. E. Chen and R. E. Parent, "Shape Averaging and Its Application to Industrial Design," *IEEE Transactions on Computer Graphics and Applications,* 11, pp. 47-54, 1989

[8] B. Sinclair, A. Hannam, A. Lowe, and W. Wood, "Complex Contour Organization for Surface Reconstruction," *The International Journal of Graphics,* 13, pp. 311-319, 1989.

[9] T. Agui, K. Arai, and M. Nakajima, "Restoration of An Object From its Complex Cross-Sections," *SPIE Proceedings* 1092, pp. 406-415, 1989.

[10] A. Shaw and E. L. Schwartz, "Construction of Polyhedral Surface from Serial Sections : Exact and Heuristic Solutions," *SPIE Proceedings* 1092, pp. 221-233, 1989.

[11] D. Myers, S. Skinner and K. Sloan, "Surfaces from Contours," *ACM Transactions on Graphics,* Vol. 11, No. 3, pp. 228-258, July 1992.

[12] A. Goshtasby, D. A. Turner, and L. V. Ackerman, "Matching of Tomographic Slices for Interpolation," *IEEE Transactions on Medical Imaging,* Vol. 11, No. 4, pp. 507-516,1992.

[13] S. P. Raya and J. K. Udupa, "Shape-Based Interpolation of Multidimensional Objects," *IEEE Transactions on Medical Imaging,* Vol. 9, No. 1, pp. 32-42, March 1990.

[14] G. T. Herman, J Zheng, and C A. Bucholtz, "Shape-Based Interpolation," *IEEE Computer Graphics & Applications,* Vol. 12, No. 3, pp. 69-79, May 1992

[15] W.-C. Lin, C.-C. Liang, and C.-T. Chen, "Dynamic Elastic Interpolation for 3-D Medical Image Reconstruction from Serial Cross-sections," *IEEE Transactions on Medical Imaging,* Vol. 7, pp. 225-232, September 1988.

[16] C.-C. Liang, W.-C. Lin, and C.-T. Chen, "Intensity Interpolation for Serial Cross Sections," *SPIE Proceedings* 1092, pp. 60-66, 1989.

[17] D. J. Burr. "Elastic Matching of Line Drawings," *IEEE Transactions on Pattern Analysis and Machine Intelligence*, Vol. *PAMI-3*, No. 6, pp. 708-713, November 1981.

[18] D. J. Burr. "A Dynamical Model for Image Registration," *Computer Graphics Image Processing*, Vol. 15, pp. 102-112, 1981.

[19] D. Vandermeulen, "Methods for Registration, Interpolation and Interpretation of 3-Dimensional Medical Image Data for Use in 3-D Display, 3-D Modeling and Therapy Planning," Catholic Univ. Leuven, Ph.D. Diss. April 1991

[20] G. Wolberg, *Digital Image Warping*, IEEE Computer Society Press, 1990.

[21] T. Beier, and S. Neely, "Featured-Based Image Metamorphosis," *Computer Graphics*, Vol. 26, No. 2, pp. 35-42, July 1992

[22] R. W. Parrott, M. R. Stytz, P. Amburn, and D. Robinson, "Towards Statistically Optimal Interpolation for 3-D Medical Imaging," *IEEE Engineering in Medicine and Biology,* pp. 49-59, 1993

[23] M. Kass, A.Witkin, and D. Terzopoulos, "Snake: Active Contour Models," *International Journal of Computer Vision*, Vol. 1, pp. 321-331, 1987.

[24] L. D. Cohen, "On Active Contour Models and Balloons," *Computer Vision Graphics Image Processing: Image Understanding*, Vol. 53, pp. 211-218, March 1991.

[25] L. D. Cohen, and I. Cohen, "Deformable Models for 3D Medical Images Using Finite Elements and Bloons," *Proceedings of IEEE Conference on Computer Vision Pattern Recognition*, pp. 592-597, 1992.

[26] L. D. Cohen, and I. Cohen, "A Finite Element Method Applied to New Active Contour Models and 3D Reconstruction from Corss Sections," *Proceedings of the Third International Conference on Computer Vision*, Osaka, Japan, pp. 587-591, 1990.

[27] C. A. Davatzikos, and J. L. Prince, "Segmentation and Mapping of Highly-Convoluted Contours with Application to Medical Images," *Proceedings of IEEE Acoustic, Speech, and Signal Processing*, pp. 569-571, 1992.

[28] C. A. Davatzikos, and J. L. Prince, "Adaptive Active Contour Algorithm for Extracting and mapping thick contours," *Proceedings of IEEE Conference on Computer Vision Pattern Recognition*, pp. 524-529, 1993.

[29] M. O. Berger, and R. Mohr, "Toward Autonomy in Active Contour Models," *Proceedings of the 10th International Conference on Pattern Recognition*, pp. 847-851, 1990.

[30] W. C. Lin, R. Lin, C. C. Liang, and C. T. Chen, "Regularized Active Contour Models," *SPIE Proceedings* 2622, pp. 824-835, 1995

[31] M. Shapira and A. Rappoport, "Shape Blending Using the Star-Skeleton Representation," *IEEE Computer Graphics and Applications*, pp. 44-50, Mar. 1995

Appendix: intensity filling algorithm

The process of calculating each pixel value in the interpolated image is as follows:

For each regions R in the image to be interpolated (Depth-first tree traversal order)

    For each pixel X in the region R but not in the children regions of the region R

$$SUM\_A = SUM\_B = (0,0)$$
$$WSUM = 0$$

For each contour line segment P_iQ_i on the interpolated contours on R's parent branch and direct children branches

    calculate u,v based on P_iQ_i

    calculate X_{ai} based on u,v, and $P_{ai}Q_{ai}$ (P_iQ_i's corresponding line segment on contours of Image_A)

    calculate X_{bi} based on u,v, and $P_{bi}Q_{bi}$ (P_iQ_i's corresponding line segment on contours of Image_B)

    $dist$ = shortest distance from X to P_iQ_i

    $weight = (a + dist)^{-b}$

    $SUM\_A \mathrel{+}= X_{ai} * weight$

    $SUM\_B \mathrel{+}= X_{bi} * weight$

    $WSUM \mathrel{+}= weight$

$X_{ai} = SUM\_A\ /\ WSUM$

$X_{bi} = SUM\_B\ /\ WSUM$

$$\text{Interpolated\_Image}(X) = \frac{W_1}{W_1 + W_2} * \text{Image\_A}(X_{ai}) + \frac{W_2}{W_1 + W_2} * \text{Image\_B}(X_{bi})$$

Author Index

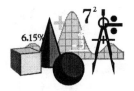

NOTES

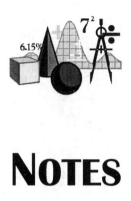

NOTES

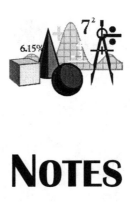

NOTES

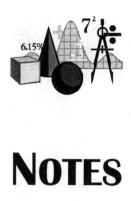

NOTES

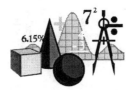

NOTES

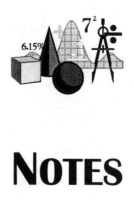

NOTES

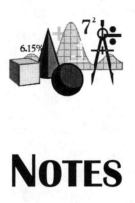

NOTES

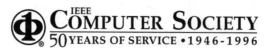

IEEE
COMPUTER SOCIETY
50 YEARS OF SERVICE • 1946-1996

http://www.computer.org

Press Activities Board

IEEE Computer Society Press Publications

The world-renowned Computer Society Press publishes, promotes, and distributes a wide variety of authoritative computer science and engineering texts. These books are available in two formats: 100 percent original material by authors preeminent in their field who focus on relevant topics and cutting-edge research, and reprint collections consisting of carefully selected groups of previously published papers with accompanying original introductory and explanatory text.

Submission of proposals: For guidelines and information on CS Press books, send e-mail to csbooks@computer.org or write to the Acquisitions Editor, IEEE Computer Society Press, P.O. Box 3014, 10662 Los Vaqueros Circle, Los Alamitos, CA 90720-1314. Telephone +1 714-821-8380. FAX +1 714-761-1784.

IEEE Computer Society Press Proceedings

The Computer Society Press also produces and actively promotes the proceedings of more than 130 acclaimed international conferences each year in multimedia formats that include hard and softcover books, CD-ROMs, videos, and on-line publications.

For information on CS Press proceedings, send e-mail to csbooks@computer.org or write to Proceedings, IEEE Computer Society Press, P.O. Box 3014, 10662 Los Vaqueros Circle, Los Alamitos, CA 90720-1314. Telephone +1 714-821-8380. FAX +1 714-761-1784.

Additional information regarding the Computer Society, conferences and proceedings, CD-ROMs, videos, and books can also be accessed from our web site at www.computer.org.